Ultrasonography in Ophthalmology 15

Documenta Ophthalmologica Proceedings Series

VOLUME 61

The titles published in this series are listed at the end of this volume.

Ultrasonography in Ophthalmology XV

Proceedings of the 15th SIDUO Congress, Cortina, Italy 1994

Edited by
G. Cennamo and N. Rosa

Springer-Science+Business Media, B.V.

Library of Congress Cataloging-in-Publication Data is available.

Ultrasonography in ophthalmology 15 / edited by G. Cennamo.
p. cm. -- (Documenta ophthalmologica. Proceedings series ; v. 61)
Proceedings of the XV SIDUO Conference held in 1994 in Cortina d'Ampezzo.
ISBN 0-7923-4464-2 (HB)
1. Ultrasonics in ophthalmology--Congresses. 2. Eye--Ultrasonic imaging--Congresses. I. Cennamo, G. (Giovanni) II. SIDUO Congress (15th : 1994 : Cortina d'Ampezzo, Italy) III. Series.
[DNLM: 1. Eye Diseases--ultrasonography--congresses. 2. Eye--ultrasonography--congresses. 3. Ultrasonography--methods--congresses. W3 DO637 v.61 1997 / WW 143 U47 1997]
RE79.U4U424 1997
617.7'1543--dc21
DNLM/DLC
for Library of Congress 97-231

ISBN 978-94-010-6450-7 ISBN 978-94-011-5802-2 (eBook)
DOI 10.1007/978-94-011-5802-2

Printed on acid-free paper

Contents

ANTERIOR EYE SEGMENT

VITREORETINAL DISORDERS

ORBITAL AND PERIORBITAL TUMORS

EXTRAOCULAR MUSCLES AND ORBITAL DISORDERS

INSTRUMENTATION AND TECHNIQUES

OPTIC NERVE DISORDERS

1. DENOMINAZIONE DELLA SPECIALITÀ

INDOCOLLIRIO® (Indometacina) 0,1%

2. COMPOSIZIONE QUALITATIVA E QUANTITATIVA IN PRINCIPI ATTIVI ED ECCIPIENTI

- Un flacone con liofilizzato contiene: Principio attivo: Indometacina mg 5,00. - Eccipienti: Destrano mg 20,00; Acido borico mg 28,10; Borace mg 5,10;
- Un flacone con solvente contiene: Acido borico mg 99,75; Borace mg 7,45; Metil p-idrossibenzoato mg 2,50; Polietilen glicole 400 mg 1242,50; Edetato bisodico mg 2,50; Acqua purificata q. b. a 5 ml.

3. FORMA FARMACEUTICA

Collirio da instillare nel fornice congiuntivale.

4. PROPRIETÀ FARMACOLOGICHE, TOSSICOLOGICHE E FARMACOCINETICHE

L'INDOCOLLIRIO® 0,1% è un antiinfiammatorio non steroideo in soluzione. Inibisce la sintesi delle prostaglandine oculari a livello di iride, corpo ciliare, congiuntiva, limitando cosi l'effetto infiammatorio a carico di tali strutture. Gli studi di farmacocinetica sull'INDOCOLLIRIO® hanno consentito di individuare le concentrazioni di indometacina che, somministrate nel segmento anteriore dell'occhio, risultano efficaci nell'inibizione della sintesi prostaglandinica. La presentazione del preparato sotto forma di soluzione assicura, inoltre, una buona tollerabilità locale e, in particolare, corneale.

5. INFORMAZIONI CLINICHE

5.1. Indicazioni terapeutiche

Prevenzione dell'insorgenza della miosi intraoperatoria nel corso di interventi di cataratta. Prevenzione dei processi infiammatori conseguenti ad interventi chirurgici di cataratta e del segmento anteriore dell'occhio.

5.2. Controindicazioni

L'INDOCOLLIRIO® 0,1% è controindicato in pazienti che presentino ipersensibilità all'indometacina, al conservante e a qualsiasi componente del prodotto. Essendo stato accertato che il farmaco viene assorbito sistemicamente sia pure in modo esiguo, si raccomanda una particolare attenzione in caso di somministrazione del collirio a pazienti che presentino ipersensibilità accertata (broncospasmi) ai salicilati o ad altri antiinfiammatori non-steroidei.

5.3. Effetti indesiderati

Occasionalmente dopo l'instillazione si puo avvertire un lieve bruciore o una sensazione di calore.

5.4. Speciali precauzioni d'uso

Il prodotto non deve essere usato dopo 15 giorni dalla prima apertura e ricostituzione dei componenti. Si raccomanda di non usare lenti a contatto durante il trattamento.

5.5. Uso durante la gravidanza e l'allattamento

Nelle donne in stato di gravidanza e nell'allattamento il prodotto va somministrato nei casi di effettiva necessità, sotto il diretto controllo del medico.

5.6. Interazioni con altri medicamenti ed interazioni di altro genere

Non sono note particolari interazioni nell'uso topico.

5.7. Posologia e modo di somministrazione

Instillare il collirio nel fornice congiuntivale inferiore dell'occhio secondo prescrizione medica. - Nella prevenzione dell'insorgenza della miosi intraoperatoria nel corso di interventi di cataratta, instillare 1 goccia ogni 30 minuti nelle due ore precedenti l'intervento chirurgico. - Nelle prevenzioni dei processi infiammatori conseguenti a interventi chirurgici di cataratta e del segmento anteriore dell'occhio, instillare 1 goccia, da 4 a 6 volte al giorno prima dell'intervento chirurgico, 1 goccia ogni 30 minuti nelle due ore precedenti e, successivamente, 1 goccia 4 volte al giorno fino a completa scomparsa della sintomatologia. - La durata del trattamento non dovrebbe superare il mese.

5.8. Sovradosaggio

Non sono stati mai segnalati casi di sovradosaggio.

5.9. Avvertenze speciali

Non essendo stata accertata l'efficacia e la sicurezza nei bambini, se ne sconsiglia l'uso in pediatria. - Il prodotto, se accidentalmente ingerito o se impiegato per lungo periodo a dosi eccessive, può determinare fenomeni tossici. Esso va quindi tenuto lontano dalla portata dei bambini. - Non deve essere comunque impiegato nei bambini sotto i tre anni di età.

5.10. Effetti sulla capacità di guidare veicoli ed usare macchinari

Non esistono controindicazioni.

6. INFORMAZIONI FARMACEUTICHE

6.1. Incompatibilità

Non note.

Depositato presso il Ministero della Sanità in data: 12.07.1996

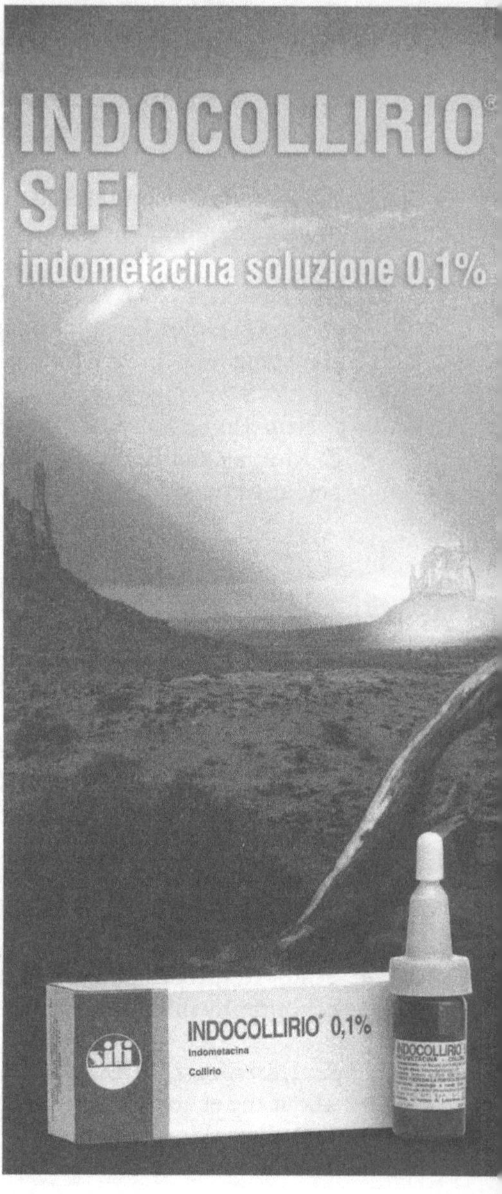

6.2. Periodo di validità

Il collirio con confezionamento integro, conservato al riparo dalla luce, h una validità di 18 mesi. - Il collirio ricostituito e pronto per l'uso non dev essere usato 15 giorni dopo la prima apertura.

6.3. Precauzioni particolari per la conservazione

Conservare al riparo dalla luce.

6.4. Natura e capacità del contenitore

Il solvente è contenuto in un flacone in polietilene a bassa densità da 5 ml. Il liofilizzato è contenuto in un flacone in vetro ambra di tipo I.

6.5. Ragione sociale sede del titolare dell'Autorizzazione all'Im missione in Commercio

S.I.F.I. S.p.A. Via N. Coviello, 15/B - Catania.

6.6. Numero di AIC e data di prima commercializzazione

028718017 - 15/02/1995

6.7. Eventuale tabella di appartenenza

Nessuna.

6.8. Regime di dispensazione al pubblico

Da vendersi solo dietro presentazione di ricetta medica.

Introduction

When in the early 60s echography was introduced into the field of ophthalmology, very few ophthalmologists realized the enormous potential of this procedure, the fundamental impact it would have on our branch of medicine or the innovations it would spawn. From its hesitant beginnings, echography has led to revolution in the field of ophthalmology and to our way of examining, treating and monitoring patients affected by eye disorders. This technique has brought untold benefits to patients worldwide.

A crucial element in fostering the advance of the application of ultrasound in ophthalmology has been and is the biannual conference of the Societas Internationalis pro Diagnostica Ultrasonica in Ophthalmologia (SIDUO), and incidentally, the Latin name reflects the wish of the founding members that SIDUO be truly international, and even though the instruments and apparatus used in the discipline are highly innovative, the underlying philosophy is one that traces back to Hippocrates, i.e., the healing of man and the improvement of man's quality of life. The first SIDUO conference was held in 1964 in Berlin. Since that first conference, SIDUO has grown in size and in influence, and when in 1994 SIDUO convened for the second time in Italy, at Cortina D'Ampezzo, more than 200 ophthalmologists attended the meeting and more than 100 presentations were made. A notable feature of the Cortina meeting was the high number of young ophthalmologists that attended, which bodes very well for the vigorous future of ultrasound diagnostics in ophthalmology. When organizing the XV SIDUO Conference we tried to provide space also for last minute, "hot topics", i.e., new data or findings that, although still preliminary, appeared to hold promise, or that could be useful for delegates. This proved to be a worthwhile strategy because it encouraged researchers to present data that although not definitive would be of interest to participants.

In summing up the XV SIDUO conference, four major points emerge: (1) standardized echography has become an essential diagnostic procedure in ophthalmology; (2) an enormous breakthrough in ophthalmology was made with the use of endovenous contrast medium to enhance the echo signal; this new procedure promises to open up new areas to ophthalmic echography; (3) high frequency probes, which allow the visualization and study of the entire anterior segment of the eye, is pushing back the frontiers of ultrasound diagnostics; (4) communication among ophthalmologists is improving as the result of the evolution of an "ultrasound diagnostic language".

G Cennamo and N. Rosa (eds.), Ultrasonography in Ophthalmology 15, pp. xiii–xiv.

This proceedings volume contains practically all the work presented at the XV SIDUO Conference; only about 10% of delegates failed to submit manuscripts. The text starts with two invited lectures and is divided into nine sections (Posterior Eye Segment, Intraocular Tumors, Anterior Eye Segment, Vitreoretinal Disorders, Orbital and Periorbital Tumors, Extraocular Muscles and Orbital Disorders, Axial Eye Length Biometry and IOL Calculations, Instrumentation and Techniques, and Optic Nerve Disorders.

The Jules Françoise Lecture at Cortina was delivered by Professor Roberto Sampaolesi who gave a masterly talk on his long experience in using echometry to diagnose and treat congenital glaucoma in infants and children. Professor Sampaolesi's work in this field dates back to 1960, and his exhaustive, well structured article contains some interesting illustrations, including two early figures taken from Seefelder and Wolfrum. Professor Sampaolesi concludes that in children, the optic nerve fibers start deteriorating as soon as ocular hypertension occurs, while the visual field starts to deteriorate ten years later. Consequently, patients affected by congenital glaucoma must be given surgery as soon as the condition is diagnosed.

Rolf Schurmann, one of the invited speakers, provides an introduction to the use of echo enhancers, which is just beginning to be used in patients in whom Doppler signals are weak. As the technique is refined even further, it is predicted that echo enhancers will become a standard feature in ultrasound diagnostics in ophthalmology.

A vast range of topics are covered in the individual sections: from bacterial contamination of ultrasound probes to spectral maps, from intraocular tumors obtained with a new imaging technique to rhabdomyosarcoma, from the color Doppler technique to echographic diagnosis of acute retinal necrosis.

In conclusion, this proceedings volume reviews the latest understanding in ultrasound diagnostics in ophthalmology, highlights clinical resuls and provides a balanced overview of how standardized echography is being used today.

I would like to extend my thanks to the Organizing Secretariat of SIDUO XV and to the Scientific Committee, in particular Professor Antonio Rossi for his invaluable encouragement and advice in the months preceding the meeting. I gratefully acknowledge the enthusiastic assistance of my collaborators, in particular Dr Nicola Rosa, at the University of Naples Federico II, who provided the intellectual substrate necessary to organize a meeting of this scale. A last word of thanks goes to Jean Gilder who diligently edited the text.

Finally, I am pleased to acknowledge the excellence of the work of the authors of this volume. It has been very rewarding for me to interact with many friends and colleagues and I am pleased to have had the opportunity of establishing new relationships and consolidating earlier ones.

Giovanni Cennamo

1. Congenital glaucoma. The importance of echometry in its diagnosis, treatment and functional outcome

R. SAMPAOLESI
(Buenos Aires, Argentina)

Abstract

Echometry is the most important parameter for the early diagnosis of congenital glaucoma and its follow-up. When signs and symptoms of glaucoma are observed, abnormal echometric results with respect to age confirm the diagnosis even when intraocular pressure (IOP) values are normal. Anesthetic agents affect IOP readings but not axial length values, which is why echometry is the most important parameter in deciding whether to operate. In the follow-up echometry is also the most important parameter in deciding reoperations in cases of abnormal axial length growth, even when IOP readings are apparently normal.

Visual field defects in reoperated patients, manifested as diffuse damage (scotomas are not found) are well correlated with axial length values, i.e., the higher the axial length values, the more severe the visual field defects.

Optic nerve examination with confocal laser tomography also shows that the higher the axial length values, the more severe the optic nerve alterations represented by the enlargement of the Elschnig ring.

Finally, because ocular hypertension leads to visual field defects, which in 85% of cases appear 5–10 years after the onset of ocular hypertension, congenital glaucoma has a good prognosis provided that it is diagnosed early, with the aid of echometry and tonometry, and surgery is performed immediately. Our 28 years of experience with a group of 60 operated patients confirms this concept; indeed, all the patients are well integrated in society, some of them have even undertaken university studies, and they have good visual fields and binocular vision.

Introduction

I am deeply grateful to the Executive Committee of SIDUO for having appointed me Jules François Memorial Lecturer. This is a great honor, and I am delighted to have this opportunity of paying tribute to my friend Jules

G Cennamo and N. Rosa (eds.), Ultrasonography in Ophthalmology 15, pp. 1–47.

François who was a remarkable figure: an outstanding scientist and upright, humane personality. I am also pleased with the results of my assessment of the children I operated on from 10 to 28 years ago. The majority of cases have maintained a good visual function with one or more operations thanks to the early and accurate diagnosis achieved by echometry. What is even more satisfying is that they have become useful and well-integrated members of society.

In dealing with the topic of primary congenital glaucoma as a whole, I shall focus on the remarkable value of echometry in its diagnosis, follow-up and assessment of functional results.

I would like to thank my son, Juan Roberto Sampaolesi, for his valuable contribution to the study of the optic nerve in congenital glaucoma.

Definition of primary congenital glaucoma

In primary congenital glaucoma there is detention in the development of the chamber angle which leads to obstruction of the aqueous humor outflow pathways. This, in turn causes an increase in IOP, followed by increased axial length and corneal enlargement, which, if not arrested by surgery, leads to damage of the optic nerve, visual field and visual acuity. Figures 1a and b are two old pictures of Seefelder and Wolfrum (1906) [1] showing that in cases of congenital glaucoma, the development of the chamber angle stops and remains as it was at the seventh month of intrauterine life. The remaining mesodermal tissue impedes aqueous humor inflow to Schlemm's canal.

The incidence of congenital glaucoma in relation to other types of glaucoma is small: 0.008% (8 cases each 100,000 children) [2]. In 80% it is bilateral, 70% of cases occur in males, and it is the most frequent cause of early blindness of congenital origin.

I shall deal exclusively with cases with an onset from birth to 24 months of age. These are *primary congenital glaucomas* with definite clinical features, evolution and pathological anatomy. Glaucomas associated with ocular and systemic malformations are a separate group. Prognosis depends on the time elapsed between the occurrence of the first clinical manifestations and surgery. This is why immediate surgical treatment is crucial, and why echometry is of great help, especially in some cases of doubtful diagnosis. *Abnormal axial length growth is the indicator for surgery even when tonometric values are doubtful.*

My research on congenital glaucoma falls into three periods:

1960–1970:	Intraocular pressure: normal and pathological
1970–1980:	Echometry in the diagnosis and follow-up
1980–1990:	Functional results in operated primary congenital glaucomas
1992–1994:	Optic disk changes in congenital glaucoma with confocal tomography (studied with the Heidelberg Retina Tomograph) of the optic nerve head.

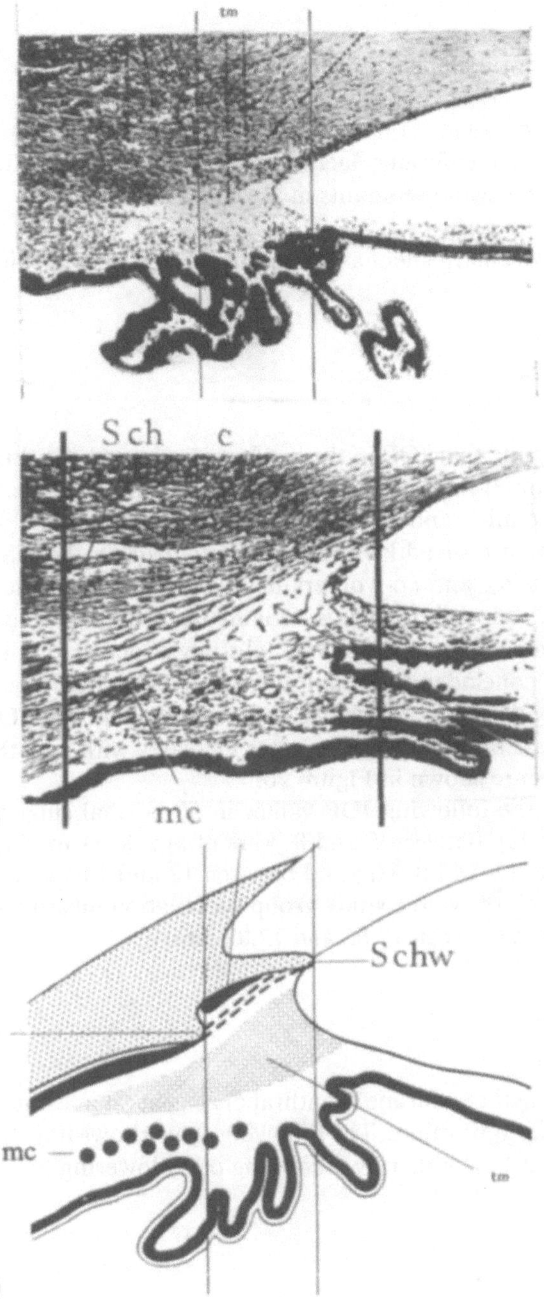

(a)

(b)

(c)

Fig. 1. Histologically, the chamber angle in congenital glaucoma has the same appearance as that of the normal chamber angle at seven months of gestation. a) chamber angle of a seven-month-normal fetus [1]; b) chamber angle in congenital glaucoma; c) sketch representing a and b (tm: mesodermal tissue, mc: ciliary muscle, Sch: Schlemm's canal, Schw, Schwalbe's line). (Figures a and b reproduced from Seefelder and Wolfrum)

Symptoms and signs of congenital glaucoma

Symptoms: Photophobia; epiphora; blepharospasm; frequent sneezing.

Signs: Hazy cornea; enlarged cornea (>11 mm); anterior embryotoxon; tears in endothelium and in Descemet's membrane; **increased axial length**; reversible disk cupping; pathological mesodermal remnants in the chamber angle.

In 1970 we added axial length enlargement as an important sign of congenital glaucoma.

Intraocular pressure

In 1967 I showed for the first time that IOP in the newborn and up to the third year of age has a mean of 10 mmHg, and not 15 mmHg as found in adults [3]. In the American continent, Carvalho and Calixto, in 1969, were the first to confirm this finding [4], followed by Radtke and Cohan, in 1974, in the USA [5]. More recently, in 1992 Tucker and co-workers have also confirmed these results [6], as have Tarkkanen, Reibaldi, Fledelius, Goldmann, Dominguez and others in Europe. Ytterborg, in 1960, in an experimental study of ocular rigidity in the eyes of dead newborns, concluded that the IOP in newborns should be 5 mmHg lower than in adults [7]. Figure 2a shows the normal range for IOP between birth and the sixth year of age. This parameter increases with age; the values of age-matched subjects are shown in Figure 2b.

In 1984, Borrone obtained the following IOP values in 50 normal subjects between 5 and 15 years of age [8]: between 5 and 8 years of age: 8–11 mmHg; between 9 and 11 years of age: 12–14 mmHg; and between 12 and 15 years of age: 15–17 mmHg. Then he took the whole study group (population mean) and he found the mean ($\bar{X}$) IOP to be between 11.65 and 12.02 mmHg.

Anesthetic agents used

In our research we have used methoxyflurane (Penthrane) as general anesthetic agent because it does not modify IOP values. The following chart shows how the different anesthetic agents affect IOP, either by increasing or by lowering it.

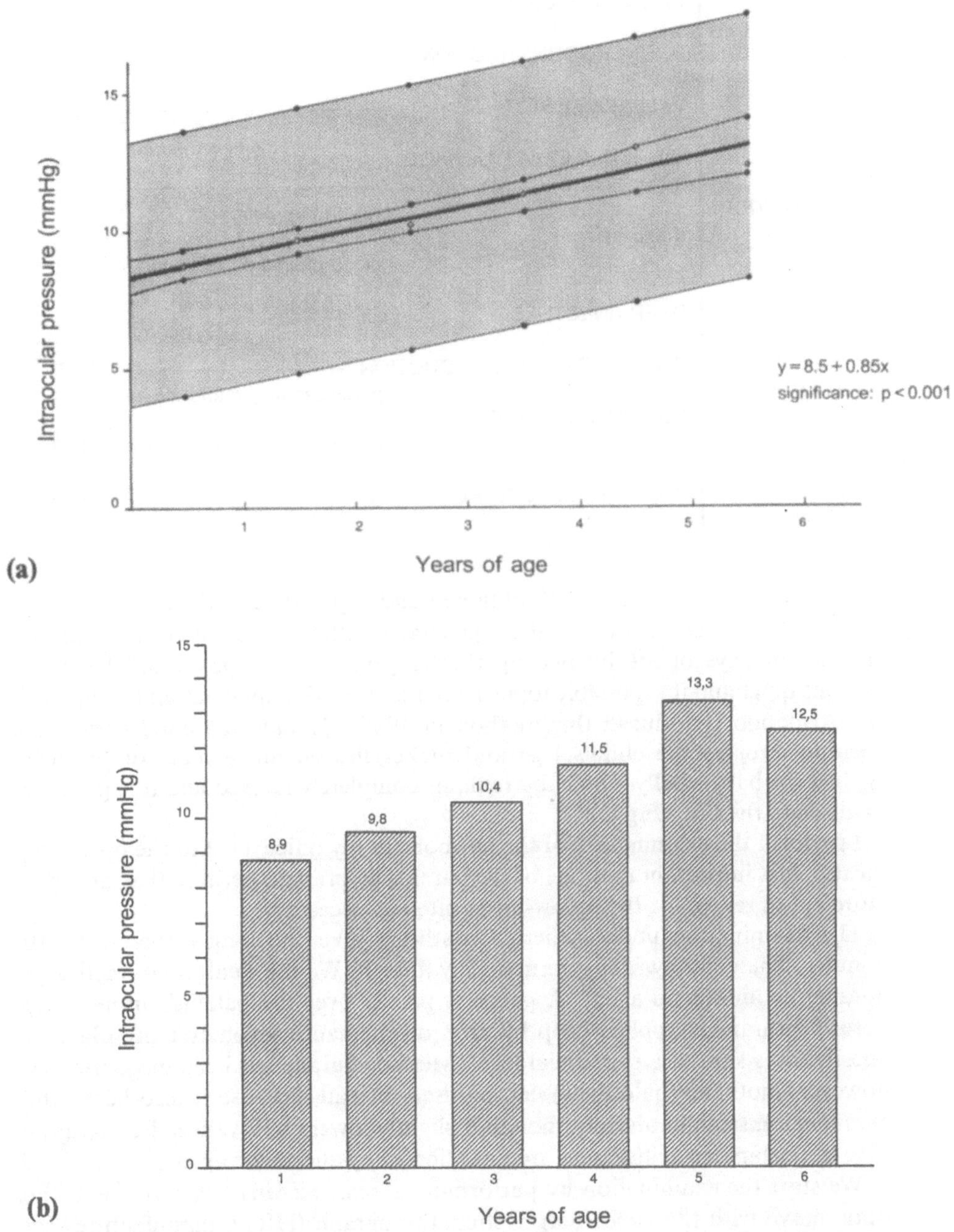

Fig. 2. **Normal IOP in children up to 5 years of age.** a) The regression line (thick line) shows the annual increase in IOP values from birth to 5 years of age. This chart is useful for physicians and they must have it at sight when measuring the IOP under general anesthesia in a child. For example, at 6 months of age, the maximum possible IOP value is 14 mmHg. b) IOP values in the different age-matched groups

ETHER	BRONCHIAL SECRETION ↓ BRONCHOCONSTRICTION ↓ VALSAVA TEST	——> IOP
BARBITURATES	DIFFICULT EXACT DOSAGE: If insufficient	——> IOP
	If excessive	respiratory deficiency ↓ blood pressure reduction —< IOP
INTUBATION	DEEP ANESTHESIA ↓ BLOOD PRESSURE REDUCTION	——< IOP
	SUCCINYLCHOLINE	paralyzes respiratory movements ↓ blood pressure increase ——> IOP
HALOTHANE (Fluothane)	BLOOD PRESSURE REDUCTION	——< IOP

I confirmed the values of IOP obtained under general anesthesia by measuring the IOP of the same baby without general anesthesia. This can be done in the first fifteen days of life by placing the baby in the fetal position. The baby remains quiet and it is possible to measure the IOP with applanation tonometry. Dr. Armando introduced this method in 1967. He puts the child in a fetal position, crosses the child's legs and makes flexion movements of the legs against the baby's belly. The baby remains completely relaxed and it is possible to measure the IOP (Fig. 3).

I perform the examination of the newborn in my office, next to the operating theatre. It is important that one of the parents be present, because they are then more apt to return for the follow-up as often as necessary.

The examination under general anesthesia takes no longer than 7 to 10 minutes. The child awakens immediately after it. We use Penthrane (methoxyflurane) as anesthetic agent. A gauze is placed over the patient's mouth and nose. Penthrane is applied drop by drop on the gauze (open system). General anesthesia is kept at a superficial level. Methoxyflurane has been discontinued, however fluothane (halothane) can be used instead, because it also keeps the eyes looking straight ahead although it slightly lowers IOP values. Echography is so important since its values are not affected by anesthetic agents.

We start the examination by performing a *confocal laser tomography* of the optic nerve with the Heidelberg Retina Tomograph (HRT), manufactured by Heidelberg Engineering, while the pupil is undilated. The measurement takes 1.6 seconds and 32 optic disk images separated from each other by 50 μ are obtained.

We then perform *skiascopy* followed by direct or indirect ophthalmoscopy. The anesthetist seats the child on his lap in front of the slit lamp and because the

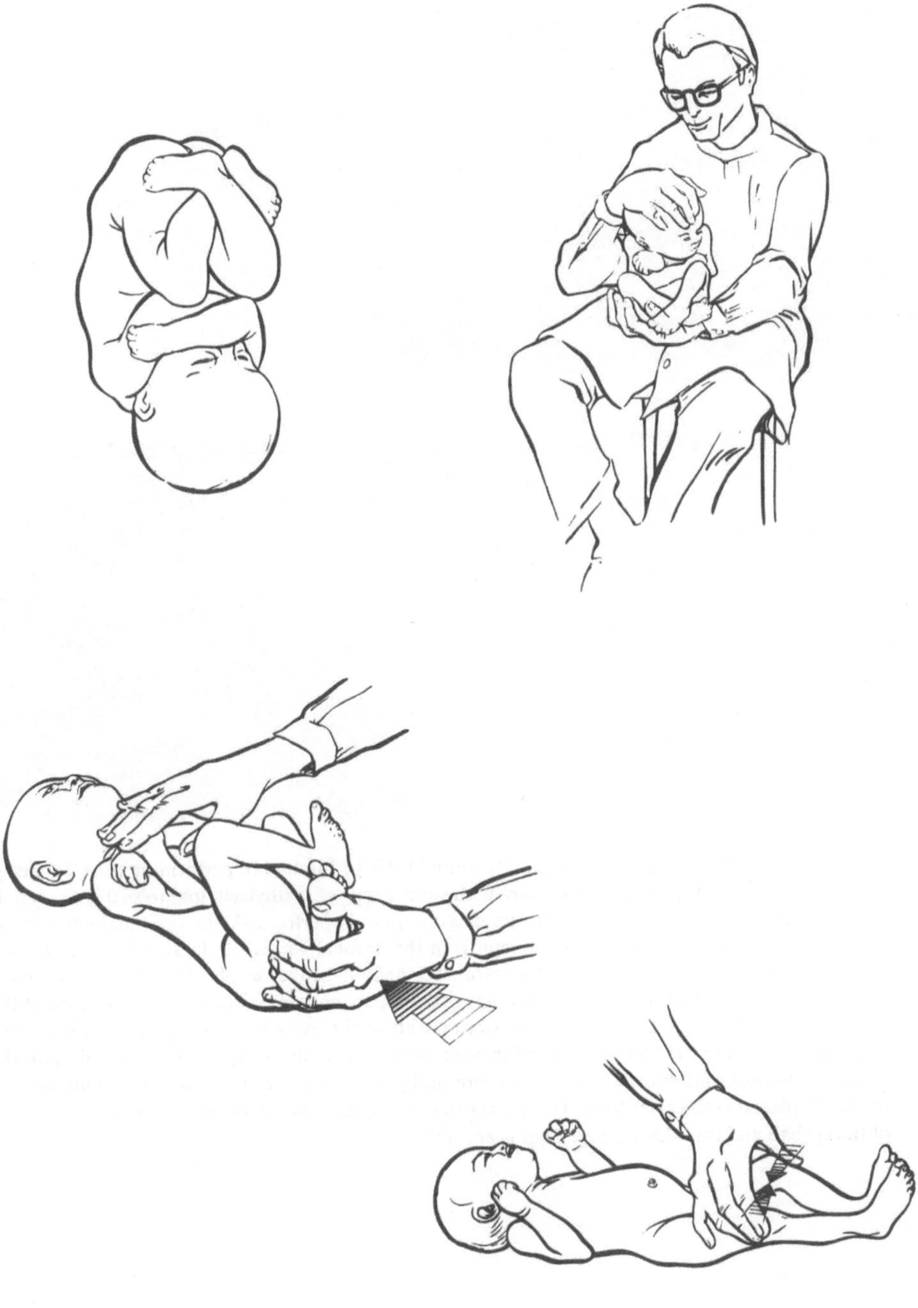

Fig. 3. **IOP measurement without general anesthesia (Dr Armando's method).** The physician puts the baby in fetal position, crosses his legs and makes flexion movements of the legs against the baby's belly

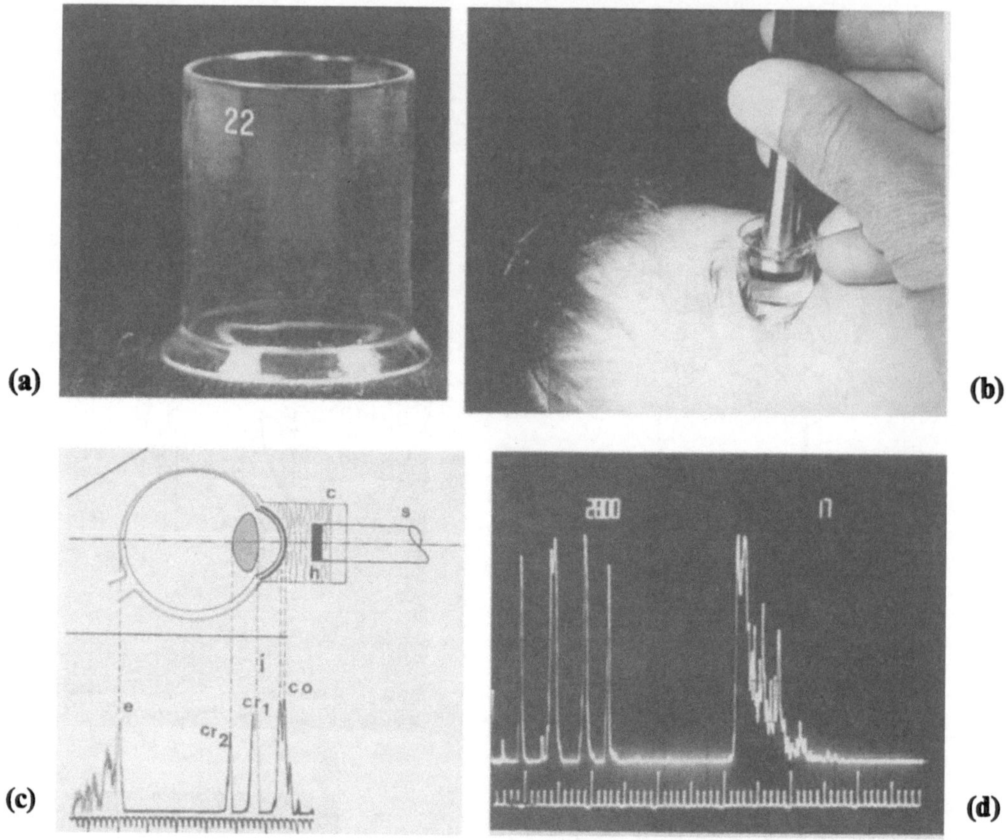

Fig. 4. a) Plastic cylinder for echometry (Ossoinig Shell). b) Method of performing the echometry. The plastic cylinder is placed on the sclera with some drops of methylcellulose to seal it off well. It is filled with saline solution and when the measurement is performed, the proximal edge of the probe must be separated by at least 0.5 cm from the corneal vertex. c) the sketch correlates the method of measurement with the echogram obtained; s: probe, c: plastic reservoir, h: saline solution within the reservoir, with the echogram below, co: cornea, i: iris, cr1: anterior face of the lens, cr2: posterior face of the lens, e: posterior wall of the eyeball. d) echogram obtained. The most important point is that at 17 dB of measurement sensitivity the spikes corresponding to the anterior and posterior corneal surface, anterior and posterior face of the lens, retina, choroid and sclera are placed at the same level. This means that the probe is perpendicular to the posterior face of the eyeball and that the measurement is accurate

baby's head is small a device is added to the chin holder to lift the patient's head.

The ophthalmologist first examines *the anterior segment*, and then he measures the *IOP with applanation tonometry.* The IOP is measured three times in each eye to obtain the mean value, as specified by Goldmann. Penthrane, like fluothane, maintains the eye looking straight ahead, so the IOP can be easily measured.

The examination continues with *gonioscopy*, performed with the three-mirror Goldmann's lens manufactured by Haag Streit and especially designed for babies. One has a diameter of 10 mm, and the other, 11 mm. We take a *goniophotograph* by fitting a camera without a lens directly to the microscope, with a ring I designed many years ago. We use a 160-ASA film for artificial light, without flash. The exposure time ranges from 0.30 to 0.15 seconds. We lay the baby down and we measure the *horizontal diameter of the cornea* because the vertical diameter changes in relation to the development of the anterior embryotoxon, which is generally present. The last step of the examination is *echometry.*

Diagnosis by echometry

Gernet and Hollwich, in 1969, were the first to measure axial length in cases of congenital glaucoma [9]. In 1970 I started measuring the axial length with echometry, first in children with normal eyes and then in children with congenital glaucomas. I found that echometry was a particularly useful parameter when IOP values were doubtful because they were borderline. This led us to undertake a systematic study of ocular echometry in normal children to determine the mean values and their spread according to age. Unlike IOP readings, axial length is not influenced by general anesthesia.

For echometry, we use a Kretz 7200 apparatus with a 10-MHz probe or an Okukretz unit. We use an immersion device consisting of a plastic cylinder fitted to the sclera (Fig. 4b) manufactured by Hansen Ophthalmic Development Laboratory (Iowa City; Ossoinig scleral shell no. 20) (Fig. 4a) in which we first instill four drops of methylcellulose 2.5% with a viscosity of 4000 centipoises to seal off the scleral contact area. The cylinder is then filled with isotonic saline solution. Methoxyflurane used as anesthetic agent allows perfect centering of the eye with the child in a supine position; a perfectly centered eye is an absolute prerequisite for correct measurement.

The probe is put into the cylinder, approximately 5 mm from the cornea; the cornea must not be touched. We obtain echograms at tissue sensitivity and at *measuring sensitivity.* Four echograms of each eye are performed (Figs. 4c and d).

At the 1974 Glaucoma Symposium held in Wurzburg I first drew the attention to the extraordinary value of echometry in the diagnosis of congenital glaucoma, as a better parameter than IOP [10]. Other papers followed [11–16]. Then, Reibaldi [17], Betinjane [18,19], Tarkkanen [20] and Fledelius [21]

Table 1. Echometric and IOP values in a 3-month-old male infant (case 1- s.m.)

Date	Corneal diameter	IOP	Anterior Cornea	Vitreous chamber	Cornea	body	Axial length
			Echometry				
October 1978	12	10	.54	3.45	3.69	12.26	20.29
	12.5[a]	29	.78	3.06	3.94	13.02	21.15
December 1978	12	8	.54	3.45	3.69	13.41	21.44
	12.5	8	.54	3.06	3.94	12.64	20.53
February 1979	13.5[a]	25	.54	3.83	3.28	13.79	21.71
	12.5	12	.54	3.06	3.69	12.64	20.29
May 1979	13.5	10	.54	3.83	3.69	13.79	22.20
	12.5	10	.54	3.06	3.69	12.64	20.29

[a]Trabeculotomy

[b]The underlined figures indicate echometric values permitting the diagnosis of congenital glaucoma

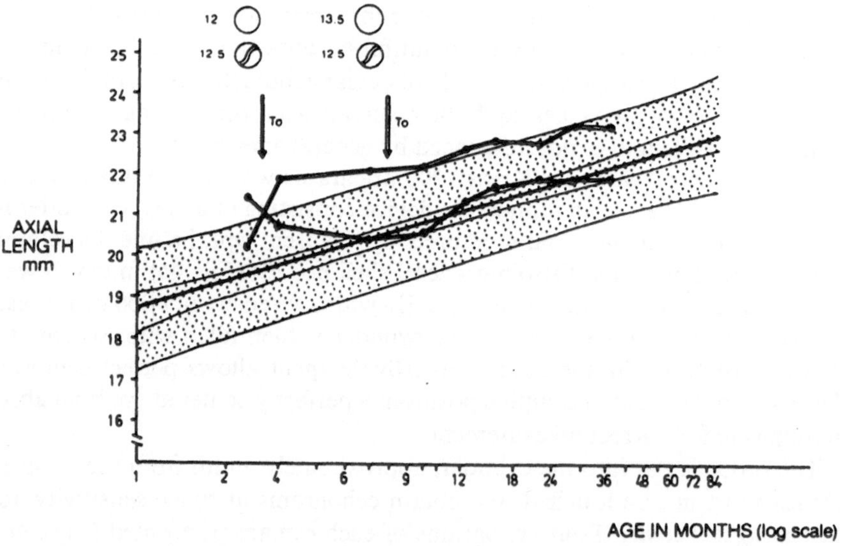

Fig. 5. Case 1: = right eye; - left eye. The arrows indicate surgery; *To*, trabeculotomy. The circles indicate cornea with or without tears in Descemet's membrane and endothelium. The numbers close to the circles are the corneal diameters in millimeters

demonstrated the value of echometry in the early diagnosis of congenital glaucoma and its advantages over tonometry. The following is an example of the value of echometry in the diagnosis of congenital glaucoma.

A 3-month-old boy came for consultation in October 1978 with symptoms of unilateral infantile congenital glaucoma. The corneal diameter was 12 mm in the right eye and **12.5** mm in the left eye (abnormal eye); the IOP, upon examination under general anesthesia, was 10 mmHg in the right eye and **29** mmHg in the left eye. The left cornea was edematous and was 0.78 mm thick, while the cornea of the normal contralateral eye was 0.54 mm thick. Table 1 shows that both vitreous and axial length were significantly larger than those of the normal eye. Successful trabeculotomy was performed in the abnormal eye. Two months later, in December 1978, the patient was brought back for examination and *his IOP was 8 mmHg in both eyes, while the corneal diameter had not changed. Nevertheless, both the vitreous and axial length of the normal eye had become larger than those of the operated eye. However, in the absence of symptoms, ocular hypertension and optic nerve damage, we decided not to operate.*

Two months later, all the parameters of the operated eye were normal, while the IOP of the previously healthy eye was 25 mmHg and the vitreous and axial length values were not only higher than those of the operated eye but also higher than those found in December; the cornea had grown from 12 mm to 13.5 mm.

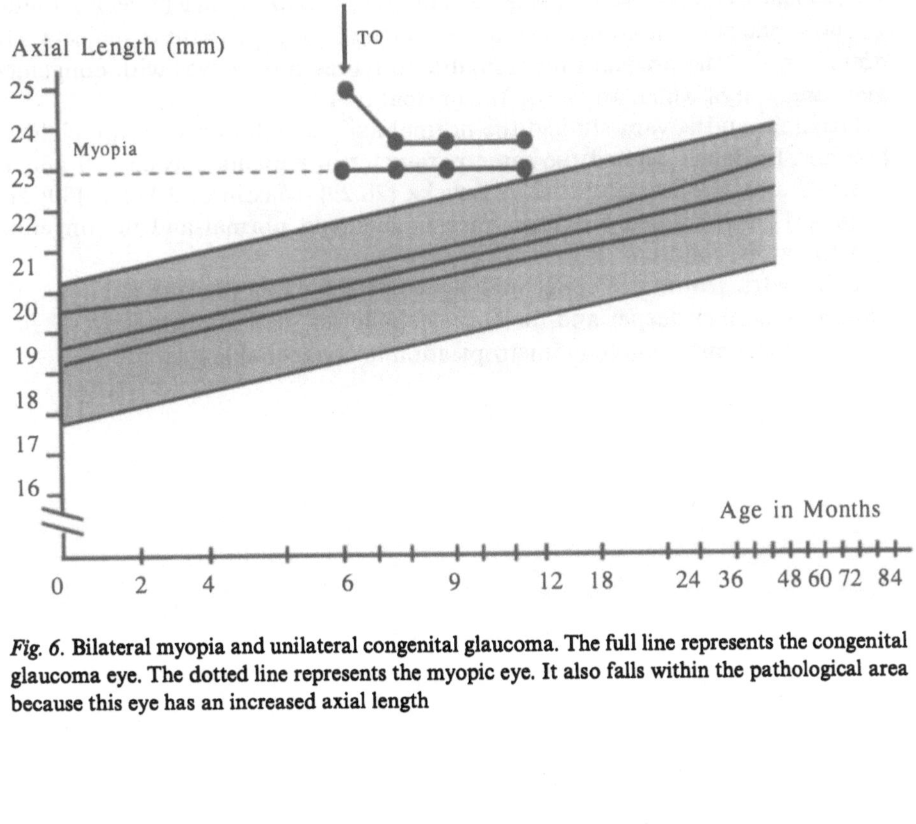

Fig. 6. **Bilateral myopia and unilateral congenital glaucoma. The full line represents the congenital glaucoma eye. The dotted line represents the myopic eye. It also falls within the pathological area because this eye has an increased axial length**

We decided to operate immediately. As shown in Figure 5 and Table 1, the IOP returned to normal values and the rapid increase of echometric values stopped with time. When the baby was 18 months of age these values were normal. His family was sure of the success of the treatment, but we know that the second eye should have been operated on when the child was 4 months old instead of when he was 7 months old.

When a child has bilateral myopia, axial length values fall within the abnormal range both in the normal and glaucomatous eye. Figure 6 shows that after trabeculotomy the axial length decreases because myopic eyes are very elastic. In non-myopic eyes with congenital glaucoma there is always a slight lowering of axial length values, but this decrease is not as great as that observed in myopic eyes.

Therefore, the question of a mistaken diagnosis arises: can axial length values lead to a diagnosis of congenital glaucoma when the child has congenital myopia? The answer is that children with congenital myopia are not brought for consultation by their parents because they do not have signs and symptoms of glaucoma.

Axial length according to age in normal and in congenital glaucomatous eyes

We studied 100 normal eyes in children up to 84 months of age (7 years). Figure 7a shows the correlation between the axial length and age in these subjects. The dotted area is the normal range. Figure 7b represents 79 eyes with congenital glaucoma, all of which are above the normal range.

Grignolo and Rivara studied the normal axial length in premature children [22] and Fledelius studied the same parameter in patients between 10 and 18 years of age [23]. Larsen [24–27]. Luyckx [28,29], Massin and Pellat [30] and Prahs [31] also studied biometric measurements in normal and in congenital glaucomatous children.

Echometric features in congenital glaucoma show that the lens is thinner, the anterior chamber deeper and the cornea shallower than in normal eyes. These three factors contribute to emmetropization in congenital glaucoma.

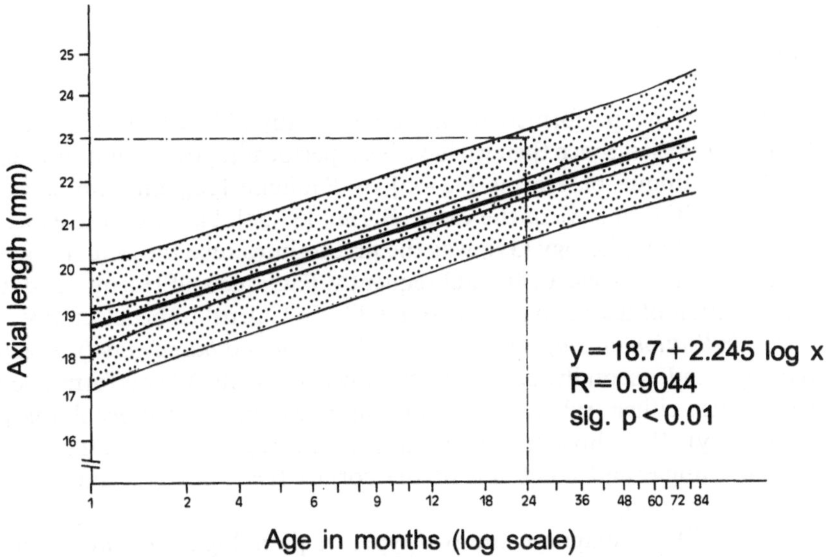

(a)

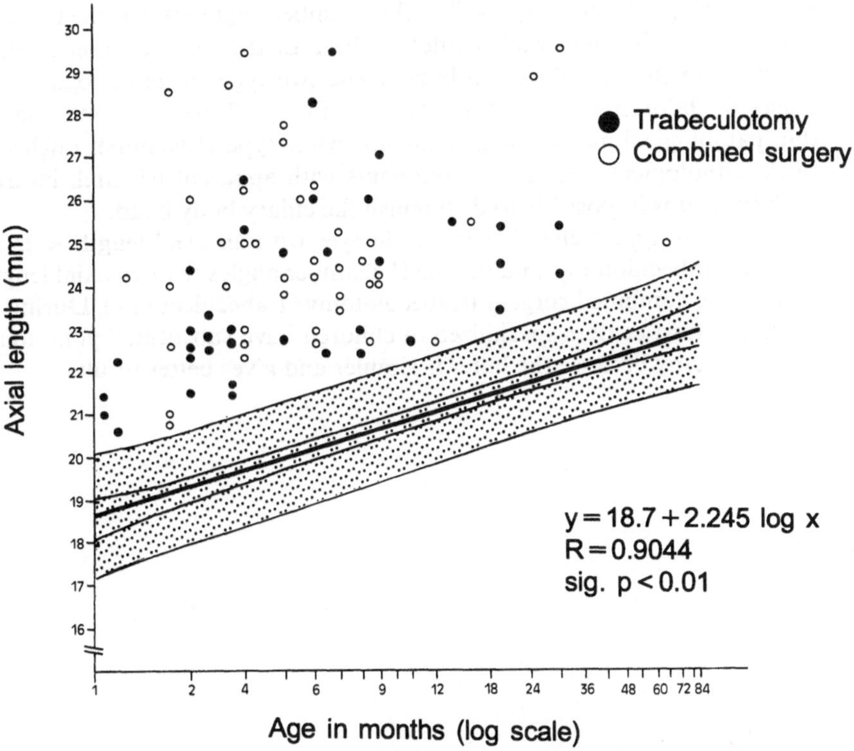

(b)

Fig. 7. a) Correlation between axial length and age in 100 normal eyes. Normal range band. The dashed line encloses a rectangle covering up to 24 months. Pure congenital glaucomas are enclosed by this area. b) Seventy-nine eyes with congenital glaucoma all placed outside and above the normal range band. Only four of the total 79 eyes belonged to children over 24 months of age.

Surgery

Up to 1968, we performed Barkan's goniotomy [32], which was successful in 65% of the cases. Since then we have been performing trabeculotomy, according to the technique of Harms [33–35] or Paufique [36], and we succeeded in regulating IOP in 98% of the cases. Burian [37,38], based on the experience of Dellaporta in pathology [39], was the first to introduce trabeculotomy, but this technique was not successful. Subsequently, Paufique and Harms introduced the modification of dissecting a scleral flap like in Cairns' trabeculectomy.

The indication for surgery in congenital glaucoma is based mainly on echometric readings, and, secondly, on tonometric measurements. We perform two surgical techniques: either trabeculotomy or combined surgery (trabeculotomy+trabeculectomy). We chose the technique according to echometry, tonometry, chamber angle and condition of the cornea (tears in Descemet's membrane and endothelium).

To be able to diagnose the two types of pathological chamber angles in a baby, one must know the appearance of a normal chamber angle in adults and in babies (Fig. 8). The outer wall of the chamber angle is the same in adults and in babies, but the inner wall is different, because the surface mesenchymal layer is not completely developed in babies. The two types of pathological chamber angles in children are: type I and type II (Fig. 9). Type I chamber angles have thin pathological mesodermal remnants, while type II chamber angles present thick pathological mesodermal remnants with apparent iris high insertion. In both types it is impossible to distinguish the ciliary body band.

In cases of type I chamber angles in eyes with an axial length <23 mm we perform trabeculotomy, and in type II chamber angles with an axial length >23 mm we use combined surgery (trabeculotomy+trabeculectomy). During the last 25 years, most centers specialized in children have substituted goniotomy with trabeculotomy because the latter is simpler and gives better results.

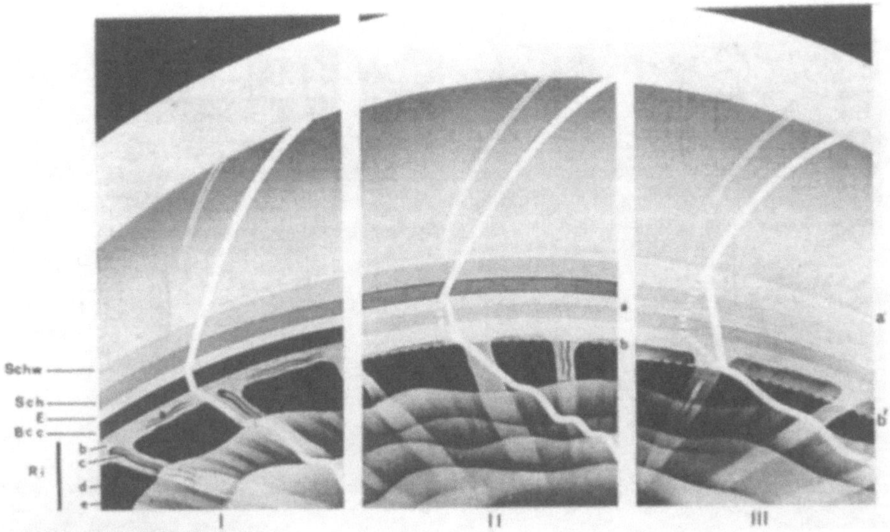

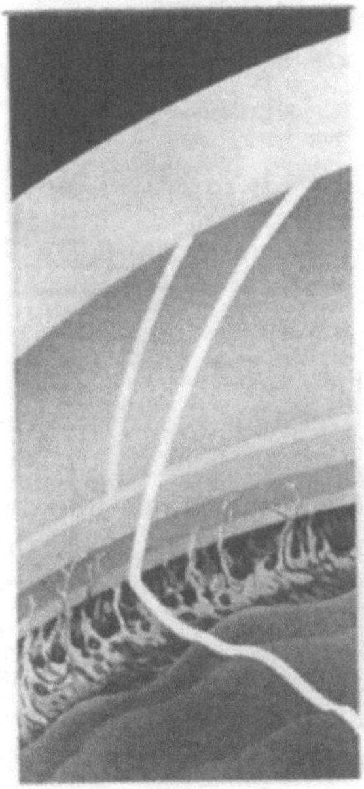

Fig. 8. **Variations of the normal chamber angle during the first year of age.** Schw: Schwalbe's line. Sch: Schlemm's canal. E: scleral spur. Bcc: ciliary body band. Ri: iris root. b, iris root portion corresponding to the circulus arteriosus iridis, c, avascular cord. e, iris epithelial pigmentary layer
I, chamber angle with no Barkan's membrane. II, persistence of Barkan's membrane from a to b. III, persistence of Barkan's membrane from a' to b'. IV, persistence of normal mesodermal remnants in children

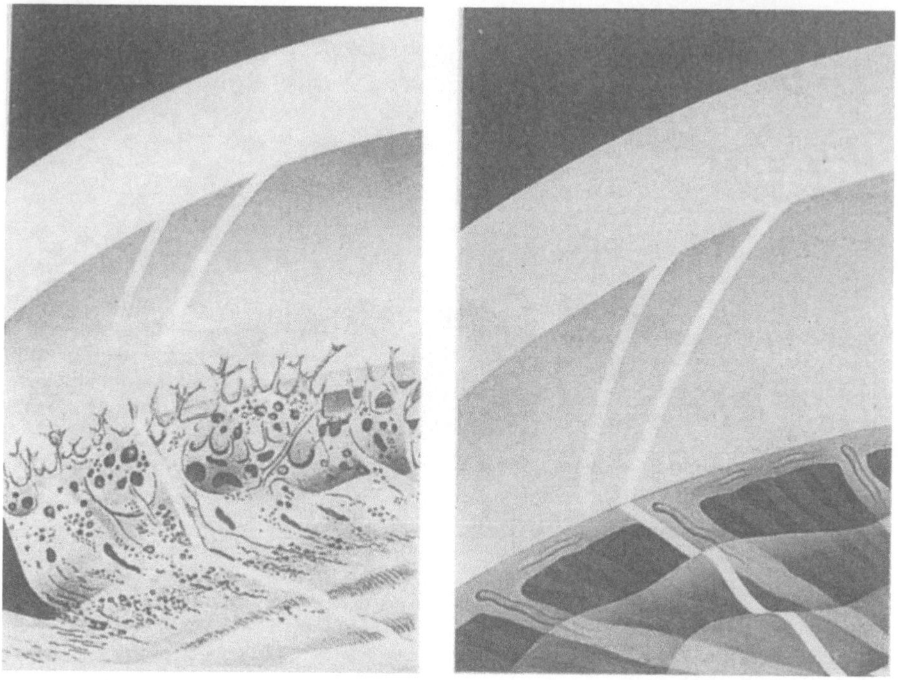

(a) (b)

Fig. 9. **Persistence of pathologic mesodermal remnants.** a) Type I chamber angle. b) Type II chamber angle. Apparent high insertion of the iris

Trabeculotomy

Based on our experience with Harms' and Paufique's technique (Figs. 10a and b), the key factor in trabeculotomy is locating Schlemm's canal [40]. Once the scleral flap has been performed, by means of transillumination (Misky's maneuver), the edges of the chamber angle are clearly visible. Consequently, the incision can be correctly placed, i.e., exactly at the limit between light and shadow, at the center. The incision is oval-shaped, made up of two triangles, a black one at the top and a nacreous one below. The black triangle corresponds to Schlemm's canal. The trabeculotome must be introduced at this level. The trabeculotome enters Schlemm's canal, breaks through its inner wall, the trabecular meshwork and the pathological mesodermal remnants, to enter into the chamber angle.

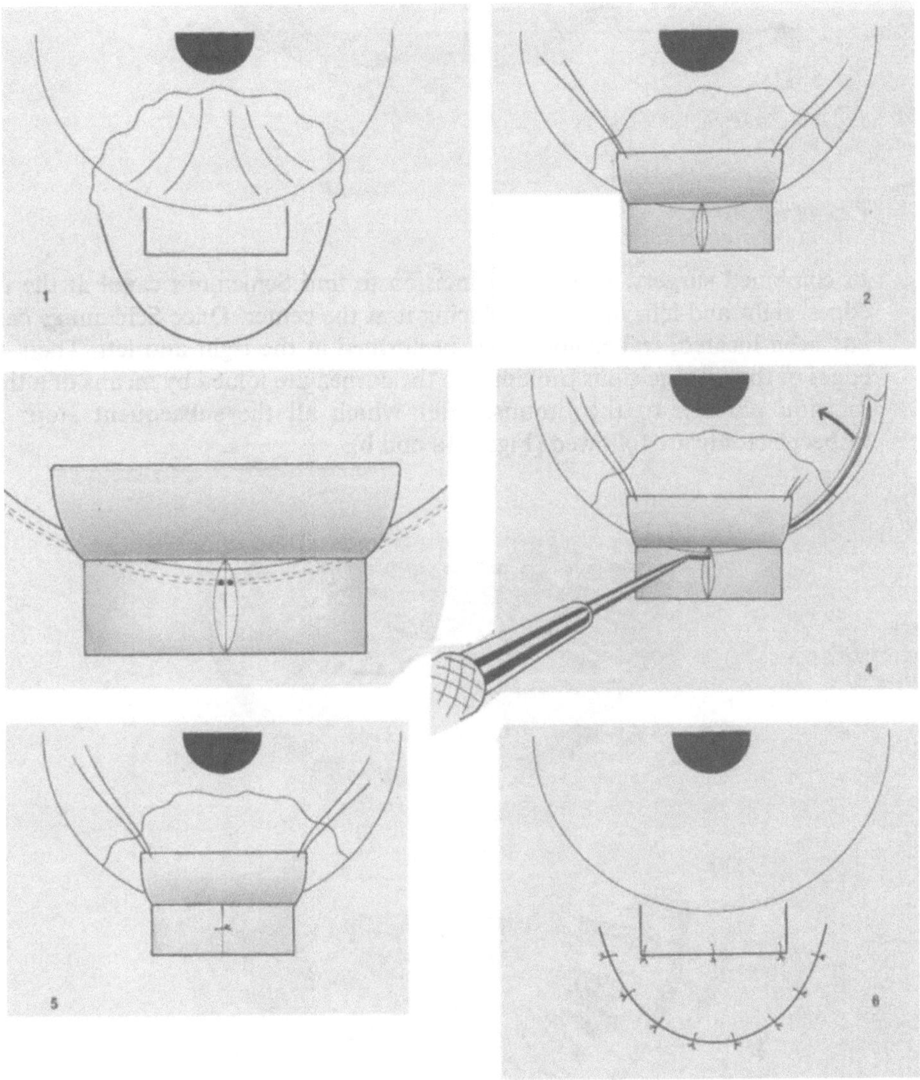

(a)

Fig. 10. **Trabeculotomy according to Harms' or Paufique's technique.** (a) 1, conjunctival flap. 2, scleral flap. 3, scleral incision perpendicular to the limbus. Location of Schlemm's canal. 4, Introduction of the trabeculotome. The same is performed at the left side. 5, closing of the scleral incision. Closing of both conjunctival and scleral flaps 6. The only difference between Harms' and Paufique's techniques is the kind of trabeculotome used. b) In the incision made to find Schlemm's canal, a superior dark triangle with its base downwards, and a white-nacreous triangle of base upwards, can be clearly seen. The dark triangle corresponds to Schlemm's canal and the nacreous one to the spur's fibers

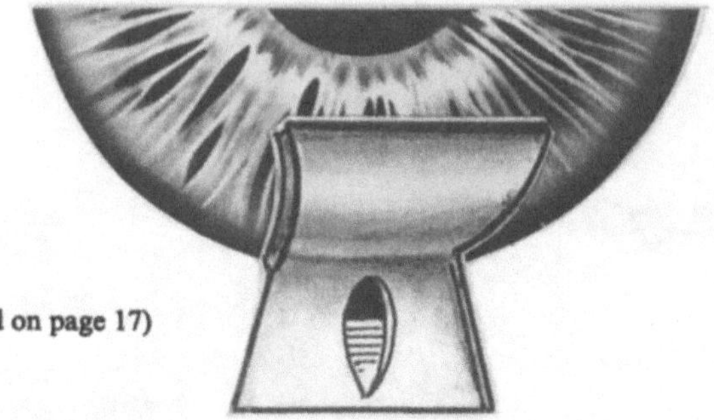

Fig. 10b. (see legend on page 17)

Combined surgery

In combined surgery, I make the incision to find Schlemm's canal at the two edges, right and left, instead of placing it at the center. Once Schlemm's canal has been located, trabeculotomy is performed at the right and left. Then, the edges of the two incisions proximal to the cornea are joined by means of a third incision parallel to the limbus, after which all the subsequent steps for trabeculectomy are followed (Figs. 11a and b).

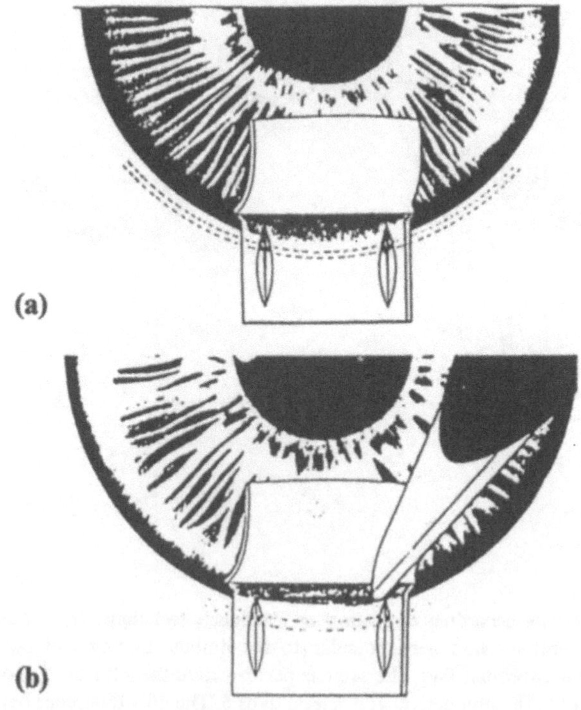

Fig. 11. **Combined surgery:** trabeculotomy+trabeculectomy. a) Once Schlemm's canal has been found, two trabeculotomies are performed; the one on the right is made through the incision on the right, and the one on the left, through the incision of the left. b) An incision parallel to the limbus joining the two proximal edges at the limbus of the incisions described in a) are performed, then penetrating into the anterior chamber

Echometry in the follow-up

In 1974, Buschmann and Bluth [41,42] were the first to conduct a follow-up of congenital glaucomas with echometric measurements. Echometry is very useful in the follow-up of congenital glaucoma, particularly when reoperation is required. There are four types of post-surgical evolution (Fig. 12). 1) The axial length does not increase, and, with time, falls within the normal range of growth; it is the best evolution one can expect. 2) The axial length continues to increase and deviates even further from the normal range; this is the worst type of evolution, and invariably requires reoperation. 3) The axial length continues to increase parallel to the normal range; reoperation is required in all such cases. 4) The fourth type of evolution, which was described by Massim and Pellat [30], is when the axial length remains for some time at pathological levels running parallel to the normal range, after which it increases sharply and returns parallel to the normal band. Also these cases must be reoperated even when the IOP is normal.

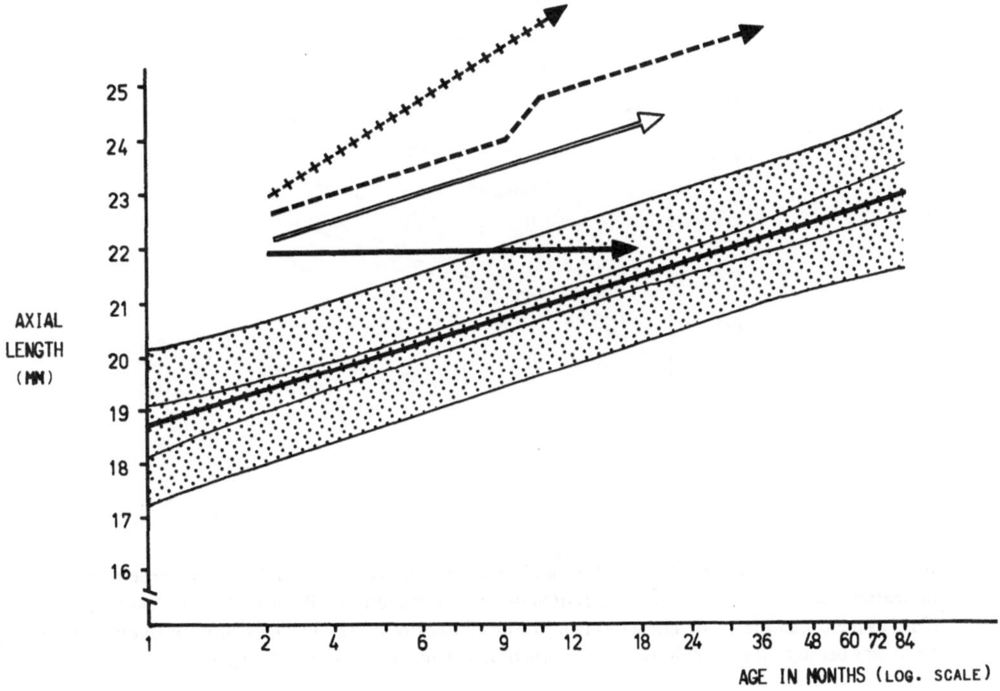

Fig. 12. Four different types of axial length evolution in congenital glaucoma

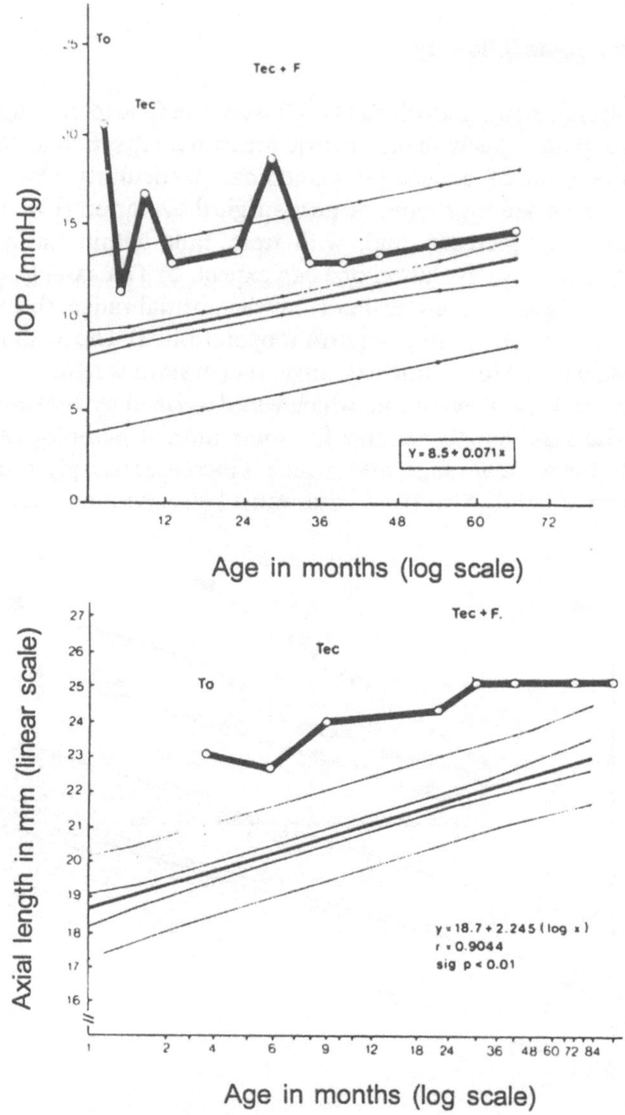

Fig. 13. **a and b) The evolution of IOP and axial length are well correlated. In these cases the indication for surgery is very easy. c) IOP values in the evolution fall within the normal range but close to the upper limits. d) The axial length started to grow markedly at six months of age but the child was brought for consultation at 2 years of age, when he underwent surgery**

When the axial length continues to grow and the IOP rises to pathological values, as shown in the case illustrated in Figures 13a and b, the indication for surgery is very simple, but in cases like that of Figures 13c and d, when the IOP stays just within the upper values of the normal range, echometry is of great value in deciding whether or not to reoperate. Carvalho *et al.* [43] also studied

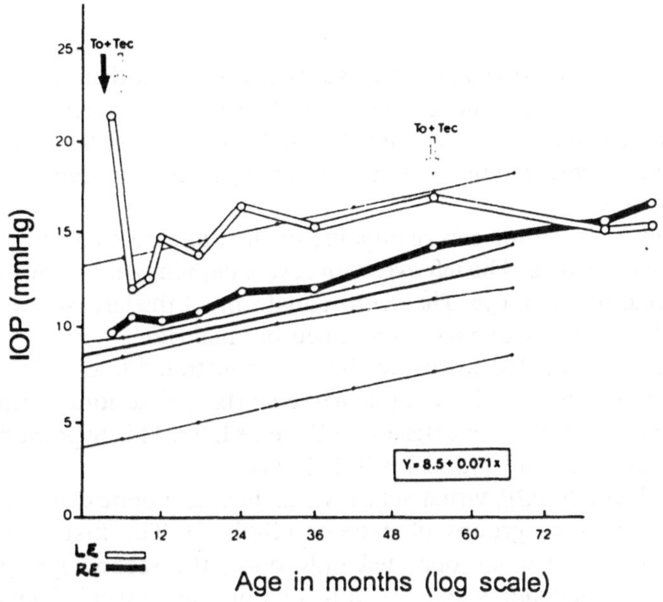

(c)

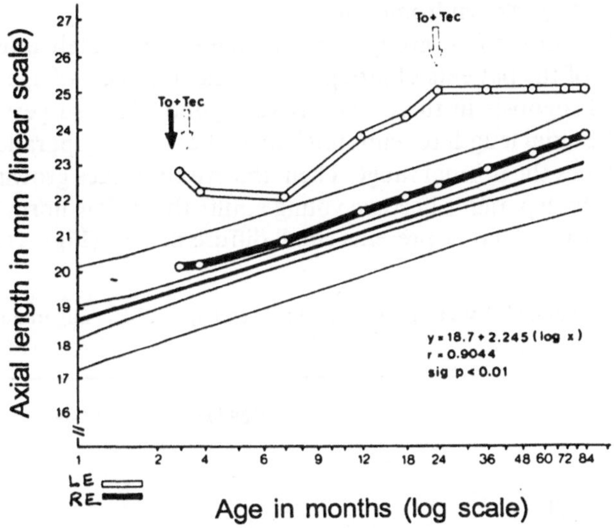

(d)

Fig. 13 (cont).

the results of goniotomy and trabeculotomy.

The following is a case in which echometry saved the eye of an 8-month-old child with congenital glaucoma just in time (Fig. 14). Right IOP stabilized between 10 and 15 mmHg by the time the child was 10 years old, while the axial length ceased enlarging at 24 mm. Left IOP stabilized between 15 and 20 mmHg, while at 18 months of age left axial length had increased 1 mm; at 2 years it continued to enlarge and when the child was 4 years old, axial length had reached 26 mm. Surgery was indicated but it was not performed until the patient was 6 years of age. At 10 years of age, the patient had a visual acuity of 20/30 in both eyes, and a myopia of –6 in his left eye and –3 in his right eye. Both eyes had a normal visual field and his optic nerve was normal in the right eye and severely damaged in the left eye, as revealed by confocal laser topography.

Figure 15a, shows severe cupping of the optic disk and Fig. 15b, the fellow normal optic disk. The left eye, with severe cupping, had a much larger cupping area than the right eye. The neuroretinal ring of the left eye was barely present, while the right eye had a complete neuroretinal rim.

Studies conducted worldwide have demonstrated that in 85% of cases, once the IOP has increased, the optic nerve starts to deteriorate immediately, while the visual field starts to deteriorate 10 years later. This hypothesis was proposed by Goldmann and Leydhecker in 1959 [44,45].

Axial length, IOP, visual acuity, visual field and optic disk configuration were studied in three groups of patients (Table 2). The first group consisted of congenital glaucomas operated only once, the second group of reoperated congenital glaucomas and the third one of late congenital glaucomas, goniodysgenesis, Rieger's syndrome, etc.

The babies of the first group were operated immediately after diagnosis was made. 95% of the patients of group 1 were under 2 years of age, and 50% under 2 months. Prognosis in these cases is very good when surgery normalizes the IOP and the axial length remains unchanged but running parallel to the abscissa until it reaches the normal range. Then, the eye continues growing like a normal one; when these patients become young adults the disk is normal and the visual field is almost normal or presents small diffuse defects (Figs. 16a, b and c).

Table 2. Axial length, IOP, visual acuity, visual field and optic disk configuration in three groups of patients

	No	Age (ys.)	Male	Female
Group 1 Primary congenital Glaucomas operated once	19	12-28	13	6
Group 2 Reoperated primary Congenital Glaucomas	12	7-22	10	2
Group 3 Goniodysgenesis	29	11–23	15	14
Total	60	7–24	38	22

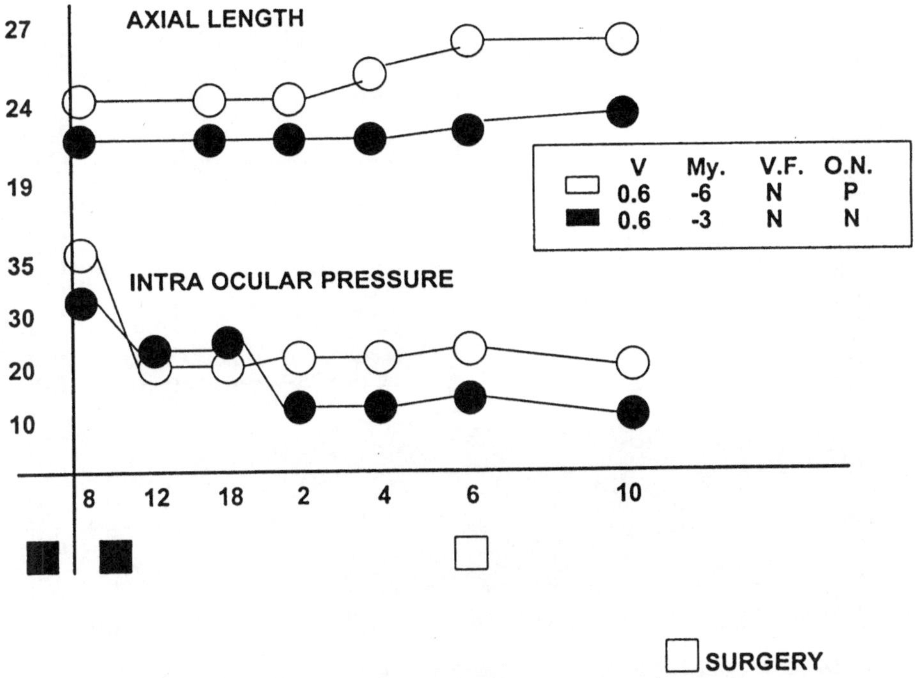

Fig. 14. **Importance of echometry in the follow-up.** In the ordinate, on the upper left, axial length in mm; on the lower right, IOP in mmHg. In the abscissa, age in months (8, 12, 18) and in years (2, 4, 6, 10). The gray circles represent the left eye which regulated its IOP and kept the normal growth of its axial length. The white circles represent the right eye, which presented IOP values near the normal ones while the axial length climbed to pathological values: 27 mm. The squares below indicate two trabeculotomies performed at 8 months of age and one combined surgery (trabeculotomy+trabeculectomy) at 6 years. V.F.: visual field, normal in both eyes; My: myopia, 6 in the reoperated eye and 3 in the eye operated once; V: visual acuity, with the same values in both eyes; O.N.: optic nerve, normal in the left eye and with typical glaucomatous cupping in the right eye. The figure shows that both visual acuity and visual field are normal in spite of the evolution, while the optic nerve is severely damaged in the reoperated eye

In the second group, one or more reoperations were necessary because surgery failed to regulate the IOP and the axial length continued to grow. In these cases, if not operated as many times as is necessary to regulate their IOP, when they become young adults, their optic disks have concentrical glaucomatous cupping and the visual field presents a larger diffuse defect (Figs. 17a, b and c).

The third group (late congenital glaucoma, Rieger's syndrome and goniodysgenesis) consisted of children older than 5 years of age, whose sclera was no longer elastic and even if they were hypertensive, their axial length remained normal.

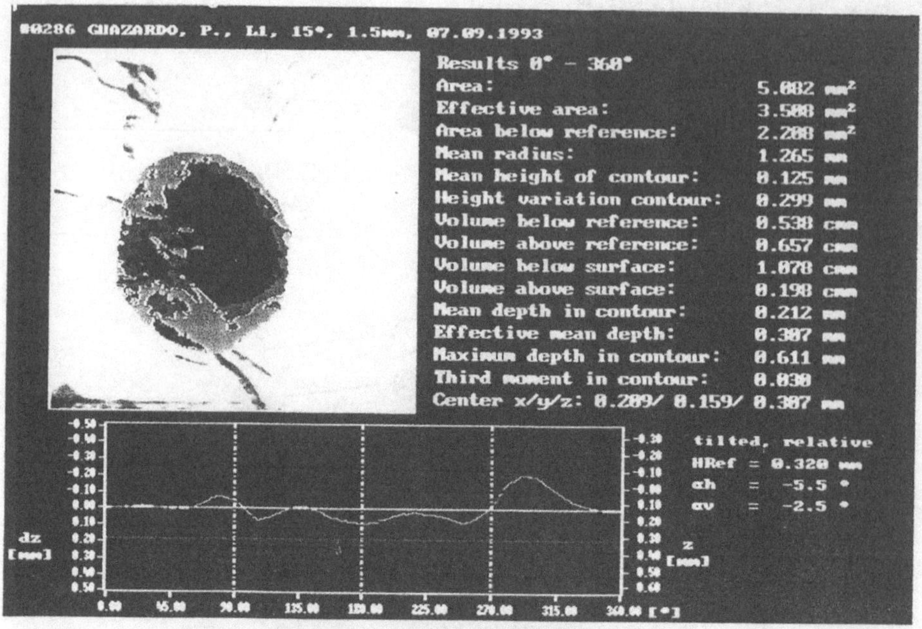

(a)

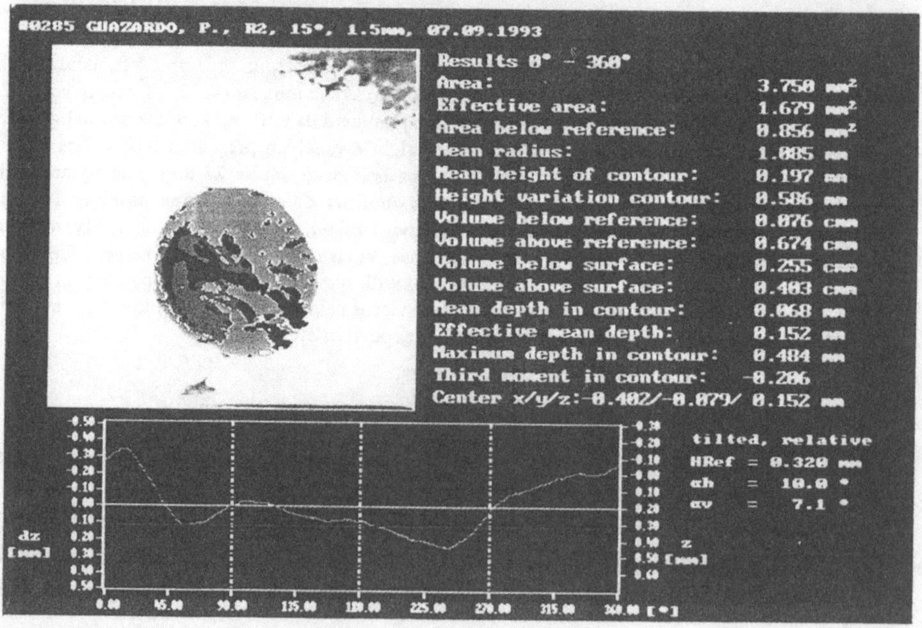

(b)

Fig. 15. Confocal tomography of the optic disk of the patient of figure 14. a) Image of the optic disk. In light and dark gray, neuroretinal rim; in black, optic disk cupping. The optic disk cupping is very large and the neuroretinal rim is very thin. b) The dark area is the small cupping. The neuroretinal rim is almost normal, nevertheless it was slightly damaged and it is thin in the inferior temporal part

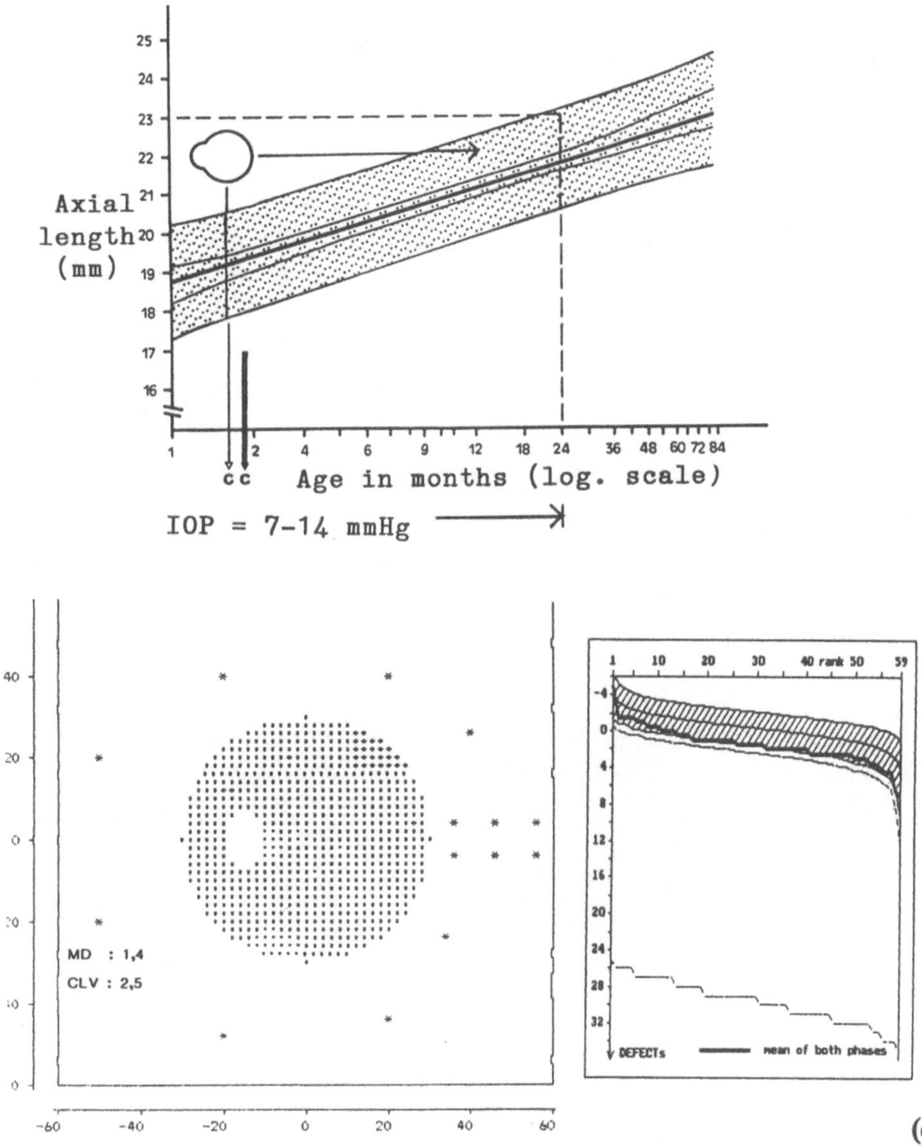

(a) (b) (c)

Fig. 16. a) Normal range band of axial length growth, with the eye of a child consulting within the first month of age represented (abscissas). This child had an axial length of 22 mm (ordinates). The arrow running parallel to the abscissa indicates the time when surgery was performed, and the arrow coming from the eye and running parallel to the ordinate indicates the axial length follow-up, which did not grow and at 9 months of age fell within the normal range band. The dashed line, joining 22 mm of length with 24 months of age shows that all the children underwent surgery before 24 months of age and that the axial length was not higher than 23 mm. During these 24 months of age normal IOP values ranged between 7 and 14 mmHg. b) Normal visual field (grey scale) with the visual indices. c) Bebie's curve

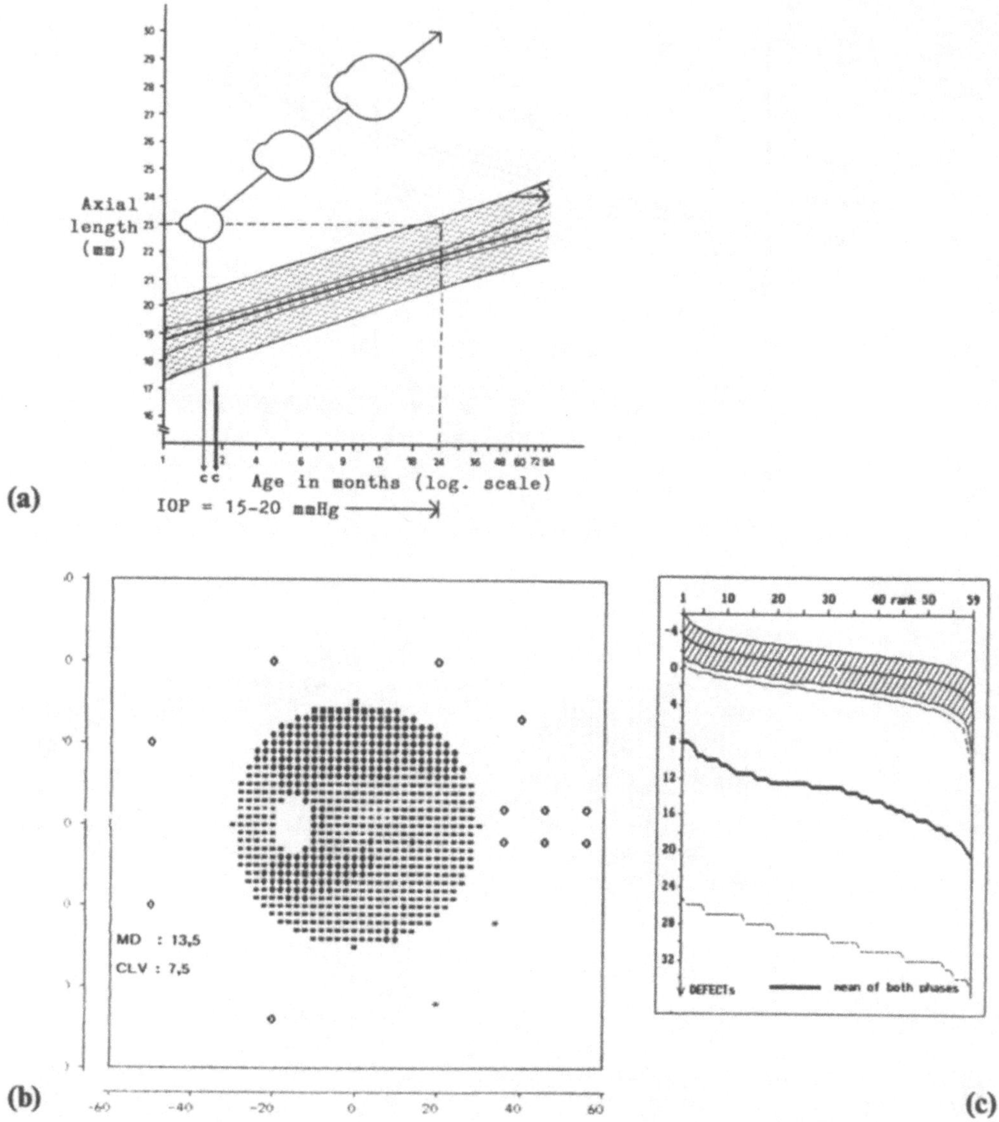

Fig. 17. **Typical follow-up of group 2.** a) Follow-up of the axial length and representation of how the eye continues to grow after surgery. b) Visual field. Grey scale presentation evidencing deteriorated MD values and normal CLV values. c) Bebie's curve showing more clearly the behaviour of MD and CLV and the presence of a typically diffuse defect

Axial length. After surgery, group 1 remained at the values reached before surgery; in group 2 (reoperated cases), the axial length was longer, and in group 3 (late congenital glaucomas, Rieger's syndrome and goniodysgenesis) it fell within the normal range, because the sclera does not enlarge after 5 years of age (Fig. 18).

Refraction. In group 2 the eyes were highly myopic, group 1 was mildly myopic and in group 3 the eyes were almost emmetropic (Fig. 19).

Visual acuity. The best visual acuity was found in group 3, and the worst in group 2. In group 1, it was substantially good, except in those cases arriving late to consultation (Fig. 20). When the axial length was higher than 27 mm, the visual acuity decreased substantially. Our findings are consistent with those of Vidic and Lerchner [46]. Visual acuity also depends on the location of the tears in the endothelium and Descemet's membrane. If tears are central, the visual acuity is 20/60, if they are peripheral, it is 20/50 and if there are no tears, it is 20/20 or 20/25. Tears in endothelium and Descemet's membrane affected visual acuity, particularly in group 2. In severe cases, when tears are located at the center of the cornea, a perforating corneal graft later supplemented by refractive surgery is required.

Visual field. We compared differential light sensitivity perimetry and high-pass resolution perimetry in the three groups. These two techniques had previously been studied in adults [47–50], but not in children with congenital glaucoma.

As we reported at the IPS Meeting held in Malmö in 1990 [51], diffuse damage was the only defect observed in children who received surgery for congenital glaucoma; the visual field was studied with the Octopus 2000 equipment. From 10 to 28 years after surgery visual field examinations were performed with the Octopus 1-2-3 apparatus (Interzeag, program G1, 59 locations within 30 degrees of the visual field) and Ophthimus High-Pass Resolution Perimetry (HighTech Vision, Malmö, version 2.0) (50 locations are measured within the central 30 degrees of the visual field).

We compared the results obtained with both instruments by means of the PeriData program, so as to correlate the mean defect (MD) and corrected loss variance (CLV) of the Octopus PeriData with those of the Ophthimus HighTech Vision PeriData, and then to study the means and standard deviations of both parameters in order to make a statistical analysis to find the significance.

In this study, Pearson's correlation coefficient was calculated between mean defect and neural capacity (NC), mean defect and global deviation (GD), and corrected loss variance and local deviation (LD) in the three groups. Neural capacity is an index estimating the total number of functioning retinal ganglion cells.

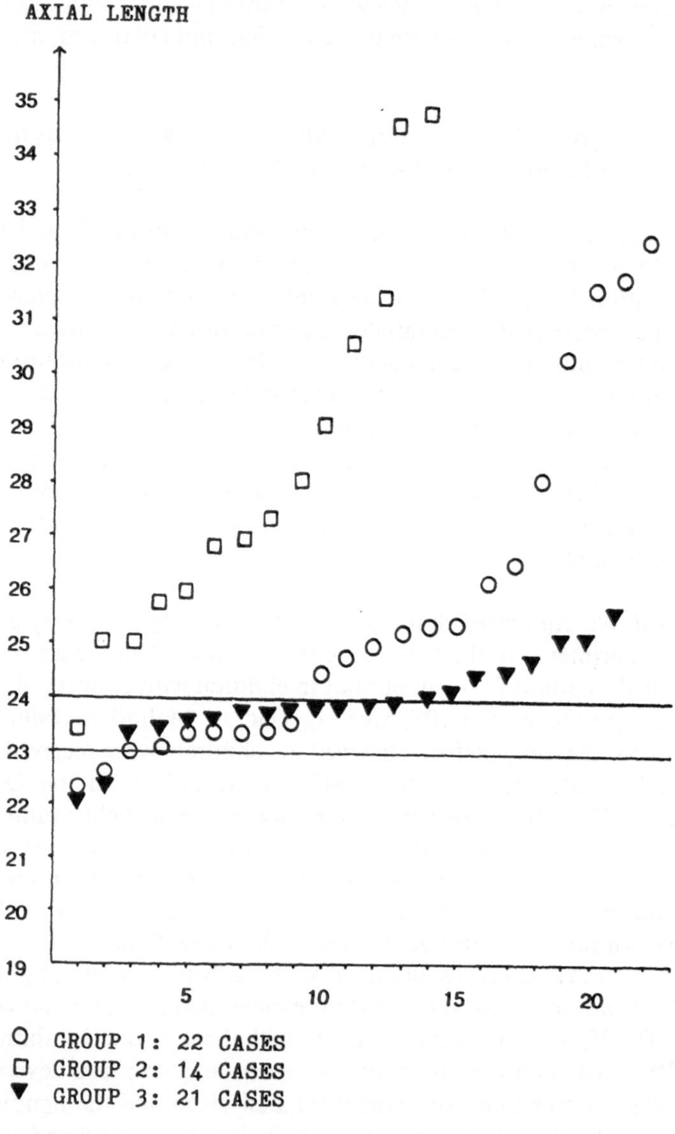

Fig. 18. **Axial length of the 3 groups.** Group 1: primary congenital glaucoma operated once. Group 2: reoperated primary congenital glaucoma. Group 3: goniodysgenesis. On the ordinate: axial length in mm. On the abscissa: number of cases. Between the two horizontal lines: normal axial length in mm

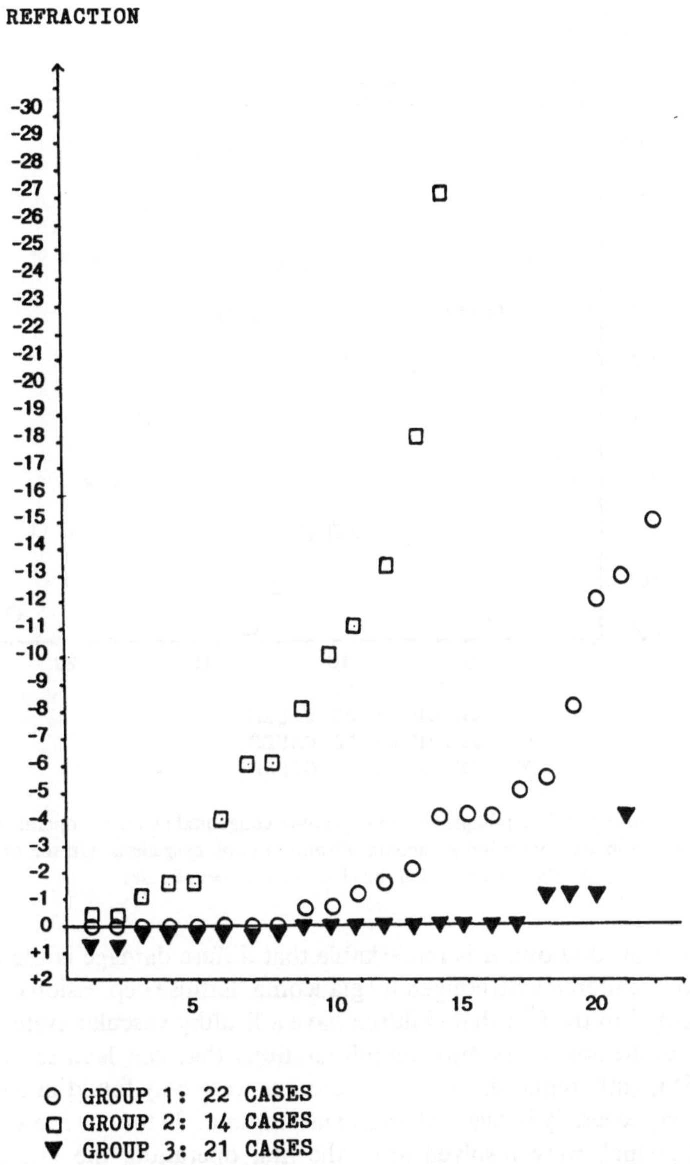

Fig. 19. **Refraction of the 3 groups.** Group 1: primary congenital glaucoma operated once. Group 2: reoperated primary congenital glaucoma. Group 3: goniodysgenesis. On the ordinate: refraction in diopters. On the abscissa: number of cases

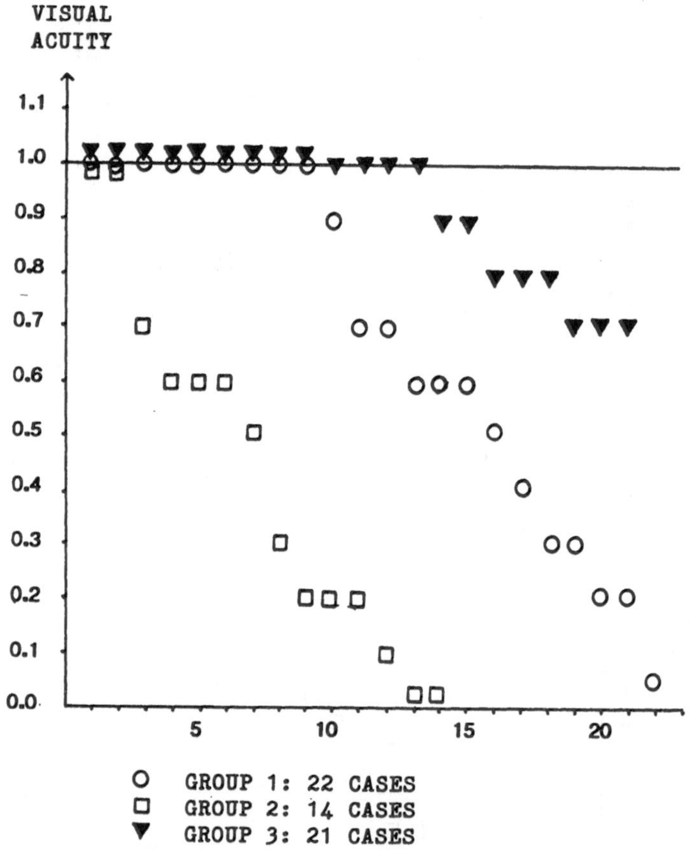

Fig. 20. **Visual acuity of the 3 groups.** Group 1: primary congenital glaucoma operated once. Group 2: reoperated primary congenital glaucoma. Group 3: goniodysgenesis. On the ordinate: visual acuity according to the Snellen chart. On the abscissa: number of cases

As mentioned above, it is remarkable that diffuse damage is the only defect observed in children with congenital glaucoma. Diffuse depression can probably be attributed to the fact that children have a healthy vascular system, and thus the risk of hemorrhages and microinfarctions that can lead to scotomatous defects is greatly reduced. Macular scotomas were only found in children with amblyopia, generally in eyes with an axial length of 30 mm or more. In cases of group 1, which were resolved after the first operation, the visual field was generally normal or had a mild diffuse depression. In group 2 (reoperated cases), the diffuse depression was more severe.

We have studied 50 eyes of 30 patients belonging to the three groups with and without optic disk glaucomatous damage who were followed-up in the Glaucoma Clinic of the Department of Ophthalmology of the University of Buenos Aires, Argentina.

Mean defect and global deviation. In group 1 MD and GD were significantly correlated: $\boldsymbol{r=0.80, p<0.001}$ (Fig. 21). The correlation was not significant in groups 2 and 3.

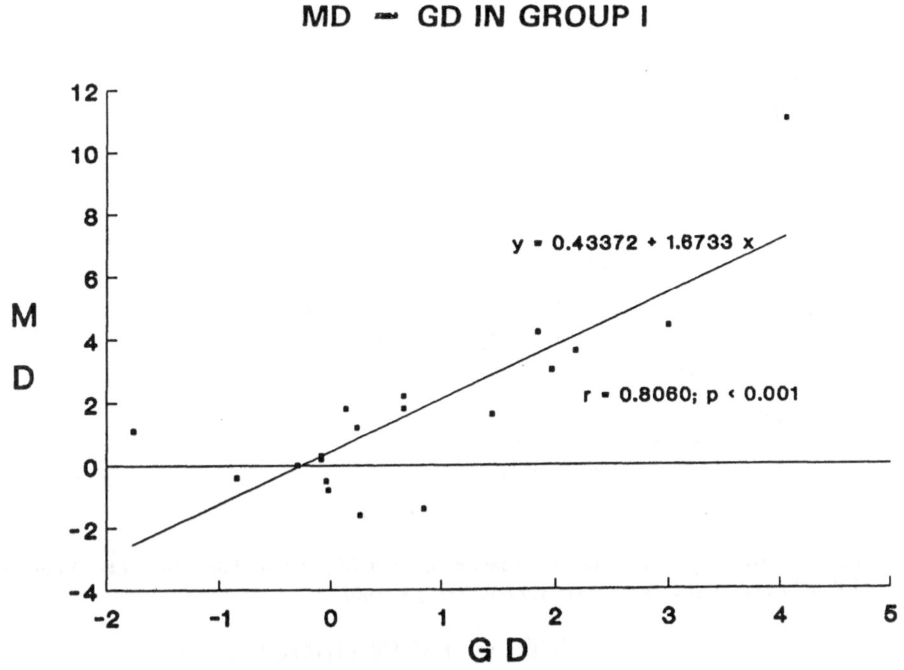

Fig. 21. **Relationship between mean defect (MD) and global deviation (GD).** In group 1: MD-GD: correlated significantly: $r=0.8060; p<0.001$

Corrected loss variance and local deviation. In group 1 CLV and LD were significantly correlated: $\boldsymbol{r=0.78, p<0.001}$ (Fig. 22). The two parameters were not correlated in group 2, and the correlation was fairly significant in Group 3: $\boldsymbol{r=0.45, p<0.01}$.

Mean defect and neural capacity. In group 1 there was a significant correlation between MD and NC: $\boldsymbol{r=0.78, p<0.001}$ (Fig. 23). The correlation was not significant in group 2, and fairly significant in group 3: $\boldsymbol{r=0.42, p<0.02}$. However, when we tried to correlate the MD and NC of the three groups together, we found two groups of cases: one located far from the zero line and the other clustering around. The correlation is not represented by a straight line but by a curve (Fig. 24), which means that in many cases the MD is normal but the NC is not. The correlation between these two indices is far from perfect. In my opinion, these different methods of psychophysical tests measure different aspects of the visual field system.

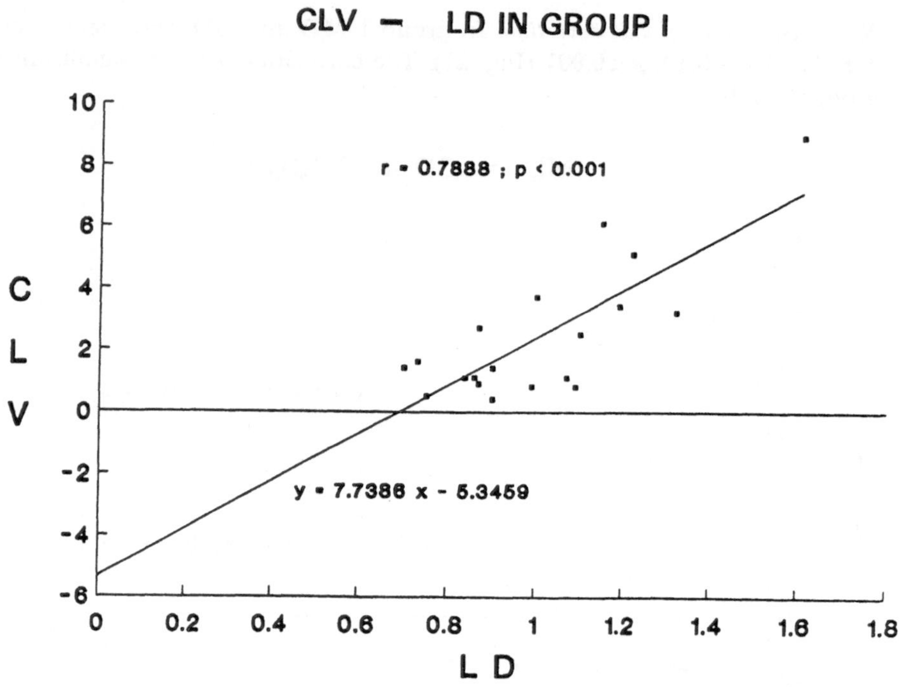

Fig. 22. **Relationship between corrected loss variance (CLV) and local deviation (LD).** In group 1, CLV and LD correlated significantly: $r = 0.7888$; $p < 0.001$

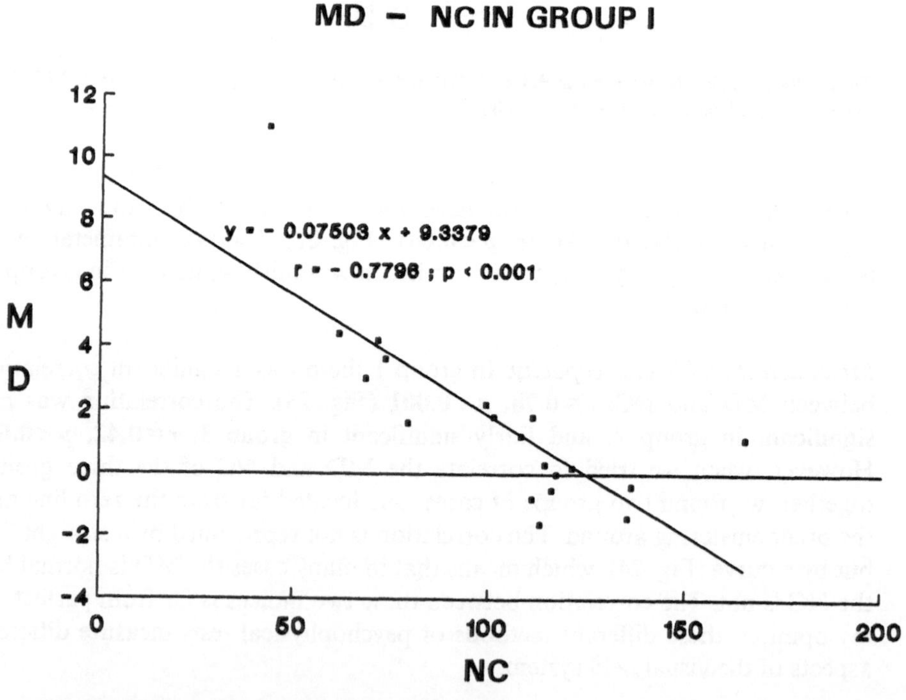

Fig. 23. **Relationship between mean defect (MD) and neuroretinal capacity (NC).** The first group correlated significantly: $r = 0.77796$; $p < 0.001$

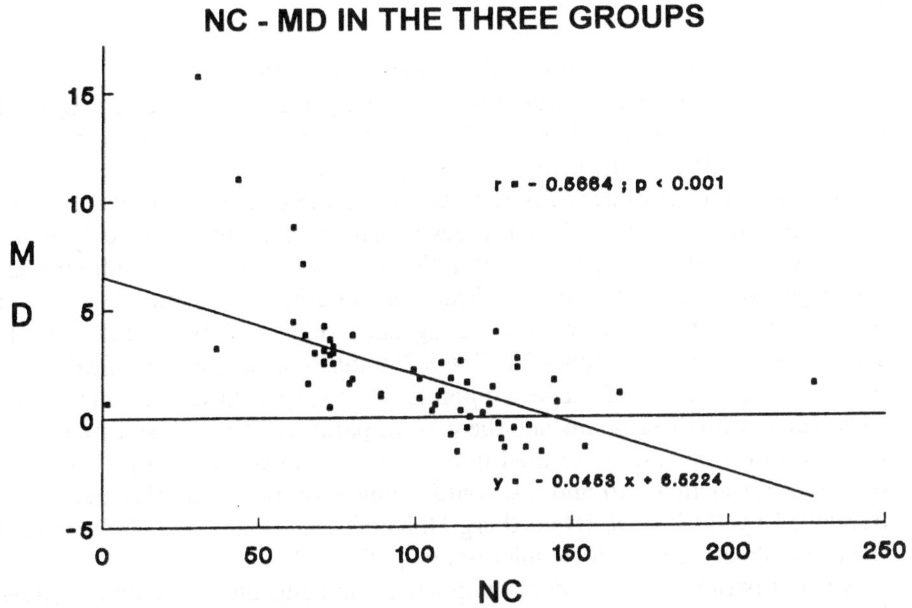

Fig. 24. **Correlation between mean defect (MD) and neural capacity (NC) of the three groups together.** When we tried to correlate the MD and NC of the three groups together we found two groups of cases; one located far from the zero line and the other, surrounding it. The correlation is not represented by a straight line but rather by a curve. This means that in many cases the MD is normal but the NC is pathological. The correlation between these two indices is far from perfect

As far as we are aware, we were the first to study the visual field in children with differential light sensitivity perimetry (Octopus 2000 and 1-2-3 perimeters) and with high-pass resolution perimetry. Both perimeters gave reliable results in children between 5 and 10 years of age. To be sure of the accuracy of our results, we used a reliability factor of below 10. Both perimetric methods showed the absence of scotomas in the visual fields of children. The only visual field damage that can be found in children was diffuse sensitivity depression, i.e., pathological mean defect values.

In conclusion, both differential light sensitivity perimetry and high-pass resolution perimetry can be used to examine the visual field in children from 5 to 8 years of age. Before starting the examination the children are allowed to become acquainted with its functioning. Our experience shows that high-pass resolution perimetry is very useful in children: they accept the examination better because it is easier and it takes only 6 minutes per eye.

With both perimetric methods the only defect found is diffuse sensitivity loss. In cases with normal MD values, high-pass resolution perimetry also revealed abnormal NC. Therefore, the indices of the two methods reflect different aspects of the condition of the visual field system.

Optic nerve

In the three groups we studied the optic disks with the Heidelberg Retina Tomograph (HRT) manufactured by Heidelberg Engineering (Interzeag). The equipment has a laser supplier (He Ne Laser long wave = 632.8), a laser camera which receives the energy of the laser supplier and generates the laser beam, a monitor and a control panel. A joystick moves the camera, thus changing the direction of the laser beam. The joystick is placed on a table with a chin-holder and a forehead-holder like those of a slit lamp. With the pupil undilated and under general anesthesia with Penthrane or Halothane, 32 planes of the optic nerve with a 50-μm interval separating each other can be obtained in 1.6 seconds. Each of these planes has 256 × 256 pixels which, if multiplied by 32, means a total of 2,097,152 reported points. The topography of the optic nerve is thus rebuilt with these points and the various parameters can be assessed. Three image acquisitions are performed in each eye, the mean is obtained (standard deviation lower than 30) and the contour line is drawn on it. This device was developed by Burk *et al.* (Heidelberg University, Germany) [52–54] exploiting the principle of laser confocal microscopy [30].

A list of parameters, in order of importance in congenital glaucoma is shown in Table 3.

I shall now describe the alterations found in each parameter for each group, compared with the parameters of a group of 108 normals, ranging from 10 to 25 years of age (Figs. 25 and 31).

Rim volume. Group 1 (glaucomas operated only once) and group 3 (late congenital glaucomas) had a rim volume *lower than* normal values and higher than the one found in group 2 (reoperated congenital glaucomas). Group 2 was exposed to ocular hypertension for the longest time; therefore, it had the lowest rim volume values. Because rim volume and cup volume are part of the same volume separated by the reference plane, this reduction in the rim volume is invariably associated with an increase in cup volume.

Cup volume. Cup volume was the most altered in group 2, the one with the longest exposure to ocular hypertension. The cup volume was *12 times higher* than the normal value, while groups 1 and 3 had only triple the normal value.

Rim area. Group 1 had higher rim values compared with normal values, and groups 2 and 3 had values slightly lower than normal. This is due to the enlargement of the disk area.

Cup area. Group 2 had a cup area four times greater than normal values and groups 1 and 3, twice and a half the normal values.

To understand these findings better, one should consider what happens in congenital glaucoma as compared with glaucoma in adults. Because ocular

Table 3. Optic nerve head parameters in congenital glaucoma (version 1.11)

1. Rim volume
2. Cup volume
3. Rim area

Basic parameters in 360 degrees
4. Cup area
5. Third moment (cup shape measure)
6. Maximum depth in contour
7. Mean RNFL thickness
8. Height variation contour

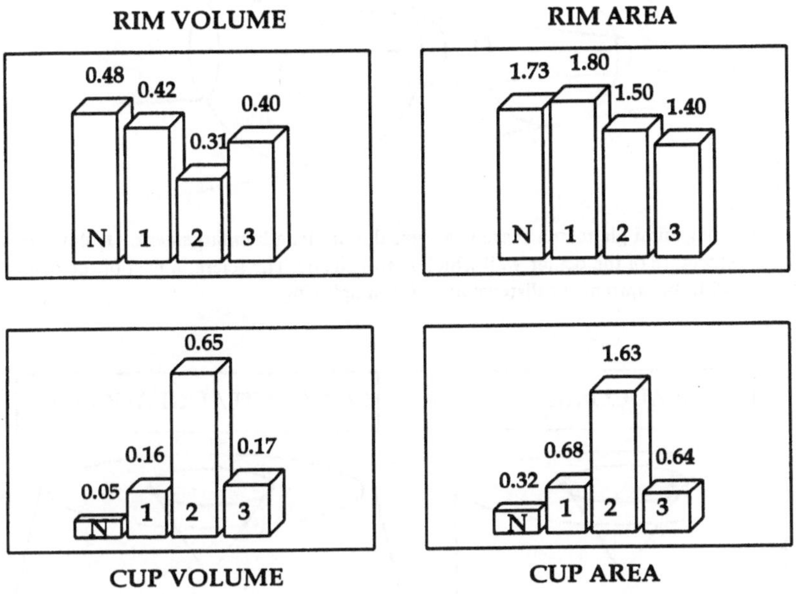

Fig. 25. In group 2 the rim volume is greatly reduced while in groups 1 and 3 it is slightly lower than normal values.
Cup volume: Group 2 is 12 times higher than the normal values. Group 1 and 3 just triple this value
Rim area: Group 1 is higher than normal values and group 2 and 3 are slightly lower than this value (this is due to the enlargement of the disk area)
Cup area: Group 2 is 4 times greater than normal value, and group 1 and 3 is 2 times higher than this value

hypertension in adults occurs when the eye is no longer distensible, the increase in IOP does not affect the size of Elschnig's ring. In congenital glaucoma there is a typical axial length enlargement. Ocular hypertension affects the structures of the ocular wall, which is still elastic. The sclera, a part of the ocular wall, is distended, with the consequent distension of Elschnig's ring. As already mentioned, axial length enlargement of the eye was associated with an increase in volume, especially in reoperated primary congenital glaucomas (group 2) (Fig. 26). Distension of the ocular wall was much less in group 3 (late congenital glaucomas) because ocular hypertension took place after 5 years of age (the limit for ocular distensibility); it was also less in group 1 because the IOP was regulated immediately after the first surgery.

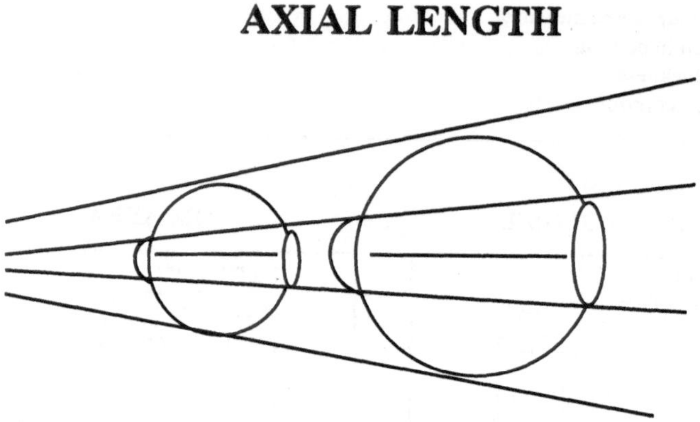

Fig. 26. In congenital glaucoma there is a typical axial length enlargement. Ocular hypertension affects the structure of the ocular wall which is still elastic. The sclera, a part of the ocular wall, is distended, with the consequent distension of Elschnig's ring

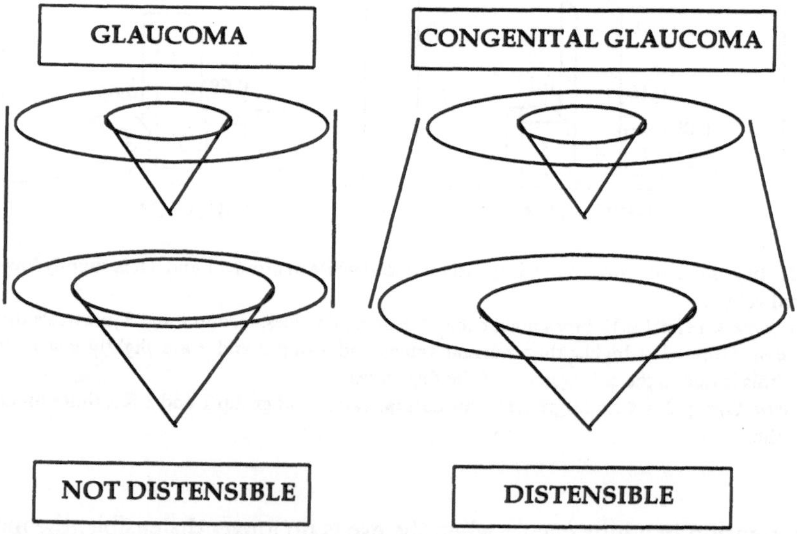

Fig. 27. Left: glaucoma in adults. The eye is not distensible. In the upper part: normal optic disk. In the lower part: optic disk in glaucoma. The Elschnig ring does not distend. When the cup area increases the neuroretinal ring is reduced.
Right: congenital glaucoma. In the upper part: normal optic disk. In the lower part: optic disk in congenital glaucoma. The cup area also increases, because the Elschnig ring distends. They have a large neuroretinal rim area due to the distension of the total disk area

Figure 27 illustrates the enlargement process that brings about an enlargement of Elschnig's ring, and consequently, an increase of the disk area. In adults, Elschnig's ring does not distend. When the cup area increases, the neuroretinal rim area is reduced. However, in children, the cup area also increases, because Elschnig's ring distends. Children have a large neuroretinal rim area due to the distension of the total disk area.

As the eye enlarges due to ocular hypertension in the three axes (x, y, z), the optic disk not only enlarges in axis z but also in axes y and x. Figure 28 shows the normal surface compared with that of the three groups. The surface in group 1 is larger than normal, and it is even larger in group 2; the surface of group 3 is the same as the normal one. The surface of the neuroretinal rim in groups 1, 2 and 3 is almost the same (due to the enlargement of the axial length, which results in a larger total area of the optic nerve head).

Figure 29 shows the values of the surface of the disk area, rim area and cup area in the three groups. In group 2 the disk area is significantly increased as well as the cup area.

Cup shape measure (Fig. 30). The cup shape measure in groups 1 and 3 were consistent with the mean normal values, while in group 2 the value was more than twice greater than the standard deviation.

Maximum cup depth. As explained above, groups 1 and 3 had a normal maximum cup depth, while it was double the normal value in group 2 (Fig. 30).

Mean RNFL thickness. This parameter was normal in groups 1 and 3 while in group 2 the thickness of the retinal fiber layers decreased beyond half the normal value (Fig. 30).

Height variation contour. This parameter was normal in all three groups. This suggests that there is no localized depression of the contour line in any quadrant or octant (absence of scotomatous defects in congenital glaucomas) (Fig. 30).

As mentioned above, although the mean RNFL thickness decreased in all groups (much more in group 2), the height variation contour was normal in all three groups. This finding is due to the fact that there was no localized damage of the retina but there was always a general decrease in thickness (Fig. 31).

In open angle glaucoma of adults, unlike the situation in groups 1–3, the height variation in contour is pathological, while the mean RNFL thickness also decreases (Fig. 32).

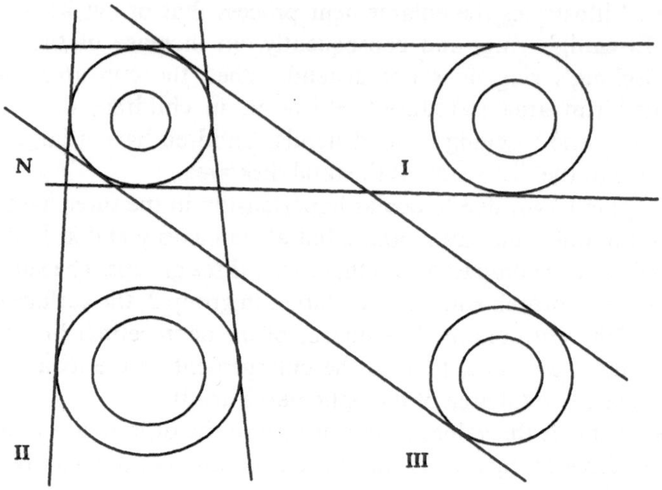

Fig. 28. **The normal surface of the disk N is compared with the surface of the disk of group 1, 2 and 3. Group 1 has a larger surface than the normal. Group 2 has the largest surface, and group 3 has the same surface as the normal one**

PARAMETERS CORRELATION BETWEEN
NORMAL & CONGENITAL GLAUCOMA
OPTIC NERVE HEAD

PARAMETER	NORMAL	Group 1	Group 2	Group 3
• DISK AREA	2.05	2.47	3.14	2.09
• RIM AREA	1.74	1.79	1.50	1.40
• CUP AREA	0.32	0.68	1.63	0.64

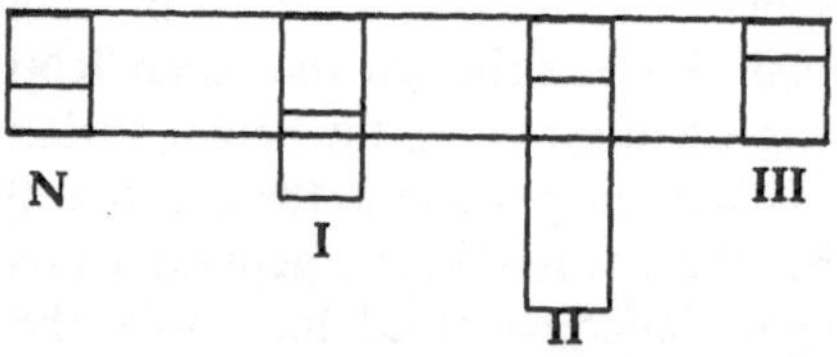

Fig. 29. **Values of the surface of the disk area, rim area and cup area in the three groups**

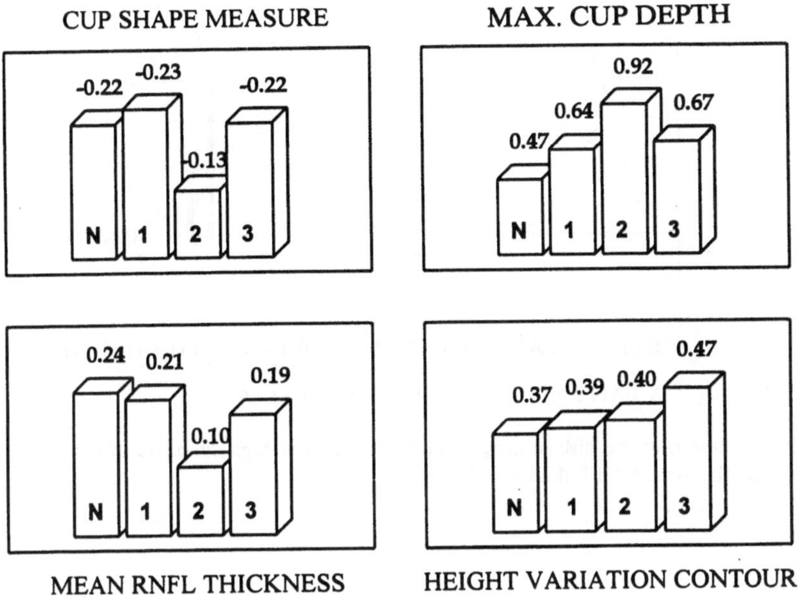

Fig. 30.
Cup Shape Measure: Group 2 has a pathological value greater than twice the standard deviation while groups 1 and 3 are normal.
Max. Cup Depth: Group 2 has double the normal value and groups 1 and 3 fall within the normal range
Mean RNFL Thickness: Group 2 decreases to half the normal value while groups 1 and 3 are normal.
Height Variation Contour: The three groups are normal. This suggests that there is no localized depression of the contour line (absence of scotomatous defects in C.G.)

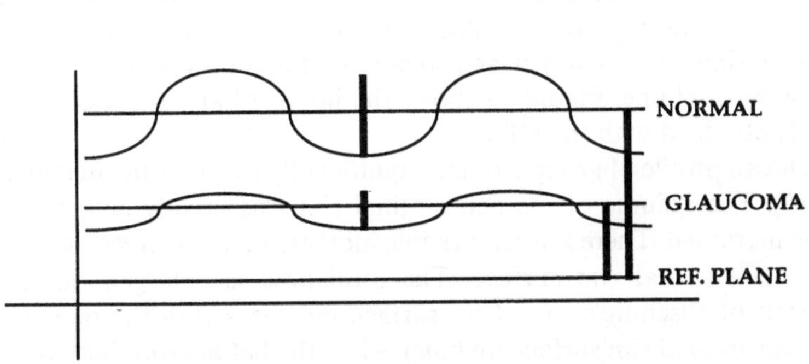

- HEIGHT VARIATION CONTOUR DECREASES
- MEAN RNFL THICKNESS DECREASES

Fig. 31. Evolution of the disk in glaucoma. The high variation of contour decreases, and the mean retinal nerve fiber layers (RNFL) thickness decreases

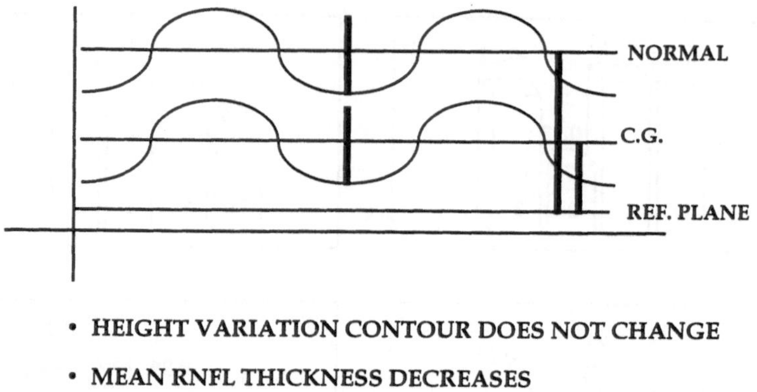

Fig. 32. Evolution of the disk in congenital glaucoma. The high variation of contour does not change and the mean RNFL thickness decreases

Profiles

Based on the different parameters of the optic nerve head and the data obtained with the HRT (software 1.11), we constructed the mean profile of the optic nerve head in each group with the Turbocad software package (version 2.0). To compare the findings to the mean profile of a normal disk, we studied a normal group of 108 subjects aged between 9 and 25 years.

Figure 33 shows the mean profile of group 1 as compared with the profile of the normal optic nerve. These profiles are almost the same because, as surgery regulated the IOP within a short time, the optic nerve did not suffer. A comparison of their surfaces shows that the increase in the total area is due to an increase in the cup area and not to a reduction in the neuroretinal rim area. Elschnig's ring became larger and, therefore, the total disk area became larger than the normal one. Figure 34 shows the image of an optic disk belonging to group 1, obtained with the HRT.

The mean profile of group 2 differs significantly from the normal mean profile (Fig. 35). The volume of the neuroretinal rim was greatly decreased and cup volume increased. There is a remarkable increase in cup surface and a reduction in the neuroretinal rim surface. The total area is enlarged due to a large distension of Elschnig's ring. Cup surface increases with the reduction of the tilted neuroretinal rim surface (in blue), while the flat neuroretinal rim (in green) remains almost unchanged. According to our experience with the evolution of open angle glaucoma in adults, when the red area of the cup fills the tilted neuroretinal rim area and overlaps the flat neuroretinal rim area, localized fiber defects leading to visual field scotomas, appear. This does not occur in children because the flat neuroretinal rim remains unchanged. Figure 36 shows the image of an optic disk belonging to group 2, obtained with the HRT.

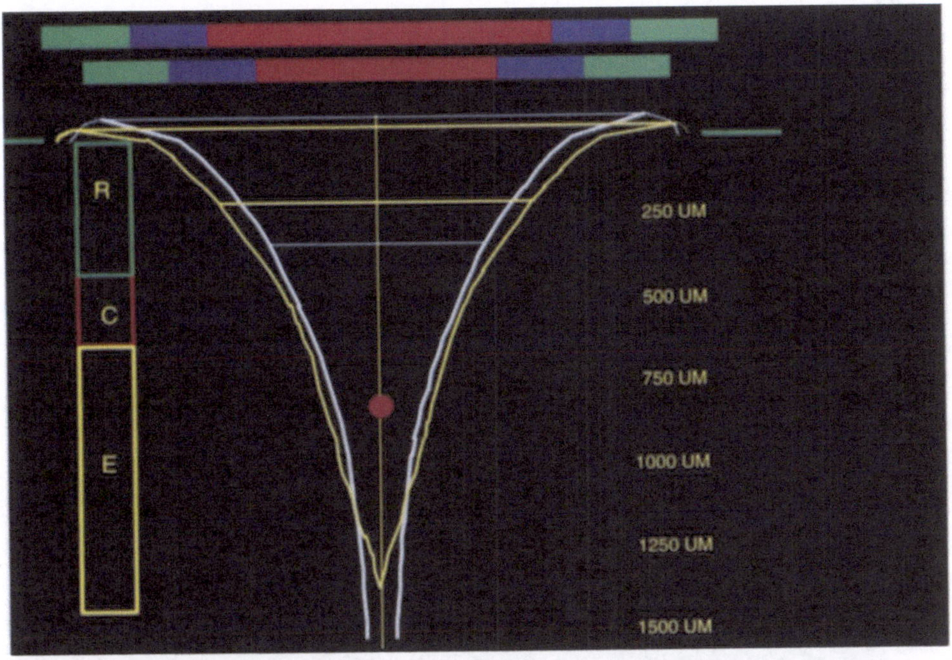

Fig. 33. Mean profile of group 1 is compared with the profile of the normal group. These profiles are almost the same because, as surgery succeeded to regulate the intraocular pressure quickly, the optic nerve did not suffer. Horizontal line: green: flat neuroretinal rim; blue: tilted neuroretinal rim; red: cup. Vertical line: R: retina, C: choroid, E: sclera (Violet profile: normal profile; yellow profile: profile of group 1)

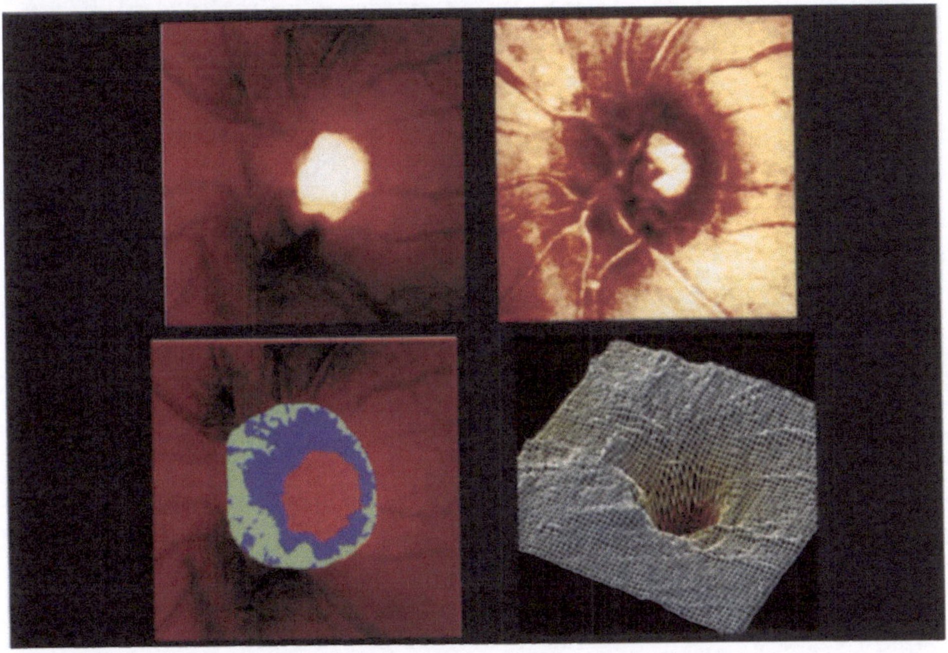

Fig. 34. Example of the Heidelberg retina tomograph (HRT) of a patient of group 1. Upper side left: topographic image. Upper side right: reflectivity image. Lower side left: green: surface of the neuroretinal rim; blue: neuroretinal tilted plane; red: surface of the cup. Lower right: three-dimensional image

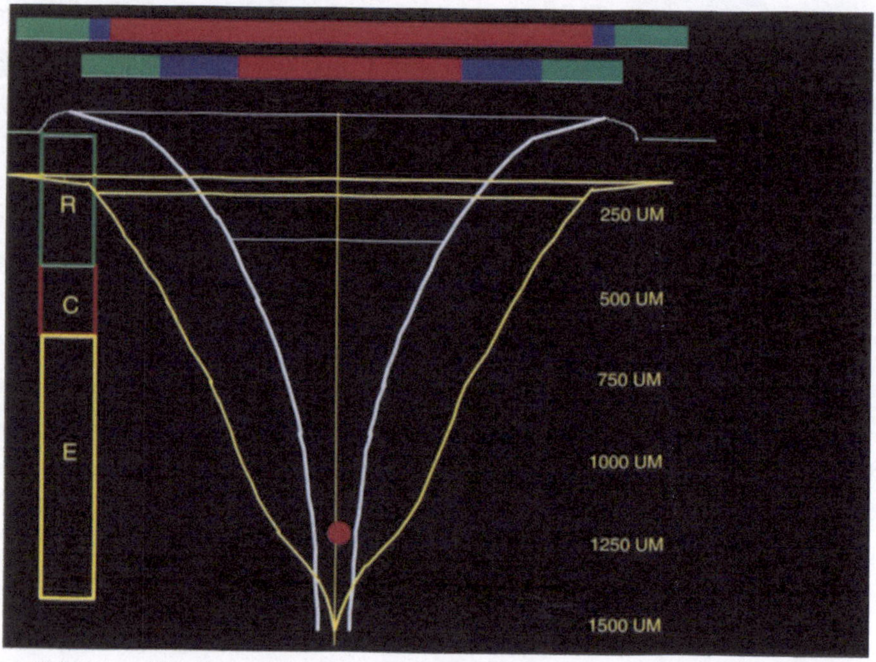

Fig. 35. Mean profile of group 2 is compared with the profile of the normal group. This group differs significantly from the normal mean profile. It shows a great increase in the cup volume. Horizontal line: green: flat neuroretinal rim; blue: tilted neuroretinal rim; red: cup. Vertical line: R: retina, C: choroid, E: sclera (Violet profile: normal profile; yellow profile: profile of group 2)

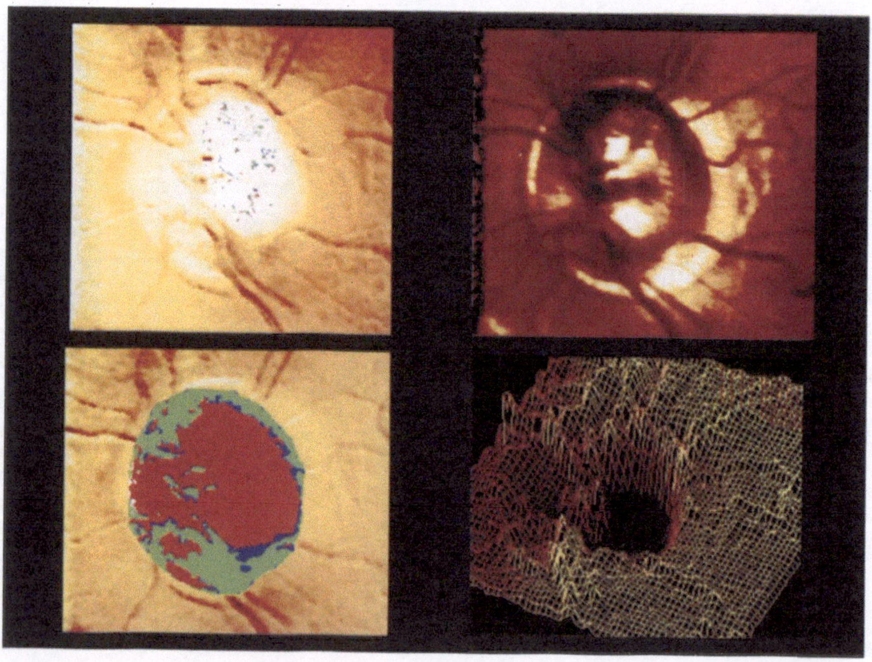

Fig. 36. Example of the Heidelberg retina tomograph (HRT) of a patient of group 2. Upper side left: topographic image. Upper side right: reflectivity image. Lower side left: green: surface of the neuroretinal rim; blue: neuroretinal tilted plane; red: surface of the cup. Lower right: three-dimensional image

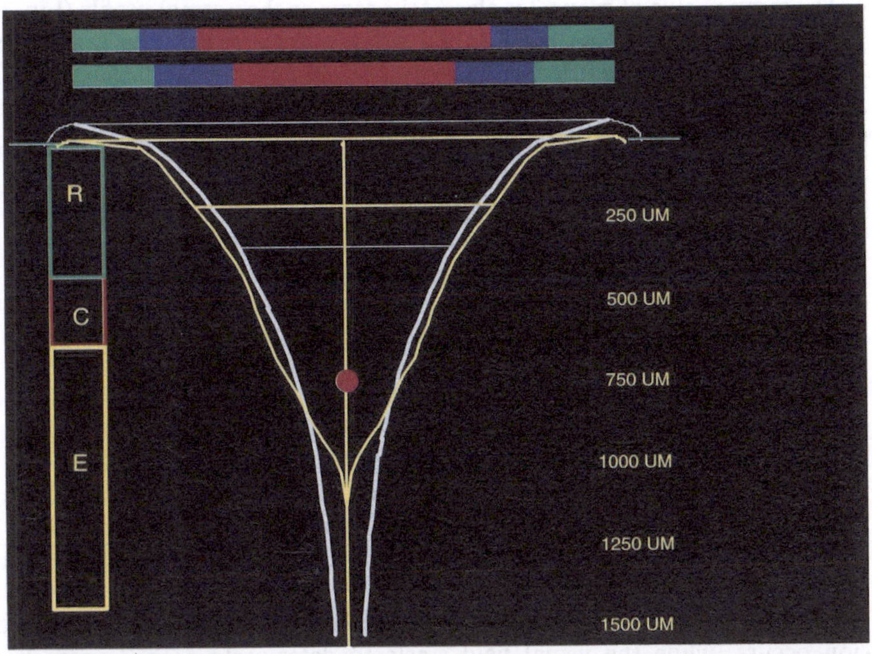

Fig. 37. Mean profile of group 3 is compared with the profile of the normal group. Unlike the two other groups, the total disk area (G + B + R) is the same as the normal one. Horizontal line: green: flat neuroretinal rim; blue: tilted neuroretinal rim; red: cup. Vertical line: R: retina, C: choroid, E: sclera (Violet profile: normal profile; yellow profile: profile of group 3)

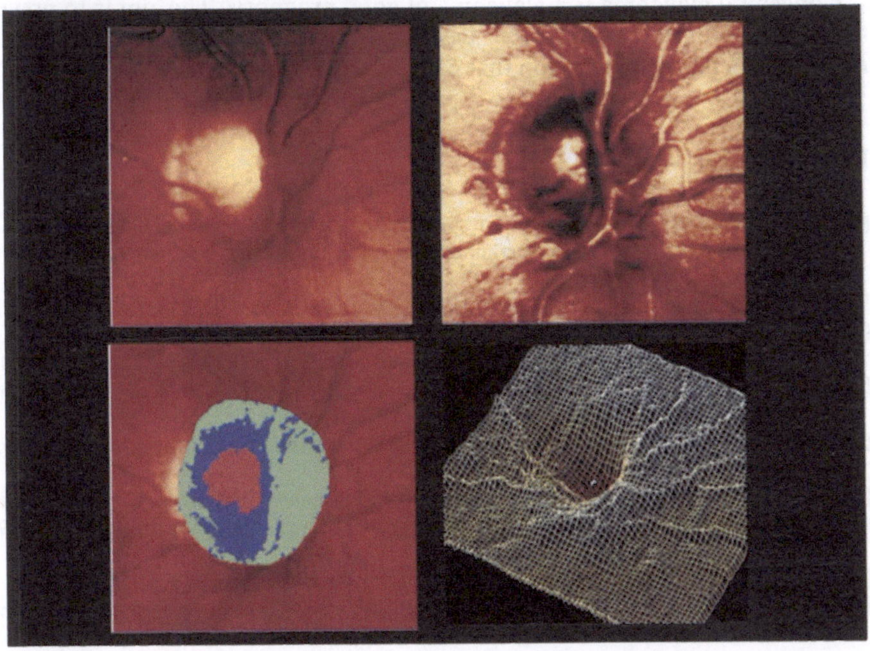

Fig. 38. Example of the Heidelberg retina tomograph (HRT) of a patient of group 3. Upper side left: topographic image. Upper side right: reflectivity image. Lower side left: green: surface of the neuroretinal rim; blue: neuroretinal tilted plane; red: surface of the cup. Lower right: three-dimensional image

47The mean profile of group 3 is almost the same as the normal profile (Fig. 37). Unlike in the two other groups, the total disk area is the same as the normal one. *There is no Elschnig's ring distension because ocular hypertension begins only after 5 years of age.* This behavior is the same as that of glaucoma in adults, where the cup area enlargement is proportional to the neuroretinal rim area reduction. The neuroretinal rim volume is smaller than that of group 1.

The red point of each graph indicates the end of the cup and the beginning of the hyaloid duct (with a surface of 62 μ). In group 3, unlike in groups 1 and 2, it remains almost normal and it is not posteriorly displaced because the eye is no longer elastic. Figure 38 shows an optic disk belonging to group 3, obtained with the HRT.

Conclusion

Leydhecker and Goldmann's hypothesis that the optic nerve deteriorates many years before the occurrence of visual field damage is now being confirmed by clinical evidence. In 85% of cases, about 10 years elapse between optic nerve deterioration and visual field damage [44,45].

In children, the optic nerve starts deteriorating as soon as ocular hypertension occurs, while the visual field starts to deteriorate 5 to 7 years later. Therefore, patients affected by congenital glaucoma must be subjected to surgery as soon as the condition is diagnosed, and if, despite surgery, the axial length continues to grow, it is necessary to reoperate.

Congenital glaucoma is a glaucoma of good prognosis. The aim is to prevent the optic nerve head from further deterioration. This is achieved by surgery to reduce the ocular hypertension that causes the eye enlargement.

References

[1] R. Seefelder and G. Wolfrum. Zur Entwicklung der vorderen Kammer und des Kammerwinkels beim Menschen nebst. Bemerkungen über ihre Entstehung bei Tieren. Graefes Arch. Ophthalmol. 1906;430–451.

[2] R. Miller. Genetic aspect of glaucoma. Trans. Ophthalmol. Soc. U.K. 1962;425–432.

[3] R. Sampaolesi, R.Y. Reca and A. Carro A. Presion ocular en el niño hasta los 5 años bajo anestesia con Pentrane (Metoxifluorane). Buenos Aires, Arch. Oftalmol. 1967;42:180–185.

[4] C. Carvalho and N. Calixto. Semiologia do glaucoma congenito. XV Cong. Bras. Ophthalmol., Porto Alegre. 1969;105–174.

[5] N.D. Radtke and B.E. Cohan. Intraocular pressure measurement in the newborn. Amer. J. Ophthalmol. 1974;78:501.

[6] S.M. Tucker, R.W. Enzenauer, A.V. Levin, J.D. Morin and J. Hellmann. Corneal diameter, axial length and intraocular pressure in premature infants. Ophthalmology 1992;99:1296–1300.

[7] J. Ytterborg. On scleral rigidity. Oslo: Oslo Univ. Press, 1960.

[8] R.N. Borrone. Presion ocular en niños de 5 a 15 años. Buenos Aires, Arch. Oftalmol. 1984;59:219–234.

[9] H. Gernet and F. Hollwich. Oculometrie des kindlichen Glaukoms. Ber. Dtsch. Ophthalmol. Ges. 1969;69:341–348.

[10] R. Sampaolesi, R. Recar and E. Armando. Normaler Intraocularer Druck bei Kindern bis zu 5 Jahren mit und ohne Allgemeinnarkose: Seine Wichtigkeit für die Frühdiagnose des angeborenen Glaukoms. Glaucoma Symposium (Würzburg, Germany). 1974;278–289.

[11] R. Sampaolesi. Ocular echometry in the diagnosis of congenital glaucoma. Ophthal. Proc. Series 1981;29:177–189.

[12] R. Sampaolesi and R. Carusso. Ocular echometry in the diagnosis of congenital glaucoma. Arch. Ophthal. 1982;100:574–577.

[13] R. Sampaolesi. Ocular echometry in the diagnosis of congenital glaucoma and its evolution. In G.K. Krieglstein and W. Leydhecker (eds), Glaucoma Update II. Berlin, Heidelberg: Springer-Verlag, 1983;175–184.

[14] R. Sampaolesi. Echométrie oculaire, un noveau paramètre dans le diagnostic et le contrôle de l'évolution du glaucome congénital. Bull. et Mem. S.F.O. 1984;95:401–409.

[15] R. Sampaolesi. Congenital glaucoma. Long-term results of surgery. In G.K. Krieglstein (ed.), Glaucoma Update III. Berlin, Heidelberg: Springer-Verlag, 1987;154–161.

[16] R. Sampaolesi. Echometry in congenital glaucoma: long-térm results after 10 to 17 years of surgery. Ultrasonography in Ophthalmol. Dordrecht: Kluwer Academic Publishers, 1990;12:181–191.

[17] A. Reibaldi. Biometric ultrasound in the diagnosis and follow-up of congenital glaucoma. Ann. Ophthalmol.1982;707.

[18] C. Carvalho and A.J. Betinjane. Valores da biometria ultrasonografica obtidos em olhos normais de pacientes ate 18 meses de idade. Rev. Bras. Oftalmol. 1980;39:479–482.

[19] A.F. Betinjane. Contribũao ao estudo da biometria ultrasonografica no glaucoma congenito. Tese Doc. Livre Fac. Med. USP, 1982.

[20] A. Tarkkanen, R. Uusitalo, J. Mianowicz. Ultrasonographic biometry in congenital glaucoma. Acta Ophthalmol. 1983;61:618–623.

[21] H.C. Fledelius. Personal communication.

[22] A. Grignolo and A. Rivara. Biometry of the human eye from the sixth month of pregnancy to the tenth year of life (measurements of the axial length, retinoscopy, total refraction, corneal lens refraction). In Diagnostica ultrasonica in Ophthalmologia. Brno: Univ. J.E. Purkyne 1968;251–257.

[23] H.C. Fledelius. Eye size of the premature infant around presumed ter. Ultrasonography in Ophthalmology. Dordrecht: Kluwer Academic Publishers, 1990;12:165–172.

[24] J.S. Larsen. The sagittal growth of the eye. I. Ultrasonic measurement of the depth of the anterior chamber from birth to puberty. Acta Ophthalmol. 1971;49:239–262.

[25] J.S. Larsen. The sagittal growth of the eye. II. Ultrasonic measurement of the axial diameter of the lens and the anterior segment from birth to puberty. Acta Ophthalmol. 1971;49:427–440.

[26] J.S. Larsen. The sagittal growth of the eye. III. Ultrasonic measurement of the posterior segment (axial length of the vitreous) from birth to puberty. Acta Ophthalmol. 1971;49:441–453.

[27] J.S. Larsen. The sagittal growth of the eye. IV. Ultrasonic measurement of the axial length of the eye from birth to puberty. Acta Ophthalmol. 1971;49:873-886.

[28] J. Luyckx. Mesure des composantes optiques de l'oeil du nouveauné pour échographie ultrasonique. Arch. Ophthalmol. 1966;26:159–170.

[29] J. Luyckx and Y. Delmarcelle. Contribution of ultrasonography to the study of microcornea and megalocornea. In K.A. Gitter, A.K. Keeney, L.K. Sarin and D. Meyer (eds), Ophthalmic Ultrasound. St. Louis: The C.V. Mosby Co., 1969;149–157.

[30] M. Massin and B. Pellat. Ultrasonic biometry in congenital glaucoma, a clinical study – Personal communication. 1982.

[31] B. Prahs. Des mesures biométriques dans les glaucomes congénitaux primaires. Bull. et Mem. S.F.O. (Congrès) 1981;405–409.

[32] O. Barkan. New operation for chronic glaucoma: restoration of physiological function by opening Schlemm's canal under direct magnified vision. Amer. J. Ophthalmol. 1936:19:951–966.

[33] H. Harms. Glaukom-Operationen am Schlemm'schen Kanal. Sitzungsber. der 114. Versammlung des Vereins RheinWestf. Augenärzte, 1966.

[34] H. Harms. Trabeculotomy results and problems. Adv. Ophthalmol. Basel, New York: Karger. 1970;27:95–96.

[35] H. Harms and R. Dannheim. Trabeculotomy. Results and problems. Microsurgery in glaucoma, 2nd. Internat. Symp. Ophthalmol., Microsurgery Study Group, Bürgenstock 1968. Adv. Ophthalmol. Basel, München, New York: Karger, 1970;22:121–131.

[36] L. Paufique, P.H. Sourdille and A.H. Ortiz-Olmedo. Technique et résultats de la trabéculotomy ab externo dans le traitement du glaucoma congénital. Bull. et Mem. S.F.O., 1969. Paris: Masson et Cie, 1970;54–65.

[37] H.R. Burian. A case of Marfan's syndrome with bilateral glaucoma. With description of a new type of operation for developmental glaucoma (trabeculotomy ab externo). Amer. J. Ophthalmol. 1960;50:1187–1192.

[38] L. Allen and H.M. Burian. Trabeculotomy ab externo. A new glaucoma operation. Technique and results of experimental surgery. Amer J. Ophthalmol. 1962;53:19–26.

[39] A. Dellaporta. Evaluation of anterior and posterior trabeculodyalisis. Amer J. Ophthalmol. 1959;48:294–309.

[40] H. Minsky. Proc. XVI Int. Congress of Ophthalmology, London, 1950. 1951;2:928-937. Ref. Ophthal. Lit. 1950;4:4074.

[41] W. Buschmann and K. Bluth. Regelmäbige echographische Messung der Achsenlänge des Auges zur Kontrolle der Druckregulierung bei Hydrophthalmie. Klin. Mbl. Augenheilk. 1974;165:878–886.

[42] W. Buschmann and K. Bluth. Eine echographische Methode zur Verlaufskontrolle angeborener Glaucome. Graefes Arch. Ophthalmol. 1974;192:313–329.

[43] C.A. Carvalho, A.J. Betinjane and M.L. Camargo. Results of goniotomy and trabeculotomy as the initial surgical procedure in the treatment of congenital glaucoma. In G.K. Krieglstein and W. Leydhecker (eds.), Glaucoma Update. Berlin: Springer-Verlag. 1979;33–38.

[44] H. Goldmann. Some basic principles of simple glaucoma. Part II. Am. J. Ophthalmol. 1959;48:213.

[45] W. Leydecher. Zür verbreitung des Glaucoma Simplex in der scheinbar gesunder Augenartzlich nicht behandelten Bevölkerung. Doc. Ophthalmol. Proc. 1959;13:359.

[46] B. Vidic and H. Lerchner. Biometrische Langzeitergebnisse bei Glaukom im Kindessalter. Fortschr. Augenheilk. 1990;87:25–27.

[47] P. Wanger and H.E. Persson. Pattern-reversal electroretinograms and high-pass resolution perimetry in suspected or early glaucoma. Ophthalmology 1987;94:1098–1103.

[48] F. Dannheim, F. Abramo and D. Verlohr. Comparison of automated conventional and spatial resolution perimetry in glaucoma. In A. Heijl (ed.), Perimetry Update. Amsterdam: Kugler Publishers, 1989;383–392.

[49] B.J. Lachenmayr, S.M. Drance, G.R. Douglas and F.S. Mikelberg. Light-sense, flicker and resolution perimetry in glaucoma: a comparative study. Graefes Arch. Ophthalmol. 1991;229:246–251.

[50] Y. Kono, M. Maeda, T. Yamamoto and Y. Kitazawa. A comparative study between high-pass resolution perimetry and differential light sensitivity perimetry in glaucoma patients. In R. Mills (ed.), Perimetry Update. Amsterdam: Kugler Publishers, 1993;409–413.

[51] R. Sampaolesi and J.F. Casiraghi. Computerized visual fields in pediatric glaucoma. Perimetry update 1990-1991. In R. Mills and A. Heijl (eds). Kluger and Ghedini. 455–464.

[52] R.O.W. Burk, K. Rohrschneider, H. Noack, H.E. Volcker and G. Zinser. Analysis of three-dimensional optic disk topography by laser scanning tomography. Parameter definition and evaluation of parameter inter-dependence. In J.E. Nasemann and R.O.W. Burg (eds). Scanning laser ophthalmoscopy and tomography. München: Quintessenz, 1990;161–176.

[53] R.O.W. Burk, K. Rohrschneider, H. Noach and H.E. Volcker. Volumetrische Papillenanalyse mit Hilfe der Laser scanning-Tomographie-Parameterdefinition und Vergleich von Glaucom- und Kontrollpapillen. Klin. Mbl. Augenheilk., 1991;198:522–529.

[54] R.O.W. Burk, K. Rohrschneider, F.E. Kruse and H.E. Volckr. Laser scanning Tomographie der Papille. In E. Gramer (ed.), Glaukom – Diagnostik und Therapie. Internationales Glaukomsymposium Würzburg 1988. Stuttgart: Enke, 1990;113–119.

Prof. Dr. Roberto Sampaolesi
Parana 1239-1°– A
(1018) Buenos Aires
Argentina

2. Characteristics and diagnostic potential of echo enhancers based on galactose

R. SCHÜRMANN
(Berlin, Germany)

Abstract

The first echosignal enhancing agents have been approved by health authorities. Most agents are based on microbubbles because of the unique acoustic properties of the latter. The increase in echogenicity can be exploited for B-mode scans as well as for Doppler examinations. Contrast-enhanced B-mode imaging is well established in right-heart echocardiography using agitated solutions. Inherent limitations of the home-made agents can be overcome by the use of a "right-heart" agent such as Echovist, after i.v. injection the blood becomes temporarily visible. Transpulmonary stability of contrast agents is required for opacification of the left heart cavities.

For Doppler sonography, the situation is different. In cases of sufficient signal intensity, there is, in general, no need to use echo enhancers. However, they can improve the diagnosis in cases in which Doppler signals are insufficient. The intravenous injection of Levovist leads to a strong increase in the intensity of the Doppler signal in the entire vessel system ('blood pool echo-enhancement'). Further, vessels will be displayed which in the precontrast scan are hidden due to attenuation, unfavourable angles and/or borderline low vessel diameters. Overall, confidence in the related Doppler diagnosis is expected to increase substantially. Colour Doppler imaging of vascularity, particularly of tumour lesions, appears promising for the display of vasculature in order to aid visual detection of abnormalities.

Key words: Echosignal enhancer, ultrasound contrast agents, contrast sonography, Echovist, Levovist

Introduction

Gaseous bubbles with microscopic diameters, 'microbubbles', are extremely effective scatterers of ultrasound as known since the pioneer work by Gramiak [1] and Meltzer [2]. Because of their unique acoustic properties, microbubbles play a key role in the basic mode of action of sound enhancing agents. However, single microbubbles, without any additional protection against gas diffusion

G Cennamo and N. Rosa (eds.), Ultrasonography in Ophthalmology 15, pp. 49–56.

(between gas bubble and carrier fluid with respect to blood serum), exhibit a very short lifetime of only a few seconds [3]. This is one of the reasons for frequently described problems of reproducibility and efficacy using homemade 'contrast agents', like agitated saline or sonicated X-ray contrast media. Despite these disadvantages they are still used for contrast echocardiography of the right heart chambers.

The last couple of years have brought about substantial advances with the first industrial sound enhancing agent being approved by health authorities. This agent is the galactose microparticle agent SH U 454 (Echovist, Schering AG Berlin, Germany), which was introduced to the market in Germany in October 1991 and since then in various other countries. Echovist was developed for echocardiographic examinations in cases of right heart abnormalities (B-mode and colour-Doppler) [4] as well as for hysterosalpingo-contrast sonography ('HyCoSy') for evaluation of Fallopian tube patency in infertile women [5].

More agents are in late phases of clinical development or have been approved recently. One is the albumin microsphere agent (Albunex®, Molecular Biosystems) developed for B-mode echocardiographic exams of the left heart [6]. Another is a derivative of Echovist with transpulmonary stability, the galactose-based agent Levovist (code name SH U 508 A) for B-mode echocardiography and Doppler echo-enhancement of the blood pool [7].

Thus, reproducible microbubble echoenhancers are available for clinical routine. Contrast related ultrasound technology will be an innovative focus of the coming years.

Principles of echosignal enhancement

Basically, ultrasound contrast agents are media that are administered into the vascular system or into body cavities thereby changing the acoustic properties of the body region under investigation. The acoustic parameters which affect tissue imaging by conventional sonographic units are backscatter, attenuation and velocity of sound. Of these, enhancement of backscatter is the most important factor since echosignal enhancing agents introduce acoustic inhomogeneities caused by microstructures (scatterers). Free gas bubbles, encapsulated gas bubbles and colloidal suspensions represent different types of scattering media [8].

Beyond simple scattering, gas bubbles may oscillate and, in particular, resonate and thus dramatically increase the echogenic effects [3]. For air bubbles with several microns of diameter, the resonance frequencies in blood are within the range of diagnostic US frequencies. Their resonance properties may be specifically evaluated by ultrasound devices of the future with 'harmonic imaging' techniques.

Another important precondition for efficacious echosignal enhancement is a sufficient pressure stability under static conditions (elevated or decreased ambient pressure) as well as under cyclic pressure variations (e.g. in arteries).

The increase in echogenicity caused by ultrasound contrast agents can be exploited for B-mode scans as well as for Doppler examinations. However, in patients with poor image quality of the baseline scan ('precontrast'), the B-mode image quality and consequently the diagnostic improvement of the contrast injection may be limited. Generally, the overall noise level in the B-mode image can not be expected to change significantly with the injection of a contrast agent and will remain almost as poor as it was at baseline.

For Doppler sonography, the situation is different. In cases of sufficient signal intensity, there is in general no need to use echoenhancers. However, echoenhancers may improve the diagnosis in patients with inadequate Doppler signals at routine sonography. The intravenous injection of a galactose-based contrast agent leads to a strong increase in the Doppler signal intensity of about 15 to 25 dB using microbubble concentrations that are hardly or even not visible by B-mode. This is due to the sensitivity difference between B-mode and Doppler mode of about 30 dB or more.

Furthermore, additional vessels will be displayed which in the precontrast scan are hidden due to attenuation, unfavourable angles and/or borderline low vessel-diameters. Overall, confidence in the related Doppler diagnosis is expected to increase substantially after echosignal enhancement.

Physico-chemical characteristics of saccharide-based contrast agents

The underlying principle of Echovist (SH U 454) and Levovist (SH U 508 A) is identical: galactose microparticle granules manufactured in a sophisticated, sterile production process are suspended shortly before use by shaking in a galactose solution (Echovist) or sterile water (Levovist). After injection of the suspension, the blood becomes temporarily echogenic during transit of the bolus until these acoustic microstructures have dissolved in the blood stream.

The granules consist of numerous tiny galactose crystalline particles. A microparticle granule is shown in Figure 1. In the case of Echovist, these microparticles consist of galactose alone which is a known nutritive monosaccharide. In the case of the transpulmonary derivative SH U 508 A (Levovist), these microparticle granules contain as an additive 0.1% of physiologic palmitic acid.

The median diameter of the Echovist D-galactose microparticles is 2 m, 99% < 12 m [9]. 99% of the microparticles of Levovist are < 8 m. The total amount of air per 1 g microparticles lower than 100 µl in both agents.

Before use the granules have to be shaken for 5–10 seconds with an appropriate volume of aqueous galactose solution (Echovist) or sterile water (Levovist). A milky suspension of galactose microparticles in a galactose solution is created after disaggregation of the granules. The solid surfaces of the microparticles permit bubble formation and act as stabilising sites. In addition, the size of the microparticles helps to select bubbles of a certain diameter range.

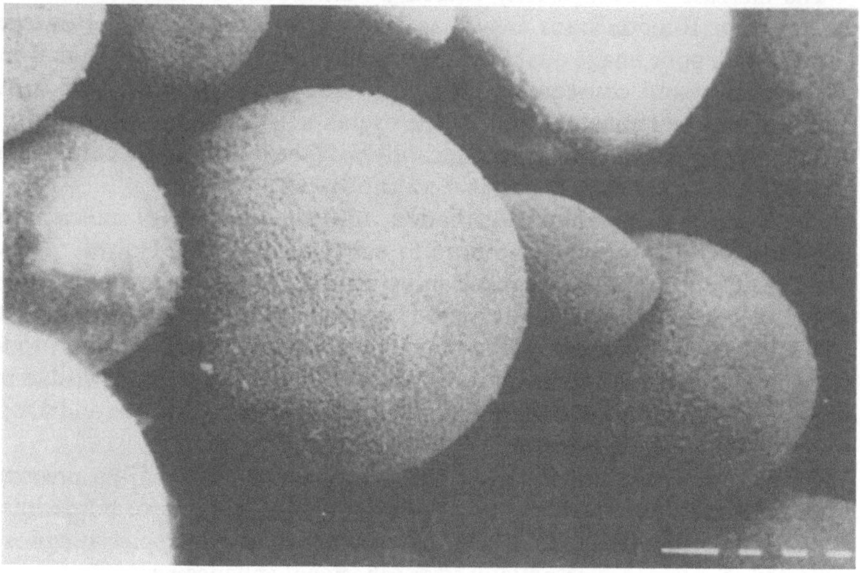

Fig. 1. Electron microscopic view of microparticle granules of Echovist

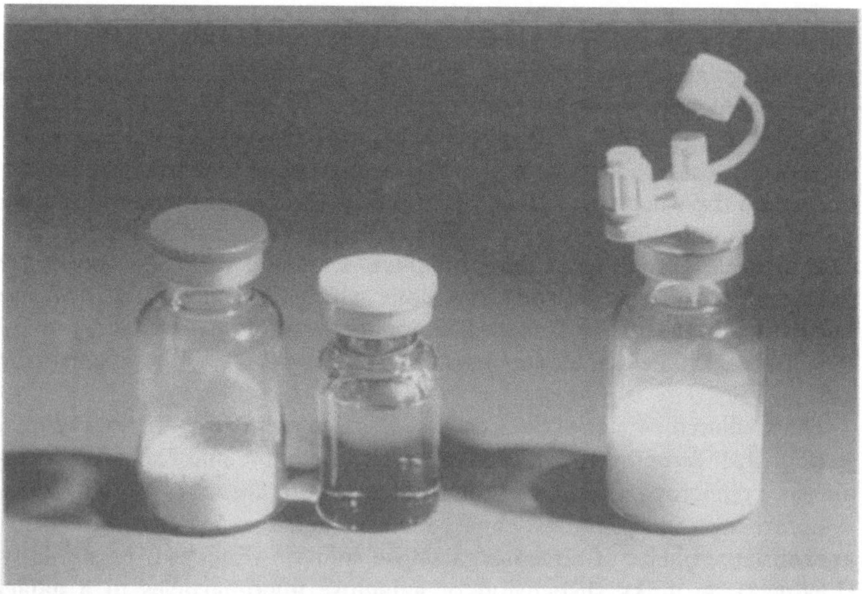

Fig. 2. Echovist suspension fluid (left vial), microparticle granules (middle), and Echovist suspension (right vial) with mini-spike

Figure 2 shows the vial with Echovist granules (left vial), the suspension fluid, 20% galactose solution W/V, (middle) and the milky-white suspension containing scattering microbubbles (right) which is ready for use. Different concentrations of scattering microbubbles can be obtained by varying the volume of the added suspension fluid. Depending on the indication and the imaging modality (B-mode or Doppler), clinically adequate concentrations of Echovist are 300 and 200 mg microparticles per 1 ml suspension. For Levovist, the maximum concentration is 400 mg/ml.

Pharmacodynamics and degradation of Echovist and Levovist

After intravenous injection, the agents lead to a reproducible, dose-dependent increase in backscatter from the blood ('echogenicity') until the acoustic active microstructures of the suspension dissolve in the blood stream. The non-transpulmonary agent Echovist dissolves after mixing and dilution with the venous blood before it reaches the left heart. The scattering microbubbles of the transpulmonary derivative Levovist predominantly dissolve later in the vascular bed. With concentrations of 300 or 400 mg/ml administered intravenously, the echogenicity increase in the left heart cavities exceeds the B-mode grey levels of the myocardium ('contrast echo'). In the following arteries, the echogenicity decreases, but it is still sufficient to lead to an effective increase in Doppler signal intensity.

After intravascular dissolution of the acoustic microstructures, the remaining galactose is transported insulin-independently to its physiological sites of degradation, primarily the liver. Galactose is a non-toxic monosaccharide and has no known allergenic potential.

For many years, intravenous injections of galactose in high dosages (e.g. 0.5 g/kg body weight) have been used for liver function tests [10]. These injections are well tolerated even in cases of liver diseases. Galactosaemia is a contra-indication for the application of galactose contrast agents. This condition can easily be ruled out by the patient's history.

Palmitic acid is administered in a total dose which is 20 times lower than the amount of free fatty acids already present in the body.

Indications for echosignal enhancers

B-mode imaging

Contrast-enhanced B-mode imaging is well established in right-heart echocardiography using agitated solutions. Inherent limitations of the homemade agents (e.g. lack of stability, reproducibility of echogenicity and variability of bubble-size) can be overcome by the use of a 'right-heart' agent like Echovist. After intravenous peripheral injection the blood becomes temporarily visible

[11]. Thus, shunt flow through atrial or ventricular defects can be diagnosed. Especially, small right-to-left shunts, in particular patent foramen ovale, are domains for the use of right-heart agents.

Echocontrast agents may be used as indicators for echogenic demarcation of body cavities. After transcervical administration, the uterine cavity can be echogenically delineated and tubal patency can be evaluated by visualisation of flow in the Fallopian tubes ('hysterosalpingo-contrast sonography') [5].

Transpulmonary stability of contrast agents is required for opacification of the left heart cavities. B-mode contrast echocardiography with Levovist improves the endocardial delineation in suboptimal stress echocardiography [12] and the detection of left-to-right shunts or thrombi.

Doppler sonography

For right heart Doppler echocardiography, the use of Echovist increases substantially the sensitivity of blood flow detection [13]. This results in a better visibility of formerly poorly demonstrated shunts or of valvular incompetence, particularly in patients with low Doppler signal-to-noise ratios (e.g. caused by attenuation due to obesity or emphysema).

Noisy Doppler recordings of continuous wave or colour Doppler echocardiography of the left heart chambers can be considerably improved by Levovist. The detection and severity grading of mitral insufficiency or aortic stenosis can be improved in patients with insufficient precontrast scans [14].

After passing the left heart cavities, the increase in echogenicity caused by stabilised microbubbles of Levovist is still sufficient for a strong enhancement of vascular Doppler signals in the entire vessel system ('blood pool echo-enhancement'). Thus, diagnostic benefits can be expected in patients with suboptimal Doppler signal intensities in all parts of the body, e.g. vessels of head and neck, renal arteries, the portal system, or peripheral arteries [15,16]. The Doppler signal enhancement compensates for attenuation in the patient or unfavourable imaging conditions. However, after enhancement clinically important differences may occur e.g. due to missing or reduced peak velocities in the noisy precontrast registrations. In this case, the high intensity recording properly reflects the haemodynamics.

Colour Doppler examination of tumor vascularity is a new area currently under intensive research regarding clinical relevance [17]. Tumours are known to secrete neoangiogenesis factors. The resulting neovascularisation is characterised by abnormal vessels with disorderly arrangement, size and wall structure, sometimes with connections between adjacent arteries and arteriovenous shunt flow which are characterised by elevated blood flow velocities. Blood flow mapping as well as the reliable demonstration of either the absence of vessels or the lack of demonstrable blood flow are diagnostic signs of equal importance.

Similar information can only be obtained by selective X-ray angiography; however, because of its invasiveness, it became a routine procedure in the assessment of tumours only in specialised diagnostic areas. Furthermore, angiography does not provide the additional information on flow velocities which is a specific advantage of the Doppler technique.

Vascularity imaging by colour Doppler is usually to be performed with settings of maximum sensitivity of the sonographic unit. This is necessitated by the small size of the vessels, low blood flow velocities, multiple orientations of flow and attenuation of signals on their way to the transducer.

All these factors are related finally to the signal-to-noise ratio. Contrast enhancement can be expected to be a major contribution for further clinical development in imaging of vascularity. First results of contrast-enhanced colour Doppler imaging of focal liver lesions, female breast and brain tumours have been published [18–20].

Results of a multicentre trial with Levovist

A total of more than 1200 patients were included in a European phase III clinical multicentre trial. The aim of the trial was to prove the diagnostic efficacy and safety of Levovist. Only patients with diagnostically insufficient Doppler signal intensity at routine Doppler echocardiography, vascular Doppler, or colour Doppler imaging of vascularity were included. In more than 95% of the patients Doppler signal enhancement was achieved, even in peripheral parts of the vasculature. Thus, the echo-enhancing properties as a 'blood pool agent' were confirmed. It was possible to establish a diagnosis by contrast Doppler sonography in patients who otherwise would have undergone more invasive procedures. The diagnostic confidence, evaluated by a rating scale (range 0–100), increased from 31.024.3 (prevalue) to 79.819.9 (after Levovist; mean value standard deviation). The repeated intravenous injections were well tolerated. No specific risk was found for patients of any disease group. The data obtained in the various diagnostic areas have been presented at an investigators' meeting [21].

References

[1] R. Gramiak and P.M. Shah. Echocardiography of the aortic root. Invest. Radiol. 1968;3:356–366.

[2] R.S. Meltzer, G. Tickner, T.P. Sahines and R.L. Popp. The source of ultrasound contrast effect. J. Clin. Ultrasound 1980;8:121–127.

[3] N. de Jong, F.J. Ten Cate, C.T. Lancée, J.R.T.C. Rodand and N. Bonn. Principles and recent developments in ultrasound contrast agents. Ultrasonics 1991;29:324–330.

[4] H. Becher and R. Schlief. Improved sensitivity of colour doppler by SH U 454. Am. J. Cardiol. 1989;64:374–377.

[5] S. Campbell, T.H. Bourne, S.L. Tan and W.P. Collins. Hysterosalpingo contrast sonography (HyCoSy) and its future role within the investigation of infertility in Europe. Ultrasound Obstet. Gynecol. 1994;4:245–253.

[6] S.B. Feinstein, J. Cheirif, F.J. Ten Cate, P.R. Silverman, P.A. Heidenreich, C. Dick, R.M. Desir, W.F. Armstrong, M.A. Quinones and P.M. Shah. Safety and efficacy of a new

transpulmonary ultrasound agent: initial multicenter clinical results. J. Am. Coll. Cardiol. 1990;16:316–324.

[7] R. Schlief, R. Schürmann, Th. Balzer, J. Petrick, A. Urbank, M. Zomack and H.P. Niendorf. Diagnostic value of contrast enhancement in vascular Doppler ultrasound. In N.C. Nanda and R. Schlief (eds), Advances in echo imaging using contrast enhancement. Dordrecht/ Boston/London: Kluwer Academic Publishers,1993;309–323.

[8] J. Ophir and K.J. Parker. Contrast agents in diagnostic ultrasound. Ultrasound Med. Biol. 1989;15:319–333.

[9] T. Fritzsch, B. Maaß, B. Müller, C. Schöbel, J. Siegert and K. Stevens. Composition and tolerance of galactose-based echo contrast media. In H. Katayama and R.C. Brash (eds), New dimensions of contrast media. Tokyo: Excerpta Medica Ltd., 1991:156–162.

[10] G. Marchesini, A. Fabbri, E. Bugianesi, G.P. Bianchi, E. Marchi, M. Zon and E. Pisi. Analysis of the deterioration rates of liver function in cirrhosis, based on galactose elimination capacity. Liver 1990;10:65–71.

[11] D. Rovai, M. Lombardi, G. Cini, M.A. Morales, M. Colonna, G. Bechelli, P. Marino, L. Zanolla, M.A. Prioli, G.L. Nicolosi, D. Pavan, D. Sanuttini, S. Iliceto, M. Izzi, P. Rizzon and A. L'Abbate. Echocardiographic contrast imaging of the human right heart: a multicenter study of the efficacy, safety, and reproducibility of intravenous SH U 454. J. Clin. Ultrasound 1991;19:523–530.

[12] K. Schröder, H. Völler, R. Agrawal, R. Schlief and R. Schröder. Improved border delineation in suboptimal stress echocardiography by the new left heart contrast agent SH U 508 A. J. Am. Coll. Cardiol. 1992;19(3):175A.

[13] H. Becher and R. Schlief. Improved sensitivity of colour doppler by SH U 454. Am. J. Cardiol. 1989;64:374–377.

[14] H. v. Bibra, H. Becher, C. Firschke, R. Schlief, H.P. Emslander and A. Schömig. Enhancement of mitral regurgitation and normal left atrial color Doppler flow signals with peripheral venous injection of a saccharide-based contrast agent. J. Am. Coll. Cardiol. 1993;22(2):521–528.

[15] K. Rosenkranz, W. Zendel, R. Langer, T. Heim, P. Schubeus, A. Scholz, R. Schlief, R. Schürmann and R. Felix. Contrast-enhanced transcranial Doppler US with a new transpulmonary echo contrast agent based on saccharide microparticles. Radiology 1993;187:439–443.

[16] U. Bogdahn, G. Becker, R. Schlief, J. Reddig and W. Hassel. Contrast-enhanced transcranial color-coded real-time sinography. Stroke 1993;24:676–684.

[17] D.O. Cosgrove, J.C. Bamber, J. Davy, J.A. McKinna and H.D. Sinnett. Colour Doppler signals from breast tumours. Radiology 1990;176:175–180.

[18] E. Leen, W.J. Angerson, H.W. Warren, P. O'Gorman, B. Moule, E.C. Carter and C.S. McArdle. Improved sensitivity of colour Doppler flow imaging of colorectal hepatic metastases using galactose microparticles: a preliminary report. Br. J. of Surg. 1994;81:252–254.

[19] V.F. Duda, G. Rode and R. Schlief. Echocontrast agent enhanced color flow imaging of the breast. Ultrasound Obstet. Gynecol. 1993;3:191–194.

[20] U. Bogdahn, T. Fröhlich, G. Becker, A. Krone, R. Schlief, J. Schürmann, P. Jachimczak, E. Hofmann, W. Roggendorf and K. Roosen. Vascularization of primary central nervous tumors: detection with contrast-enhanced transcranial color-coded real-time sonography. Radiology 1994;192:141–148.

[21] R. Schlief. Diagnostic potential of I.V. contrast enhancement in various areas of cardiovascular Doppler ultrasound - efficacy results of a multinational clinical trial with the galactose-based agent SH U 508 A. (Abstracts of a one day investigators' meeting from January 30, 1993 in Berlin, Germany). Echocardiography 1993;10(6):665–682.

Clinical Development Diagnostics
Schering AG
Müllerstr. 170–178
D-13353 Berlin, Germany

Posterior eye segment

3. New generation echography and macular edema

T. AVITABILE, F. MARANO, S. FARO and A. REIBALDI
(Catania, Italy)

Abstract

Macular edema can occur in such disorders as diabetes mellitus, pars planitis and cataract, and as a complication of vitreo-retinal surgery. Because these conditions often give rise to severe opacification of the ocular media, we conducted a study, using traditional and new B-scan echographic equipment, to ascertain whether macular involvement could be foreseen. We focused our attention on diffuse and cystoid macular edema, and also studied the condition of the vitreous above the posterior pole. In our paper we compared the echographical images with the fluorescein angiograms. In this manner macular edema can be recognized also in cases of unclear ocular media.

Key words: Macular edema, B-scan echography, high resolution scan

Introduction

Ophthalmic disorders that involve a disruption of either the inner or the outer blood-retinal barrier at the posterior pole are often associated with macular edema. Initially, the edema is diffuse, and can become cystoid with time. The tendency to become cystoid is increased at the macula but may occur in any part of the fundus [1]. Diseases such as diabetes mellitus, vein occlusion, aphakia or pseudophakia, uveitis, retinal detachment, choroidal tumors and hypertension can cause macular edema.

Cystoid macular edema (CME) is characterized by spaces filled with increased extracellular fluid in the outer plexiform and inner nuclear retinal layers [2]. These cysts often surround the fovea and central cysts are not uncommon. If the underlying disease persists the cysts can result in the formation of a lamellar, or a full thickness macular hole. Other authors reported histopathologic changes in patients affected by macular edema consisting of swelling and degeneration of the Müller cells [3].

The clinical examination of retinal thickening in patients with macular edema is generally performed using either the slit lamp and a fundus contact lens or the slit lamp and a +60, +78 or +90 diopter aspheric lens. Fluorescein angiography is also an essential step in the evaluation of macular edema. Each of these

G Cennamo and N. Rosa (eds.), Ultrasonography in Ophthalmology 15, pp. 59–63.

techniques provides contributory data only when the media are clear. Echography, having an axial resolution of 0.15 mm with the 10 MHz A-scan mode and 0.2 mm with the 10 MHz B-scan mode, could be used to evaluate the retinal contour and to quantify the retinal thickness. However, with the advent of commercially available computerized equipment the macular structure can be studied in greater detail, which is important in the case of such small lesions.

The aim of this study was to describe the echographical changes observed in patients affected with diffuse and cystoid macular edema using the new computerized echographic B-scan system (Sonovision STT-100) in comparison with other equipment (Ophthascan S).

Patients and methods

We studied 25 eyes of 25 patients selected from 500 subjects who underwent fluorescein angiography at our Department from December 1992 to December 1993. All patients had angiographic signs of macular edema, the media were clear, four eyes were pseudophakic and one was aphakic. None had undergone laser treatment.

Among these 25 patients: 11 were affected by background diabetic retinopathy, 4 were pseudophakic, 3 had branch retinal vein occlusion, 2 had uveitis, 2 idiopathic CME, 1 Irvine-Gass Syndrome, 1 hypertensive retinopathy, and 1 choroidal tumor (hemangioma).

We examined each eye at the slit lamp using a +90 diopter aspheric lens and stereo fundus color photography (Zeiss 40 SL/P Photo Slit Lamp, Canon Fundus Camera CF-60U) was taken. Echography was then performed using two different apparatuses: Sonovision STT-100 and Ophthascan S. Both instruments are equipped with a 10 MHz B-scan probe; an 8 MHz A-scan probe is available with the Ophthascan S to perform standardized echography. To evaluate the macular region we used both the horizontal axial and the vertical transverse B-scan approaches. Standardized A-scan was performed with the Ophthascan S by placing the probe at the nasal limbus. The Sonovision STT-100 'high resolution scan' was particularly useful during real time echography. This increases the size of the B-scan image by 50% and simultaneously increases the data acquisition resolution along the ultrasound beam by 50%. It also doubles the number of lines in the sector. Images were stored on a floppy disk for subsequent study. When processing the images we eliminated all the ultrasound echoes below the selected level so as to visualise better the border of the lesion.

We measured the thickness of the lesion from the vitreoretinal echoes that correspond with its inner surface, to the highest spike from the sclera. We used the A-scan trace extracted from the frozen video B-scan image. The amplitude of the A-scan trace is fixed with the 'gain' setting of the frozen B-scan image. We elected to measure the lesions from the video B-scan image because we could be certain of measuring from the highest part of the edematous retina at the posterior pole.

We graded the fluorescein angiograms on a scale of 0 to 4, using a system described by [4], modified by Spaide in 1993 [5]:

- grade 0: no leakage;
- grade 1: patchy incomplete perifoveal leakage;
- grade 2: mild 360° perifoveal leakage;
- grade 3: moderate 360° perifoveal leakage (with perifoveal hyperfluorescence approximately 1 disc diameter);
- grade 4: severe perifoveal leakage (hyperfluorescence greater than 1½ disc diameters).

Results

We analyzed only the first fluorescein angiography performed at our Department. The fluorescein agiograms obtained from the 25 patients were graded as follows: 3 patients: grade 4; 10 patients: grade 3; 6 patients: grade 2; and 6 patients: grade 1. The shape and the border of the lesion were evaluated from fundus color stereo photography.

Echography showed retina thickening in the macular region in 12 patients. According to the CME angiographic grading, 3 were of grade 4, 8 were grade 3, and only 1 was grade 2. Retinal thickening was not found in the echographic images of the posterior pole of two patients with grade 3, five patients with grade 2, and in all the patients graded 1.

The following findings were obtained among the eyes with echographic alterations (retina thickening): a) An irregular morphology of the interface between vitreous and retina (which reflects an alteration of the inner surface of the retina). This aspect was found in four eyes (one grade 2, and three grade 3); b) A small dome-shaped lesion corresponding to the angiographic image of the perifoveal leakage. This was found in six eyes (five grade 3, and one grade 4); c) A dome-shaped lesion with a small central hole corresponding to the angiographic image of the perifoveal leakage, probably due to the image of the intraretinal cysts (the last two eyes graded 4). This finding is probably not the result of the single cyst, but it could be the echographic image of different confluent cysts; d) A maximal thickness of 2.19 mm.

Among the 25 eyes with macular edema studied by echography, the vitreous body was found to be completely attached to the retinal surface in 14 eyes. Partial peripheral vitreous detachment, with an adherence at the posterior pole in 9 eyes. Finally, posterior vitreous detachment was detected in two eyes.

Discussion

Macular edema is the most frequent cause of visual loss in patients with background diabetic retinopathy [6]. It also occurs in a variety of other common ocular disorders (diabetes mellitus, vein occlusion, uveitis, retinal detachment, choroidal tumors) and as a complication of intraocular surgery (cataract extraction, retinal detachment surgery).

Usually, when the ocular media are clear the macula examination is performed with the three mirror contact lens (Goldmann lens), +90/+78/+60 diopters aspheric lens and fluorescein angiography. In the case of a complication like vitreous hemorrhage, vitreous opacity or secondary cataract, echography is the technique of choice to study the macular region. Because cystoid macular edema is a frequent finding in various disorders that cause ocular media opacities, and 40% of eyes with macular edema are affected by retinal thickening of the center of the macula [7], a detailed echographic study could predict eventual macular involvement.

With the 10 MHz-B-scan probe, echography lacks specificity and diagnosis can be difficult [8]. In particular, it can be difficult to distinguish between dome-shaped lesions from age-related macular degeneration, which show a multi-layered highly reflective structure on A-scan and irregular echographic structures on B-scan; macular hemorrhagic disciform lesions; pigment epithelial detachments; drusen, focal choroidal hemorrhages; and intraocular tumors [9].

The first step in cases of such small, highly specific lesions is to consider the patient history and to perform a complete ophthalmic examination. Subsequently, an echography should be performed with the computerized B-scan equipment, which allows the lesion to be defined in greater detail, in order to search for a dome-shaped lesion with a thickness less than 2.2 mm, the eventual presence of a central hole, any irregularities of the retinal surface. Only grade 4 or 3 macular edema can be detected with echography. Because these findings are only suggestive of, rather than specific for, cystoid macular edema the patient should undergo serial examinations, and the fellow eye should also be examined.

In agreement with earlier findings, we found that the vitreous body was attached to the macular region in almost all our patients (22/25). Only in 2 patients was the posterior vitreous completely detached. Furthermore, the degree of macular thickness is strongly correlated with visual acuity [10]. Recently Spaide *et al.* [5] confirmed this finding and reported that the extent of foveal edema is strictly related to the changes in architecture, with subsequent reduced function. They also found a low correlation between the fluorescein angiographic grade and visual acuity, because the amount of foveal edema is not strictly related to the lateral extent of fluorescein leakage as determined by conventional fluorescein angiography. In this light, we suggest echography could be an useful tool with which to predict visual acuity before treatment, particularly in the presence of secondary cataract or vitreous hemorrhage.

Hopefully, new commercially available instruments with a high frequency (20 MHz or more) and sophisticated computerized programs will be developed that will improve axial and lateral resolution. The advent of such equipment will probably increase the number of correct diagnoses in such a minute and frequent lesion.

References

[1] A.C. Bird. Retinal edema. Introduction to the first international cystoid macular edema symposium. Surv. Ophthalmol. 1984;28 suppl.:433–436.

[2] J.D.M. Gass, D.R. Anderson and E.B. Davis. A clinical, fluorescein angiographic, and electron microscopic correlation of cystoid macular edema. Am. J. Ophthalmol. 1985; 100:82–86.

[3] B.S. Fine and A.J. Brucker. Macular edema and cystoid macular edema. Am. J. Ophthalmol. 1981;92:466–481.

[4] K. Miyake. Prevention of cystoid macular edema after lens extraction by topical indomethacin. (I) A preliminary report. Albrecht von Graefes Arch. Klin. Exp. Ophthalmol. 1977;203:81–88.

[5] R.F. Spaide, L.A. Yannuzzi and L.J. Sisco. Chronic cystoid macular edema and predictors of visual acuity. Ophthalmic Surgery 1993;24:262–267.

[6] G.H. Bresnick. Background diabetic retinopathy. In S.J. Ryan (ed.), Retina. St. Louis: The C.V. Mosby Company, 1989;327–366.

[7] R. Klein, B.E.K. Klein, S. Moss, M.D. Davis and D.L. DeMets. The Wisconsin epidemiologic study of diabetic retinopathy, IV. Diabetic macular edema. Ophthalmology 1984;91:1464–1474.

[8] O. Berges and E. Nau. High resolution B mode echography and colour Doppler (CDFI) of the macula. Acta Ophthalmologica 1992;204 suppl.:74-75.

[9] S.F. Byrne and R.L. Green. Ultrasound of the Eye and Orbitr. Mosby Year Book. St. Louis: The C.V. Mosby Company, 1992.

[10] R.B. Nussenblatt, S.C. Kaufman, A.G. Palestine, M.D. Davis and F.L. Ferris. Macular thickening and visual acuity. Measurement in patients with cystoid macular edema. Ophthalmology. 1987;94:1134–1139.

T. Avitabile
Institute of Ophthalmology
Catania University
Via Bambino 32
Catania, Italy

4. Chorioretinal folds and tumors: echographic study

N. ROSA, G. CENNAMO, A. LA RANA and A. PASQUARIELLO

(Naples, Italy)

Abstract

Chorioretinal folds are undulations of the choroid, Bruch's membrane and the overlaying retina. These can be idiopathic, but because orbital tumors and several other lesions could produce this picture, an echographic examination of the orbit should be performed in all these cases. We describe 55 patients with retinochoroidal folds and orbital tumors. The pathogenesis of these folds with or without an orbital tumor, and the role of the echographic examination are discussed.

Key words: Standardized echography, fluorescein angiography, chorioretinal folds, intraorbital tumors

Introduction

Chorioretinal folds were long considered typical of an orbital tumor. However, other causes of chorioretinal folds are: pseudotumor, mucoceles, Graves' ophthalmopathy, orbital cellulites, postoperative orbital edema, papilledema, papillitis, hyperopia, macular degeneration, hypotony, congenital, trauma, choroidal tumors, scleritis, uveitis, sinusitis, choroiditis, retinal detachment, scleral buckle, serous or hemorrhagic choroidal detachment, uveal effusion, vascular occlusion and bone compression of the globe [1]; chorioretinal folds can also be idiopathic.

Due to the wide variety in the pathogenesis of this disease, we used standardized echography to evaluate the frequency of the tumors that can cause these folds.

Material and method

We made a retrospective study of the orbital diseases examined over the last 20 years in our echographic service, to detect the frequency of chorioretinal folds related to the various orbital lesions and to establish the echographic features that could be used to diagnose chorioretinal folds.

G Cennamo and N. Rosa (eds.), Ultrasonography in Ophthalmology 15, pp. 65–67.

Results

Fifty-five patients had choroidal folds associated with an intraorbital tumor: 24 were due to cavernous hemangiomas (43.6%), seven to lacrimal gland tumors (12.7%), five to optic nerve meningiomas (9.1%), four to vascular tumors (7.3%), four to mucoceles (7.3%), two to metastasis (3.6%), two to sinus diseases (3.6%), two to dermoid cysts (3.6%) and five to different tumors (9.1%). Among these patients, 37 (67.3%) had tumors inside the muscle cone, and 18 (32.7%) outside. In these cases with chorioretinal folds, echography showed a flattening of the ocular wall, with retinochoroidal thickening.

Discussion and conclusion

Chorioretinal folds are wrinkles or undulations in Bruch's membrane, the retinal pigment epithelium, or inner choroid, and may involve the outer retina.

They may be uni- or bilateral and are often arranged in horizontal, parallel fashion, but may be vertical, oblique or irregular [2]. Chorioretinal folds may develop because of choroidal congestion, scleral shrinkage or folding, and contracture of Bruch's membrane [1].

Chorioretinal folds should be differentiated from retinal folds that involve only the retina. The latter are generally narrower than chorioretinal folds, cannot be demonstrated by fluorescein angiography and may be associated with epiretinal membranes, subretinal scars, subretinal neovascular membranes, uveal or scleral thickening, optic nerve diseases [1].

Fluorescein angiography is the best method to show the presence of chorioretinal folds. They appear as a series of alternating hyperfluorescent and hypofluorescent streaks. The yellow or light lines seen on ophthalmoscopy correspond to the hyperfluorescent lines and represent the peaks of the choroidal folds.

The dark lines correspond to the hypofluorescent lines and represent the valleys of the folds.

The hypofluorescent streaks might correspond to an inclination of the retinal pigment epithelium in the valleys of the folds, causing an increase in the thickness of the retinal pigment epithelium and thus blocking the underlying choroidal fluorescence. The hyperfluorescent streaks might be the result of atrophy or thinning of the retinal pigment epithelium over the peaks of the choroidal folds [2]. Another explanation for the fluorescein pattern could be a partial collapse of adjacent blood vessels in the choriocapillaris that would produce a decreased fluorescein filling in the valley of the folds.

Fluorescein angiography detects chorioretinal folds, but is not contributory as to the underlying cause(s). Standardized echography is not very sensitive in detecting choroidal folds, but can be crucial in evaluating the pathogenesis of chorioretinal folds. Atta *et al.* [3], based on data from standardized echography, suggested that chorioretinal folds may be produced by any of the following mechanisms: 1) scleral shortening as in primary hypermetropia; 2) choroidal thickening as in scleritis; and 3) enlargement of various retrobulbar orbital structures.

It is not known how a choroidal fold is produced; it could be caused by compression of the globe or distortion of the optic nerve [4], or it may be a choroidal edema due to the compression of the ophthalmic vein by the tumor. Nevertheless, our data suggest that the echographic examination, particularly if performed with standardized echography [5,6], not only gives characteristic images of this disease, but is also an essential atraumatic method to detect and differentiate the lesions that produce this ophthalmic picture.

References

[1] A. Leahey, A.J. Brucker, E. Wyrynsky and P. Shaman. Chorioretinal folds, a comparison of unilateral and bilateral cases. Arch. Ophthalmol. 1993;111:357–359.

[2] F.E. Cangemi, C.L. Trempe and J.B. Walsh. Choroideal folds. Am. J. Ophthalmol. 1978;86:380–387.

[3] H.R. Atta and S.F. Byrne. The findings of standardized echography for choroidal folds. Arch. Ophthalmol. 1988;106:1234–1241.

[4] T.R. Friberg and A.S. Grove Jr. Choroidal folds and refractive errors associated with orbital tumors. Arch. Ophthalmol. 1983;101:599–603.

[5] R. Gallenga, G. Bellone, P.E. Gallenga and A. Pasquarelli. Ultrasonografia clinica dell'occhio e dell'orbita. Proceedings LIII SOI Congress, Malta 1971.

[6] K.C. Ossoinig. Standardized echography: basic principles, clinical applications and results. In R.L. Dallaw (ed.), Ophthalmic ultrasonography: comparative techniques. Boston: Little Brown and Co. Intern. Ophthalmol. Clinics 1979;19:127–210.

G. Cennamo
Istituto di Oftalmologia
Università di Napoli Federico II
Via S. Pansini 5
80131 Naples, Italy

5. Scleral support on progressive myopic eyes. Short-time follow-up

V. HIDASI and L. KOLOZSVÁRI[1]
(Debrecen and [1]Szeged, Hungary)

Abstract

The scleral support procedure (i.e., reinforcement) is an operation performed to stabilize the enlargement of progressive myopic eyes. We investigated visual acuity, refractive error, astigmatism and axial length before surgery and 1 week, and 1, 2, 6 and 10 months post-surgery. At the end of the follow-up average visual acuity was better than before the operation. The refraction was practically unchanged. The astigmatism gradually changed during follow-up and finally approached the preoperative condition. The average axial length was shorter at the end of follow-up than before the operation. Thus the axial shortening may be responsible for the improvement in vision; the astigmatism did not seem to influence the improvement in vision.

Key words: Scleral support, visual acuity, refraction, axial length, astigmatism.

Introduction

The scleral support procedure has been performed on progressive myopic eyes since 1954 [1] to reduce the enlargement of myopic eyeballs. The first experiment was made by Shevelev on dogs in 1930 [2]. The surgical technique and the results of this operation have been widely discussed. The aim of our work was to examine the postoperative changes of visual acuity, refractive error, astigmatism and axial length and their inter-relationship.

Materials and methods

We studied 31 eyes of 27 patients selected at random from myopic patients who had undergone surgery with scleral support in 1992. Patient age ranged from 10 to 56 years. There were 20 females and 7 males. We examined visual acuity with Kettesy's decimal table; refraction was assessed subjectively with glasses; astigmatism was measured with a Carl Zeiss 110 type keratometer or in some cases with an EyeSys photokeratoscope and the axial length with a Cooper

G Cennamo and N. Rosa (eds.), Ultrasonography in Ophthalmology 15, pp. 69–74.

Vision Digital B IV ultrasound machine using the immersion A-scan method. Examinations were performed before the operation, and 1 week and 1, 3, 6 and 10 months post-surgery. Not all patients kept each follow-up appointment. Since 1979, in our clinic we have performed scleral support on progressive myopic eyes using the Snyder-Thompson procedure [3] (Fig. 1) but with a fascia lata band [4].

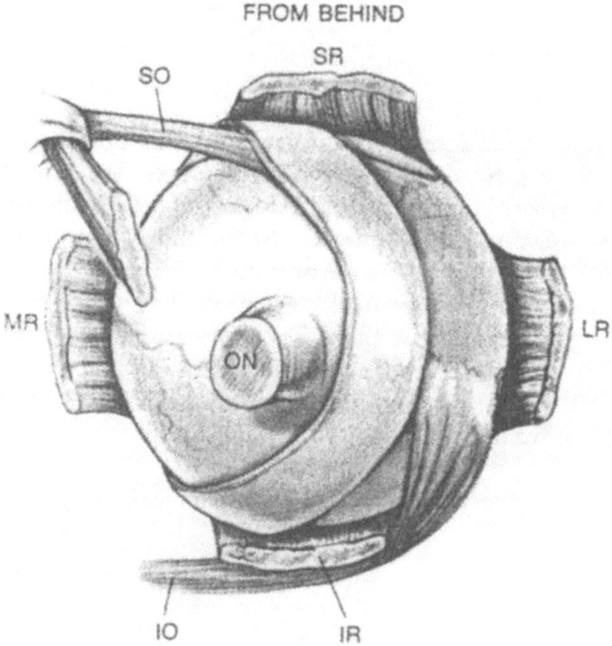

Fig. 1. Scleral support (i.e., reinforcement) according to Snyder-Thompson [3]

Results

The average visual acuity (Fig. 2) improved over starting values although the difference was not significant as compared to the starting point because of wide individual differences. In the sixth postoperative month there appeared to be an impairment; however, this may be attributable to the low number of patients. It is noteworthy that in spite of axis lengthening and the consequent increase of refractive power, visual acuity improved in the first postoperative month. We have found this to be a frequent finding also in our other patients who have undergone scleral support. The average visual acuity approached the starting point value in the tenth postoperative month, but it was still better.

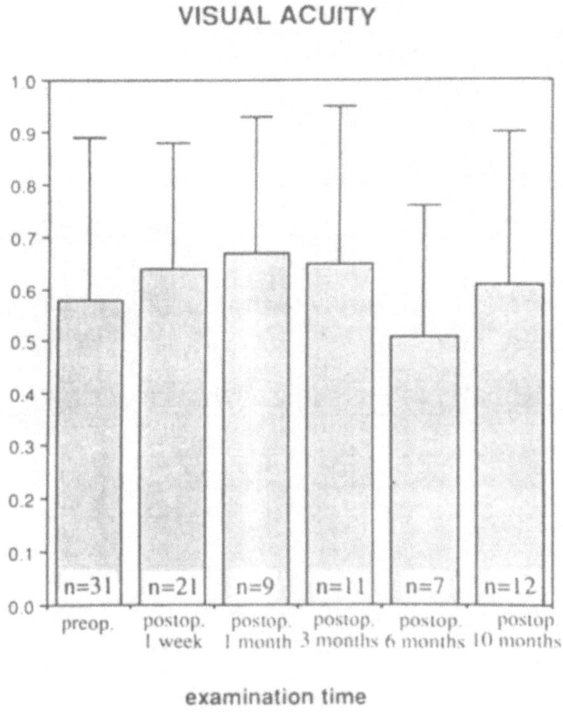

Fig. 2. Time course of visual acuity changes after scleral support

The refractive error (Fig. 3) was measured as power of the glasses that gave the best visual acuity. Apart from the first postoperative month there was no essential change of average. The impairment in the first postoperative month, however, was objectively supported by the axial lengthening.

The astigmatism (Fig. 4), measured with the Zeiss keratometer, was the greatest in the first week after surgery; this was probably due to the pressure on the bulb exerted by the swollen eyelids and orbital tissues. The increased astigmatism, however, did not result in a decrease in visual acuity. Subsequently, the value of astigmatism approached the starting point value except in the sixth month. We also measured 7 eyes with the EyeSys photokeratoscope (Fig. 5), making a total number of measurements of 22. In 21 cases the values obtained with the Zeiss equipment were higher than those obtained with the EyeSys machine, but the tendency of changes was similar in both cases. The average value of the differences of astigmatism measured with the two different machines was 0.48. There was an average difference of 8.8° between the angles of the two axes; this difference was not significant. The average axial length (Fig. 6) in the first postoperative month was longer compared with preoperative

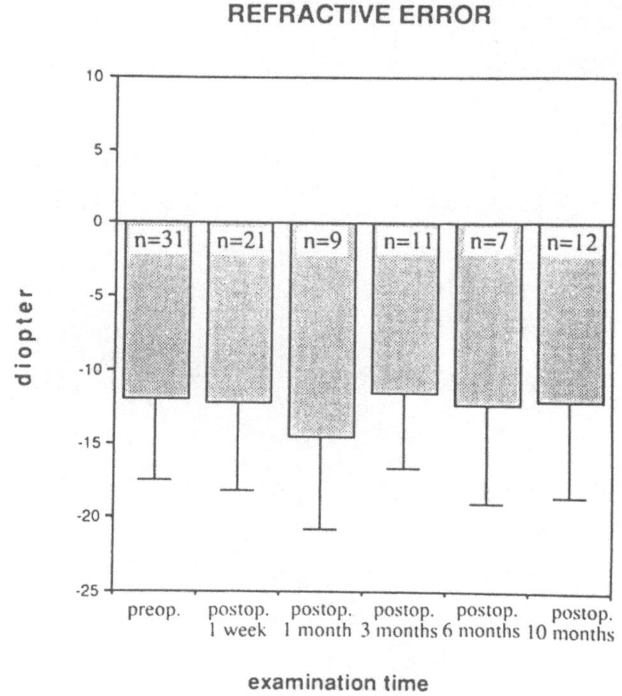

Fig. 3. Time course of refractive error changes after scleral support

values. Later, it decreased and in the tenth postoperative month in was still shorter than before surgery.

Discussion

Visual acuity in the tenth postoperative month was still better than before surgery. Refraction did not show notable changes. The axial length in the tenth postoperative month was shorter than before the operation. The axial lengthening and the consequent increase in refraction in the first month support the validity of this study. The reason for the improvement is unknown.

In conclusion, there is a correlation between axial length and refractional changes, and between axial shortening and visual improvement. The changes of astigmatism did not seem to influence the visual acuity in the present series of investigations.

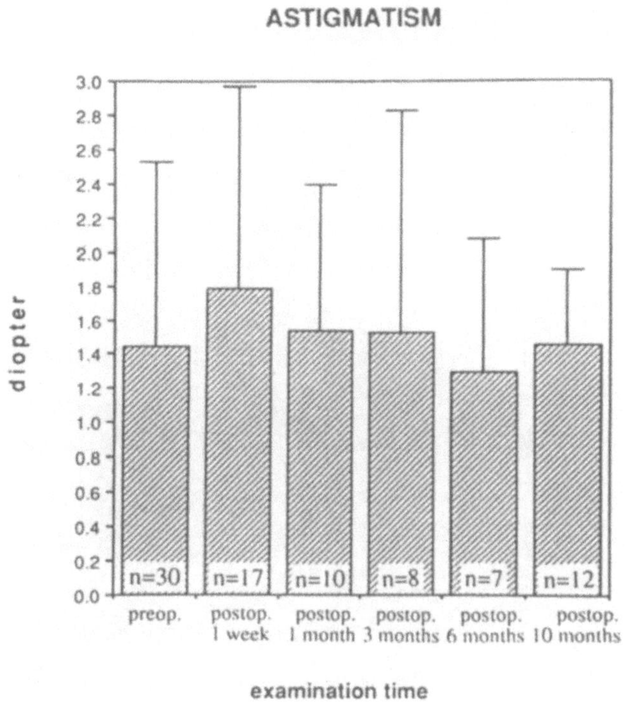

Fig. 4. Time course of astigmatism measured with the Zeiss 110 type keratometer after scleral support

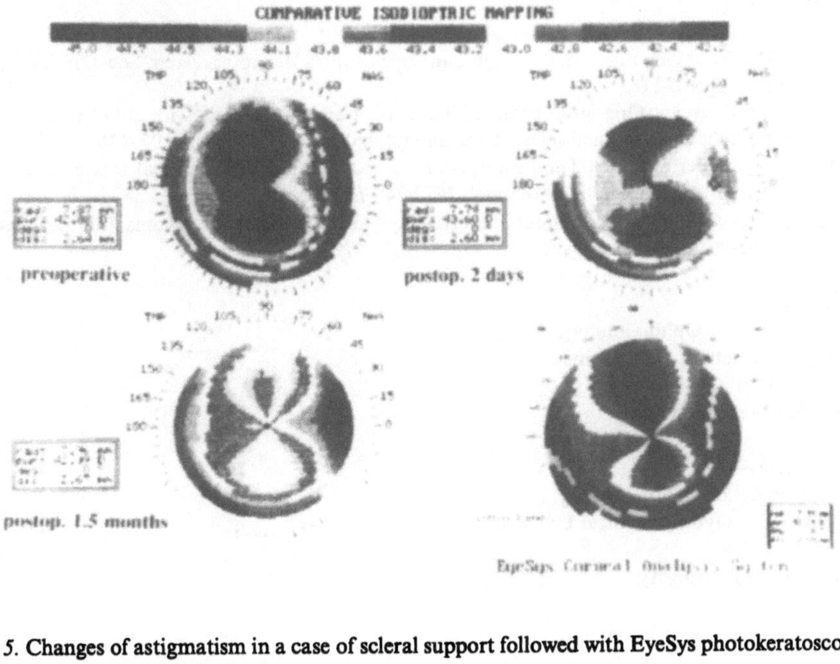

Fig. 5. Changes of astigmatism in a case of scleral support followed with EyeSys photokeratoscope (lower right: 1 year after surgery)

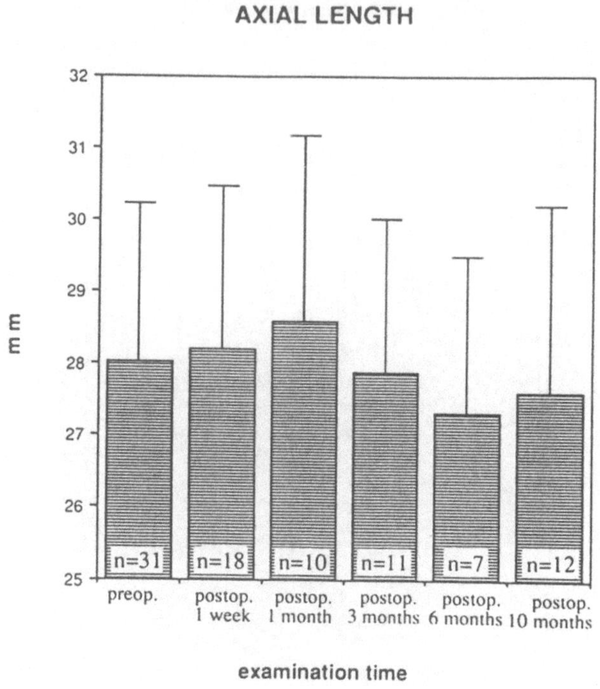

Fig. 6. Time course of axial length changes after scleral support

References

[1] J. Malbran. Una nueva orientación quirúrgica contra la miopia. Arch. Soc. Oftal. Hisp. Am. 1954;14:1167–1183.

[2] M.M. Shevelev. Operation against high myopia and sclerectasia with aid of transplantation of fascia lata on thinned sclera. Russian Ophthalmol. J. 1930;11(1):107–110.

[3] A.A. Snyder and F.B. Thompson. A simplified technique for surgical treatment of degenerative myopia. Am. J. Ophthalmol. 1972;74:273-277.

[4] Z. Nagy. Surgical procedures for arresting the progression of myopia (Surgical technik). Szemészet 1984;121:205–210.

V. Hidasi
Department of Ophthalmology
University School of Medicine
P.O. Box 30
4012 Debrecen, Hungary

L. Kolozsvári
Department of Ophthalmology
Albert Sent György Medical University
P.O. Box 407
6701 Szeged, Hungary

6. Echographical and radiological examination of intraocular calcifications

L. KOLOZSVÁRI and K. BENKŐ[1]
(Szeged and [1]Debrecen, Hungary)

Abstract

A reliable diagnosis of several intraocular disorders is possible only by means of imaging methods (traditional X-ray, computerized tomography, magnetic resonance imaging, echography). In some cases the combination of these methods is indispensable for diagnosis. The exposure of patients to irradiation and examination costs can be reduced significantly by an optimal choice of methods. We describe the possibilities of echographical and radiological differentiation of intraocular calcifications on the basis of our cases (retinoblastoma, drusen papillae, Coat's disease, astrocytoma, osteoma choroideae, cataracta luxata, phthisis bulbi, foreign body); in addition, we present our experience with these methods.

Key words: Intraocular calcifications, CT scan, echography

Introduction

Calcium may be found in the eye either as bone or as calcium salts, often phosphates, sulphates and oxalates. The origin may be neoplastic, metabolic, dystrophic or idiopathic. The majority of calcified deposits accumulates on the posterior eye segment. The differential diagnosis of calcification of the posterior globe includes the following [1]:

Calcium densities of the posterior eye segment

1. Primary neural tumors of the retina and optic nerve
   Retinoblastoma
   Optic nerve glioma
   Optic nerve meningioma

2. Glial hamartomas of the optic nerve and retina
   Tuberous sclerosis (astrocytoma)
   von Recklinghausen disease

G Cennamo and N. Rosa (eds.), Ultrasonography in Ophthalmology 15, pp. 75–82.

Drusen
Isolated

3. Vascular tumors of the retina and choroid
   Cavernous haemangioma
   Haemangioendothelioma

4. Choroidal osteoma

5. Hypercalcemic states
   Hyperparathyroidism
   Hypervitaminosis D
   Sarcoidosis
   Hypercalcaemia of chronic renal disease

6. Post-traumatic, post-inflammatory, degenerative conditions
   Phthisis bulbi
   Retrolental fibroplasia
   Coats' disease, etc.

Hypercalcemic states, post-traumatic, post-inflammatory, and degenerative conditions can also cause calcified lesions in the anterior globe: calcified cataracts, band-shaped degeneration and diffuse calcification of the cornea, different scleral deposits and so-called plaque immediately in front of the insertions of the rectus muscles [2,3].

In the last five years (1989–1993) 48 different lesions with calcification were diagnosed by means of echography at departments (Table 1). The equipment used was Cooper Vision Digital B. Some of our patients also underwent CT and MRI examinations.

Table 1. Intraocular calcifications diagnosed by echography

Diagnosis	Patient number
Retinoblastoma	31
Drusen	6
Astrocytoma (sclerosis tuberosa)	2
Osteoma	2
Phthisis bulbi	2
Cataract (luxata)	4
Foreign body	1
	48

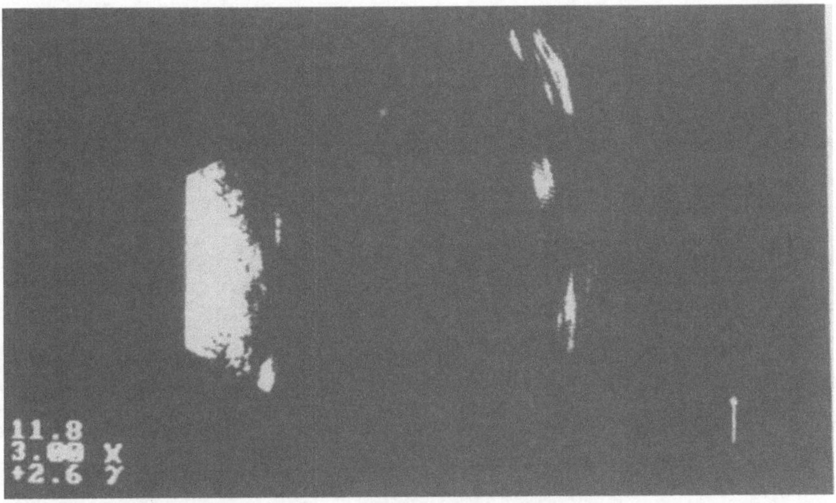

Fig. 1. **Echogram of a drusen papillae at extremely low sensitivity**

Drusen of the optic nerve head are well-delineated alterations that are high reflective even with a decreased sensitivity [2] (Fig. 1).

Astrocytoma is very similar in it's acoustic behavior to calcified hyalin bodies.

Retinoblastoma shows isolated calcified foci, or prominent irregular sonolucent masses. These signs are highly characteristic for this tumor. The expressed shadowing effect of the retinoblastoma is well known [2,4]. After any type of irradiation of the eye or after spontaneous necrosis of the tumor, a solid homogeneous calcareous mass may be present (Fig. 2).

Luxated calcified lens can occur on the retina in front of the posterior pole, or more anteriorly. Longstanding congenital, traumatic and senile cataractous lenses can calcify [3].

Osseous intraocular foreign body occurred in one of our cases (Fig. 3).

Massive gliosis is a non specific reaction of the retina to post-traumatic, post-inflammatory and degenerative conditions, representing a benign proliferation of retinal glial cells. Calcifications occur in about 50% of cases and bone formation on the metaplastic retinal pigment epithelium is common [3] (Figs. 4 and 5).

Choroidal osteoma causes elevation of the juxtapapillary retina and appears orange to orange-white with sharply defined margins. It is composed of mature

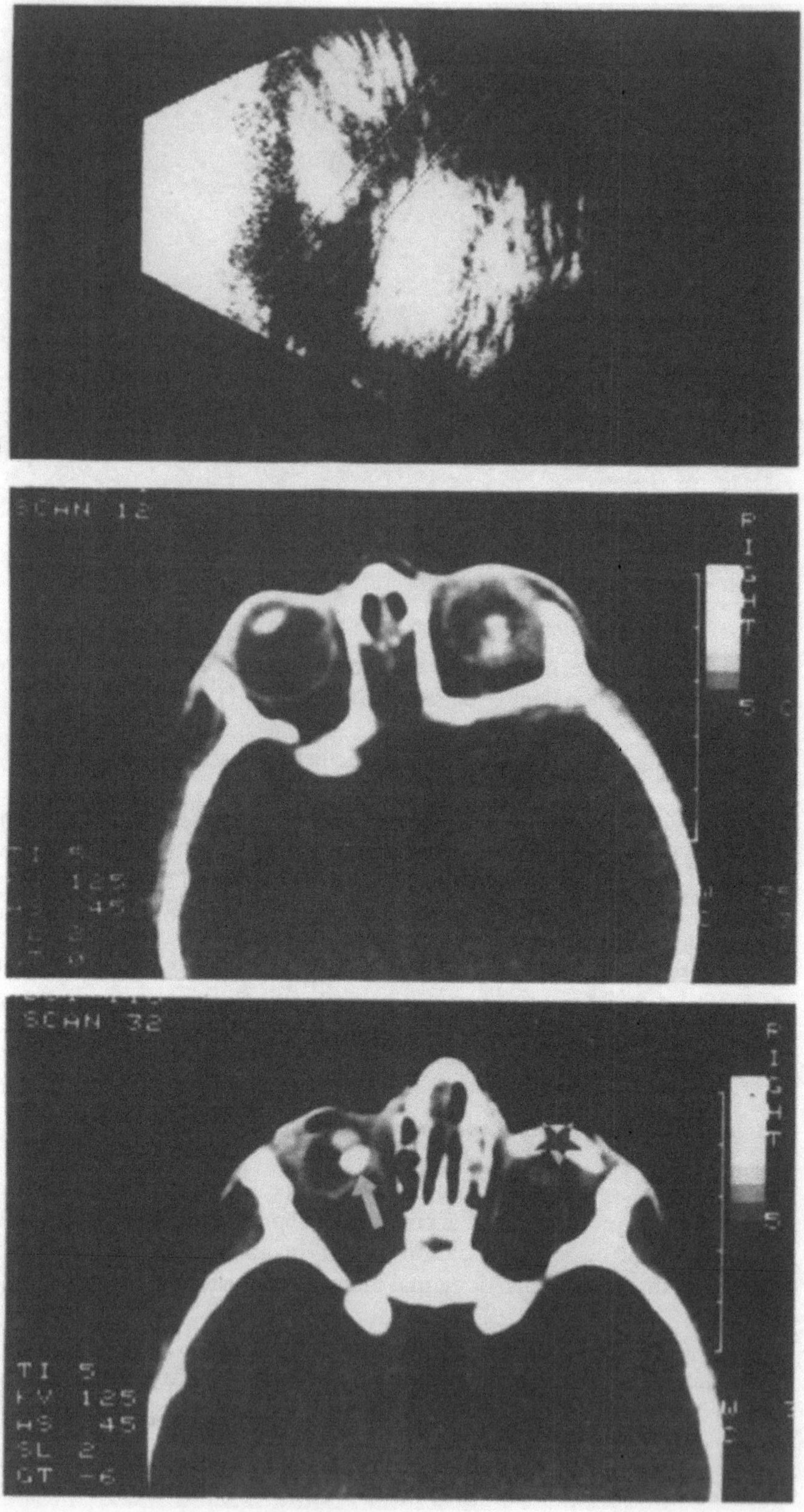

(a)

(b)

(c)

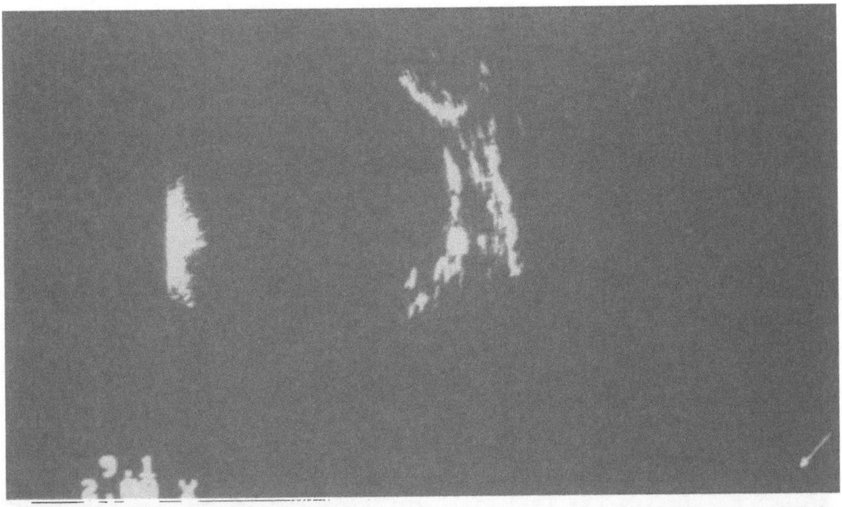

Fig. 3. Echogram of a splinter of a pig bone in front of the retina in the eye of a young butcher

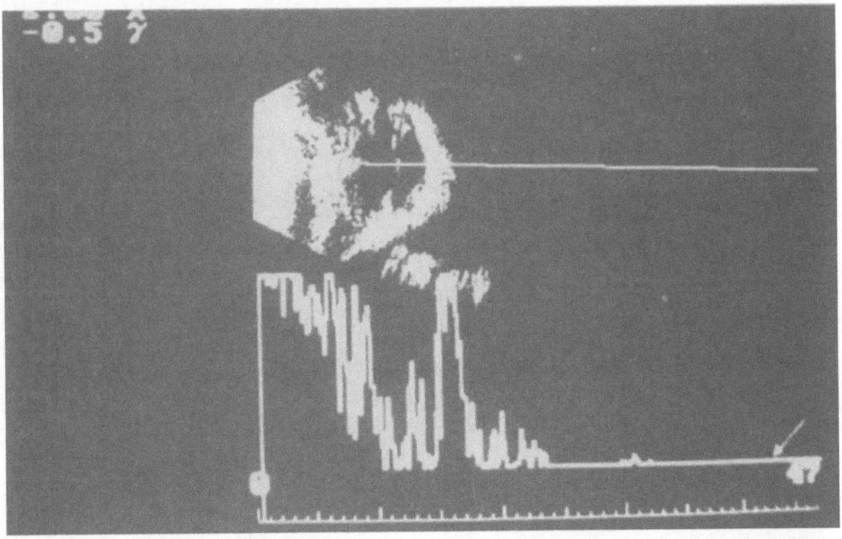

Fig. 4. High reflecting concave alteration on the posterior eye segment with shadowing effect: bone formation in a phthisic eye

---

Figure 2 (opposite)
Fig. 2a. Bilateral retinoblastoma of a 1-year-old boy. Echogram of the right eye. Marked shadowing effect behind the calcified part of the tumor
Fig. 2b. Retinal tumor in the right eye. Relative inhomogeneity in the radiolucent alteration. In this section intact left eye
Fig. 2c. Calcified tumor (arrow) after irradiation and kryotherapy in the left eye. Radiolucent formation (star) on the right already anophthalmic side: prothesis

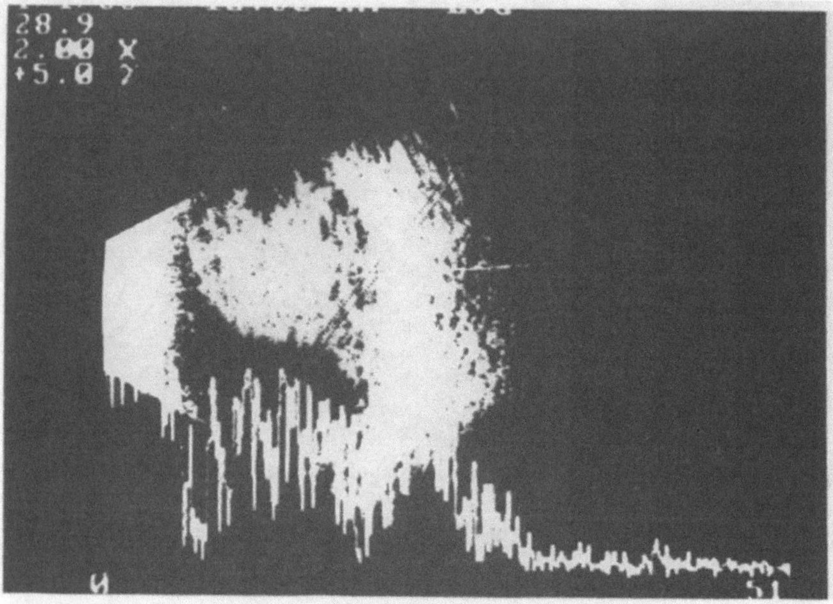

(a)

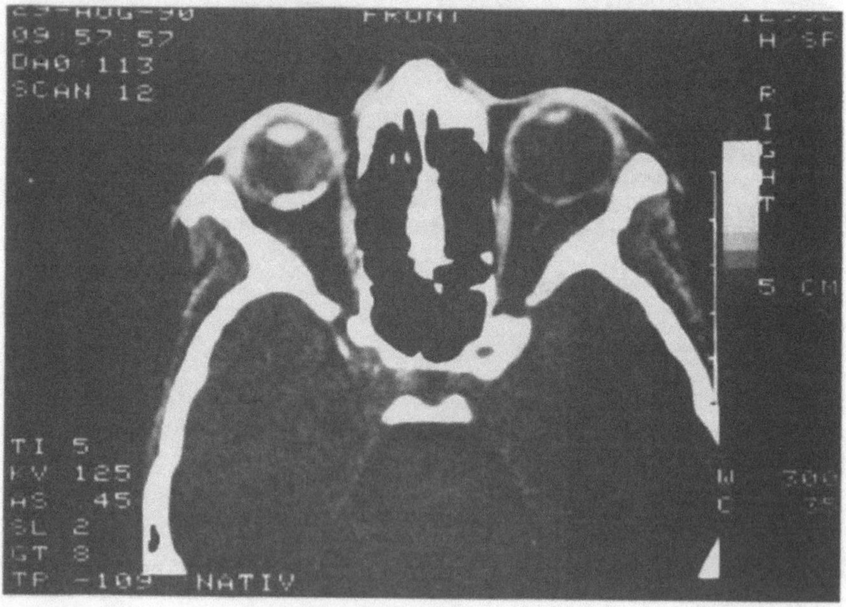

(b)

Fig. 5. Coats' disease
Fig. 5a. Slowly moving, high reflecting point-like echosources under the elevated retina in the eye of a 12-year-old girl
Fig. 5b. Radiolucent plaque in the posterior eye wall: bone formation

(a)

(b)

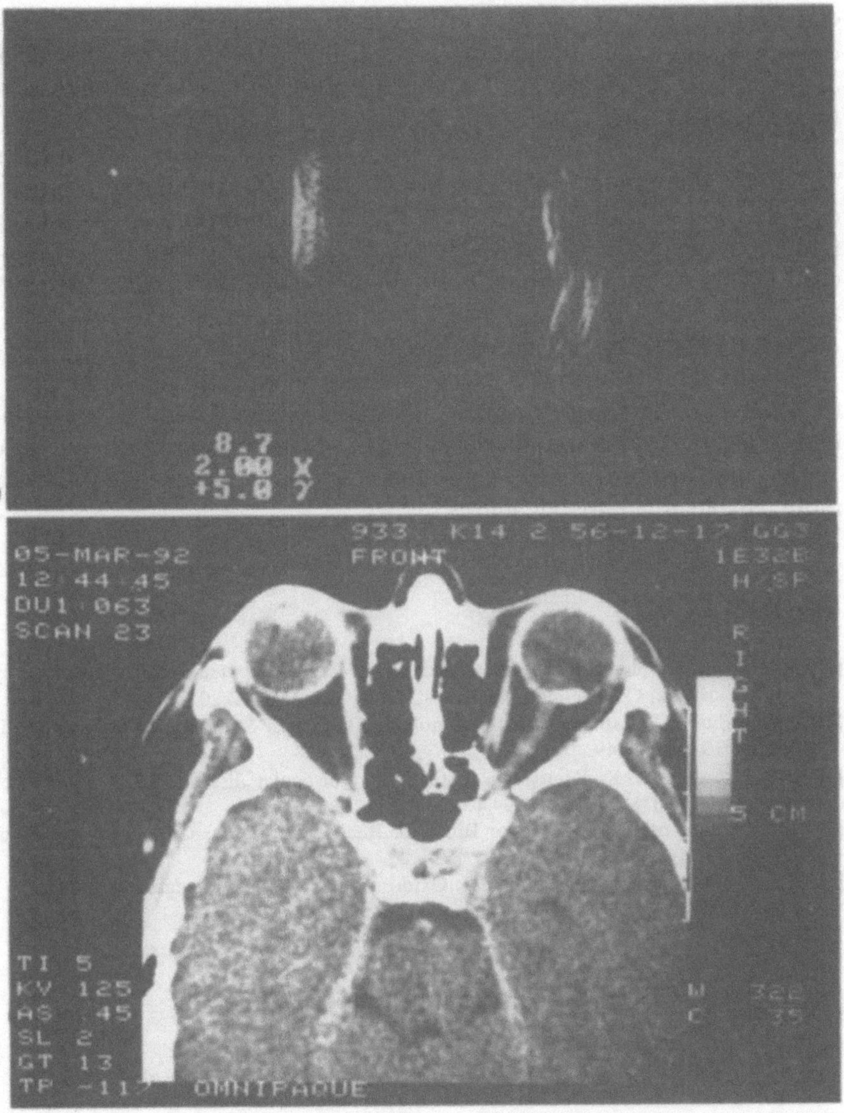

Fig. 6. Choroidal osteoma in the right eye of a 38-year-old woman
Fig. 6a. The tumor is sonolucent at a very low level of sensitivity
Fig. 6b. Osseous plaque on the posterior pole of the eye on CT scan

shadow formation (Fig. 6). The alteration affects mainly relatively young females, but can also occur in males and children [5].

Based on this experience and on the literature, echography is of great importance and our first method of choice in cases of intraocular calcifications. Only the characteristic acoustic signs together with the ophthalmoscopic picture can establish the diagnosis of drusen, astrocytoma, choroidal osteoma and secondary choroidal calcification. If needed, CT and fluorescein angiography can be helpful. Magnetic resonance imaging examinations are unnecessary in these cases.

Calcification in degenerative processes, such as Coats' disease, post-traumatic and post-inflammatory stages, phthisis bulbi etc. produces homogeneous calcified plaques in the posterior eye wall, different from the isolated deposits found in retinoblastoma. A retinoblastoma, particularly with suspected extraocular extension, indicates the CT examination. The calcified areas in the tumor are typical even with echography, but absence of such sonolucent and radiolucent areas does not exclude the retinal tumor [4].

Calcification in an adult eye can simulate an intraocular foreign body especially in the anterior sclera, but retinoblastoma should be suspected immediately in case of calcified lesions in the posterior pole of the eye of a child.

The combined use of echography, radiology and other methods will lead to a more reliable differential diagnosis.

References

[1] S.B. Hammerschlag, J.R. Hesselink and A.L. Weber. Computed tomography of the eye and orbit. Norwalk, Connecticut: Appleton-Century-Crofts, 1983;207–211.

[2] R. Guthoff. Ultrasound in Ophthalmologic Diagnosis. Stuttgart, New York: G. Thieme Verlag, 1991;146–149.

[3] A. Garner and G.K. Klintworth. Pathobiology of ocular disease. New York, Basel, Hong Kong: Marcel Dekker Inc., 1994;403.

[4] P.K. Lommatzsch. Intraokulare Tumoren. Bücherei des Augenarztes, Bd. 117. Stuttgart: Ferdinand Enke Verlag 1989.

[5] J.J. Kanski. Clinical Ophthalmology. Oxford: Butterworth-Heinemann, 1994;221.

L. Kolozsvári
Department of Ophthalmology
Albert Szent-Györgyi Medical University
P.O. Box 407
H-6701 Szeged, Hungary

K. Benkő
Dept. of Radiology
University School of Medicine
Debrecen, Hungary

Intraocular tumors

7. Echographic and immunohistochemical aspects in a case of pleomorphic adenocarcinoma of the ciliary body

A. GALANTUOMO, G. BALDI, G. NASTRI, B. PASTENA[1], S. SBORDONE, L. MANFREDONIA[1] and F. BALDI[2]

(Naples, Italy)

Abstract

The clinical and echographic distinction between a pleomorphic adenocarcinoma of the ciliary body epithelium and an uveal melanoma may be difficult. The association between adenocarcinoma of the ciliary body epithelium and ocular trauma in elderly patients has been well documented. We describe the echographic and immunohistochemical findings in a case of pleomorphic adenocarcinoma of the ciliary body in a blind eye of a 79-year-old man without signs of previous penetrating trauma.

Key words: Standardized echography, histochemistry, immunohistochemistry, pleomorphic adenocarcinoma, ciliary body

Introduction

Tumors of the neuroepithelium of the ciliary body have been classified [1] into congenital and acquired lesions and are extremely rare [2–11]. Congenital lesions occur in childhood; they include glioneuroma, medulloepithelioma, and teratoid medulloepithelioma. The second and third lesions may be benign or malignant [4,8,12–15]. Acquired tumors are most often seen in adults; they include pseudoadenomatous hyperplasia, adenoma and adenocarcinoma [14,16,17]. Among the rarest of intraocular tumors are adenocarcinomas of the nonpigmented epithelium of the ciliary body [6,9–11,18] and their incidence has been estimated at one case per year in the United States [7].

Adenocarcinomas of the ciliary body have been described as having one of four basic patterns: glandular or papillary, pleomorphic of low grade, pleomorphic with hyaline stroma, or anaplastic [9]. Clinically, they are often misdiagnosed as malignant melanomas or medulloepithelioma [8,18,19] of the ciliary body, the correct diagnosis being made after a local resection or enucleation [17]. The morphological aspect of such tumors has been well studied

G Cennamo and N. Rosa (eds.), Ultrasonography in Ophthalmology 15, pp. 85–92.

at the optic microscope and to a great extent at the electronic microscope, while the immunohistochemical aspect has been studied only in part [9,10].

Here we report the echographic and immunohistochemical characteristics of a case of pleomorphic adenocarcinoma of the ciliary body.

Case report

P.F., a 79-year-old male, came to our observation complaining of total sight reduction in the left eye, which had occurred about a month earlier. Pathological anamnesis proved negative for trauma and/or previous ocular intervention. The ophthalmoscopic examination showed, in the left eye, a globus retinal detachment affecting the temporal sectors, with the presence of rigid retinal folds. There was no evidence of retinal lacerations or holes. The retinal detachment appeared to have fairly well-defined limits and was dark grey in colour; the vitreous did not present any alterations.

The patient therefore underwent echographic examination. The echographic examination with a contact B-scan revealed a mushroom-shaped solid lesion located at ciliary body in the temporal quadrants, associated with serous retinal detachment (Fig. 1); standardized A-scan examination with the Kretz technique 7200 MA showed a solid mass lesion with a high reflectivity in the first 10

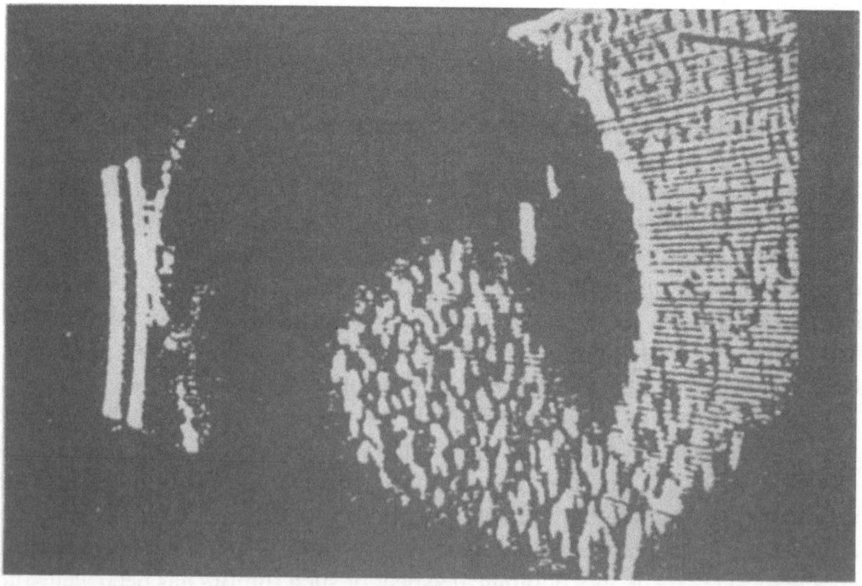

Fig. 1. Contact B-scan: mushroom-shaped solid lesion located in the ciliary body in the temporal quadrants, associated with serous retinal detachment

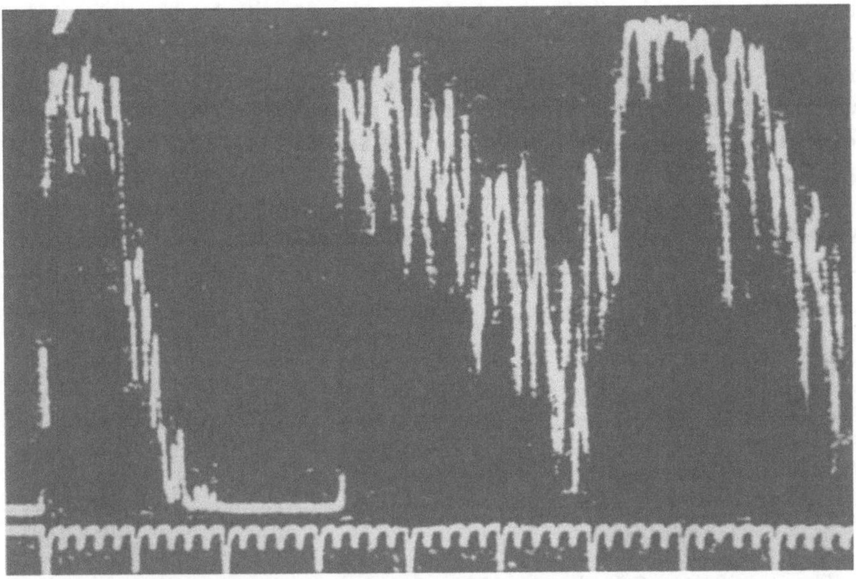

Fig. 2. **Standardized A-scan, EA 3, 30 h: solid mass lesion with high reflectivity in the first ten microseconds, followed by a medium-low reflective area. No massive scleral infiltration was found**

microseconds, followed by a medium-low reflective area. Vascularity could not be demonstrated convincingly with the A-scan unit. No massive scleral infiltration was found (Fig. 2).

A malignant melanoma in the phase of rapid growth, with a rupture of the Bruch's membrane was diagnosed. On the basis of these findings, the patient underwent enucleation of the left eye. The histological and immunohistochemical examination revealed the presence of a pleomorphic adenocarcinoma of the ciliary body.

Histology

On opening the enucleated eye, the temporal area of the ciliary body was occupied by a greyish-white mass which filled the cavity of the vitreous body and the posterior chamber. The mass extended to the choroid and retina, thereby raising these structures. The optic nerve appeared unimpaired. The ocular bulb was sectioned equatorially passing through the lesion and including the pupil, the lens, the macula and the optic nerve. The two hemispheres were fixed, one in ethyl alcohol at 70%, the other in 10% buffered formaldehyde, and then embedded in paraffin.

The sections were stained as follows: hematoxylin-eosin, hematoxylin-van

Gieson, Azan-Mallory, Gomori, PAS-Alcian blue (MacManus and Mowry) for mucopolysaccharides (before and after treatment with hyaluronidase); Luxol-fast-blue-cresil-violet for the nervous structures; and Masson-Fontana for melanin. Hsu's ABC (Vectastain) procedure was used for the immunohistochemical studies which were carried out on paraffin-embedded sections. The following monoclonal and polyclonal antibodies were used as primary anteserum:

Anteserum	Characteristics	Source
Secretory component	Polyclonal	Dako
EMA	Monoclonal	Dako
NSE	Polyclonal	Lipshaw
Synaptophysin	Monoclonal	Biogenex
Chromogranin	Monoclonal	Biogenex
S-100 protein	Polyclonal	Dako
Vimentin	Monoclonal	Dako

The specificity of the immunohistochemical methods was confirmed by the negative results obtained after removing or replacing the antesera. At the microscope the tumor was seen to originate from the nonpigmented epithelium of the ciliary body and appeared to consist of a well-differentiated adenocarcinomatous-type part and of a solid part. The adenocarcinomatous part consisted of tubules and pseudoglands covered by a cubic-cylindrical epithelium, surrounded by a more or less lax connective tissue; some papillary areas were observed. In the solid part the glandular form tended to disappear and be replaced by neoplastic cords interspersed with connective hyaline tissue; some 'washer-like' tubular formations were detected in the solid structures (Figs. 3 and 4).

The stains for mucopolysaccharides showed, also in the 'solid' areas, the presence of basal membranes and the presence of mucopolysaccharides in the glandular lumens, sensitive to hyaluronidase, which were absent from cytoplasms. Melanin was not detected in the neoplastic cells, while it was found in the remnants of the pigmented epithelium of the ciliary body. The neoplasia subsequently filtered into the retina without reaching the optic nerve. It destroyed the ciliary body and reached the innermost strata of the sclera without crossing it completely at any point. The stain for the secretory component was observed only in the areas with tubular differentiation, where it was localized in the luminal periphery or in the supernuclear region. In the same zones there was also a faint focal colouring for epithelial membrane antigen (Figs. 5 and 6).

Conversely, in the areas characterized by a solid structure we found various focal positivities for protein S-100, for Chromogranin, for neuron-specific-enolase and for synaptophysin. Vimentin was positive in all the areas of the neoplasia; the keratin, on the other hand, was negative.

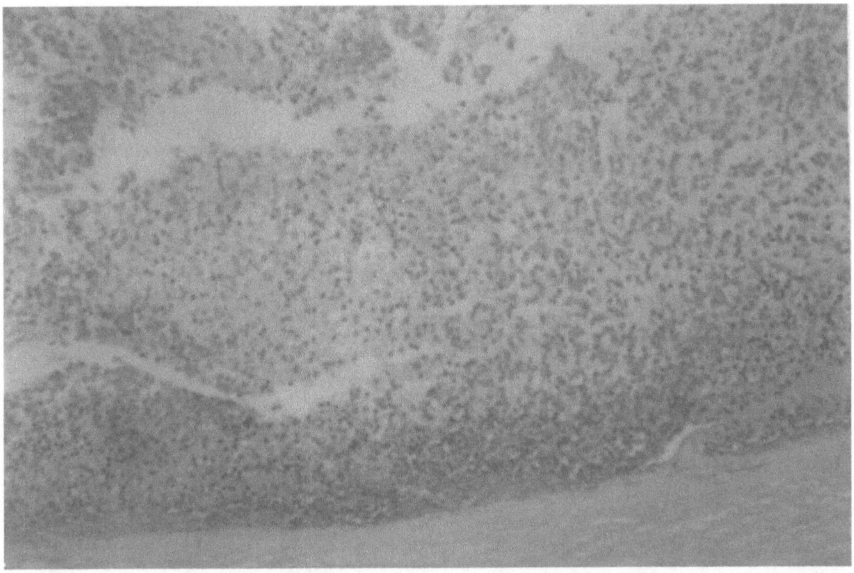

Fig. 3. Histological finding. The tumor appears to consist of a well-differentiated adenocarcinomatous part and of a solid part. Massive scleral infiltration was not found (hematoxylin-eosin × 100)

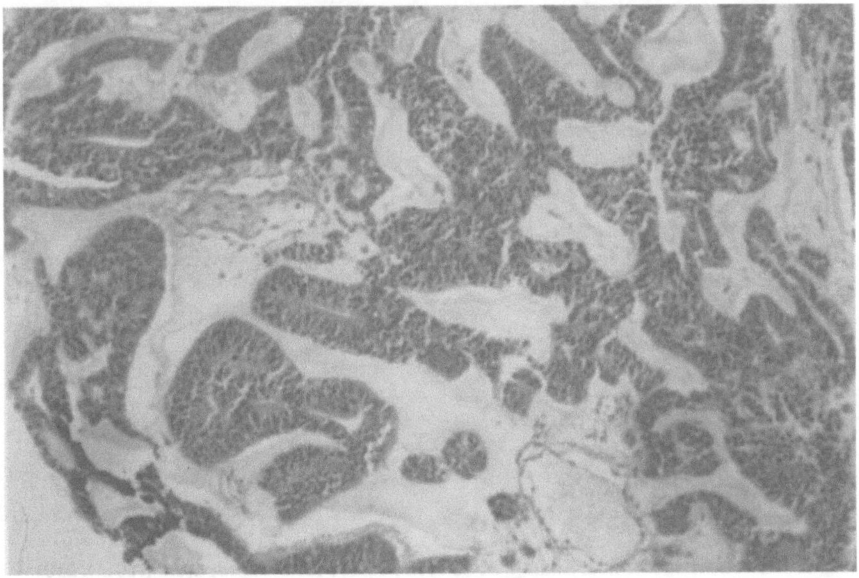

Fig. 4. Histological finding. The adenocarcinomatous part consists of tubules and pseudoglands covered by a cubic-cylindrical epithelium and surrounded by a more or less lax connective tissue (hematoxylin-eosin × 250)

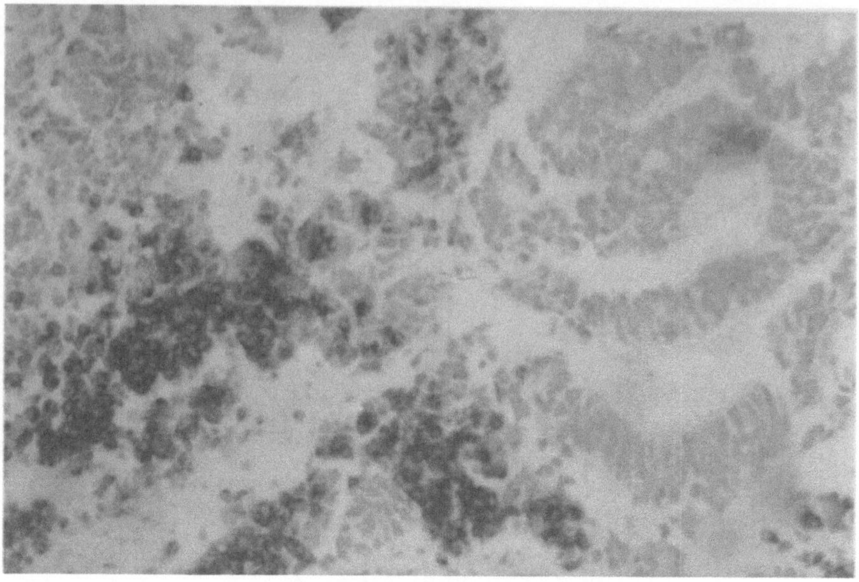

Fig. 5. Immunohistochemical finding. Glandular area positive for secretory antigen (ABC × 250)

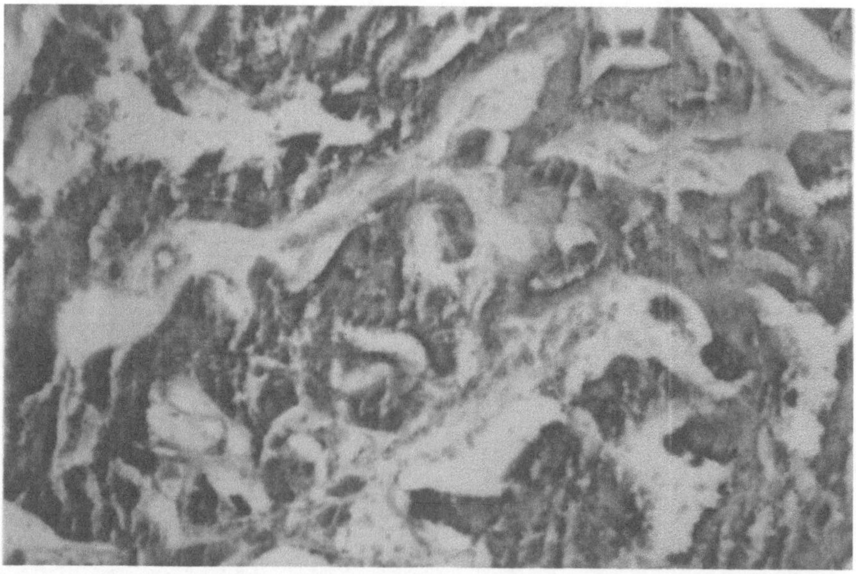

Fig. 6. Immunohistochemical finding. Solid area positive for synaptophysin (ABC × 250)

Discussion

There are very few descriptions of the echographic aspect of tumors of the ciliary body epithelium or, more generally, of the pigmented retinal epithelium [20,21]; the A- and B-scan characteristics reported previously do not differ from those typical of choroidal malignant melanoma (e.g., dome-shaped solid lesions, choroidal excavation, medium-low reflectivity).

The pleomorphic adenocarcinoma of the ciliary body examined by us appeared to be made up histologically of a well differentiated adenocarcinomatous-type part and of a solid part. The adenocarcinomatous part consisted of tubules and pseudoglands covered by a cubic-cylindrical epithelium and surrounded by a more or less lax connective tissue. In the solid part the glandular form tended to disappear and be replaced by neoplastic cords interspersed with connective hyaline tissue.

The histogenesis of the tumor under examination is related to elements still capable of epithelial and nervous differentiation; in this way the tumor would have a double cell component. The neoplastic cells proved positive for epithelial membrane antigen and for the secretory antigen in the glandular areas but not in the solid areas, where the cells were positive for chromogranin, synaptophysin, NSE and for S-100 protein. The vimentin was positive in both districts.

The histochemical and immunohistochemical findings raised the question as to whether there was a correlation between these and the preoperative echographic findings. In fact, the lesion presented two distinct areas also at the A-scan: in one area the lesion had high reflectivity, while in the other reflectivity was medium-low. The histochemical data prompted us to reevaluate this finding, which we had interpreted to be a sign of rupture of Bruch's membrane by the lesion. It could be hypothesized that the high-reflective area corresponds to the glandular part (less compact) of the tumor, whereas the medium-low reflective area corresponds to its solid part.

In any case, a preoperative echographic distinction between malignant melanoma and pleomorphic adenocarcinoma of the ciliary body is not easy and, however, does not seem to be crucial because enucleation is the treatment of choice in cases in which the tumor is advanced and widespread and the eye has become blind.

References

[1] L.E. Zimmerman. Verhoeff's 'teratoneuroma': a critical reappraisal in light of new observations and current concepts of embryonic tumors. Am. J. Ophthalmol. 1972;72:1039–1057.

[2] E. Fuchs. Wucherungen und Geschwulste des Ciliarepithelis. Albrecht von Graefes Arch. Ophthalmol. 1908;68:534–587.

[3] R.H.B. Barrow and H.B. Stallard. A case of primary melanocarcinoma of the ciliary body. Br. J. Ophthalmol. 1932;16:98–102.

[4] J.R. Wolter and B.R. James. Adult type of medullo-epithelioma of the ciliary body. Am. J. Ophthalmol. 1958;46:19–26.

[5] J.L. Harris, C.C. Gumucio and M.B. Ohanion. Adenocarcinoma of the ciliary epithelium. Arch. Ophthalmol. 1968;80:217–219.
[6] P. Kuchynka. Malignant epithelioma of the ciliary body. Ophthalmologica 1979;178:190–193.
[7] T.P. Dryia, D.M. Albert and D. Horns. Adenocarcinoma arising from the epithelium of the ciliary body. Ophthalmology 1981;88:1290–1292.
[8] I.S. Jain, A. Gupta and J. Ram. Adenocarcinoma of ciliary epithelium in a young boy. Ann. Ophthalmol. 1987;19:236–237.
[9] M. Rodrigues, A. Hidayat and J. Karesh. Pleomorphic adenocarcinoma of the ciliary epithelium simulating an epibulbar tumor. Am. J. Ophthalmol. 1988;106:595–600.
[10] H.E. Grossniklaus, L.E. Zimmerman and M.L. Kachmer. Pleomorphic adenocarcinoma of the ciliary body. Immunohistochemical and electron microscopic features. Ophthalmology 1990;97:763–768.
[11] C.E. Margo and H.L. Brooks. Adenocarcinoma of the ciliary epithelium in a 12-year-old black child. J. Pediatr. Ophthalmol. Strabismus, 1991;28(4):232–235.
[12] N. Hausmann and F.H. Stefani. Medulloepithelioma of the ciliary body. Acta Ophthalmol. 1991;69(3):398–401.
[13] H.L. Hennis, R.A. Saunders and J.A. Shields. Malignant teratoid meduloepithelioma of the ciliary body. J. Clin. Neuro-ophthalmol. 1990;10(4):291–292.
[14] J.M. Rohrbach, K.P. Steuhl and H.J. Thiel. Cyst and Fuchs' adenomas of the pars plicata corporis ciliaris. Degeneration products due to different ciliary body functions? Klin. Monatsbl. Augenheilkd. 1991;198(3):195–200.
[15] M. Wakakura and W.R. Lee. Ultrastructural pleomorphism in meduloepithelioma of the ciliary body: a comparative study of tumor cells and fetal ciliary epithelium. Jpn. J. Ophthalmol. 1990;34(3):364–380.
[16] R. Haddad and H. Slezak. Benign adenoma of the ciliary epithelium with tumor seeding. Ophthalmologica 1979;78:67-71.
[17] W.E. Lieb, J.A. Shields, R.C. Eagle, D. Kwa and C.L. Shields. Cystic adenoma of the pigmented ciliary epithelium. Clinical, pathologic and immunohistopathologic findings. Ophthalmology 1990;97:1489–1493.
[18] J.J. Papale, K. Akiwama, T. Hirose, K. Tsubota, K. Hanaoka and D.M. Albert. Adenocarcinoma of the ciliary body pigment epithelium in a child. Arch. Ophthalmol. 1984;102:100–103.
[19] M. Chang, J.A. Shields and D.L. Watchell. Adenocarcinoma of the ciliary body simulating a malignant melanoma. Am. J. Ophthalmol. 1979;88: 40–44.
[20] V. Mazzeo. Ecografia dell'apparato oculare. Milano: Fogliazza Editore, 1987;203.
[21] D. Minckler and A.W. Allen. Adenocarcinoma of the retinal pigment epithelium. Arch. Ophthalmol. 1978;96:2252–2254.

Alessandro Galantuomo, M.D.
I University of Naples
Institute of Ophthalmology,
Naples, Italy

B. Pastena
University of Naples Federico II
Institute of Ophthalmology,
Naples, Italy

F. Baldi
Institute of Pathology
University of Naples Federico II,
Naples, Italy

8. Measurement of tumour height and base diameter in choroidal melanoma. Comparison between ultrasonography and histology

G. MARCHINI, R. TOSI and C. GHIMENTON[1]

(Verona, Italy)

Abstract

Maximum tumour height and base diameter were determined in a series of 41 choroidal melanomas both *in vivo* using two-speed ultrasonography (1550 and 1660 m/sec) and on histological preparations using an optical microscope with an ocular micrometer. Tumour base was measured as the chord of a circle. The mean interval between ultrasonography and surgical enucleation was 15±9 days (range: 1 to 48 days).

The mean histological tumour height was 6.9±3.1 mm as compared to a ultrasonographically measured mean height of 8.3±3.1 mm at the speed of 1550 m/sec ($p<0.05$) and of 8.9±3.4 mm at the speed of 1660 m/sec ($p<0.01$). The mean tumour base measurement obtained histologically was 10.8±3.7 mm, versus ultrasound mean values of 12.6±3.5 mm at the speed of 1550 m/sec ($p<0.05$) and 13.5±3.8 mm at 1660 m/sec ($p<0.01$).

There was a good correlation between ultrasonographic and histological measurements at both speeds of sound both as regards tumour height ($r=0.88$; $p<0.001$) and as regards tumour base diameter values ($r=0.85$; $p<0.001$). The use of two different speeds of sound may account for maximum differences in tumour measurements not exceeding 0.9 mm, whereas the difference between histological and ultrasonographic measurements ranged from 1.7 to 2.9 mm.

Key words: Choroidal melanoma, ultrasonographic measurement, histological measurement, prognostic factors

Introduction

The size of choroidal melanomas at the time of diagnosis is an important prognostic factor because larger melanomas are associated with lower survival rates compared to smaller ones [1–3]. One of the parameters used to assess tumour size is its maximum height, although it is also routine practice to consider its maximum lateral extension (maximum diameter of the tumour

G Cennamo and N. Rosa (eds.), Ultrasonography in Ophthalmology 15, pp. 93–100.

base). In terms of tumour height measured on histological preparations, choroidal melanomas are classified as small when they measure <3 mm in height, medium-sized when they measure from 3 to 5 mm, and large when they measure >5 mm. Similarly, they are also divided into three different size categories on the basis of histological tumour base diameter measurements, namely <10 mm, 10 to 15 mm, and >15 mm.

Ultrasonography, particularly A-scan echobiometry, is the most precise method currently available for ocular measurements *in vivo* [4,5] and can be used to determine the sizes of intraocular tumours. When a choroidal melanoma is treated with conservative radiotherapy, the ultrasonographic technique is the reference method for establishing the size of the tumour. However, there is a considerable difference between ultrasonographic and histological tumour measurements: the former tend on average to be some 2 mm larger than the histological estimates [6,7]. The latter biometric studies were conducted using speeds of sound of 1500 [6] and 1550 m/sec [7], whereas, according to J.D. Coleman, the speed of sound in uveal melanoma is 1660 [personal communication].

The aim of our study was to assess the correspondence between ultrasonographic and histological measurements by comparing tumour height and base diameters in a series of 41 choroidal melanomas using ultrasound speeds of 1550 and 1660 m/sec.

Materials and methods

The case series analyzed comprised 52 patients suffering from uveal melanoma treated by enucleation after an ultrasound examination. Eleven patients were excluded because of incomplete data or because the melanomas could not be correctly measured (see procedures outlined below). Our study was therefore conducted in 41 patients (20 males, 21 females) with a mean age of 64 ± 12 years (range: 32 to 88 years) suffering from choroidal melanoma, for a total of 41 tumours, 23 of which were dome-shaped (biconvex) and 18 mushroom-shaped. The mean interval between ultrasonography and surgical enucleation of the affected eye was 15 ± 9 days (range: 1 to 48 days).

For each tumour we measured the maximum tumour height and base diameter (chord) in mm both *in vivo* by ultrasonography and on histological preparations under the optical microscope.

The ultrasound measurements were obtained with an Ophtascan S instrument (Biophysic Médical, Clermont-Ferrand) using the contact technique which allows perpendicular exploration from the side opposite to the tumour and two probes, one a focused 10 MHz B-scan probe, and the other an unfocused 8 MHz A-scan probe with a tissue sensitivity level of T = 68 dB. The ultrasound examination was conducted first in B-scan to identify the area of maximum elevation and maximum lateral extension of the tumour, and then in A-scan. Tumour height was determined with standardized A-scan after obtaining an echogram identifying the maximum elevation and complying with the perpendicularity criteria. These characteristics were guaranteed by the simultaneous presence of two echoes of maximum amplitude, steeply rising from baseline, situated at the maximum distance apart and representing the tumour and scleral surfaces. When the tumour surface spike was not distinct from the retinal spike, the latter was taken as the starting echo of the echogram. Tumour height in mm was calculated using ultrasound speeds of 1550 and 1660 m/sec.

The diameter of the tumour base, taken as the chord of a circle, was measured on a B-scan echogram that simultaneously represented the maximum lateral extension and the maximum height of the melanoma. After identifying the two outermost points of the tumour base, where the surface of the tumour comes into contact with the inner surface of the ocular wall, we used a caliper to calculate the length of the chord in relation to the maximum height in mm calculated earlier using the two speeds of sound.

For histological measurements, the enucleated eyes were prepared in the routine manner, i.e., fixation in 5% formaldehyde, dissection of the eyeball, dehydration in alcohol, embedding in paraffin, microsectioning and staining with haematoxylin and eosin. After identifying the microsection with the maximum lateral extension and maximum height, the measurements were obtained under the optical microscope using an ocular micrometer. Maximum height was measured in mm from the surface of the retina (or tumour, if distinct) to the inner surface of the sclera, whereas the tumour base diameter, taken as the length of the chord in mm, was measured after identifying the outermost points of contact between the tumour surface and the wall of the eyeball.

Student's t-test was used for the comparison of the mean ultrasonographic and histological values. The degree of correlation of the measurements obtained with the two procedures was analyzed by linear regression, calculating the coefficient of correlation r.

Results

Using a speed of sound of 1550 m/sec the ultrasonographic tumour height values were greater than the corresponding histological values in 35 melanomas, equal in 1 case and lower in 5 cases. Ultrasonographic tumour base diameter values were also higher than the corresponding histological values in 35/41 melanomas and lower in the other 6 cases.

With a speed of sound of 1660 m/sec, the ultrasonographic tumour height values were greater in 38/41 melanomas and lower in 3/41, while the ultrasonographic tumour base measurements were greater than the corresponding histological values in 39/41 cases and lower in the other 2.

Table 1 shows the ultrasonographic and histological maximum tumour height values in the 41 melanoma cases: the histological mean value was 6.9 ± 3.2 mm as against mean ultrasonographic values of 8.3 ± 3.1 mm at the speed of 1550 m/sec and 8.9 ± 3.4 mm at 1660 m/sec.

Table 1. Histological and ultrasonographic tumour height values in 41 choroidal melanomas

	Histology	Echography 1550 m/s	Echography 1660 m/s
Mean	6.9	8.3*	8.9**
SD±	3.2	3.1	3.4
CI±	1.0	1.0	1.0
Min	1.1	2.0	2.1
Max	13.4	15.5	16.6
	*$p<0.05$	**$p<0.01$	

Table 2. Histological and ultrasonographic tumour base diameters in 41 choroidal melanomas

	Histology	Echography 1550 m/s	Echography 1660 m/s
Mean	10.8	12.6*	13.5**
SD±	3.7	3.5	3.8
CI±	1.2	1.0	1.2
Min	4.2	5.5	5.9
Max	18.6	22.0	23.6
	*$p<0.05$	**$p<0.01$	

The maximum tumour base diameter values are shown in Table 2. The histological mean diameter was 10.8±3.7 mm versus 12.6±3.5 mm, as measured at the ultrasonographic speed of 1550 m/sec, and 13.5±3.8 mm, as measured at 1660 m/sec. In the case of both mean tumour height and base diameter, the differences between ultrasonographic and histological values were statistically significant ($p<0.05$ at the 1550 m/sec speed and $p<0.01$ at the 1660 m/sec speed).

The degree of correlation between US and histological tumour height measurements is illustrated in Figures 1 (1550 m/sec) and 2 (1660 m/sec), and the tumour base diameter correlations are shown in Figures 3 (1550 m/sec) and 4 (1660 m/sec). Increasing histological tumour height values are associated with a linear increase in the corresponding ultrasonographic values with a coefficient of correlation $r=0.88$ for both speeds of sound. The same is true of the tumour base diameter values, where the coefficient of correlation r is 0.85 for both speeds.

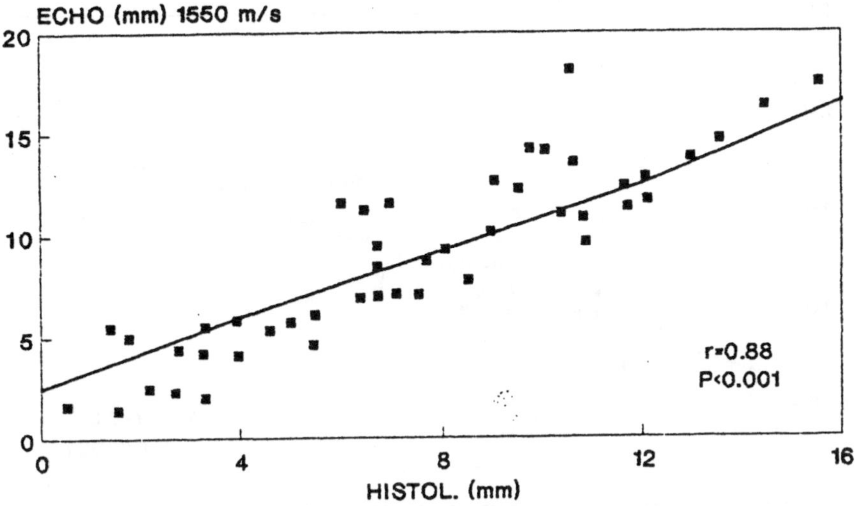

Fig. 1. Correlation between ultrasonographic and histological tumour height measurements in 41 choroidal melanomas. A speed of sound of 1550 m/sec was used for the ultrasonographic measurements

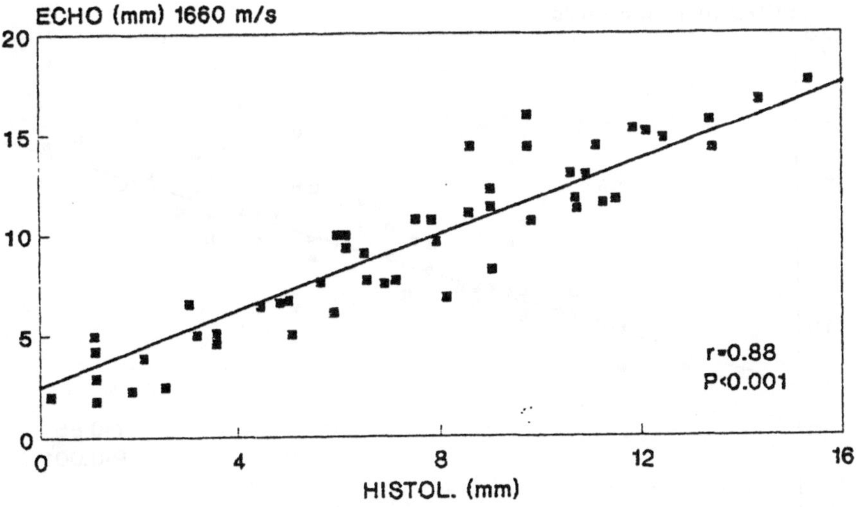

Fig. 2. Correlation between ultrasonographic and histological tumour height measurements in 41 choroidal melanomas. A speed of sound of 1660 m/sec was used for the ultrasonographic measurements

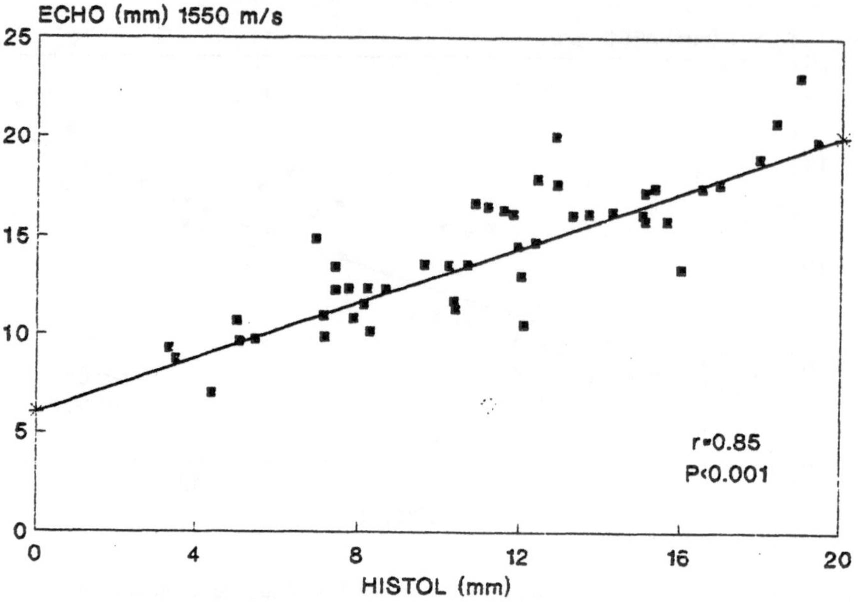

Fig. 3. Correlation between ultrasonographic and histological tumour base diameter measurements in 41 choroidal melanomas. A speed of sound of 1550 m/sec was used for the ultrasonographic measurements

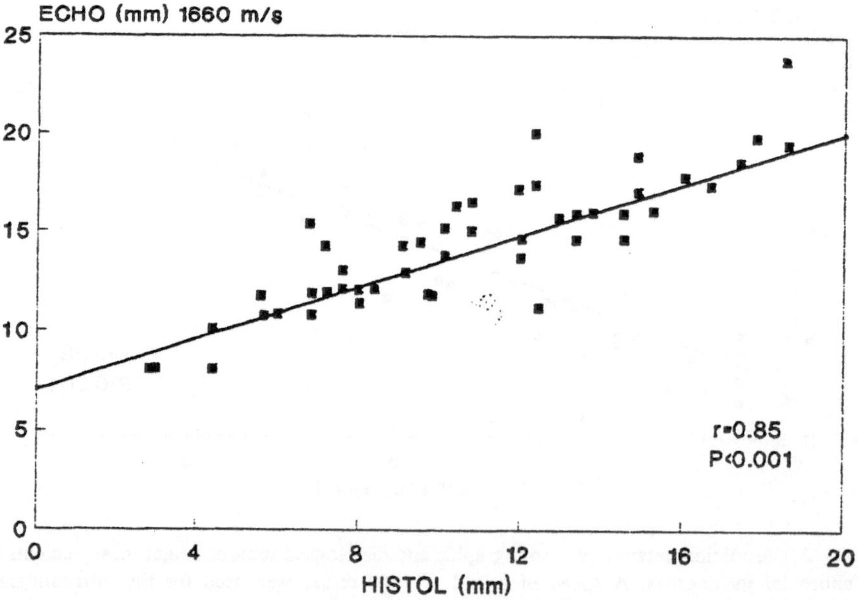

Fig. 4. Correlation between ultrasonographic and histological tumour base diameter measurements in 41 choroidal melanomas. A speed of sound of 1660 m/sec was used for the ultrasonographic measurements

Discussion

Eighty-five percent (35/41) and 95 percent (39/41), respectively, of the choroidal melanomas measured at the two speeds of sound showed higher values when measured ultrasonographically than when measured histologically. According to Nicholson *et al.* [6], this difference is probably due to a varying degree of shrinkage of the tumour induced by fixation and histological preparation. Nicholson and coworkers measured a number of tumours (6/53) on the evening before enucleation, immediately after the operation and immediately after fixation with formaldehyde, but before histological treatment. They found no appreciable difference between measurements before and immediately after enucleation. The contraction evidently takes place both during fixation with formaldehyde solution and during histological preparation of the fixed specimen. Our previous data confirm this hypothesis and appear to rule out an effect of the intra-tumoral blood volume on tissue contraction [7].

Using the equation corresponding to the straight line curve expressing the correlation between ultrasonographic and histological measurements we have calculated the equivalent ultrasonographic dimensions for the various histological magnitudes (Table 3).

Table 3. Equivalent histological and ultrasonographic measurements used to classify tumour size

	Histology	Echography 1550 m/s	Echography 1660 m/s
Tumor height			
	3	5.0	5.3
	5	6.7	7.2
Tumor base diameter			
	10	12.0	12.9
	15	16.9	17.7

In terms of maximum histological height, melanomas are regarded as small when the height is <3 mm, medium-sized when the height ranges from 3 to 5 mm, and large when the height is >5 mm, whereas the corresponding categories based on histological tumour base diame4ers are <10 mm, 10–15 mm, and <15 mm. The corresponding ultrasonographic limits calculated on the basis of our data exceed the histological values by 1.7 to 2 mm at the speed of 1550 m/sec and by 2.2 to 2.9 mm at 1660 m/sec. It should be noted that when a speed of 1500 m/sec was used, the difference between ultrasonographic and histological measurements was 2.2 mm [6].

The use of these three different speeds of sound may account for maximum differences in both tumour height and tumour base diameter measurements not exceeding 0.9 mm. Much more significant, by contrast, is the difference between histological and ultrasonographic measurements, whatever the speed adopted. This difference is important in survival studies on choroidal melanoma, when comparing conservative radiotherapies, in which the tumour size is measured ultrasonographically, with surgical enucleation, where the size of the melanoma is measured at histology. The result might, in fact, be a survival bias in favour of radiotherapy since with the two different measurement methods there might be a tendency to attribute larger tumours to the subjects treated by enucleation. It would therefore be advisable to use ultrasonographic measurements for all comparisons between different forms of therapy.

References

[1] I.W. Mc Lean, W.D. Foster and L.E. Zimmermann. Prognostic factors in small malignant melanomas of choroid and ciliary body. Arch. Ophthalmol. 1977;95:48.
[2] H.F. Shammas and F.C. Blodi. Prognostic factors in choroidal and ciliary body melanomas. Arch. Ophthalmol. 1977;95:63.
[3] I.W. Mc Lean, W.D. Foster and L.E. Zimmermann. Uveal melanoma: location, size, cell type and enucleation as risk factors in metastasis. Hum. Pathol. 1982;13:123.
[4] K.C. Ossoinig. Standardized echography. Basic principles, clinical applications and results. Int. Ophthalmol. Clin. 1979;19:127.
[5] H.F. Shammas. Atlas of ophthalmic ultrasonography and biometry. St. Louis: The C.V. Mosby Co., 1984.
[6] D.H. Nicholson, S. Frazier-Byrne, M.T. Chiu, J. Schiffman, J.R. Hughes and E.K. Novinski. Echographic and histologic tumor height measurements in uveal melanoma. Am. J. Ophthalmol. 1985;100:454.
[7] G. Marchini, C. Ghimenton, R. Tosi, G. Castagna and A. Tomezzoli. Confronto fra misurazioni ecografiche e istologiche nel melanoma coroidale. Clin. Ocul. Pat. Ocul. 1992;13:227–230.

G. Marchini and R. Tosi
Istituto di Clinica Oculistica
Università di Verona
Verona, Italy

C. Ghimenton
Servizio di Anatomia Patologica
Ospedale Civile Maggiore di Verona
Verona, Italy

9. Chorioretinal solid tumor: clinical and echographic study

A. ZANONI and L. FERRARI

(Rovereto, Italy)

Abstract

We report the case of a 66-year-old woman with a chorioretinal solid tumour that appeared to be a metastasis. It is hypothesized that the small lesion, which disappeared within 15 days, was a focal benign non inflammatory choroidal lesion.

Key words: Chorioretinal tumour, chorioretinal metastasis, echography, focal fugax choroiditis, pseudolymphoma

Introduction

Primary and secondary chorioretinal tumours can be studied with echography: only echography reveals the entity of thickness and the tissutal acoustic behavior and characteristics of the spikes in the lesion [1]. The differential diagnosis of solid chorioretinal tumours includes [2,3]: melanoma, hemangioma, metastatic tumours, hemorrhagic detachment, and macular disciform degeneration. In clinical practice we occasionally find anomalous cases, in which the clinical, instrumental and semeiological signs and symptoms are misleading and diagnosis is difficult. We present one such clinical case.

Case report

A 66-year-old woman was referred to our Division in February 1993 with blurred vision in the left eye that started 10 days earlier. The history documented in the out-patients' records was negative for eye diseases (the last examination in May 1992 showed a normal fundus in both eyes). The physical ocular examination was unremarkable in the right eye with corrected visual acuity = 20/20 and normal fundus. In the left eye corrected visual acuity = 20/20, and there was a prominent dome-shaped solid lesion light pink in colour, oval and 3 disc diameters large in the fundus along the inferior temporal vascular arcade and subretinal. The optic disc, vessel, macula and peripheral retina were

G Cennamo and N. Rosa (eds.), Ultrasonography in Ophthalmology 15, pp. 101–106.

normal. The patient was informed of the suspicion that this 'tumour' with atypical features was a solid chorioretinal malignant disease. The patient underwent laboratory analyses which were within normal limits (VES = 11; hepatic enzymes; rheumatic tests and immunoglobulin).

The visual field (Humphrey strategy full threshold programme) showed a relative scotoma in the superior nasal quadrant. The fluorescein angiography showed a rapid choroidal filling time with irregular spots and a peripheral leakage halo due to serous pigmented epithelial detachment. The "spotted" leakage increased at the late time and the retinal vessels were regular (Fig. 1).

B-scan echography showed a dome-shaped, limited, spongy, solid chorioretinal mass without shadowing or acoustic vacuoles (Fig. 2). A-scan standardized echography showed high reflectivity (80% with irregular spikes); no spontaneous vascular vertical motion of single tumour spikes; maximum thickness was 2.4 mm (Fig. 3).

We made a diagnosis of suspected choroidal metastasis. We excluded angiomas, where the reflectivity is high and regular, and the fluorescent stain rapid, but without irregular staining of the giant choroidal vessels [4].

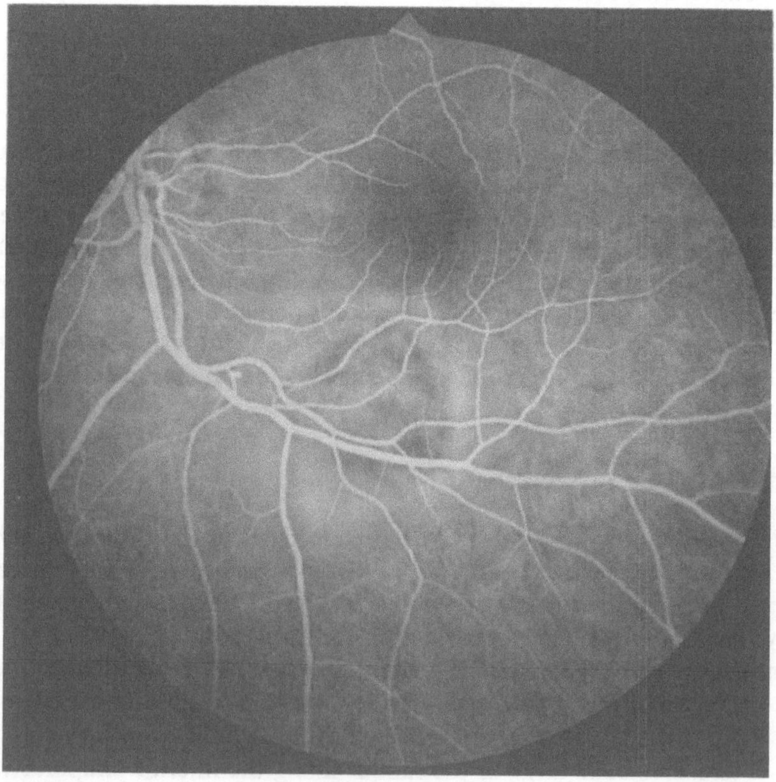

Fig. 1.

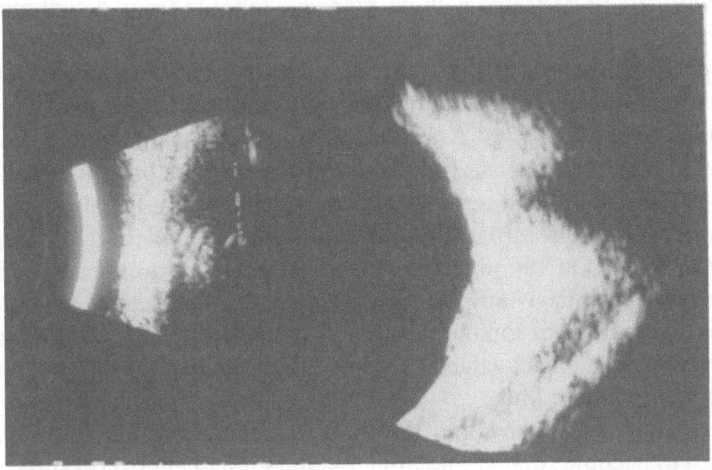

Fig. 2.

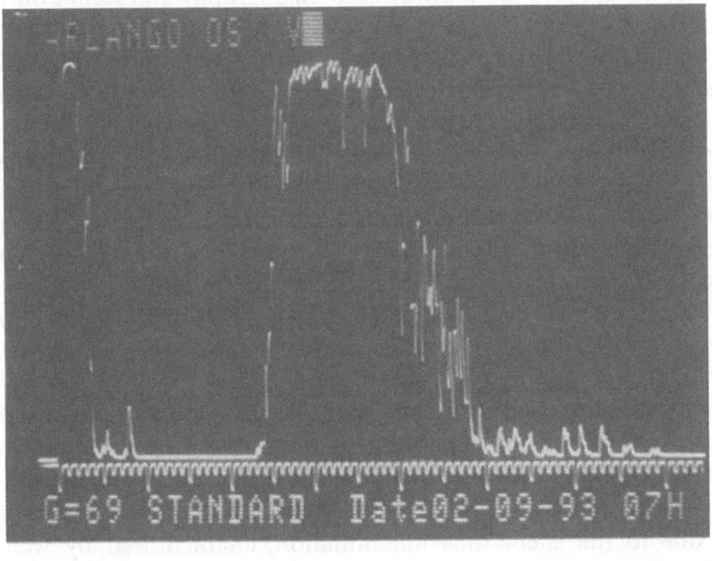

Fig. 3.

The extramacular site ruled out macular sierohemorrhagic degenerations. The melanomas of small size, also with high reflectivity, have a characteristic ophthalmoscopic pigmentation and fluorescein angiography peculiar to internal vessels [2].

The irregularity of the inner acoustic structure and the high reflectivity together with the presence of a slight adjacent retinal serous detachment, was suggestive of a chorioretinal carcinomatous metastasis [5]. The ophthalmoscopic aspect, characterized by a pinkish colour, slight blurring on the edges and the fluorescein angiographic images, supported this diagnosis.

These images could suggest a metastasis even if in the first stages, leakage is not always visible in metastasis [6,7]. Because the case-history was negative, the following examinations and tests were prescribed: thyroid, hepatic, and splenic renal echography, thyroid-parathyroid scintigraphy, total body scintigraphy, mammography, occult blood in the faeces, search for tumoural cells in the urinary sediment, alpha-1-fetoprotein and CEA. All these exams were negative. The nuclear magnetic resonance excluded a tumor. After some gadolinium administration, on the back edge of the left eye, at the level of the choroid, there was a thin hyperintense line.

After several days the size and the thickness of the examined chorioretinal area started to become smaller and after 7–8 days it had almost disappeared and was almost indistinguishable from the surrounding pinkish retinal area.

Echography did not show any solid mass or any other change in the chorioretinal outline. We did a fluorescein angiography and found only a faint spotted marbling which later gave a slight deep staining without diffusion.

A re-examination of the previous fluorescein angiography showed that the mass was not large and it was not associated with a large retinal edema as is usually seen in metastases. Metastases propagate through the blood to the choriocapillaris vessels, consequently they are positioned on the surface of the choroidal layer and more elevated, while in the present case the staining was deep. Moreover, the fluorescein normally propagates so as to involve large areas of the mass only in later stages. Here, the fluorescent staining was limited to spots, except for the peripheral diffusion in the detached epithelium of the retina. Examining the ecographical images again, we noticed that the mass split into layers, very similar to that found in cases of hemorrhagic disciform macular detachment.

We compared this splitting into layers with archival images of focal choroiditis. In 18 of our patients, none of whom had toxoplasmic choroiditis, or vitreal disorders, the echography revealed a flat or smooth dome-shaped lesion, which in most cases showed an inner split into layers, which was probably due to the edematous inflammation, characterised by well-shaped borders [8]. The split into layers can be due to bubbles of serum which, as reported elsewhere [9], often occurs in the flattened area. The case we were examining was easily echographically comparable with these images both in A-scan and in B-scan.

During the following week, without any therapy, the left eye became normal and the fundus seemed regular. Later, the only abnormal finding was a slight fluorescence due to local deep leakage without any spreading or window-shaped modification in the pigmented epithelium or in the Bruch membrane.

Discussion

A review of the literature shows that a metastasis or a hemangioma cannot disappear by necrosis without leaving any ophthalmoscopically-detectable sign. The echographic images obtained in our patient correspond to our archival data of focal choroiditis.

Does non-inflammatory choroiditis exist? Secchi *et al.* [10] reported evidence for this pathology. In our opinion, the most feasible explanation of our case is a transitory accumulation of lymphocytes or at least of lymphocytic type cells or anyway of the white ones. Pigmented and blastic hematopoietic cells predominate in the choroid. In fact, in premature infants and the completed foetus, there is extra medulla ossium hematopoiesis in the choroid [11]. These cells accumulate in the deep choroidal area among the large choroidal vessels, in front of the lamina fusca and under the choriocapillaris, probably due to local stimuli. This group of cells, are not necessarily the result of inflammation.

In fact, besides the negative response in our patient at the inflammatory and immunologic tests (immunoglobulin, anti herpes simplex, anti cytomegalovirus, anti varicella zoster), there were no changes in the pigmented retinal epithelium or Bruch's membrana, even months later, that could suggest a choriocapillaritis or a inflammatory choroiditis. According to Hogan and Zimmerman [4]:

> "Occasional lymphomatoid tumors are seen in the eyes of patients who show no evidence of blood dyscrasia, palpable glands, or other systemic disease. Moreover the patients have remained without symptoms for years following enucleation. In many of these cases the multiplicity of cell types, and the presence of plasma cells in particular, suggest that the tumors are reactive inflammatory processes rather than neoplasms".

In the systemic or leukemic forms [12,13], excluded in this patient, the spreading is multifocal and has a typical different appearance. Mazzeo [9] reported a case of transitory choroidal accumulation which proved to be exudative choroiditis. This lesion had a high reflectivity and was linked to a minor exudative retinal detachment and disappeared in one month. These features suggest lymphoid reactive hyperplasia or pseudolymphoma [14] which rarely affects the choroid with an associated retinal detachment; there is no vitreous involvement. The instrumental tests show the homogeneity in the lesion, the clear borders and no variation in the anatomic structure of the sclera. Moreover, the lesion is susceptible to corticosteroid therapy.

These considerations lead to the assumption that our patient was affected by a disease that developed locally from proliferating cells (already existing cells) in the vessel tissue of the deep choroid of large vessels due to local stimuli.

Colleagues of the H.O. S. Raffaele (Milan), have observed similar cases, which they cured with large quantities of steroid therapy. We did not administer any therapy or in our patient, and the condition gradually improved and became normal within 15–20 days. Thus far, there has been no relapse and the patient is in good health.

This case, considered a transitory benign non-inflammatory focal choroiditis, illustrates the difficulty in making a differential echographic diagnosis of small (<4–5 mm) solid choroidal lesions, and the need for frequent check-ups to detect minute changes in the thickness and structure of the lesion. Unlike lymphoid reactive hyperplasia, non-inflammatory focal choroiditis regresses spontaneously without using corticosteroid therapy.

Obviously, a histological specimen could provide data that may clarify the pathogenesis of this disorder.

References

[1] A. Reibaldi, T. Avitabile and S. Guerriero. L'ecografia nella patologia della coroide. Clin. Ocul. e Patol. Ocul. 1984;6:18–22.

[2] C. Marchini, G. Totolo, L. Franceschetti and S. Gios. Diagnosi differenziale ecografica delle piccole neoformazioni coroideali. Clin. Ocul. e Patol. Ocul. 1990;5:327–331.

[3] G. Panzardi, M. Donati, G. Dal Pozzo and A. Mannelli. La TAC e la RMN nella diagnostica delle lesioni simulanti il melanoma della coroide. In Maccari Ed. Proc. Società Tosco Umbro Emiliana Marchigiana di Oftalmologia, Spoleto, Italy. 1991;463–470.

[4] M. Hogan and L. Zimmerman. Ophthalmic pathology, an atlas and textbook. London: W.B. Saunders Company, 1962;457.

[5] P. Perri, M. Chiarelli, P. Monari, L. Ravalli and V. Mazzeo. Aspetti ecografici delle matastasi coroideali. Nostra esperienza. Clin. Ocul. e Patol. Ocul. 1991;4:247–250.

[6] U. Menchini, A. Pece, S. Fantaguzzi and R. Brancato. Aspetti fluorangiografici delle metastasi oculari. Clin. Ocul. e Patol. Ocul. 1986;6:385–387.

[7] A. Minella, E. Merendino and B. Bagolini. Le metastasi coroidali. Ann. Oftalmol. e Clin. Ocul. 1992;118(2):133–145.

[8] S.L. Yoser, D.J. Forster and N.A. Rao. Systemic viral infections and their retinal and choroidal manifestations. Survey of Ophthalmol. 1993;5:313–352.

[9] V. Mazzeo. Ecografia dell'apparato oculare. Fogliazza Ed. 1987;219.

[10] M.S. Tognon, B. Turrini and A.G. Secchi. Le coriocapillariti: si tratta sempre di manifestazioni infiammatorie? 48th Società Oftalmologica Lombarda Congress. Boll. Ocul. 1994; Suppl. 5:185.

[11] A.B. Reese and F.C. Blodi. Hematopoiesis in and around the eye. Am. J. Ophthalmol. 1954;38:214–221.

[12] A. Colotto, C. Tamburelli, A. Giudiceandrea and G. Fadda. Interessamento oculare in corso di hairy cell leukemia. Clin. Ocul. 1990;3:203–206.

[13] L. Pierro, E. Zaganelli, L. Guarisco, E. Conforto, M. Muraglia and G. Cambri. Coinvolgimento oculare in corso di leucemia linfoblasica acuta: studio ecografico. Clin. Ocul. e Patol. Ocul. 1993;2:110–112.

[14] G. Alfieri, S. Brogelli, M. Allegranti, S. Di Lollo and S. Dini. Linfoma e pseudolinfoma. Tumori intraoculari. Florence: Medical Books, 1990.

Adriano Zanoni
U.S.L. C 10 Vallagarina
Ospedale di Rovereto
Divisione Oculistica
Rovereto, Italy

10. Uveal melanoma conservative surgery: echography pre- and post-surgery

L. SABETTI, M.G. SERRA, N. FURCESE and E. BALESTRAZZI
(L'Aquila, Italy)

Abstract

The aim of this study is to provide indications for conservative surgery of uveal melanoma. A-B scan ultrasonography provides accurate information not only on the site and the size of the melanoma and the involvement of neighbouring tissues, but also on the post-surgical evolution. Between January 1988 and December 1993 we used echography to study 31 patients who subsequently underwent localized surgical resection.

The echographic diagnosis was confirmed in most cases during surgery, and the tumour tissular rating was confirmed in 93.5% of cases. Frequent echographic examinations during post-surgical follow-up showed hemovitreous, cataract, choroidal detachment, retinal detachment, bulbar phthisis and recurrences. Ultrasonography is the most effective diagnostic means both in the pre-surgical phase, as an aid in selecting therapy, and in the post-surgical phase where it alerts the physician to possible complications.

Key words: Echography, choroidal melanoma, local resection

Introduction

Up to about 20 years ago the only surgical therapy of all uveal melanomas was enucleation. The prognosis *quoad vitam* for this destructive treatment was about 50% after 10–15 years [1]. In the last 20 years, conservative surgical (local resection) and parasurgical (radiation or laser therapy) treatments were proposed to save the bulbar integrity, if not the visual function [2]. Conservative surgery of melanomas localized in the iris, ciliary body and anterior choroid, and less than 14 mm in size, have a good prognosis *quoad vitam* with a good anatomical and functional outcome.

Echography combined with clinical data (ophthalmoscopy and biomicroscopy) provides the information necessary for a correct pre-surgical indication for this treatment. The site, the size, the tissutal type and the macroscopic involvement of the neighbouring structures can be investigated in detail with ultrasounds (Fig. 1). Echography is also useful in post-surgical controls to

G Cennamo and N. Rosa (eds.), Ultrasonography in Ophthalmology 15, pp. 107–112.

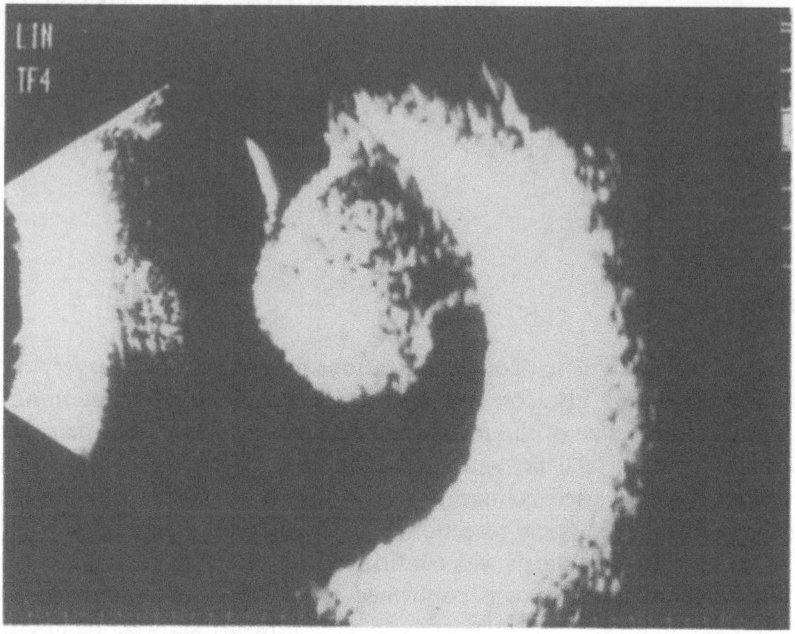

Fig. 1. B-scan of choroidal melanoma with rupture of Bruch's membrane

predict the anatomical outcome of the treatment and possible complications of surgery (hemovitreous, vitreo-retinal tractions, retinal detachment, choroidal detachment, bulbar phthisis and recurrence).

The aim of this study was to investigate the correspondence between the echographic and histological measurement of the size of the neoformations and the complications resulting from conservative surgery of the tumours.

Material and methods

Between January 1988 and December 1993, 31 patients affected by uveal melanoma (14 males, 17 females), with an age range between 24 and 65 years (means 54.8 ± 6.2), were examined by ocular echography, before undergoing localized resection of the neoformation. The intraocular neoplasia was in the anterior choroid in 20 cases (64.5%), in the ciliary body in 9 cases (29%) and in the iris in the last 2 cases (6.5%).

Echography was performed with an A-scan standardized Ophthascan S 'mini A', a B-scan Sonomed B-3000 and a B-Scan Humphrey 635. The B-scan examination was carried out using the immersion technique, which is the best procedure for studies of neoplasias located in the iris or the ciliary body. For all examinations, we used a sequence of parallel scans of 1 mm each in both the frontal and sagittal planes. With this technique, one may visualize the complete structure and shape of the neoformation and calculate the 'linear' measurement of each part of the neoplasia as well as its total volume.

During the post-surgical controls, every 6 months for a period of 5 years, the patients underwent a complete ocular examination, an ocular and orbital echography, an hepatic echography, serum liver enzyme test and a clinical examination. In addition, once a year for 5 years the patients underwent chest X-ray, brain and eye magnetic resonance imaging (MRI), bone scintigraphy and abdominal echography. In cases of suspected recurrence we carried out immunoscintigraphy and fluorangiography.

Results

The comparison between the pre-surgical echographic data and the histological results showed that the tissutal diagnosis of melanoma was correct in 93.5% of the cases (29/31). In the other two cases (6.4%) the echographic tissutal diagnosis of a possible melanoma, which presented an anomalous behaviour, i.e., the presence of a capsule, a large internal non-reflective space and a small part with low reflectivity, was invalidated by the histological diagnosis, in both cases, of neurilemmoma of the ciliary body.

The sizes of the neoformations, measured after histological fixing and section, were lower than the echographic values; the difference between the two techniques was within 1.5 mm in 90.4% of the eyes (28/31); in two eyes (6.4%) it was within 2.5 mm, and in the last eye (3.2%) within 3 mm.

Post-surgical complications were easily identified if hemovitreous, vitreo-retinal tractions, retinal detachment, bulbar phthisis were present singly. In cases (4 eyes of 31, 12.8%) in which various complications were present together, it was more difficult to evaluate the echographic pattern. Two cases which presented severe oedema of the choroid with choroidal detachment and a hemovitreous, were completely resolved, with a good anatomical and functional outcome. The most difficult diagnosis concerns the choroid. In fact, in the first post-surgical controls it is frequent to find a choroidal reaction characterized by oedema with the formation of swellings or a real detachment.

In all cases, at the site of the surgical excision we found a highly reflective zone (100%), which caused acoustic shadowing of the posteriorly-situated structures, which resembled an intraocular foreign body but without ringing (Fig. 2). During the following echographic controls, this portion decreased in reflectivity, however it remained overloaded for a long period (6–12 months), after which the reflectivity decreased to the level of the neighbouring structures (ocular wall).

The persistence of choroidal detachment, with involvement of the ciliary body, together with retinal detachment, can determine the formation of a bulbar phthisis which is indicative of a poor anatomical and functional outcome, and it

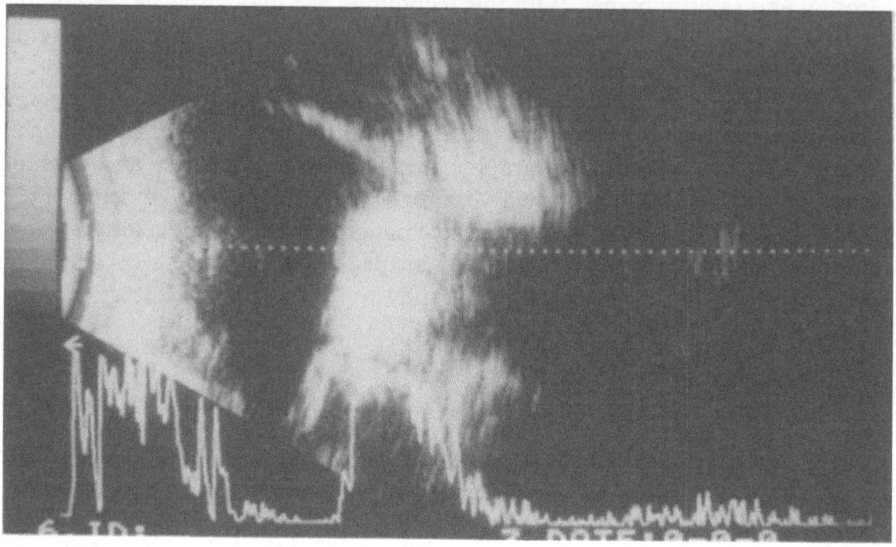

Fig. 2. High reflectivity of the site of excision

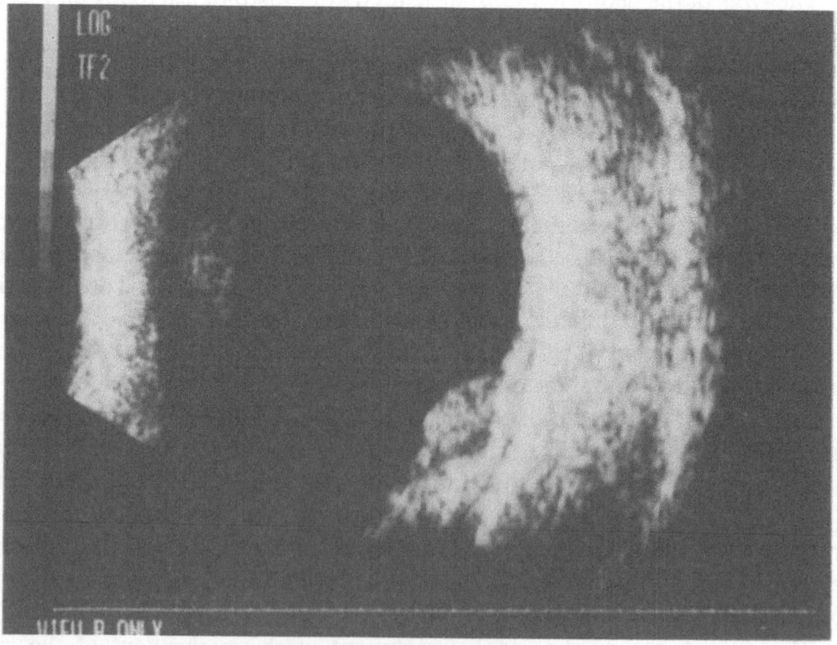

Fig. 3. B-scan image of a recurrence of choroidal melanoma

becomes very difficult to detect signs of recurrence. In our study there were only three cases of this complication. In two cases, ocular echography showed a recurrence of the choroidal melanoma (Fig. 3).

The site of the neoformations was distant from the primary lesion and the scar. The echographic characteristics of the neoplasia were the same as those of a primary melanoma of the choroid.

Conclusions

The difference between histological and echographic values [3–6] can be due, in our experience, to two factors: 1) the histological fixing and manipulation, which can cause alterations of the neoformation section; and 2) the echographic examination.

At this point, we must consider such aspects as the problem of the corrected velocity of the ultrasounds in the tumour, and also the possible formation of a shadow on the posteriorly-located structures and the distortion of the curvatures, e.g., a concave surface appears more concave than it really is [7]. Moreover, the A and B-scan display only plane images of the eye, on two orthogonal axes (x, y) which does not permit a tridimensional evaluation. The representation of the tumour on three orthogonal axes (x, y, z) (which gives a tridimensional image) could permit also precise sectioning for histological purposes.

'Linear' measurements do not evaluate either the physiological curvature of the eye or the pathological morphology of the neoplasia. In fact, this measurement represents only the chord of an arc, and in order to obtain the real values of the curvature one must apply the mathematical formula:

$$MD = \frac{MB \times MB}{MC}; \qquad \sin\alpha = \frac{MB}{OB}; \qquad AB = \frac{2\alpha}{360} \times 2\pi r$$

These measurements, even if numerous and repeated, cannot exactly correspond to the measurement that results from histological section.

A more precise evaluation of the neoformation size can be achieved only by considering the total volume of the neoplasia. The echographic aspect becomes even less accurate when various complications coexist so that all internal structures are no longer distinct. In such cases, echography alone does not allow for precise evaluation.

Echography has allowed us to follow-up the different complications consequent to the sclero-uveo-tumorectomy and to evaluate the outcome of therapy. Lastly, echography was fundamental in the timely detection of complications.

References

[1] J.M. Seddon, K.M. Egan and E.S. Gragouda. Choroidal melanoma: prognosis. In S.J. Ryan (ed.), Retina. St. Louis: The C.V. Mosby Company, 1989;1.

[2] J.A. Shields, C.L. Shields and L.A. Donoso. Management of posterior uveal melanoma. Surv. Ophthalmol. 1991;36(3):161–195.

[3] D.H. Char, S. Kroll, R.D. Stone, R. Harrie and Kerman B. Ultrasonographic measurement of uveal melanoma thickness: Interobserver variability. Br. J. Ophthalmol. 1990;74(3):183–185.

[4] J.J. Augsburger, J.W. Gamel, R.S. Bailey, L.A. Donoso, J.R. Gonder and J.A. Shields. Accuracy of clinical estimates of tumor dimensions. A clinical-pathologic correlation study of posterior uveal melanomas. Retina 1985;5(1):26–29.

[5] D.J. Coleman. Echographic and histologic tumor height measurements in uveal melanoma. Am. J. Ophthalmol. 1986;101(1): 124–125.

[6] D.H. Nicholson, S. Frazier-Byrne, M.T. Chiu, J. Schiffman, J.R. Hughes and E.K. Novinski. Echographic and histologic tumor height measurements in uveal melanoma. Am. J. Ophthalmol. 1985;100(3):454–457.

[7] R. Guthoff. Ultrasound in Ophthalmologic Diagnosis. Stuttgart, New York: Georg Thieme Verlag, 1991.

L. Sabetti
Eye Clinic
Department of Surgery
University of L'Aquila
67100 L'Aquila, Italy

11. Classic and anomalous standardized A-scan patterns of choroidal nevi elevated up to 3.5 mm

D. DORO, E. MANTOVANI, M. VACCARO and E. MILIZIA
(Padua, Italy)

Abstract

High internal reflectivity and a predominantly irregular structure on standardized A-scan were the classic acoustic features encountered at first examination in nine patients with unilateral ophthalmoscopic evidence of choroidal nevus elevated from 1.6 to 3.5 mm. In all patients but one with a 3.5 mm elevated nevus, periodic fluorescein angiography and automated perimetry findings were consistent with the diagnosis of choroidal nevi located at the posterior pole or in the mid periphery. Slight or no growth was observed echographically during the follow-up (seven months to seven years) except in one eye with a solid pigmented lesion which progressively grew 1 mm and showed low reflectivity without spontaneous vertical movements or evidence of melanoma at ancillary examinations. In two other eyes the internal reflectivity of the choroidal nevus decreased gradually from high to medium. The differentiation between choroidal nevus and melanoma with standardized echography and the existence of a possible histologically intermediate lesion ('nevoma') are discussed.

Key words: Standardized echography, choroidal nevus, choroidal melanoma, choroidal 'nevoma', automated perimetry

Introduction

As Folberg [1] recently pointed out, there is experimental evidence that a spectrum of conjunctival atypical melanocytic proliferations separates benign nevi from malignant melanomas. Because uveal melanocytic proliferations are not accessible to incisional biopsy without possible disruption of vision, only two points in the spectrum of uveal tumor progression are clinically defined: nevus and melanoma. It is well known that there are specific standardized acoustic criteria [2,3] that allow the differentiation of elevated choroidal nevus from melanoma, but to our knowledge there are no reports concerning the echographic follow-up of even small series of choroidal nevi.The aims of our study were: 1) to analyze the standardized echograms of some unilateral non peripheral choroidal lesions consistent with a diagnosis of nevus; and 2) to detect possible acoustic changes during the follow-up.

G Cennamo and N. Rosa (eds.), Ultrasonography in Ophthalmology 15, pp. 113–123.

Patients and methods

Nine (seven female and two male) patients aged between 50 and 80 years (average 67 years) were referred to the Echographic Service of the University Eye Clinic of Padua with an ophthalmoscopic diagnosis of suspected unilateral choroidal elevated nevus located at the posterior pole or in the mid periphery. All patients were studied with fluorescein or indocyanine green angiography and automated perimetry. Standardized echography (Coopervision Ultrascan Digital B® and Biophysic Ophthascan 'S' mini-A) was regularly performed (every three-four months in the first year and then annually) during the follow-up that ranged from seven months to seven years.

Results

As shown in Table 1, on standardized A-scan the reflectivity of all choroidal nevi was high at the first examination, but, during follow-up, in two cases (nos. 4 and 6) the internal reflectivity decreased to a mid (Fig. 1) and in one case (no. 8) to a medium-low level. The structure was mostly regular in four nevi that were 2 mm high. A definite regular structure was detected in two eyes with choroidal nevi around 2 mm high, whereas an irregular structure was found in three eyes with choroidal nevi from 2.3 to 3.5 mm high. A focal subsurface decrease in reflectivity occurred in patients nos. 7 and 8. Contact B-scan texture, displayed at the same system sensitivity (15 dB), was full in all eyes except in patient no. 5 where a full spongy texture was noted (Figs. 2 and 3); a doubtful choroidal excavation was found in patient no. 1 (Fig. 4). The height of choroidal nevi ranged from 1.6 to 3.5 mm; two nevi (patients nos. 3 and 4) showed minimal

Table 1. Elevated choroidal nevus: echographic features

No.	Patient age	A-scan reflectivity	Structure	B-scan texture	Elevation (mm)	Follow-up (months)
1.	63	High	Regular?	Full**	1.6	12
2.	50	High	Regular?	Full	1.6	11
3.	66	High	Irregular?	Full	1.5 to 2.0*	84
4.	55	High to mid*	Regular?	Full	1.6 to 2.0*	9
5.	70	High	Regular	Full-spongy	2.0	11
6.	77	High to mid*	Regular	Full	1.9	8
7.	67	High	Irregular	Full	2.3	7
8.	77	High to mid-low*	Irregular	Full	2.1 to 3.1*	35
9.	80	High	Irregular	Full	3.5	9

*Change during the follow up; **Doubtful choroidal excavation

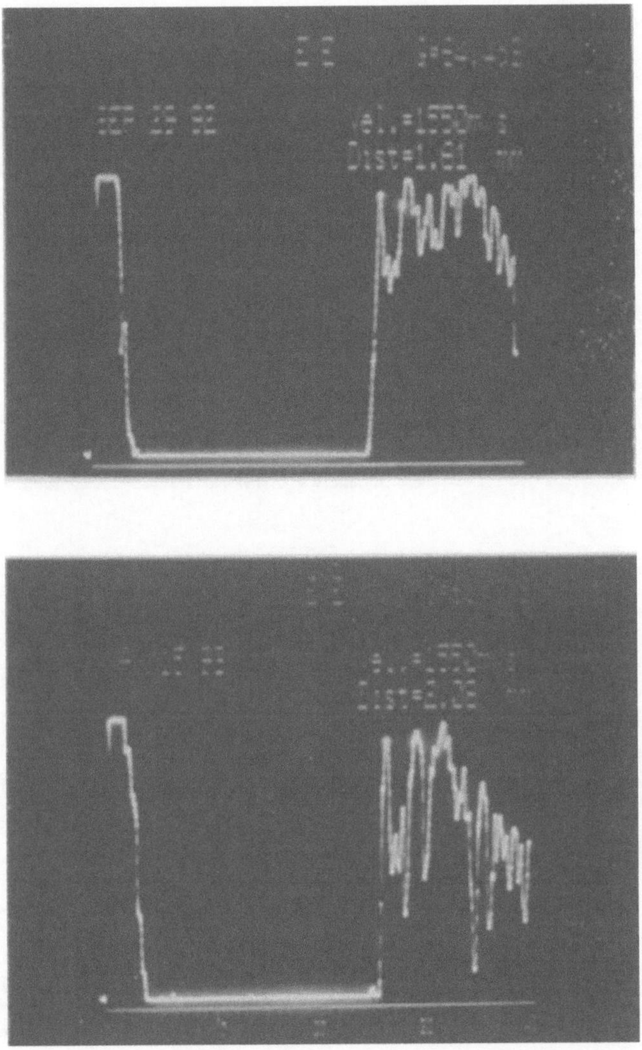

Fig. 1. Standardized A-scan echograms of a choroidal nevus showing high reflectivity (top) and decreased reflectivity (bottom) after an eight month follow-up. Note the minimal growth and regular structure

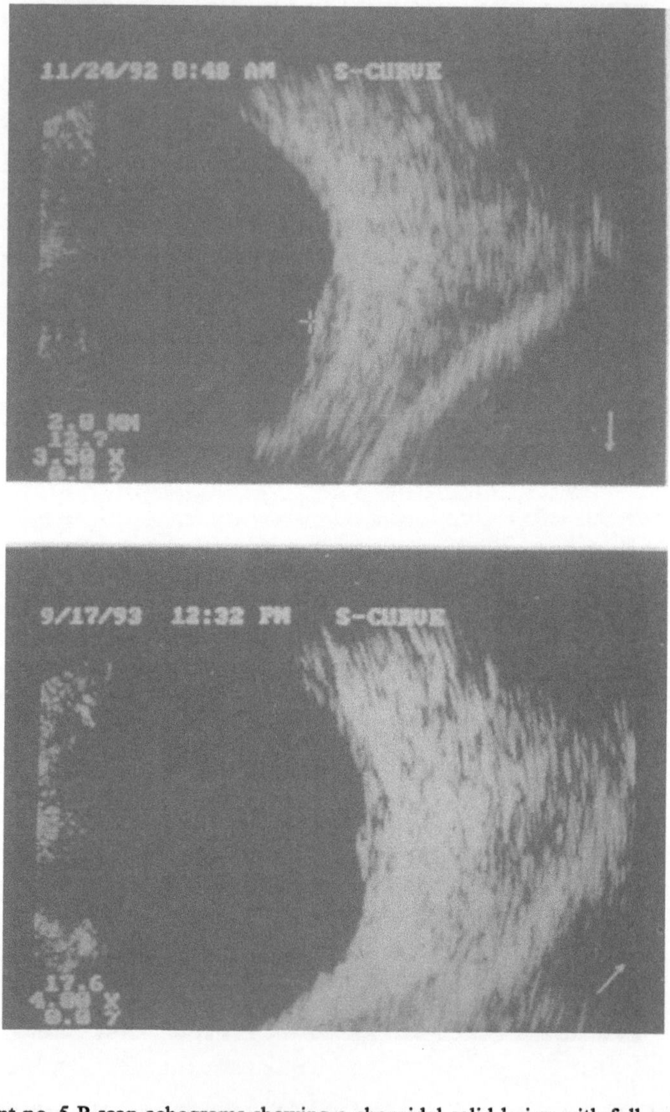

Fig. 2. Patient no. 5 B-scan echograms showing a choroidal solid lesion with full-spongy texture (top) unchanged after 10 month follow-up (bottom)

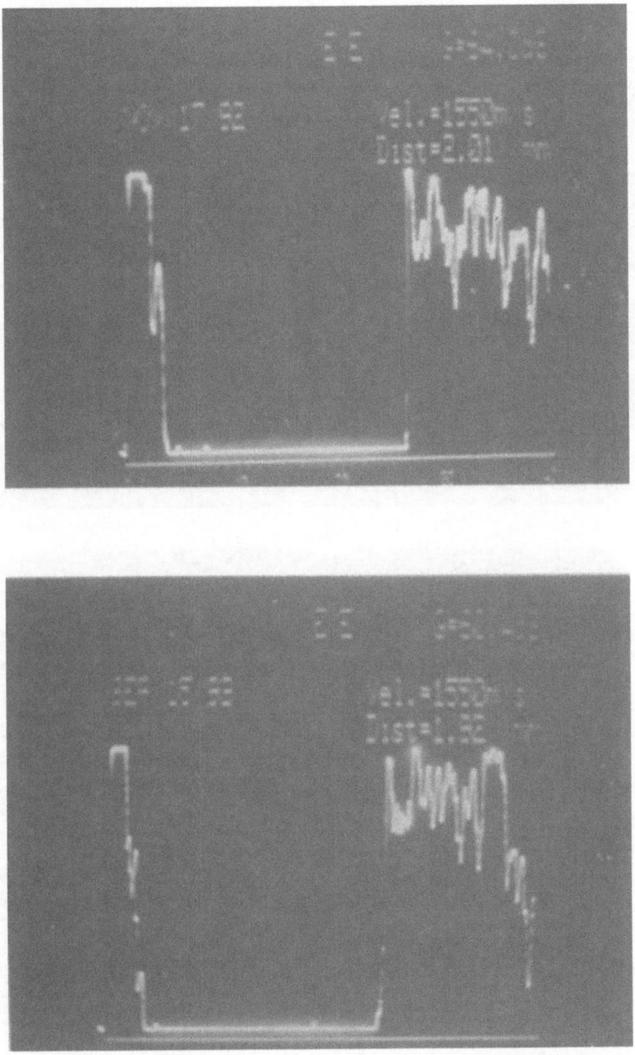

Fig. 3. Patient no. 5. High reflectivity and regular structure of a 2 mm high choroidal nevus on standardized A-scan examination in November 1992 (top) and in September 1993 (bottom)

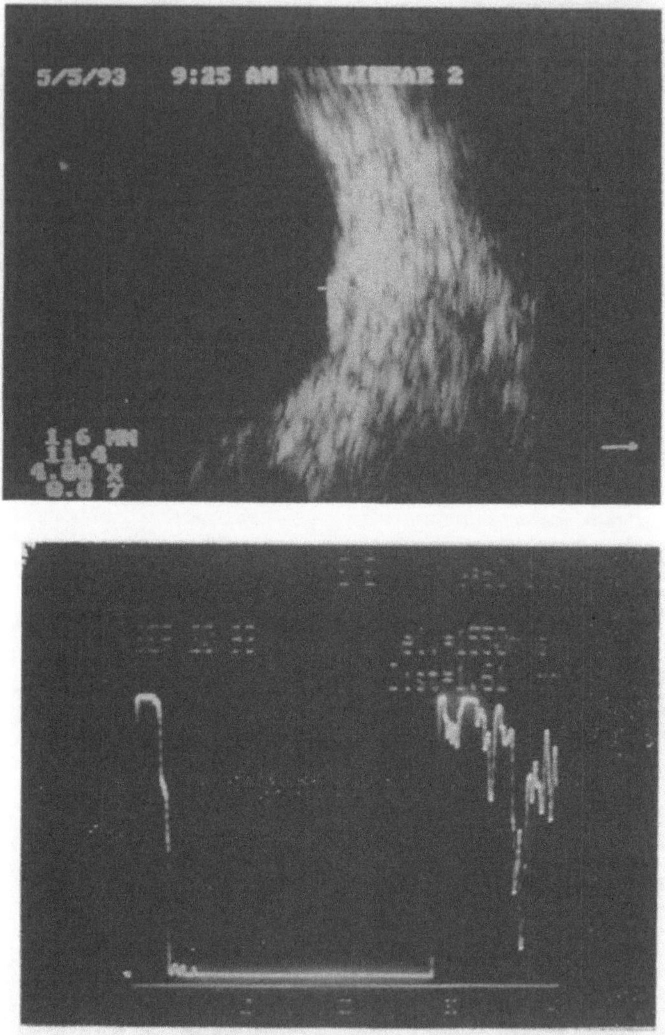

Fig. 4. Patient no. 1. Contact B-scan showing echogenic dome-shaped choroidal lesion with doubtful choroidal excavation (top). High internal reflectivity displayed on standardized A-scan (bottom)

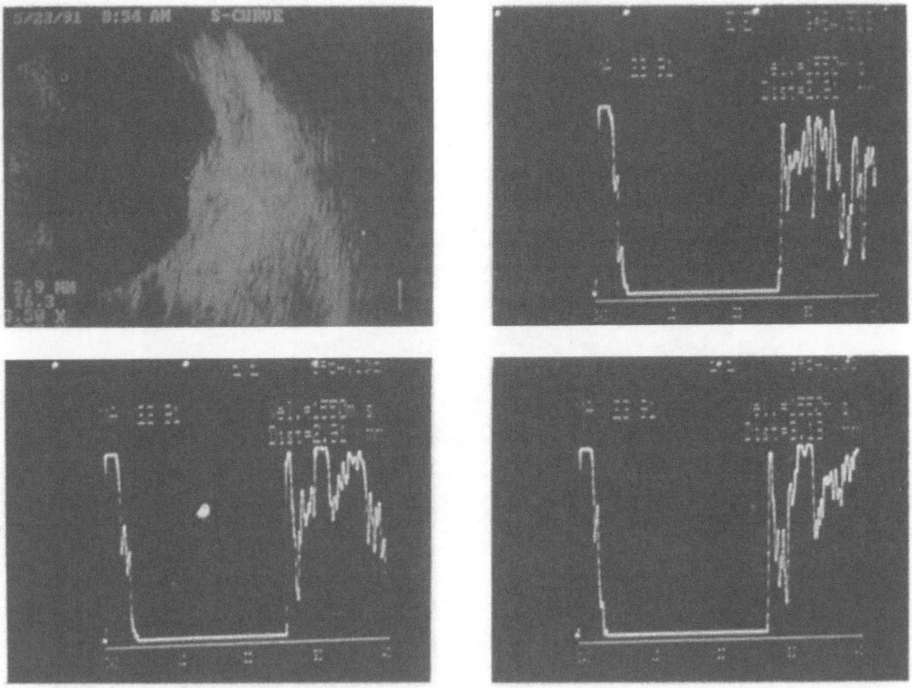

Fig. 5. Patient no. 8 May 1991. Contact B-scan showing echogenic dome-shaped choroidal lesion (top left). With different standardized A-scan projections high (top right), medium-high with a focal subsurface decrease (bottom left) and low (bottom right) reflectivity can be displayed

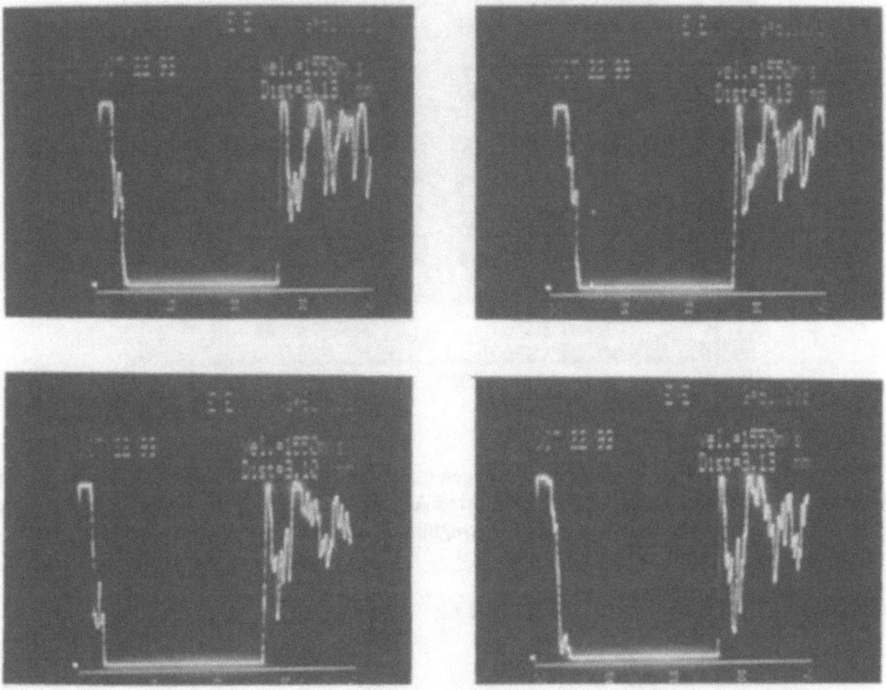

Fig. 6. Patient no. 8. October 1993. Similarly to findings shown in Fig. 5, the reflectivity of the choroidal lesion was variable on standardized A-scan: medium-high (top right), medium (top and bottom left) or low to medium (bottom right). Maximal elevation remained 3.1 mm

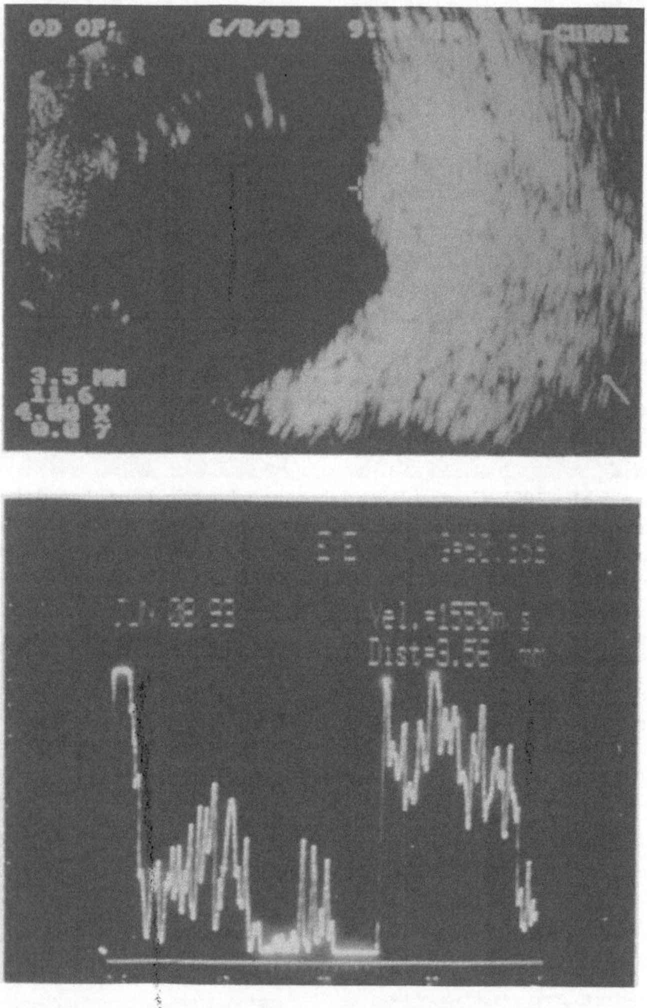

Fig. 7. Patient no. 9. Contact B-scan: echogenic elevated choroidal lesion with full texture and evidence of asteroid hyalosis (top). Standardized A-scan: vitreous mostly medium reflective echoes and high reflective choroidal lesion with irregular structure; maximal elevation from retina to inner sclera is 3.5 mm

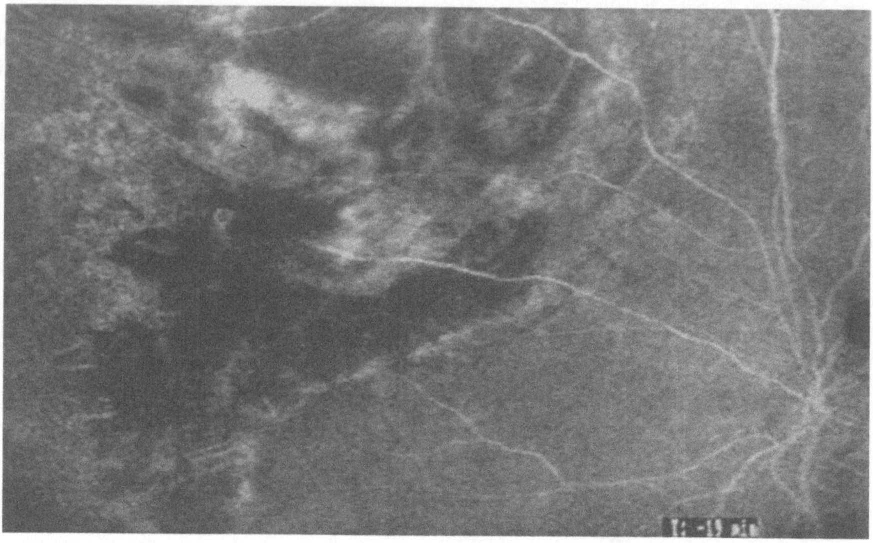

Fig. 8. Patient no 9. Fluorescein angiography of the left eye with scanning laser ophthalmoscopy. In the arterovenous phase the choroidal lesion located supero-nasally to the optic disc shows patchy hyperfluorescence (from choroidal vessels?) that increased in later angiograms

growth and one (patient no. 8) a growth of 1 mm during the follow-up. Spontaneous vertical movements of the internal echo-spikes were not detected in any choroidal nevus.

In patient no. 8 unilateral choroidal nevus with typical drusen was diagnosed ophthalmoscopically and confirmed by fluorescein angiography in 1983. In 1990 standardized echography revealed a 2.1 mm high reflective lesion and in May 1991 a lesion that reached a maximum height of 3.1 mm; no further growth was detected in the follow-up. The internal reflectivity ranged from high to low according to different A-scan projections both in May 1991 (Fig. 5) and in October 1993 (Fig. 6); the internal structure was predominantly irregular.

In patient no. 9 the reflectivity of the choroidal lesion during the nine month follow-up remained high with an irregular structure and the maximal height remained 3.5 mm (Fig. 7).

Fluorescein angiography in all patients and indocyanine green angiography (in patients nos. 1, 3 and 8) were consistent with the diagnosis of choroidal nevus; in patient no. 9 the results did not rule out a choroidal melanoma (Fig. 8). Automated perimetry (Humphrey 30-2 and 30/60-2 programs combined) failed to show localized areas of decreased sensitivity in eight out of nine eyes; only in patient no. 9 was there a marked retinal decrease in the area corresponding to the choroidal tumor.

Discussion

Our echographic results are essentially in accordance with the echographic findings in choroidal elevated nevi reported by Ossoinig and Lohmeyer [3]. High internal reflectivity was the classic standardized A-scan pattern encountered at the first examination in all our patients with unilateral choroidal nevus, and in two cases there was a focal subsurface decrease in reflectivity. However, in two nevi with minimal or questionable (less or equal to 0.5 mm) growth during the follow-up, the internal reflectivity decreased from high to medium. In nevi elevated more than 2 mm the internal structure was irregular, but in less elevated nevi the structure was or seemed rather regular, a feature reported by other authors [4]. In our series we confirm the lack of spontaneous vertical movements [3,5]. At the same system sensitivity setting, full texture on contact B-scan was constant in virtually all our cases; however, in our experience, eyes with this acoustic sign must be carefully evaluated with standardized A-scan examination.

Patients nos. 8 and 9 are of special interest. In patient no. 8 the remarkable decrease in reflectivity of a choroidal tumor discovered ten year before and followed-up echographically for three years with evidence of a growth of 1 mm may indicate a change to a low-grade malignancy; however, fluorescein and indocyanine green angiography and automated perimetry ruled out a diagnosis of choroidal melanoma. In patient no. 9 the doubtful angiographic and perimetric [6] results do not coincide with standardized echography examination typical for an elevated choroidal nevus. To our knowledge, this is probably the most elevated nevus reported in the echographic literature.

Unfortunately, echographic and clinical features intermediate between choroidal nevus and melanoma cannot be confirmed by incisional biopsy, but these two intriguing cases (patients 8 and 9) may represent an example of slow progression of choroidal nevus towards melanoma, a clinical, but not histologically verified condition that Char [7] has termed 'nevoma'.

References

[1] R. Folberg. Tumor progression in ocular melanomas. J. Invest. Dermatol. 1993;200:3265–3315.

[2] K.C. Ossoinig. Standardized echography: basic principles, clinical applications and results. Intern. Ophthalmol. Clinics 1979;19:107–210.

[3] K.C. Ossoinig and M. Lohmeyer. Choroidal nevi: diagnosis with standardized echography. In R. Sampaolesi (ed.), Ultrasonography in Ophthalmology 12. Dordrecht: Kluwer Academic Publishers, 1990;173–180.

[4] G. Marchini and R. Tosi. Echographic differential diagnosis of small choroidal solid lesions. In P. Till (ed.), Ophthalmic Echography 13. Dordrecht: Kluwer Academic Publishers, 1993;313–317.

[5] S.F. Byrne and R.L. Green. Ultrasound of the Eye and Orbit. St. Louis: Mosby Year Book, 1992;179–180.

[6] D.H. Abramson. Computerized visual field of choroidal melanomas. Glaucoma 1988;10:29–48.
[7] D.H. Char. Inter. Symp. on Intraocular Tumors in The Adult; Therapeutic Choices. Padua, Italy, April 23–24, 1993.

Daniele Doro
Institute of Ophthalmology
University of Padua
Padua, Italy

12. Choroidal hemangioma in the posterior pole: management and follow-up in a clinical case

L. FERRARI and A. ZANONI
(Rovereto (TN), Italy)

Abstract

A particular clinical case of choroidal hemangioma in a 50-year-old male is reported. He was referred to us for an ocular trauma (contusion) in the left eye with a suspected chorio-retinal tumour in the posterior pole erroneously diagnosed as a subretinal hematoma. Fluorangiographic imaging and echographic scanning revealed a cavernous choroidal hemangioma. This diagnosis was confirmed in the follow-up of the patient. We emphasize the primary role of echography in the diagnosis of choroidal tumours, especially in the case of cavernous choroidal hemangioma.

Key words: Ocular contusion, chorio-retinal solid detachment, fluorescence angiography, A- and B-scan echography, choroidal cavernous hemangioma

Introduction

Cavernous hemangioma is the third most frequent primitive choroidal tumour, after the benign and malignant melanotic tumours, naevi and melanomas [1]. It is a relatively rare tumour and in about 65% of cases it is isolated, while in the remaining 35% it is associated to the Sturge Weber syndrome [2–5].

The isolated hemangioma is generally of the cavernous type and it is not a malignant tumour; it has a typical histologic internal structure that reflects the particular echographic acoustic signals. Capillary hemangioma, on the contrary, is more frequently associated with the Sturge Weber syndrome and it is prevalently intrachoroidal and flat without a solid elevated retinal detachment.

Cavernous choroidal hemangioma is usually monolateral, although it can be bilateral. The posterior pole is the typical site, and it is more frequently temporal; it is never pre-equatorial or on the equator [3,4]; there are no significant sex differences, nor it is peculiar to a particular age group. Ophthalmoscopy and biomicroscopy show a typical dome-shaped solid retinal detachment, variable in diameter, size, thickness and colour (from white-gray to pink-orange); an associated serous retinal detachment and a cystoid maculopathy can also be found in these patients [2]. These objective clinical signs are

G Cennamo and N. Rosa (eds.), Ultrasonography in Ophthalmology 15, pp. 125–131.

not sufficient for diagnosis; indeed, diagnosis can only be made with fluorescein angiography (FA) and even better with green indocyanine angiography (ICGA) [1,2,6], associated with A- and B-scan echography [2–4,7,8], and acoustic tissue typing (ATT) [9]. Computerized tomography, magnetic nuclear resonance [1] and ERG with EOG [2] are further aids for the diagnosis.

The angiographic data for hemangioma can be similar to those observed in cases of choroidal melanoma. The typical angiography [1,2,6,10] has the following characteristics: 1) Early injection of the vascular network of the tumour in the choroidal time (claw- or network-like). 2) An increase of fluorescence during the retinal arterial and the initial venous times (the fluorescence is initially unhomogeneous due to the asynchronous filling of the lacunar spaces of the tumour, and it becomes more regular as staining increases; the outline of the fluorescence can be well-defined or blurred, depending on the conditions of the pigmentary epithelium near the tumour). 3) A progressive late increase in the staining, with a sponge-like final picture, due to the leakage of fluoresceine into the retina [2,6].

Pigmentary spots can appear over the hemangioma and cause a typical blocking of fluorescence in the late time of angiography. Therefore, a relative hypofluorescent area may appear near the hyperfluorescent area of the tumor [2], as observed in our patient. There may also be a typical 'strip-like' picture caused by a pigmentary epitheliopathy that results in a fluorescent strip from the lower edge of the hemangioma to the lower peripheral retina (sub-retinal fluid which, because of the force of gravity, 'slides' towards the lower retina) [6].

Green indocyanine angiography allows us to define the choroidal hemangioma. In fact, green indocyanine does not pass through the choroidal vessel wall and this gives typical filling images of the vascular choroidal tumors. Then, using infra-red light, it is possible to bypass the pigmentary epithelium barrier; therefore ICG-angiography is the best echographic technique for the diagnosis of choroidal hemangioma [1,2,6]. This technique yields a typical picture that allows us to differentiate choroidal hemangioma from the other choroidal tumors: a massive, fast, regular and progressive injection that is of maximal intensity during the venous time of the angiogram [6]. The choroidal melanoma never stains in this fashion [1].

Therefore, fluorescein angiography is not suitable for the diagnosis of isolated choroidal hemangioma. If, as in our case, ICG angiography is not available, ocular echography must be used. The echographic findings of the choroidal cavernous hemangioma are well known [3,4,8]; they are reported in the Table 1 and lead to the correct diagnosis in 100% of cases.

We report a particular case of cavernous choroidal hemangioma, and highlight the fundamental role played by echography in the diagnosis of this clinical case.

Table 1. Echographic findings of cavernous choroidal hemangioma [7].

A-scan	B-scan
Solid tumor	Dome-shaped
High internal reflectivity (85-100%)	High echogenic structure
Regular structure	No shadowing
	No choroidal excavation

Clinical case and methods

In July 1989 a 50-year-old male was referred to us for deterioration of sight in the left eye, which was apparently related to an ocular trauma, but in the same eye there was a previous sight deficiency of uncertain origin to which he attached no importance. We had no other information about the sight and ocular conditions of this patient.

In the right eye the visual acuity was 20/20 with 0.5 sph.; adnexes, anterior chamber, lens and fundus were within normal limits; intraocular pressure (IOP) was normal. In the left eye the visual acuity was about 20/2000 not improved with correction; there was a lid hematoma with a mild ocular inflammatory reaction (pericheratic hyperemia, with bleeding Tyndall in the anterior chamber), but IOP was normal. The ophthalmoscopic examination showed a slight hemovitreous with some hemorrhages and post-traumatic ischemic edema areas especially in the peripheral nasal retina. The most important finding in the left eye fundus was a large, apparently solid, retinal detachment, located in the posterior pole temporal to the macular side, between the vascular arches. It was about 4–5 optic disk diameters, pink-orange coloured, with subretinal red dark areas (hemorrhages) and large pigmentary spots over the retinal layers in the centre (Fig. 1). In the periphery of the solid detachment, resembling a serous retinal detachment, there was a diffuse retinal edema.

Based on the data from ophthalmoscopy and the biomicroscopy, we suspected the trauma was unrelated to solid detachment because it did not resemble the typical post traumatic intraocular lesions described for the chorioretina [11]. The patient was admitted to our Ophthalmological Operative Unit for further examinations. Several days later there was an improvement in the hemovitreous and in the ischemic edema. Vision did not improve because the solid retinal detachment involved the macular area. The patient underwent FA and ocular echography.

Fluorescein angiography showed a solid choroidal mass, below and temporal to the macula, with its own vascularization, characterized by early injection in the choroidal phase; fluorescence staining progressively increased, and stabilized in the late phases. During the angiogram hypofluorescence areas were

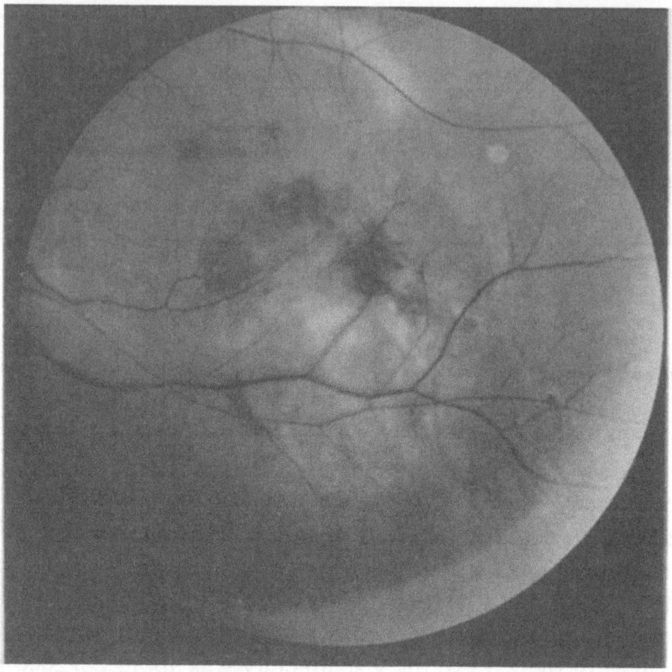

Fig. 1.

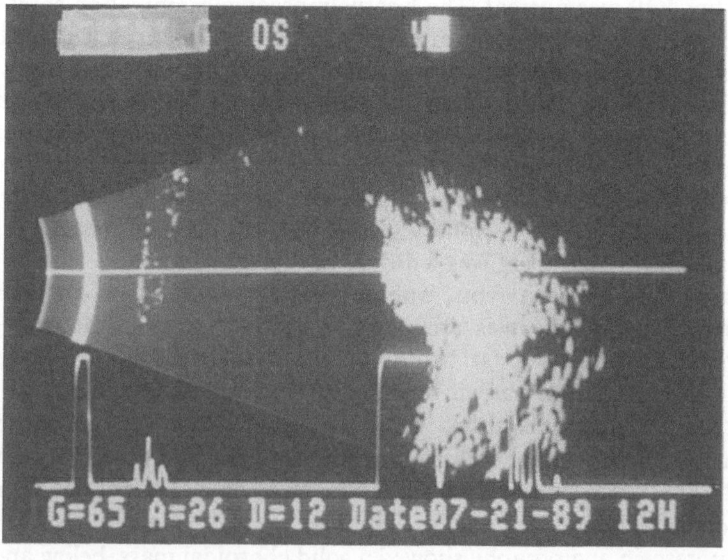

Fig. 2.

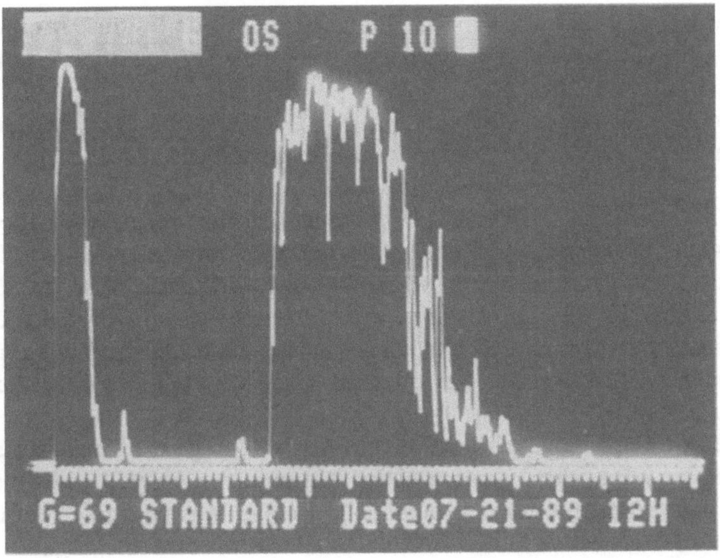

Fig. 3.

observed at the site of the lesion; some appeared only in the initial stage, while others lasted throughout the angiography: the latter were more evident in the late phases of the angiography and caused fluorescence blocking (deep hemorrhages and superficial hyperpigmented irregular spots). There was also an area of relative hypofluorescence all around the lesion, which was more evident in the central time of the angiogram.

Echography was performed with the contact technique with a 10 MHz focused B-scan probe and an 8 MHz non-focused A-scan probe also at T = 69 dB, using the Ophthascan S echograph.

The B-scan did not reveal echographic signs of hemovitreous. In the posterior pole, there was a dome-shaped regular retinal detachment, near the macula; it had a solid aspect, high reflectivity and a homogeneous internal structure, combined with a serous retinal detachment, peripheral to this lesion. Internal acoustic vacuoles, choroidal excavation with shadowing, or choroidal thickening were not found (Fig. 2). Standardized A-scan confirmed the solid lesion; it showed high internal reflectivity (90–100%), clear spikes and regular structure. The maximal measured thickness was = 3.4 mm (Fig. 3).

Discussion

The ophthalmoscopy and the biomicroscopy confirmed a mild post traumatic intraocular lesion, which cleared up in a few days.

The solid retinal detachment could not be attributed to the ocular trauma, because it was unlike the typical choroidal traumatic lesions. Moreover, the ophthalmoscopic appearance (colour and pigmentary superficial spots) could suggest choroidal melanoma.

Other possible causes of the retinal solid detachment could be age related macular degeneration (ARMD), choroidal metastasis, or choroidal hemangioma.

The FA excluded the ARMD, because of the absence of the typical detachment of the pigmentary epithelium and the subretinal neovascularization; in addition, the patient was too young to have this kind of disorder and there was no lesion in the controlateral eye. Fluorescence angiography does not discriminate between choroidal metastasis and choroidal hemangioma. However, because the lesion was not of recent date, we excluded the possibility of metastasis.

Therefore, the echography was critical for the diagnosis, and the use of the 'echographic algorithm', proposed by Marchini *et al.* [12] as a diagnostic echographic procedure for choroidal solid lesions, was particularly useful. The high internal reflectivity, the lack of stratification and the regular internal structure, obtained by A-scan together with the B-scan data indicated choroidal hemangioma rather than a metastasis, and excluded a purely traumatic cause and the other possible causes of solid retinal detachment [13].

To confirm diagnosis, we followed-up this lesion using ophthalmoscopy, biomicroscopy, angiography and echography.

We scheduled FA and echography after 15 days, echography alone after 1 month, and FA and echography after 3 and 6 months. All these examinations confirmed the angiographic and echographic results reported above. In particular, the thickness of the solid detachment did not change, and the other echographic parameters, evaluated with A- and B-scan were unchanged.

After this follow-up, the patient was examined with FA and echography at six-month intervals.

Because the choroidal hemangioma was very widespread and involved the macular area, laser treatment was not advisable, also because the lesion was not of recent date, and thus not amenable to laser therapy. Indeed, smaller hemangiomas can be treated by laser photocoagulation [5,14], while radiotherapy is more appropriate for larger lesions [14].

Conclusion

Two considerations may be drawn from this study and from other reports [4,12]. The first is that echography plays a fundamental role in the diagnosis of retinochoroidal solid detachments. In fact, only echography can quantify the entity of the solid detachment seen with ophthalmoscopy and biomicroscopy and yields data about tissular differentiation using A- and B-scan techniques, and ATT. The second is that the echographic features of choroidal hemangioma are so well-defined as to allow a correct diagnosis in about 100% of the cases [3–5].

References

[1] G. Panzardi, M.C. Donati, G. Dal Pozzo and A. Mannelli. La TAC e la RMN nella diagnostica delle lesioni simulanti il melanoma della coroide. S.T.U.E.M.O. Congress, Spoleto, Italy. 1991;463–470.

[2] G. Brancato, G. Lodato and G. Cascio. La diagnostica dell'emangioma coroidale, Boll. Oculistica 1987;66(2):163–173.

[3] V. Mazzeo. Ecografia dell'apparato oculare. Testo-Atlante. Milano: Fogliazza Ed. 1987.

[4] V. Mazzeo, P. Perri, L. Ravalli, R. Monari and M. Chiarelli. Angioma cavernoso della coroide: nostra esperienza. Clin. Ocul. e Patol. Ocul. 1992;4:220–222.

[5] J.A. Shields. Tumors of the uveal tract. T.D. Duane (ed.), Clinical Ophthalmol., vol. 4. Philadelphia: Harper and Row Publ., 1987;1–13.

[6] A. Giovannini. Diagnostica angiografica dell'angioma della coroide. LXI S.O.I. Congress, Rome, Italy. Bologna: Nuova Casa Editrice "L. Cappelli", 1981;203–209.

[7] L. Pierro, E. Zaganelli, L. Guarisco, E. Conforto, M. Muraglia and G. Cambri. Emangioma capillare e cavernoso del disco ottico: studio ecografico e istopatologico. Clin. Ocul. e Patol. Ocul. 1993;2:107–109.

[8] H.J. Shammas. Atlas of ophthalmic ultrasonography and biometry. St. Louis: The C.V. Mosby Co., 1984;78–79.

[9] L. Falco, N. Passarelli, S. Esente, S. Fanfani and S. Utari. Possibilità diagnostiche dell'Angiodinografia (Color Doppler Imaging) e dell'Acoustic Tissue Typing (Ecografia B Scan assistita da computer) nella diagnostica dei tumori intrabulbari. Convegno S.T.U.E.-M.O., Spoleto. Bologna: Nuova Casa Editrice "L. Cappelli", 1991;395–403.

[10] H. Schatz, T. Burton, L. Yannuzzi and M. Rabb. Interpretazione fluorangiografica del fondo oculare. Palermo: Medical Books, 1984;480–486.

[11] C. Sborgia, S. Santoro, A. La Tegola and T. Micelli Ferrari. Traumatologia della coroide. Clin. Ocul. e Patol. Ocul. 1987;3: 229–232.

[12] G. Marchini, G. Totolo, L. Franceschetti and S. Gios. Diagnosi differenziale ecografica delle piccole neoformazioni coroideali. Clin. Ocul. e Patol. Ocul. 1990;5:327–331.

[13] E. Mantovani, L. Bergamo, E. Milizia and D. Doro. Follow-up ecografico di un'emorragia sottoretinica spontanea. Clin. Ocul. e Patol. Ocul. 1993;2:67–69.

[14] C. Blodi. Vascular anomalies of the fundus. Clinical Ophthalmology. T.D. Duane, Philadelphia: Harper and Row Publ., 1987;3:1–10.

Luciano Ferrari
Divisione Oculistica
Ospedale di Rovereto
USL C 10 Vallagarina
Rovereto (TN), Italy

13. An atypical intraocular tumor: echographic study

G. CENNAMO, N. ROSA, A. MELE,[1] P. DE ROSA[1] and A. LA RANA

(Naples, Italy)

Abstract

Standardized echography can detect and differentiate intraocular tumors with a great accuracy. However, these tumors may present atypical characteristics. Here we describe a patient with a black mass on the skin of his nose, and retinal detachment due to a solid lesion in his left eye. The echographic characteristics of this lesion and the differential diagnosis with other tumors are discussed.

Keywords: Standardized echography, mushroom lesion, metastasis

Introduction

Standardized echography is a safe and reliable method for the detection and differentiation of ocular and orbital diseases [1]. In the case of ocular tumors, malignant melanomas can be distinguished from other intraocular benign and malignant tumors [2,3]. Here we describe a clinical case that presented an atypical feature.

Clinical case

A 64-year-old white male was referred to our eye department for a progressive loss of vision in his left eye. His examination showed a large pigmented lesion on the skin of his nose, 2 centimeters in diameter. The right eye was normal with a 20/20 corrected visual acuity. The left eye showed no light perception, and congestion of the episcleral vessels in the nasal side; the vitreous was not very clear. His left eye fundus examination revealed a total retinal detachment. A solid mass underneath the retinal detachment was suspected and an echographic examination with standardized echography was performed.

A-scan examination showed a lesion with a fairly regular structure, medium low reflectivity with sound attenuation and spontaneous fast movements due to internal vascularization. B-scan examination showed a mass with a characteristic mushroom shape. A diagnosis of malignant melanoma was made and the

G Cennamo and N. Rosa (eds.), Ultrasonography in Ophthalmology 15, pp. 133–135.

left eye of the patient was enucleated, and the cutaneous neoplasm was excised.

The histological examination of the cutaneous neoplasm showed the presence of a basal cell carcinoma. The histopathological examination of the eye showed a metastatic lesion, with gland-like structure. A total body examination revealed a prostatic carcinoma as the primary site.

Discussion and conclusion

Standardized echography is a safe and effective method for the differentiation of intraocular tumors. At standardized echography, choroidal metastatic tumors show an irregular structure with a high to medium reflectivity related to the macroscopic structure of the tumor, due to the connective tissue that irregularly separates different areas of neoplastic cells. In B-scan the metastatic tumors appear as a flat, concave wax-like lesion [4].

Metastatic lesions with a regular structure, and low to medium reflectivity have been described [4]. The low reflectivity of these tumors are probably related to scarce connective tissue and a prevalence of neoplastic cells due to a fast growth; these tumors have a poor life prognosis.

A mushroom shape, due to the rupture of Bruch's membrane, is considered typical for a malignant melanoma [5]. However, a few mushroom shape lesions that were not malignant melanomas have been described. Kerman *et al.* in 1987 [6] described three mushroom-shaped lesions that were not malignant melanomas: one astrocytoma of the ciliary body, a presumed metastatic carcinoma from a parotid gland and a retinoblastoma. Schuttermann *et al.* [7] described a benign adenoma of the retinal pigment epithelial cells that was mushroom-shaped. It was considered benign because no infiltration in the choroid was found, but it was obviously destructive to the eye.

According to Apple [8], Bruch's membrane often ruptures due to pressure from the underlying neoplasm. In the early stages of the disease, Bruch's membrane prevents the growth of the tumor, and when it ruptures the tumor can easily expand through the breach. At the site of the rupture, there is a collar button or purse-string constriction that causes vasodilatation in the tumor vessels at the apex of the mass, and consequently, the tumor assumes a mushroom-shape configuration.

Malignant melanomas that rupture Bruch's membrane tend to be highly aggressive and show cytologic changes characteristic of more malignant forms. Therefore, the mushroom shape is suggestive of an accelerated growth pattern.

Consequently, because malignant melanomas grow faster than other intraocular tumors this explains why a mushroom shape is considered typical for this lesion.

The only other lesions that can present such or even faster growth are the low reflective metastatic lesions.

In conclusion the case reported here indicates that even if a mushroom-shaped lesion is considered typical for a malignant melanoma, it could be caused by different diseases, but it does however suggest an aggressive growth pattern.

References

[1] K.C. Ossoinig. Standardized echography: basic principles, clinical applications and results. Intern. Ophthalmol. Clin. 1979;19:4.

[2] N. Rosa, G. Cennamo and F. Tranfa. Comparison between echographic and histologic findings in choroidal malignant melanomas. Acta Ophthalmol. 1992;99(204):102.

[3] G. Cennamo and N. Rosa. Ruolo dell'ecografia standardizzata nella diagnosi differenziale degli pseudomelanomi. Proc. International Symposium on Intraocular Tumors. Florence, 2–4 February 1990.

[4] G. Cennamo, N. Rosa, T. Foà and A. Mele. Metastatic choroidal lesions: a retrospective study. Proc. 13th SIDUO Congress, Doc. Ophthalmol. Proc. Series 55. In P. Till (ed.), Ophthalmic Echography. 1990:13:277–283.

[5] R. Green. Echographic diagnosis of large choroidal melanomas. Proc. 9th SIDUO Congress, Doc. Ophthalmol. Proc. Series 38. In J.S. Hillman and M.M. Le May (eds), Ophthalmic Ultrasonography. 1983.

[6] B.M. Kerman and M.L. Fishman. Non malanomatous collar button tumors. Proc. 10th SIDUO Congress, Doc. Ophthalmol. Proc. Series 48. In K.C. Ossoinig K.C. (ed.), Ophthalmic Echography. 1987;413–416.

[7] J. Schuttermann and U. Axelsson. A mushroom shaped pigmented pseudomelanoma (case report). Proc. 11 SIDUO Congress, Doc. Ophthalmol. Proc. Series 51. In J.M. Thijssen, J.S. Hillman, P.E. Gallenga and G. Cennamo (eds). Ultrasonography in Ophthalmology. 1988;11:185–187.

[8] D.J. Apple and M.F. Rabb. Clinicopathologic correlation of ocular disease. II Ed. St. Louis: The C.V. Mosby Co., 1978.

Giovanni Cennamo
Istituto di Oftalmologia
Università di Napoli Federico II
Via S. Pansini 5
80131 Naples, Italy

[1]Divisione di Oculistica
Ospedale Cardarelli
80131 Naples, Italy

14. Choroidal osteoma – clinics and ultrasonography

L. HENČ -PETRINOVIĆ, I. DEKARIS, J. BUDIŠIĆ[1] and
L. RITZ-MUTEVELIĆ[1]
(Zagreb, Croatia)

Abstract

The cause of sudden visual acuity reduction in one eye in a young white female, with a picture of an extensive central chorioretinitis, was identified by means of ultrasonography. Visual acuity (0.1) was obscured by a central relative scotoma in the right eye. Ophthalmoscopy revealed a pink oval macular lesion, surrounded by an atrophic rim, involving also the peripapillary region. Fluorescein angiography presented initial hypofluorescence followed by patchy hyperfluorescence in the central part of the macular lesion, corresponding to the subretinal neovascular membrane in the right eye. No pathology was found in the left eye. Computerized tomography showed a bony plaque at the posterior pole of the right eye and no alteration in the left.

The ultrasonographic picture showing a characteristic highly reflective lesion in the chorioretinal layer, 10 mm in diameter and 3 mm thick, casting a shadow on all posteriorly-situated structures, helped distinguish between inflammatory and tumours changes at the posterior pole. Parabulbar corticosteroid therapy every day for two weeks resulted in regression of the exudative component, as shown on the control angiography. The improvement of the visual acuity was only partial (0.3).

Key words: Choroidal osteoma, echography, fluorescein angiography

Introduction

After Gass and his associates [1] described the typical clinical, histological, angiographic, ultrasonographic and radiographic features of choroidal osteoma, this rare intrabulbar lesion is being recognized more often [2–4]. Mostly monocular, this benign tumor appears in both eyes in about 25% of patients [5, 6]. Most affected persons are white adult females, although the lesion has also been described in children [5,7,8] as well as in elderly male patients [9]. Choroidal osteoma has usually been reported in healthy persons without any medical or ocular history apart from an osteoma associated with fatal systemic disease in an 11-year old black boy [7]. The patients are visually asymptomatic

G Cennamo and N. Rosa (eds.), Ultrasonography in Ophthalmology 15, pp. 137–145.

until the occurrence of degeneration of overlying pigment epithelium. Subretinal neovascularisation complicates the course [5,7,8]. Complete absence of subjective symptoms is in contrast with the extent of a yellow-white placoid choroidal mass in the juxtapapillar and macular region. Echography is the best method with which to identify the nature of such subretinal lesions and to differentiate this benign tumor from more sinister tumors as well as from post-traumatic and post-inflammatory secondary ossification of diseased or disorganized ocular tissues [9–11].

We report a case of monocular choroidal osteoma complicated by subretinal neovascularisation in a young female. Fluorescein angiographic and ultrasonographic follow-up was sufficient to establish final diagnosis.

Case history

A 23-year-old female experienced sudden reduction of central visual acuity (0.1) of her right eye with positive central scotoma. She had no medical or ocular history that suggested the triggering factor. At the initial examination of her right eye a sharply demarcated, slightly prominent reddish-orange choroidal lesion was observed in the juxtapapillar and submacular region. The pigment epithelium was reduced, so that well-defined scalloped margins of the plaque contrasted with surrounding area. The retinal vasculature and optic disc were unaffected. The macular region was partially occupied by a grayish subretinal neovascular membrane. Her left eye was without any pathological changes.

Fluorescein angiography performed at this time revealed initial hypofluorescence replaced soon by patchy hyperfluorescence and late diffuse staining of the area occupied by the choroidal osteoma with secondary changes of the retinal pigment epithelium. The subretinal neovascular membrane was demonstrated by early lacy macular hyperfluorescence and late diffuse subretinal leakage. Some empty vascular channels were recognized within peripheral parts of hyperfluorescent plaque of the choroidal osteoma. Small scattered hyperfluorescent dots outside the neovascular membrane, demonstrating pigment epithelium defects, were also visible (Figs. 1 and 2).

Ultrasonography (Nidek 3000) confirmed the suspicion that the lesion was a choroidal osteoma. The osseous nature of the tumor was demonstrated by high reflectivity spikes (100%) on A-scan examination detectable even with reduced sensitivity of the system and by ultrasound absorption causing acoustic shadowing of orbital tissues posterior to the tumor. With B-scan ultrasonography, a mildly elevated highly reflective lenticular plaque, obscuring distal structures was detected. Some reverberation was detected on the edges of the osseous plaque (Fig. 3).

A radiopaque lesion with a bony density was revealed by computed tomography on the posterior pole of the right eye, corresponding to the location of the tumor. The ERG curve of the right eye was reduced with b-wave amplitude being half of the value of the left eye.

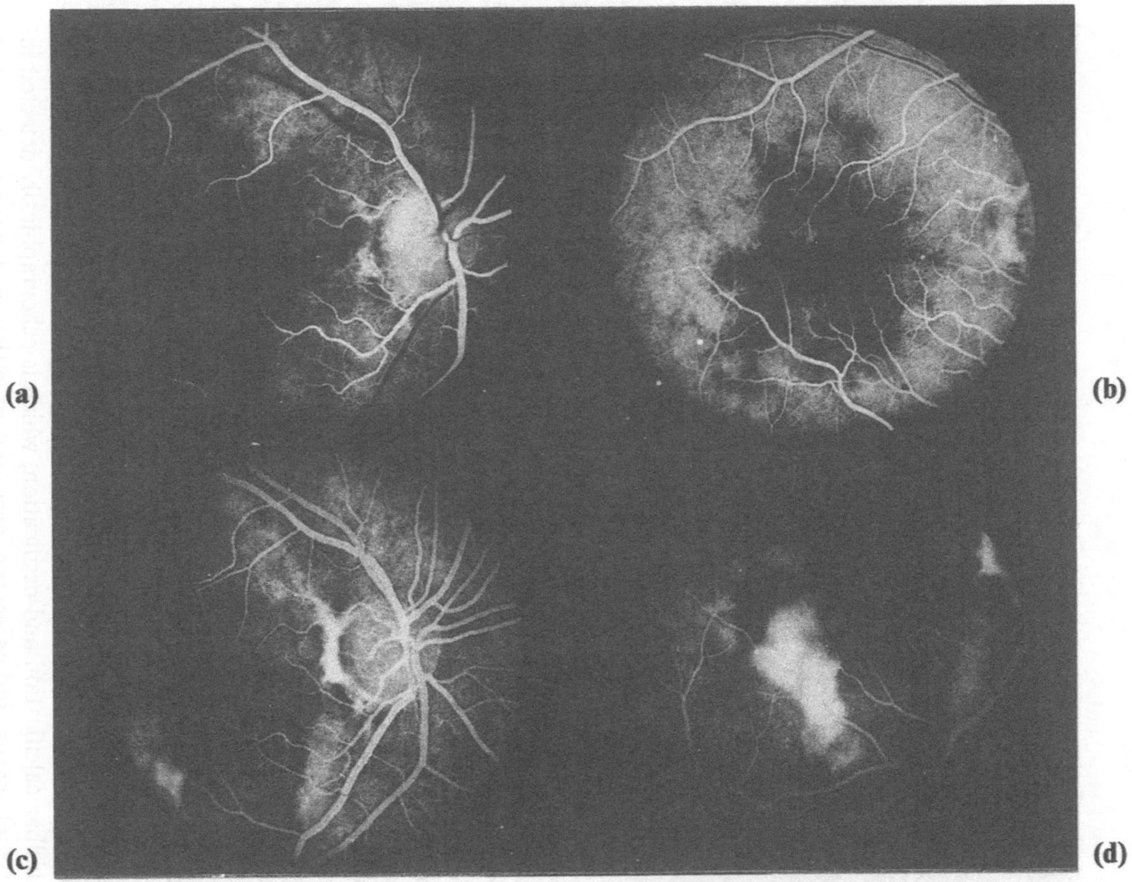

Fig. 1. Fluorescein angiography of choroidal osteoma of the right eye in four phases: a) early retinal with patchy hyperfluorescence of the choroidal osteoma on the posterior pole; b) mid retinal phase, with diffuse hyperfluorescence; c) hyperfluorescent margins of osteoma; d) neovascular subretinal membrane in the macular region

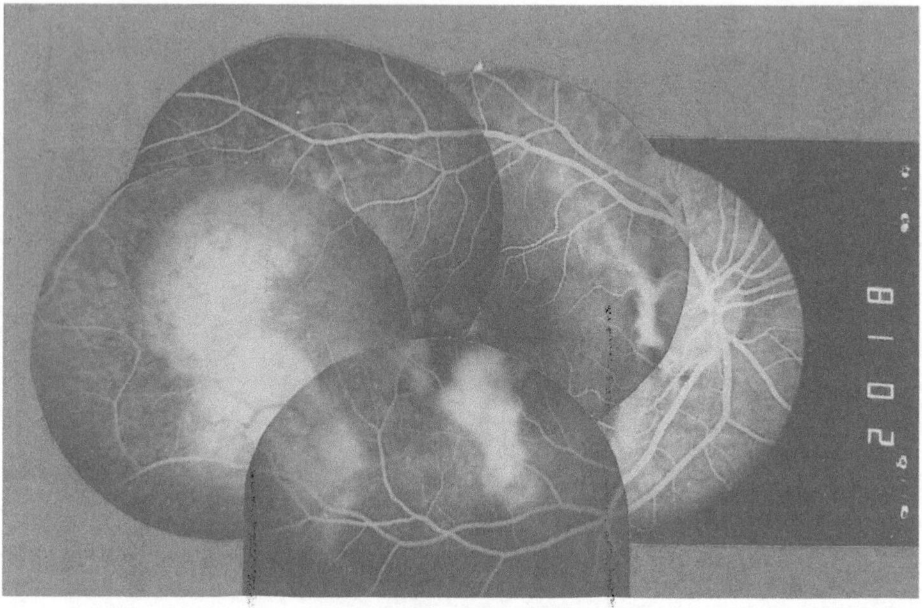

Fig. 2. Composed picture of fluorescein angiography of the choroidal osteoma occupying posterior pole of the right eye

Secondary exudative maculopathy was treated by corticosteroids topically and retrobulbary (Dexamethasone 40 mg every day for two weeks). No laser treatment was applied due to central location of the subretinal neovascular membrane. Only partial amelioration of visual acuity (0.3) together with resorption of the subretinal exudation was achieved after 2 months (Fig. 4). Control ultrasonography demonstrated no changes either in the extent, or in the reflectivity of the osseous lesion in the posterior pole.

Discussion

Ultrasonography is a relevant diagnostic technique with which to clarify the nature of many chorioretinal diseases that show a peculiar fundoscopic picture. Intrabulbar calcification and ossification, which is echographically detected in some such cases, indicates the presence of either a primary congenital choristoma or a secondary process of calcification. Secondary choroidal ossification is triggered by chronic intraocular changes and involves not only the peripapillary region as in primary osteoma, but also other sites where a rich vascular supply is present. Ultrasonography in such cases with severe inflammation, and such traumatic changes as long-standing retinal detachment is

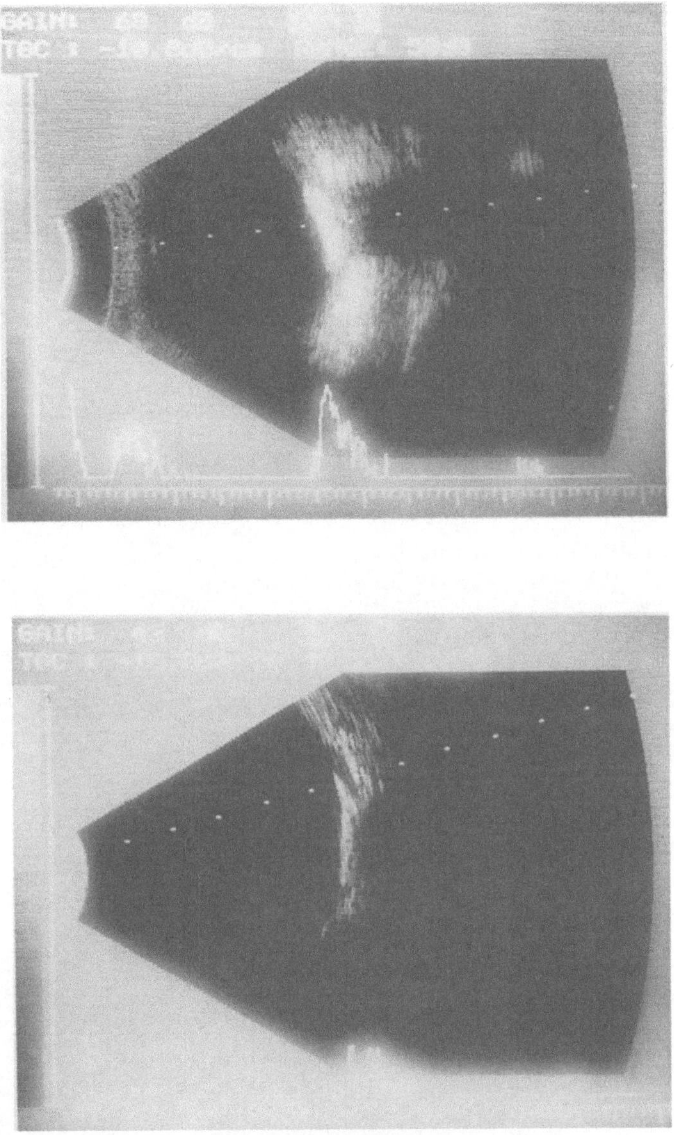

(a)

(b)

Fig. 3. Ultrasonography of the choroidal osteoma showing 100% reflectivity and shadowing of the distal orbital structures: a) at higher system sensitivity and b) at reduced sensitivity

(a) (b)

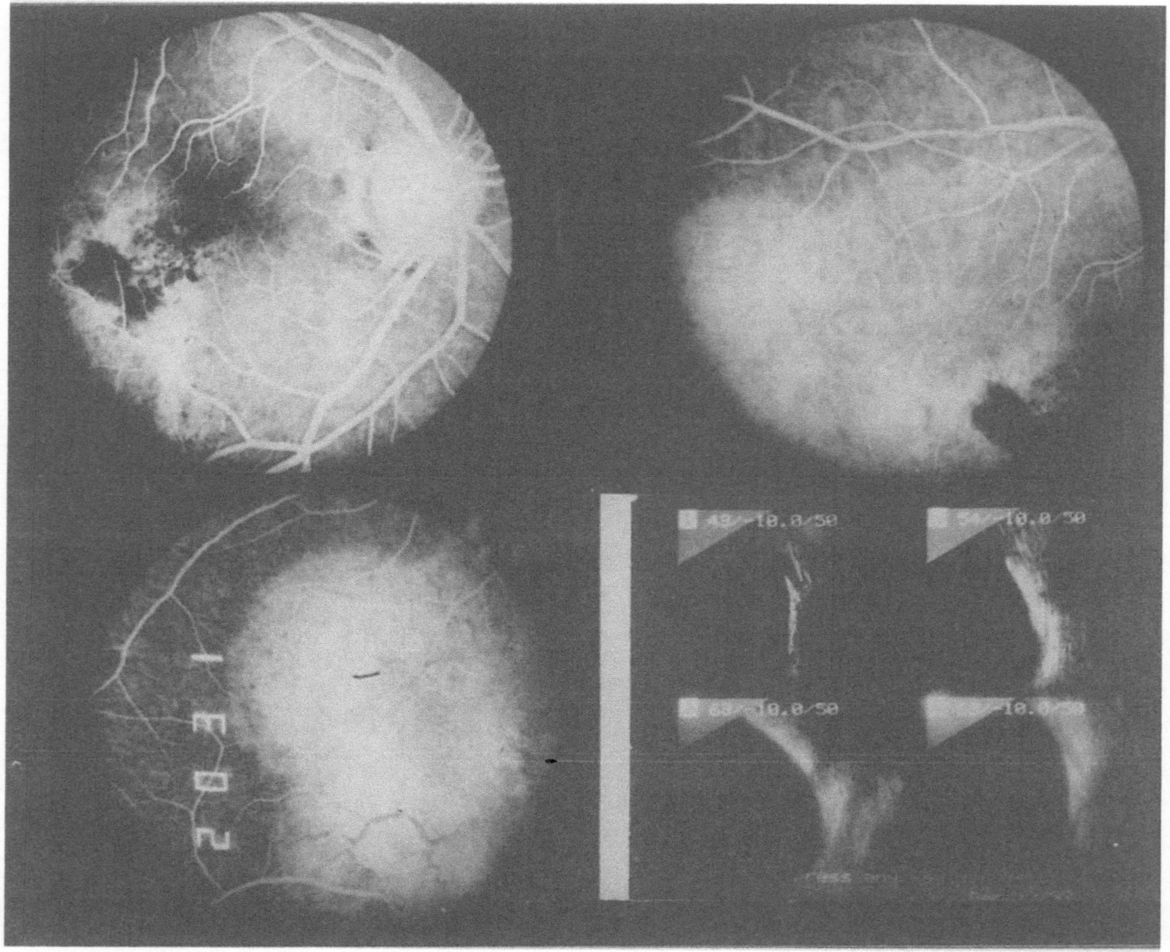

(c) (d)

Fig. 4. Control after two months: fluorescein angiography (a,b,c) with reabsorbed subretinal neovascular membrane and ultrasonography without further changes (d)

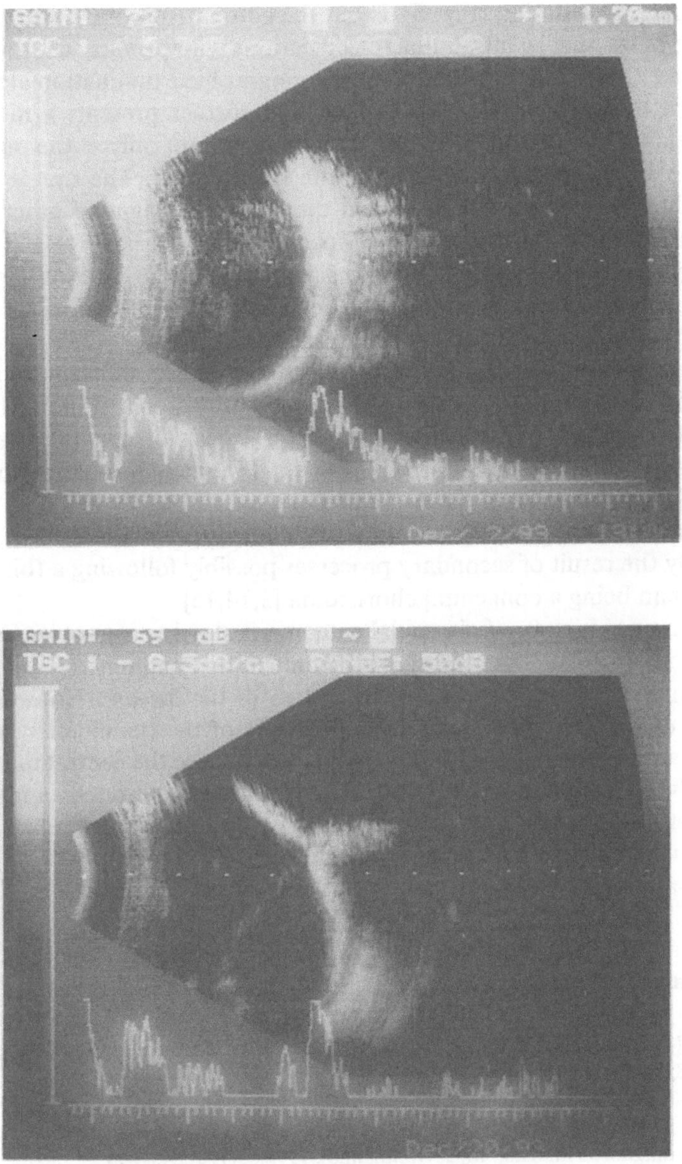

Fig. 5. Two cases of secondary intrabulbar calcification with highly reflective posterior bulbar wall and total shadowing of the distal structures

characteristic with a broad highly reflective area in B-scan examination and overloaded echo-spikes casting a shadow on posteriorly-situated orbital tissue on A-scan presentation (Fig. 5). From the comparison of the ultrasonographic pictures of secondary intrabulbar calcifications with primary choroidal osteoma described above, it appeared that ultrasonographic examination alone might be sufficient to discern these two entities. The former presents a more irregular arrangement of the calcium deposits that spread not only at the posterior pole, but also in the peripheral parts of the background. The eye is often either microphthalmic or buphthalmic and there are also signs of other intrabulbar changes (retinal detachment, vitreal opacities etc.).

Doppler ultrasonography gives no signals in cases of intrabulbar ossification due to lack of blood flow. This method can help discern this kind of tumor from those that have a rich blood supply [12].

Although clinical and ultrasonographic pictures are sufficient for diagnosis of choroidal osteoma, computed tomography can be contributory, but it is not necessary, particularly because it entails the risk of general anesthesia and represents a radiation hazard in children [8]. Magnetic resonance does not show the typical negative image of the bone [3,13].

It has been suggested that cases of primary osteomas of the choroid are probably the result of secondary processes possibly following a (birth-) trauma, rather than being a congenital choristoma [3,14,15].

The natural history of choroidal osteoma is slowly progressive [16], however our follow-up period was too short to confirm this finding.

No medical therapy can alter the course of the disease. However, there are reports of regression and even disappearance of the tumor after laser therapy [17]. Laser treatment is not indicated in cases where the central macular region is involved. We tried to decrease submacular exudation by means of local corticosteroid therapy (retrobulbar Dexamethasone at 40 mg for two weeks), with partial success: exudation was reabsorbed, but the extent of the osseous lesion remained the same.

References

[1] J.D.M. Gass, R.K. Guerry, R.L. Jack and G. Harris. Choroidal osteoma. Arch. Ophthalmol. 1978;96:428.

[2] T.O. Coston and C.P. Wikinson. Choroidal osteoma. Am. J. Ophthalmol. 1978;86:368–372.

[3] P.A. Bloom, J.D. Ferris, A. Laidlaw and P.R. Goddard. Appearances of choroidal osteomas with diagnostic imaging. Br. J. Ophthalmol. 1992;65(778):845–848.

[4] S.J. Rose, J.F. Burke and R.J. Brockhurst. Argon laser photoablation of a choroidal osteoma. Retina 1991;11(2):221–223.

[5] E. Eting and H. Savir. An atypical fulminant course of choroidal osteoma in two siblings. Am. J. Ophthalmol. 1992;113:52–55.

[6] G.C. Brown and C.L. Shield. Choroidal osteoma. In S.J. Ryan (ed.), Retina. St. Louis, Baltimore, Toronto: The C.V. Mosby Co., 1989;1:749–755.

[7] L.B. Kline, H.W. Skalka, J.D. Davidson and F.J. Wilmes. Bilateral choroidal osteomas associated with fatal systemic illness. Am. J. Ophthalmol. 1982;93:192–197.

[8] A. Stanovsky. Standardized A-scan diagnosis of bilateral choroidal osteoma in a 4, 5 year-old girl. In P. Till (ed.), Ophthalmic Echography. 13 Dordrecht: Kluwer Academic Publishers, 1993;273–276.

[9] U. Menchini, G. Davi, L. Pierro, L. Guarisco, A. Cascavilla and R. Brancato. Bilateral choroidal osteoma in an aged patient. J. Fr. Ophthalmol. 1990;13(1-2):3–9.

[10] G. Cennamo, G. Iaccarino, G. de Creccio and G. Liguori. Choroidal osteoma (osseous choristoma): An atypical case. Br. J. Ophthalmol. 1990;911(74):700–701.

[11] S.N. Trimble and H. Shatz. Choroidal osteoma after intraocular inflammation. Am. J. Ophthalmol. 1993;96:759–764.

[12] P.G. Wolf-Korman, B.A. Kormann, G.C. Hasenfratz and F.A. Spengel. Duplex and color Doppler ultrasound in the differential diagnosis of choroidal tumors. Acta Ophthalmol. 1992;204 suppl.:66–70.

[13] P. DePotter, J.A. Shields, C.L. Shields and V.M. Rao. Magnetic resonance imaging in choroidal osteoma. Retina 1991;11(2):221–223.

[14] F. Munier, L. Zografos and P. Schnyder. Idiopathic sclerochoroidal calcification: New observations. Eur. J. Ophthalmol. 1991;1(4):167-172.

[15] J.M. Rohrbach, E. Liesenhoff and K.P. Steuhl. Principles of intraocular ossification exemplified by secondary choroid ossification. Klin. Monatsbl. Augenheilkd. 1990;197(5):397–403.

[16] C.F. Zhang, P.F. Fei, F.T. Dong, P. Chen and N. Lu. Choroidal osteoma. Clinical characteristics and long-term follow-up of five cases. Chin. Med. J. (Engl.) 1990;103(3): 251-255.

[17] S.N. Trimble and H. Schatz. Decalcification of a choroidal osteoma. Br. J. Ophthalmol. 1991;75(1):61–63.

L. Henč-Petrinović
General Hospital 'Sveti Duh'
New Hospital Zagreb
Sveti Duh 64,
41000 Zagreb, Croatia

[1]New Hospital Zagreb
Aleja Izvidača
41000 Zagreb, Croatia

15. Acoustic features of two unusually elevated peripheral retinal capillary hemangiomas

D. DORO, S. LORENZINI,[1] M. VACCARO, E. MILIZIA and
E. MANTOVANI
(Padua and [1] Belluno, Italy)

Abstract

Reports on retinal capillary hemangiomas are sporadic, mainly due to rare detection, small size and peculiar ophthalmoscopical features. We performed standardized echography on 10 patients with unilateral retinal capillary hemangiomas of the peripheral retina (seven cases) or the optic disc (three cases) that were from 1 to 2.6 mm high. A predominantly medium reflectivity on standardized A-scan and an irregular dome-shape on contact B-scan were the echographic features of the two peripheral retinal capillary hemangiomas sufficiently elevated to allow echographic tissue analysis. These acoustic findings are consistent with the histopathological features of retinal capillary hemangiomas.

Standardized echography may provide useful information particularly in eyes with opaque media harbouring retinal capillary hemangioma possibly associated with exudative retinal detachment as found in one of our two unusually elevated peripheral retinal tumors.

Key words: Standardized echography, retinal capillary hemangioma, histopathology, exudative retinal detachment

Introduction

Retinal capillary hemangiomas are rare benign vascular peripheral or juxtapapillary hamartomas [1], usually inherited according to the autosomal dominant mode (with low penetrance) [2]. When associated with systemic vascular and non vascular tumors, retinal capillary hemangiomas are typical of the von Hippel-Lindau syndrome [2]. An equal sex incidence and a 30–50% bilaterality of retinal capillary hemangiomas are reported [1–3].

Retinal capillary hemangiomas are the result of a developmental anomaly of foetal vascular structures. Hemangiomas may protrude outwards (esophytic type) or inwards (endophytic type) and are usually reddish lesions. Their height at diagnosis (generally in the second to the fourth decade) ranges from 1 to 5

G Cennamo and N. Rosa (eds.), Ultrasonography in Ophthalmology 15, pp. 147–152.

mm [1,3]. Retinal capillary hemangiomas may be either asymptomatic or may cause symptoms when retinal lipid-rich exudation involves the macula or when epiretinal membranes develop.

Due to rare detection, low elevation and peculiar ophthalmoscopical features, reports of retinal capillary hemangiomas have been sporadic, and different acoustic characteristics have been described [4–8]. Here we report our series of 10 cases of retinal capillary hemangiomas sufficiently elevated to be detected by standardized echography, and describe the echographic features of the two most elevated.

Patients

Over a seven year period we evaluated echographically 10 patients who had an ophthalmoscopic and fluorescein angiographic diagnosis of unilateral endophytic retinal capillary hemangioma. As shown in Table 1, the mean age at diagnosis was 42 years (range 15 ± 76 years); right eye was affected in six cases; three patients had juxtapapillary and seven had peripheral retinal capillary hemangiomas, more frequently located in the infero-temporal quadrant (six out of seven cases). There was no sex difference (males/females ratio = 1). Two patients with peripheral retinal capillary hemangioma showed exudative localized retinal detachment (patients no. 6 and no. 10). No patient showed evidence of systemic tumors (von Hippel-Lindau syndrome); however, only half the patients have been investigated in detail.

Table 1. Clinical features of ten patients with unilateral retinal capillary hemangioma

No.	Patient		Eye	Tumor	
	ID	Age (yrs.)		Location	Elevation (mm)
1.	T.G.	51	RE	Juxtapapillary	1.0
2.	V.A.	42	LE	Juxtapapillary	1.1
3.	B.G.	67	RE	Peripheral I.T.	1.4
4.	B.C.	15	RE	Peripheral I.T.	1.4
5	L.P.	35	RE	Juxtapapillary	1.5
6.	M.L.	47	RE	Peripheral I.T.	1.5
7.	V.G.	76	LE	Peripheral I.T.	1.5
8.	C.P.	41	LE	Peripheral S.T.	1.7
9.	C.F.	31	RE	Peripheral I.T.	2.5
10.	M.L.	17	RE	Peripheral I.T.	2.6

Mean age of patients, 42 yrs
Mean elevation of retinal capillary hemangiomas, 1.6 mm
I.T., infero-temporal quadrant
S.T., supero-temporal quadrant

148Standardized echography (Coopervision Ultrascan Digital B® and Biophysic Ophthascan 'S' mini-A) was performed in all patients. The height of the three juxtapapillary retinal capillary hemangiomas ranged from 1 to 1.5 mm, whereas the height of five of the seven peripheral retinal capillary hemangiomas ranged from 1.4 to 1.7 mm; contact B-scan of these lesions revealed a full texture and a dome-shape.

Patients no. 9 and no. 10 were echographically more interesting. In patient no. 9, a 31-year-old man complaining of vague visual disturbances in the right eye, ophthalmoscopy revealed a roundish red-yellowish lesion with some satellite exudates in the peripheral infero-temporal quadrant. Visual acuity was full in both eyes and the left eye had no abnormality. A diagnosis of presumed retinal capillary hemangioma was made. Standardized echography showed a somewhat irregular dome-shaped, full texture solid lesion (contact B-scan) and medium-high reflectivity with rather regular structure and no spontaneous vertical movements; the maximal height was 2.6 mm (standardized A-scan) (Fig. 1). No ophthalmoscopical or echographic changes were observed during the eight month follow-up.

Patient no. 10 was a 17-year-old boy from Albania referred with a diagnosis of suspected choroidal melanoma of the right eye. Ophthalmological examination showed a prominent pink peripheral solid lesion and exudative retinal detachment involving the infero-temporal quadrant; macular exudates reduced vision to 20/50; the left eye was normal. B-scan showed a dome-shaped retinal tumor with full-spongy texture and a satellite retinal detachment. Medium inner reflectivity with regular heterogeneous structure and no spontaneous vertical movements was observed on standardized A-scan examination; the maximal measured height of the retinal tumor was 2.5 mm (Fig. 2). The ophthalmoscopical and echographic diagnosis was retinal capillary hemangioma. We did not have the opportunity of following-up the patient.

Discussion

Retinal capillary hemangioma is a rare disease, which is usually asymptomatic when no retinal exudation is present. The diagnosis is mainly ophthalmoscopic when media are clear and may be confirmed by fluorescein angiography. The height of retinal capillary hemangiomas is often below the lower limit of the echographic tissue differentiation [9]; thus, standardized echography may play a role only when tumors are higher than 2 mm.

To our knowledge, the only descriptions of the A-scan characteristics of peripheral capillary hemangiomas are those reported by Mazzeo [5] and by Byrne & Green [4] who found a medium to low and a medium inner reflectivity, respectively. On the other hand, Shields [8] and Moro *et al.* [6] reported some cases of juxtapapillary capillary hemangioma with high internal reflectivity, whereas Pierro *et al.* [7] reported one case with medium to low reflectivity.

In our experience, structure and internal reflectivity can be studied only in the

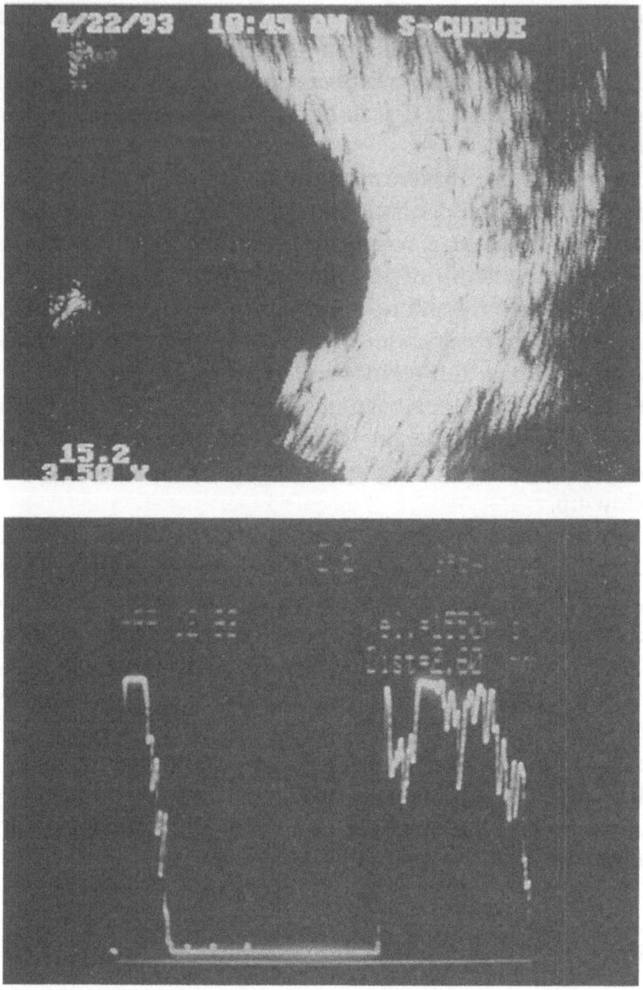

Fig. 1. **Patient no. 9. Top, longitudinal B-scan section showing the somewhat irregular dome-shaped full texture retinal tumor. Bottom, elevation of the tumors is 2.6 mm and internal reflectivity is medium-high with a rather regular structure on standardized A-scan**

case of tumors of more than 2 mm in height. A predominantly medium reflectivity with regular heterogeneous structure (standardized A-scan) and an irregular dome-shape with a full-spongy texture (contact B-scan) were the echographic features of the two peripheral retinal capillary hemangiomas that were about 2.5 mm high.

These acoustic findings are consistent with the histopathological features, i.e.,

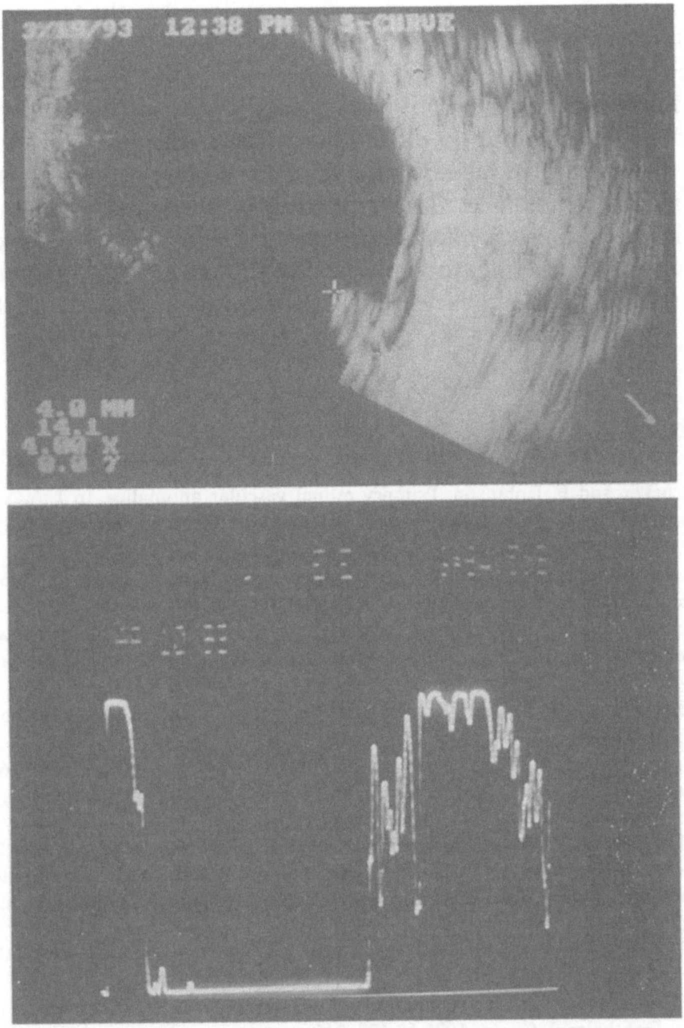

Fig. 2. Patient no. 10. Top, B-scan longitudinal section showing a dome-shaped retinal tumor with a full spongy texture and a satellite exudative retinal detachment involving the lesion. Maximal elevation measured from the tumor apex to the choroid is about 4 mm. Bottom, the shape and infero-temporal location of the lesion prevented optimal perpendicularity of standardized A-scan beam; note the medium inner reflectivity with regular heterogeneous structure; the measured elevation of the retinal capillary hemangioma alone is 2.5 mm

proliferation of endothelial cells, pericytes, glial cells and varying degrees of fibrous tissue replacing the neurosensorial retina, with cystoid spaces in the outer plexiform layer and possible exudative detachment with lipids in the subretinal space [10]. The varying degree of fibrous tissue may account for the discrepancy in the internal acoustic reflectivity found in the few cases reported and the lack of fast blood flow explains why we did not find spontaneous vertical movements of the inner echo-spikes.

The differential diagnosis of retinal capillary hemangioma by means of standardized echography is difficult because of the low elevation and the location (peripheral or juxtapapillary) of the lesion. However, in eyes with opaque media, a medium reflective small dome-shaped subretinal mass lesion located in the peripheral infero-temporal quadrant without choroidal excavation and spontaneous vertical movements should alert the physician to the possibility of retinal capillary hemangioma with or without satellite retinal exudative detachment.

References

[1] A. Brucker and F. Robinson. Primary retinal vascular anomalies. In L.A. Yannuzzi (ed.), Macular area photocoagulation. Retina. Philadelphia: J.B. Lippincott Co., 1989; suppl.:115–133.

[2] P. Hardwing and D.M. Robertson. von Hippel-Lindau disease: a familial, often lethal, multi-system phakomatosis. Ophthalmology, 1984;91:263–270.

[3] W.H. Annesley Jr., B.C. Leonard, J.A. Shields and W.S. Tasman. Fifteen year review of treated cases of retinal angiomatosis. Trans. Am. Acad. Ophthalmol. Otolaryngol. 1977;83: 446–453.

[4] S.F. Byrne and R.L. Green. Ultrasound of the eye and orbit. St. Louis: Mosby Year Book, 1992;181–184.

[5] V. Mazzeo. Ecografia dell'apparato oculare. Milano: Fogliazza editore, 1987;161–163.

[6] F. Moro, D. Doro and S. Piermarocchi. Optic disc capillary hemangioma: Fluorangiographic and echographic study of two cases. Proceed. Retina Workshop (Florence, May 2–3 1986). In Ghedini, Retinal Diseases. Amsterdam, Milano: Kugler Publishers (ed.), 1987;2:285–291.

[7] L. Pierro, L. Guarisco, E. Zaganelli, M. Freschi and R. Brancato. Capillary and cavernous hemangioma of the optic disc: Echographic and histological findings. Acta Ophthalmol. 1992;70(204):102–106.

[8] J.A. Shields. Diagnosis and management of intraocular tumors. St. Louis: C.V. Mosby Co., 1983;534–566.

[9] K.C. Ossoinig. Standardized echography: Basic principles, clinical applications and results. Intern. Ophthalmol. Clinics 1979;19:107–210.

[10] D.H. Nicholson, W.R. Green and K.R. Kenyon. Light and electron microscopy study of early lesions in angiomatosis retinae. Am. J. Ophthalmol. 1976;82:193–204.

Daniele Doro
Institute of Ophthalmology
University of Padua
Via Giustiniani, 2
I35128-Padua, Italy

[1]Department of Ophthalmology
Hospital of Belluno
Belluno, Italy

Anterior eye segment

16. A new apparatus for the study of anterior segment disorders: the ultrasound biomicroscope

T. AVITABILE, V. RUSSO, M.C. SORCE and A. REIBALDI

(Catania, Italy)

Abstract

We used the Humphrey Ultrasound Biomicroscope (UBM) system 840 to study various disorders of the anterior segment of the eye. Such images could not be obtained with earlier equipment because of poor resolution power. This UBM system, using a 50 MHz probe, has a lateral and axial resolution of about 50 μ, which allows us to visualize disorders still at an early phase. By viewing a part of the anterior segment in cross-sections, one may evaluate, in the presence of opaque media, the relations between the various parts of the anterior segment and determine the correct position of an intraocular lens, the increase of a ciliary body tumor or the evolution of corneal lesions such as Descemet's membrane detachment. Indeed, thanks to its high resolution power, this equipment allows us to perform very accurate biometries in all these disorders and to measure the angles formed by different structures of the anterior segment, by means of software.

Key words: Anterior segment, biomicroscopy, echography, ultrasound biomicroscopy (UBM)

Introduction

Ultrasonography has always played a secondary role in the study of pathologies of the anterior segment with transparent media in that this part of the eye is easily accessible to other semeiotic investigations. However, ultrasonography has always been considered to play a fundamental role in the presence of opaque media or in assessing the nature of tumors of the iris and ciliary body. To be amenable to tissutal diagnosis, these tumors must measure at least 1–5 mm. The ultrasonic biomicroscope (UBM) was a breakthrough in this field. Using probes with a frequency ranging from 50 to 100 MHz, it provides us with information, even in transparent media, on some eye structures unobtainable by any other semeiotic technique and comparable only with the optical microscope on fixed histological pieces [1].

G Cennamo and N. Rosa (eds.), Ultrasonography in Ophthalmology 15, pp. 155–162.

Materials and methods

Since May 1993 we have had the opportunity of testing an ultrasonic biomicroscope made by Humphrey under the trademark "UBM System 840", at the Ultrasonography Centre of the Institute of Ophthalmology of the University of Catania. The equipment consists of a central unit connected by means of a metal arm to a large probe that contains the mechanism allowing the crystal to oscillate. The crystal is contained in a small metal cylinder which is screwed to the bottom of the probe and is not equipped with a protective device so as to avoid attenuation of the ultrasounds which at such high frequencies is very strong. The crystal in our equipment had an emission frequency of 50 MHz, but the equipment can be connected to 62 and 80 MHz crystals. With this equipment we examined approximately 200 patients affected by a variety of disorders [7].

Examinations are carried out with the patient lying down on the bed after the eye has been anaesthetised with a surface anaesthetic. Then a small plastic cup, filled with a coupling substance (gel or water), is placed over the patient's open eye. Before starting the examination it is important to make sure that there is gel or water in the cylinder containing the crystal. This is confirmed by horizontal emission echoes on the video.

Software included with the UBM releases a series of sound impulses when the probe is too close to the cornea (about 1 mm), and it blocks the crystal's movement. After UBM, no patient showed corneal abrasions upon examination with the slit lamp and the fluorescein test.

Results

Conjunctiva

Because the conjunctiva is a surface structure, it can be studied by means of higher frequency probes, i.e., from 80–100 MHz. With a 50 MHz probe we obtained interesting results from the study of conjunctival blebs after trabeculectomy and Holmium laser sclerostomy. In the case of trabeculectomy, with the two-dimensional image of the bleb obtained with UBM, one may evaluate the bleb contents and, by means of biometry, measure its height and surface area.

The scleral flap can also be clearly viewed with UBM as can the iridectomy; in this context UBM produces images never seen with any other technique. The UBM may be useful in assessing the clinical trend of a conjunctival bleb following subconjunctival injections of antimetabolites, especially after an holmium laser sclerostomy.

Cornea

The study of the cornea with UBM is best carried out with 80–100 MHz probes because the axial resolution is directly proportional to the emission frequency. From Pavlin's studies [1,2] the cornea, with these types of probe, seems to be divided into four layers and not in five, as one would expect. The first is the epithelial layer which is fairly thin and has a slightly irregular and uneven surface. The irregularity and unevenness increase significantly in cases of oedema, which also determines an increase in thickness of the first layer.

With 80–100 MHz probes, Bowman's membrane is visible under the epithelial layer. It appears as a highly reflective continuous line because of several interfaces within it [1,2]. These two layers are not always clearly distinguishable with a 50 MHz probe, and can be better identified by carrying out signal post-processing with a PCX graphic imaging program and by Palette printing.

The corneal stroma, on the other hand, is uniform with a medium to low reflectivity due to its regular internal lamellar structure. On the contrary, the sclera, because of the irregular arrangement of its fibrils, is highly reflective.

The fourth layer is represented by Descemet's membrane and the endothelium, which cannot be visualized as two distinct layers and therefore appears as a highly reflective continuous line behind the stroma.

The corneal disorders in which the use of this method has played a decisive part in performing or confirming a diagnosis are few because the cornea is easily studied with other semeiotic investigations. In three cases of perforating lesions with a very small foreign body in the anterior segment occurring from 3 to 6 months before the UBM examination, it was possible to exclude the presence of tiny foreign bodies and to diagnose detachment of Descemet's membrane. In these cases the corneal wound was clearly visible. In cases of epithelial corneal oedemas there are various degrees of thickening of the first layer. In cases of oedema, the stromal layer is not only thicker but has an increased reflectivity because of the corneal lamellae imbibition.

With UBM one may perform a biometry of the thickness of the cornea, which will reveal whether a keratoconus has developed. In this case, it would be useful to be able to adjust the speed value of the ultrasounds which is 1.640 m/s in the cornea.

In the case of a transplanted cornea, the boundary between the host cornea and graft can be determined thanks to their different internal reflectivity (the host cornea is highly oedematous and is therefore more highly reflective). It is also possible to show the presence of any areas of adhesion between the iris and the transplanted cornea [1,2].

Iris

With UBM, the normal iris is a structure with areas of reflectivity ranging from low for the stroma to high for the posterior epithelium and iris muscles. UBM has provided a step forward in studies of these structures. Indeed, with 10 MHz probes, a neoplasia of the anterior segment must be at least 1–1.5 mm thick to be identified [3]. This causes difficulties, for instance, in the differential diagnosis between iris lesions occupying very little space, which can only be carried out by differentiating between the solid mass and the cystic mass, whereas tissutal diagnoses can be made in the posterior segment of the eye. In fact, whereas the cysts present no internal reflectivity, the solid lesions have a more or less echogenous appearance, and when they are barely detectable, it may be difficult to assess whether they are benign or malignant.

The role of traditional ultrasonography is therefore limited to monitoring changes in the size of the mass and to detect its extension to the ciliary bodies. Ultrasound biomicroscopy, compared to traditional ultrasonography, thanks to its extremely high resolution power enables us to define more precisely the location, size, thickness and internal structural features of even very small masses, and allows us to evaluate even minute increases in volume, which is crucial when assessing the need for surgical removal of the lesion.

From May 1993 we analyzed 14 iris neoformations: 11 of which were cystic and 3 solid. The cysts were of different sizes, thin-walled and with a very low internal reflectivity or were even anaechogenous. They often caused alterations of iris profile or a change in the angle approach, which can be studied easily with UBM and which is worth taking into account in the event of surgical or parasurgical treatment.

Compared with traditional ultrasonography, it is possible to distinguish whether the cyst develops from the anterior or posterior layer of the iris and to exclude the presence of a malignant tumor beneath the cyst. By means of appropriate software, micrometric measurements may be made of the various diameters, contrary to the standard A-scan ultrasonography which only allows anteroposterior measurements. The volume of the neoplasia can be calculated by means of mathematical formulae, thereby allowing close monitoring of the development and possible therapy.

Pavlin *et al.* [1,2] have described the ultrasonic biomicroscopic features of various solid tumors. They report that iris nevi can appear as a small moderately thickened peripheral iris lesion, not extending past the iris root, and with a distinctive anterior convex bowing. On the surface of these lesions there is sometimes a hypoechoic layer, possibly indicating that the superficial layer was involved with a tumor plaque. The characteristics they reported for iris melanoma are a more or less infiltrating single pigmented mass with an irregular surface or with a small extension thinly attached to it, probably representing a satellite localization.

According to Pavlin *et al.* [1,2] the UBM characteristics of a mixed cell melanoma differ from those of a spindle cell melanoma. The former appears as mass with an irregular internal structure, with a highly reflective region anteriorly and a weakly reflective one posteriorly. This is due to the arrangement of the tumoral cells which are less crowded anteriorly whereas they are tightly packed posteriorly. Spindle cell melanomas, on the other hand, show a lobulated internal structure with a higher reflectivity anteriorly, lower reflectivity posteriorly, and cystic spaces that may represent vascular channels.

Our experience of solid iris tumors is too limited to comment on the UBM characteristics described by Pavlin *et al.* [1,2] who also found a histological connection in the masses they examined. We had the opportunity of analysing three cases of solid iris tumors. They appeared fusiform, with a defined border, with anterior convex bowing and a hypoechoic layer on the surface, and so showed all the features of a nevi. We observed them over a period of time and their size did not change. Furthermore, thanks to the possibility of being able to copy the stored images onto a floppy disk in a .PCX format we developed a program which enables the images to be superimposed.

Once more, by studying the iris by means of UBM, one may obtain a precise measurement of the diameter of the pupil and of the thickness of the iris after using antiglaucomatous drugs in order to assess their effects from an anatomical point of view as well.

In three cases of haemophthalmus the UBM examination enabled us to identify a dialysis of the iris with crumpling of the iris, invisible under the slit lamp, thereby providing the surgeon with further information before surgery.

Ciliary body

The ciliary body is difficult to study with traditional ultrasonic techniques both because of its anterior location and its highly irregular surface. By means of the A and B-scan contact method it is visible only in its most posterior plane, and in some meridians, such as the temporal and nasal meridians, the pars plicata is also visible.

With UBM the ciliary body is low in reflectivity and varies in configuration depending on whether one is passing through a process or a valley between processes. With a 62–80 MHz probe it is also possible to distinguish the direction of the ciliary muscles.

With traditional ultrasonography it is impossible to carry out a tissutal diagnosis of ciliary body lesions especially if they are smaller than 1–1.5 mm. Ultrasound biomicroscopy has proved to be very useful in the study of both cysts and solid tumors of the ciliary body. In the case of ciliary body cysts, especially tiny ones, the orientation of the ciliary processes should be carefully examined because these can join up at the ends and look like a cyst. This can occur particularly with transversal scans, so in cases of doubt, an axial scan should be performed. In a case of a large cyst of the posterior layer of the iris studied with traditional ultrasonography, UBM revealed the presence of a small cyst of the ciliary body whose wall was in contact with that of the iridial cyst.

Solid tumors of ciliary bodies can be studied with UBM provided they are <4 mm thick. Conversely, tumors >4 mm are difficult to view completely because of sound attenuation [4–6]. In such cases it is better to resort to traditional echography which shows the relationship of large masses to other structures much better. As reported by Pavlin *et al.* [4–6], some tumors of the ciliary body are undetectable by conventional B-scan ultrasound because they cannot be differentiated from the normal ciliary body tissue in which they are embedded. The margins of ciliary body tumors could be more clearly differentiated from normal tissue on UBM compared with conventional ultrasound. Often it is possible to see at the posterior margin of the tumor a distinct border where the internal reflectivity changes. This probably represents the margin between tumor and normal ciliary body tissue [4–6].

Ciliary body detachment is also easy to assess with UBM. We have been able to detect it in two patients with aphakic glaucoma, immediately after cyclo-cryo-therapy and exactly in the areas treated. We also consider the ultrasound biomicroscope to be useful in the differential diagnosis of 'ring melanoma' and ciliary body detachment [8–13].

Retina

The ultrasound biomicroscope was designed to study disorders of the anterior segment but it also visualizes retinal periphery degenerations. To examine the retinal periphery, a larger cup should be used and the patient's eye should be turned as far back as possible.

During three examinations we detected, as an occasional finding, cystic degeneration of the retinal periphery. They appeared as a rosary whose beads, represented by cysts, were separated by areas of flat retina.

Pavlin *et al.* [2] report that with a 100 MHz probe, the retina is resolved as four distinct layers. The first corresponds to the surface/ganglion cell layer, the second to the inner nuclear layer and the third to the region of the outer nuclear layer and external limiting membrane. Below this is a line of low reflectivity corresponding to the visual processes.

Lens and intraocular lenses

The lens can be studied with UBM only in its anterior portion in that the posterior part falls outside the probe's scanning range which is about 6.5 mm with a 50 MHz probe. The alterations which can therefore be studied are above all capsular and have some forms of surface opacity. Among the patients under our observation, we identified 10 posterior synechiae causing a seclusio with a subsequent iris bombè. It was interesting to see how the morphology of the anterior chamber changed after a YAG laser iridectomy. Moreover, in case of multiple synechiae, present not only on the pupillary margin but also towards the iris root, the ultrabiomicroscopic examination enabled us to choose the place where an iridectomy would best be performed. However, the most useful applications of UBM were in viewing intraocular lens implants. It is indeed possible to evaluate, when the media are opaque, if the intraocular lens is in the sac, sulcus or anterior chamber. It is also possible in some cases to investigate the integrity of the posterior capsule after the intraocular lens implant.

Two interesting cases came to our attention, in which the ultrasonic biomicroscope provided us with important information. The first case was a patient who underwent an ECCE+IOL implant. The intraocular pressure remained high and the anterior segment was obscured by corneal oedemas.

After the UBM examination we were able to view the entrapment of the IOL in the pupillary foramen. The second case was a patient with an intraocular lens implant in the anterior chamber that caused a large conjunctival hyperaemia and corneal oedema which did not regress with therapy. The ultrasound biomicroscope examination revealed the entrapment of a loop in the sclero-corneal wound [14,15].

Conclusions

The UBM system is undoubtedly an innovation in the field of ultrasonography. It has a series of advantages. It supplies valuable information, unobtainable with any other technique, for the differentiation of small iris and ciliary body tumors. It throws some light on the physiopathogenetic mechanisms underlying some forms of high IDP. It enables quantitative gonioscopy to be performed, which allows an accurate assessment in time of the advantages of medical, surgical and/or parasurgical therapy. It enables high precision biometries to be performed.

In contrast with these qualities there are also some disadvantages. The equipment is very costly, and is therefore destined primarily for use in research work. Because of the probe size and the suspension mechanism of the arm, it is not easy to handle and requires a substantial period of training in order to obtain good quality images. The examination itself causes some discomfort to the patient both because of the positioning of the cup on the eyeball and the sight of a metal object that oscillates a few millimetres away from the cornea transmitting vibrations via the cup or the gel.

If advanced technology leads to a reduction in the cost of this type of apparatus, its routine use in clinical practice could become a reality. Indeed, when the UBM was available for our use, the number of traditional examinations with immersion technique fell drastically and the results obtained were decidedly better. In addition, because the equipment can be fitted with probes with frequencies higher than 50 MHz, the diagnostic potential may be increased even further, thereby allowing an ultrasound study of the cornea comparable in its resolution to that of the optical microscope.

References

[1] C.J. Pavlin, K. Harasiewicz, M.D. Sherar and F.S. Foster. Clinical use of ultrasound biomicroscopy. Ophthalmology 1991;98:287–95.

[2] C.J. Pavlin, M.D. Sherar and F.S. Foster. Subsurface ultrasound microscopic imaging of the intact eye. Ophthalmology 1990;97:244–250.

[3] D.J. Coleman, F.L. Lizzi and R.L. Jack. Ultrasonography of the Eye and Orbit. Philadelphia: Lea & Febiger, 1977.

[4] C.J. Pavlin, J.A. McWhae, H.D. McGowan and F. Stuart Foster. Ultrasound biomicroscopy of anterior segment tumors. Ophthalmology 1992;99:1220–1228.

[5] C.J. Pavlin, K. Harasiewicz and F.S. Foster. Ultrasound biomicroscopy of anterior segment structures in normal and glaucomatous eyes. Am. J. Ophthalmol. 1992;113:381–389.
[6] C.J. Pavlin, R. Ritch and F.S. Foster. Ultrasound biomicroscopy in Plateau Iris Syndrome. Am. J. Ophthalmol. 1992;113:390–395.
[7] R. Ritch. Plateau iris is caused by abnormally positioned ciliary processes. J. Glaucoma 1992;1:11.
[8] U. Scherer and B. Osterheld. Echographic findings in cyclitis anularis pseudotumorosa and ring melanoma of the ciliary body. Klin. Mbl. Augenheilk. 1985;197:455–456.
[9] M.D. Sherar and F.S. Foster. A 100 Mhz PVDF ultrasound microscope with biological applications. Acoustic Imaging 1988;16:511–520.
[10] M.D. Sherar and F.S. Foster. Ultrasound backscatter microscopy. IEEE Ultrasonics Symposium Proc. 1988;1:959–966.
[11] M.D. Sherar and F.S. Foster. The design and fabrication of high frequency poly (vinylidene fluoride) transducers. Ultrasound Imaging 1989;11:75–94.
[12] M.D. Sherar, B.G. Starkowski, W.B. Taylor and F.S. Foster. A 100 Mhz B-Scan ultrasound backscatter microscope. Ultrasound Imaging 1989;11:95–105.
[13] C. Tello, T. Chi, G. Shepps, J. Liebmann and R. Ritch. Ultrasound Biomicroscopy in Pseudophakic Malignant Glaucoma. Ophthalmology 1993;100,9:1330–1334.
[14] R. Tornquist. Angle closure glaucoma in an eye whit a plateau type of iris. Acta Ophthalmol. 1958;36:413.
[15] M. Wand, W. Grant, R.J. Simmons and B.T. Hutchinson. Plateau iris syndrome. Trans. Am. Acad. Ophthalmol. Otolaryngol. 1977;83:122.

T. Avitabile
Institute of Ophthalmology
Catania University
Catania, Italy

17. Correlation of corneal thickness with blood glucose control in diabetes mellitus

L. PIERRO, E. ZAGANELLI, G. CALORI,[1] X. ROBINO and R. BRANCATO

(Milan, Italy)

Abstract

The aim of this study was to investigate whether there is a correlation between corneal thickness and glycaemic control in insulin-dependent patients. Ultrasound pachymetry and blood glucose measurements were taken in 87 patients three times a day: fasting, and two and four hours after lunch. The patients were divided into three groups: 30 without retinopathy, 30 with background retinopathy and 27 with proliferative retinopathy. Thirty normal age-matched subjects were the control group. No correlation was found between pachymetry values, blood glucose and duration of diabetes in the three groups ($p > 0.05$). A significant increase in corneal thickness was found in patients with background and proliferative retinopathy compared to the others ($p < 0.01$). There were no differences in corneal thickness between background and proliferative retinopathy ($p = 0.74$).

Key words: Ultrasound pachymetry, corneal thickness, diabetes mellitus, glycaemia

Introduction

Corneal thickness is increased in insulin-dependent diabetic patients with proliferative retinopathy [1]. No data are available on the correlation between corneal thickness and glycaemic control in these patients. The aim of this study was to investigate this correlation.

Subjects and methods

A total of 87 insulin-dependent diabetic patients (52 males, 35 females) were selected from the medical and eye clinics. Exclusion criteria were: previous eye surgery; corneal lenses; ocular hypertension; pregnancy or estro-progestinic therapy; high myopia.

G Cennamo and N. Rosa (eds.), Ultrasonography in Ophthalmology 15, pp. 163–167.

Blood glucose was measured with Dextrostix, three times a day: fasting (8 am) and at intervals of 2 and 4 hours after lunch (2 pm and 4 pm). Central corneal thickness was then measured by ultrasound pachymetry (Corneo Scan II Storz) with a 20 MHz probe. The operator (L.P.) took three consecutive measurements and the most frequently frozen value (SD$<$0.001) was recorded. Both eyes were tested. After corneal investigation, the patients underwent ophthalmoscopic examination with a Goldmann lens (E.Z.).

Corneal thickness evaluation, blood glucose measurement, and the fundus examination were each performed by examiners unaware of the results obtained by the others.

The population sample was divided into three groups on the basis of retinal lesions: 1) diabetics without retinopathy (n. 30); 2) diabetics with background retinopathy (n. 30); 3) diabetics with proliferative retinopathy (n. 27).

The age range of the sample group was 20–68 years, mean 37.66 years, SD 13.32. The mean ages of each sub-group were: 1) diabetics without retinopathy 31.27$\pm$10.58 years; 2) diabetics with background retinopathy 33.90$\pm$8.81 years; 3) diabetics with proliferative retinopathy 48.59$\pm$12.12 years.

The duration of diabetes for the 87 patients ranged from 2 months to 32 years, mean 13 years. In each sub-group the mean duration was: 1) diabetics without retinopathy 94.2$\pm$69.7 months; 2) diabetics with background retinopathy 141.3$\pm$74.2 months; 3) diabetics with proliferative retinopathy 247$\pm$63.8 months.

Control corneal thickness values were obtained by measuring 30 normal age-matched subjects, selected from the out-patient eye clinic, with the same exclusion criteria (age range 20–52 years, mean 32.6$\pm$11.42).

Results

There was no significant difference between the sexes in any of the groups (t-test). Two-way variance analysis showed no differences in corneal thickness between the right and left eye, or at any of the three examination intervals in any of the three groups. No glycaemic changes were found in any of the three groups at any of the three intervals (one-way analysis). Therefore, the right eye at 8 am was chosen at random for statistical testing.

The corneal thicknesses were: control group, 0.559$\pm$0.017; diabetics without retinopathy, 0.570$\pm$0.049; diabetics with background retinopathy, 0.061 0.041; and diabetics with proliferative retinopathy, 0.604$\pm$0.023 (Table 1).

Corneal thicknesses were significantly different in the background and proliferative retinopathy groups compared with the non retinopathy group ($p<0.01$, non-paired t-Student test; Fig. 1). There was no significant difference in corneal thickness between the background and proliferative retinopathy groups ($p=0.74$).

Mean fasting blood glucose values were 178$\pm$60.77 mg/day in the group without retinopathy, 227$\pm$78.14 in the group with background retinopathy and

Table 1. Corneal thickness in the four groups studied

Subjects	Mean corneal thickness	SD
Control group (n. 30)	0.559	0.017
IDDM without retinopathy (n. 30)	0.570	0.049
IDDM with background retinopathy (n. 30)	0.601	0.041
IDDM with proliferative retinopathy (n. 27)	0.604	0.023

IDDM = insulin-dependent diabetes mellitus

141 ± 38.39 in the group with proliferative retinopathy. Mean HbAlc was 7.6 ± 1.29% for the group without retinopathy, 7.6 ± 1.18% for the group with background retinopathy, 9.0 ± 1.2% for the group with proliferative retinopathy. Mean total daily insulin dosage was 28.32 ± 14.1 IU for patients without retinopathy, 39.5 ± 9.02 IU for patients with background retinopathy, and 22.0 ± 3 IU for patients with proliferative retinopathy.

There was no correlation between corneal thickness and any of the following factors: age of the patients, HbAIc, total daily insulin dosage, blood glucose concentration and duration of diabetes for each group (multiple stepwise regression analysis).

Discussion

Previous studies on corneal thickness [1–5] were performed with an optical pachymeter. We used ultrasound pachymetry to obtain more precise results and to eliminate errors intrinsic to operator interpretation [6].

In the hypoxic conditions that may result from trauma or from any malpositioning of the corneal lenses, the epithelium metabolizes glucose anaerobically, producing more than normal amounts of lactic acid. When this diffuses into the stroma it raises the osmolarity level, and gives rise to stromal edema [4,6]. Therefore, our study expressly excluded patients with corneal lenses and those who had undergone surgery. Reports on the correlation between corneal thickness and intraocular pressure are contradictory: a slight increase in corneal thickness with increasing intraocular pressure was noted by some authors [3,5], and the opposite effect was found by others [2,7]. Thus we also excluded any patients with glaucoma.

Patients who were pregnant or were receiving estro-progestinic preparations of any type were also excluded because they present increased corneal thickness. Hormonal changes lead to retention of water in the cornea [8]. In high myopia the cornea is thinner than in normal eyes [9], consequently, we excluded patients with high myopia.

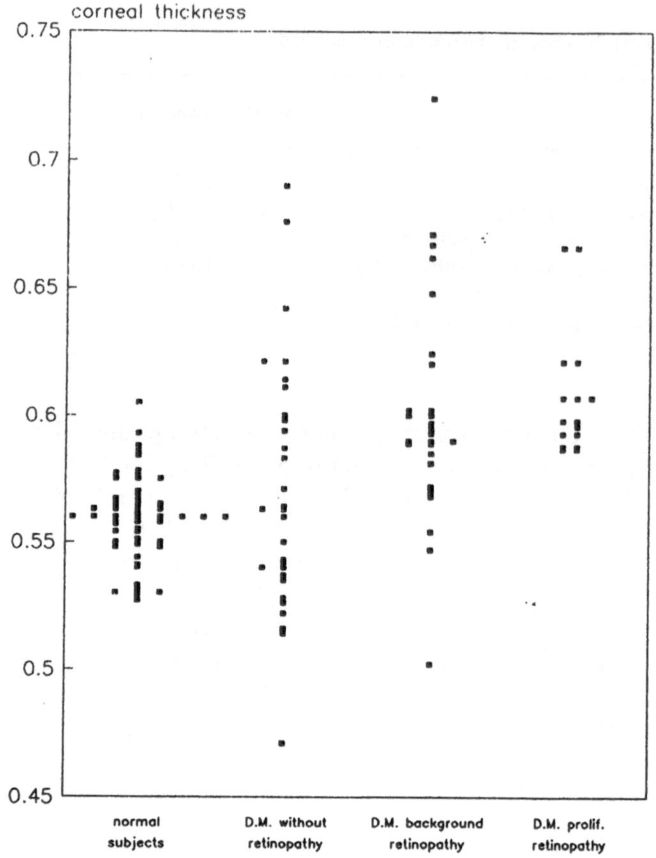

Fig. 1. The significant difference in corneal thickness in the background and proliferative retinopathy groups compared with the non retinopathy group ($p < 0.01$, non-paired Student's t test)

We included patients with proliferative retinopathy who had been treated by laser. Corneal thickness appears to be the same in patients with proliferative retinopathy who have undergone laser treatment and those who have not [1].

In contrast to previous studies [1] we found a thickening not only in patients with proliferative retinopathy but also in those with background retinopathy. Statistically, no differences were found between the proliferative and background groups ($p = 0.74$). Clearly, therefore, corneal thickness increases very early in diabetes, and could be correlated to the earliest retinal lesions. This seems to confirm the parallel behaviour of corneal thickness and retinal changes.

Like the vascular endothelium, the function of the corneal endothelium is to act as a cellular barrier. It does this by impeding the flow of aqueous humor towards the stroma and by extracting water from it, mainly by means of the sodium-potassium metabolic pump. Fluorophotometric studies have shown increased pump activity in insulin-dependent patients [10]. Patients with type I diabetes also present a reduction in cell density, with loss of hexagonal cells, which are theoretically the most stable [11]. If corneal endothelial function is impaired, corneal hydration suffers and consequently the cornea thickens [12].

Reduction of the negative charge of endothelium-aqueous humor interfaces, causes, in the corneal endothelium, the same phenomenon to occur in the avascular diabetic glomerulus [13]: reduction in the Na-K ATPase enzyme activity, with consequent alteration of bicarbonate outflow [14]. The lack of correlation between corneal thickness and the following factors: blood glucose levels at various times of day, glycosylated hemoglobin and insulin dosage casts further doubt on the role of metabolic management in the ocular complications found in diabetes.

References

[1] N. Busted et al. Clinical observations on the corneal thickness and the corneal endothelium in diabetes mellitus. Br. J. Ophthalmol. 1981;65:687–690.

[2] N. Ehlers. On corneal thickness and intraocular pressure. II: A clinical study on the thickness of the corneal stroma in glaucomatous eyes. Acta Ophthalmol. 1970;48:1107–1112.

[3] F.K. Hansen. A clinical study of the normal human central thickness. Acta Ophthalmol. 1971;48:82.

[4] M. Millidot. Effect of hard contact lenses on corneal sensitivity and thickness. Acta Ophthalmol. 1975;53:576–584.

[5] E. De Cevallos et al. Corneal thickness in glaucoma. Ann. Ophthalmol. 1976;8:177–182.

[6] R. Villasenor et al. Comparison of ultrasonic corneal thickness measurements before and during surgery in the prospective evaluation of radial keratotomy (PERK) study. Ophthalmol. 1986;93:327–330.

[7] J. Ytteborg and C.H. Dohlman. Corneal edema and intraocular pressure. II Clinical results. Arch. Ophthalmol. 1965;74:477.

[8] R.N. Weinreb et al. Maternal corneal thickness during pregnancy. Am. J. Ophthalmol. 1988;105:258–260.

[9] T. Tokoro et al. Central corneal thickness in high myopia. Folia Ophthalmol. Jap. 1971;27:610.

[10] J.H. Lass et al. Morphologic and fluorophotometric analysis of the corneal endothelium in type I diabetes mellitus and cystic fibrosis. Am. J. Ophthalmol. 1985;100:783–788.

[11] R.O. Schultz et al. Corneal endothelial changes in type I and type II diabetes mellitus. Am. J. Ophthalmol. 1984;98:403–410.

[12] B.O. Hedbys and S. Mishima. Flow of water in the corneal stroma. Exp. Eye Res. 1962;1:262–275.

[13] E. Schober et al. Glycosylation of glomerular basement membrane in type I diabetic children. Diabetologia 1982;22:485–487.

[14] J.W. Huff and K. Green. Characteristic of bicarbonate, sodium and chloride fluxes across the rabbit corneal endothelium. Exp. Eye Res. 1983;36:607–615.

Prof. R. Brancato
Department of Ophthalmology and Visual Sciences
Scientific Institute H S. Raffaele, University of Milan
Via Olgettina, 60
20132 Milan, Italy

[1]Unit of Epidemiology
H S. Raffaele, Milan, Italy

18. Two tumors of different origin in the anterior segment of a blind eye. Standardized echography with the immersion technique and histological findings

E. FRIELING and K. LÊ-RUPPERT

(Regensburg, Germany)

Abstract

A 42-year-old patient who underwent iris tumor resection 13 years ago presented with a blind, painful eye with a yellowish tumor in the anterior chamber and an epibulbar bumpy lesion. Standardized echography with the immersion technique showed the different origin of the two neoplastic lesions in the hemophthalmic eye with suspected total retinal detachment. The high reflective lesion in the anterior chamber was thought to be a part of the subluxated lens; the regular structured, low reflective epibulbar lesion was suspected to be a melanoma. Histologic and immunohistologic analysis after enucleation confirmed both diagnoses. The echographic findings and histology as well as immunohistology are described.

Key words: Standardized echography, intraocular tumor, anterior segment

Introduction

The immersion technique is an important method for echographic examination of the anterior chamber. It helps to demonstrate the tissue structures that are in direct contact with the probe. Furthermore, the waterbath shifts the focus of the B-scan transducer anteriorly from the vitreous to the anterior chamber. For the parallel sound beam of the A-scan the latter point is not important. Here we describe a case in which standardised echography performed with the immersion technique helped us to differentiate two tumors in the anterior segment of an eye.

Case report

A 42-year-old patient was referred for evaluation of a suspected tumor in the anterior segment of his left eye. In 1980 the patient had undergone iris tumor

G Cennamo and N. Rosa (eds.), Ultrasonography in Ophthalmology 15, pp. 169–177.

resection in Rumania; since that time vision had been low. During the last 3–4 months he had developed pain in his left eye and in the periorbital region.

The patient now presented with a blind left eye with marked conjunctival and epibulbar injection and a superficial and deep corneal vascularisation. There was a yellowish lesion in the temporal lower quadrant of the anterior chamber, which was partially in contact with the peripheral cornea and showed neovascularisations and hemorrhages on its surface (Fig. 1). In the inferior quadrant no iris tissue could be seen, whereas otherwise the pupil was maximally dilated. A membranous structure behind the iris hindered from visualization of the deeper structures. Covered by the lower lid there was a large, bumpy lesion under the conjunctiva (Fig. 2). The function of this left eye was 'no light perception'. The other eye was normal concerning anterior and posterior segment and visual function.

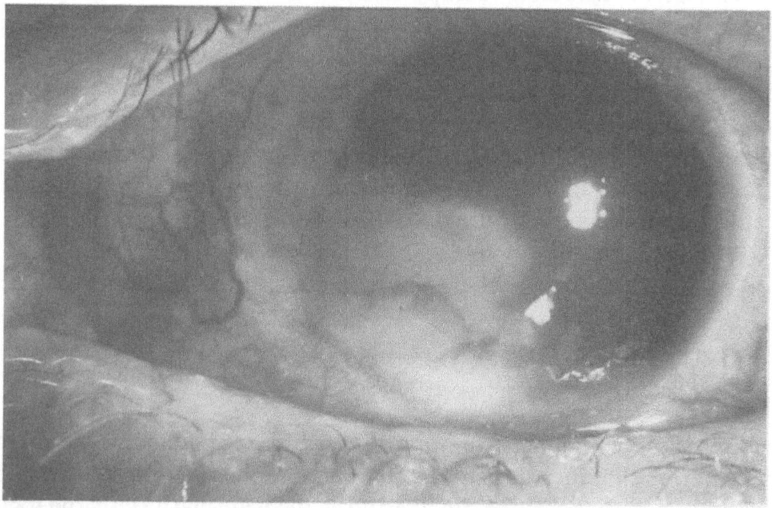

Fig. 1. Clinical aspect of the tumorous lesion in the anterior chamber

Echographic examination was performed with standardized A-scan and with B-scan echography. To obtain a better visualization of the tumors in the anterior chamber, the immersion method was performed with a contact eye cup. Echographic evaluation of the tumor in the anterior chamber with the immersion B-scan showed an oval lesion with irregular borders. It was in contact with the cornea in the lower third with membranous strands coming from the posterior segment (Fig. 3a). Furthermore, there were a few point-like, high reflective areas inside the lesion like foreign body signals.

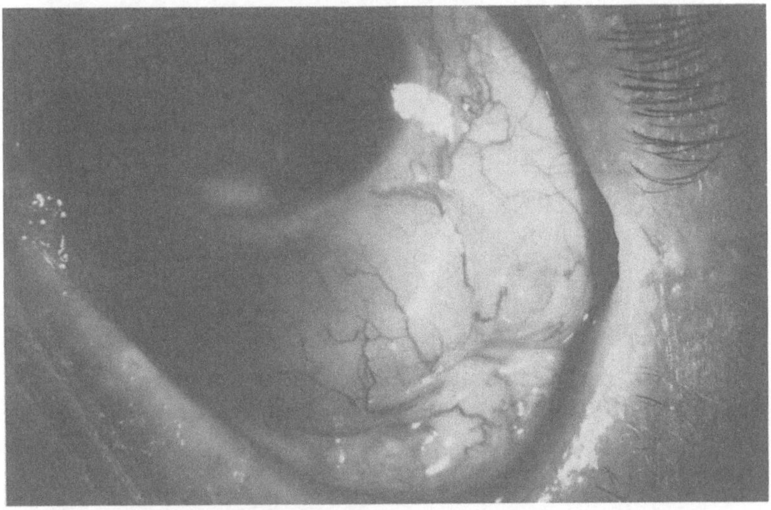

Fig. 2. Clinical aspect of the subconjunctival lesion

The standardized A-scan taken in the direction where the tumor was in contact with the cornea showed this lesion to be high reflective with fairly regular internal structure and with medium sound attenuation (Fig. 3b). These A-scan characteristics together with the calcification and the strands, which were thought to be infectious membranes, lead us to the diagnosis of a luxated lens or the remnants of a luxated lens. Other than in this location there was no structure which resembled a crystalline lens.

The second tumorous lesion under the conjunctiva was very different from the first lesion. The B-scan showed the lesion to be dome-shaped, sharply outlined, located on top of an intact sclera (Fig. 4a). With standardized A-scan the outlining structures could be distinguished; between these the lesion was low reflective (25–30%), mostly regular structured, with no sign for vascularity (Fig. 4b).

Looking at the posterior segment, an axial B-scan section showed membranous structures, which were tent-like, reaching from the upper to the lower ora serrata and to the optic disc, indicating possible total retinal detachment (Fig. 5a). The crystalline lens could not be demonstrated in the posterior segment. The vitreous space was filled with low reflective substance, fairly regularly structured indicating sanguis or inflammatory cells. When we tried to demonstrate the special maximal retinal echoes in A-scan, no 100% high spike could be obtained (Fig. 5b).

The blind, painful eye was enucleated and macroscopic sections were performed (Fig. 6). Histology revealed that the vitreous was filled with

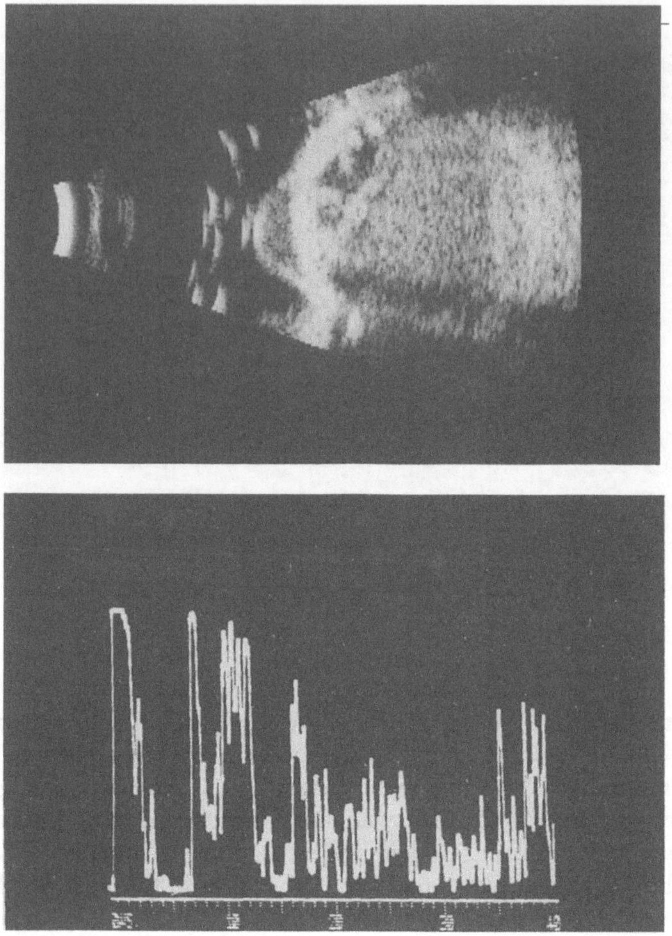

(a)

(b)

Fig. 3. B-scan (a) and standardized A-scan (b) of the lesion in the anterior chamber (immersion technique)

organized blood, the tent-like structure was shown to be the retina – as had been suspected. The retina was very atrophic in the anterior part and thickened with fibrotic changes in the posterior vitreous (Fig. 6). The white compact mass in the anterior chamber contained hyaline substance, atrophic lens capsule and point-like calcifications, so that this structure was diagnosed to be the lens (Fig. 6).

The subconjunctival lesion was round to oval shaped, macroscopically located on top of the intact sclera, without a clear sign of infiltrating the scleral structures (Fig. 7). Histologically it was composed of relatively monomorphic cells and showed a variable amount of melanin pigment, some mitotic figures and prominent nucleoli were seen in some cells (Fig. 8).

Because of the presence of numerous small capillaries within the lesion, we

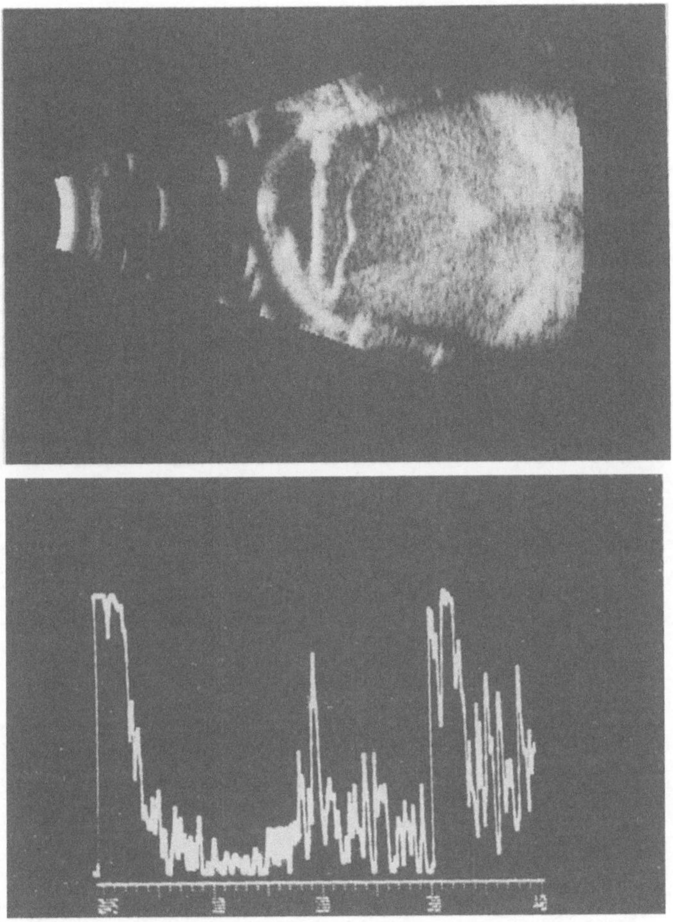

(a)

(b)

Fig. 4. B-scan (a) and standardized A-scan (b) of the epibulbar lesion (immersion technique)

performed immunohistochemical staining with Factor VIII and HMB 45. Factor VIII was negative, ruling out an hemangiopericytoma. The strongly positive reaction with HMB 45 confirmed our histological diagnosis of a malignant melanoma [1].

Most probably, this melanoma is a metastasis, originating from the iris tumor which had been resected thirteen years ago. Because of the regular, unaffected epithelium of the conjunctiva as well as the histological morphology of the tumor, a primary melanoma of the conjunctiva is very unlikely [2].

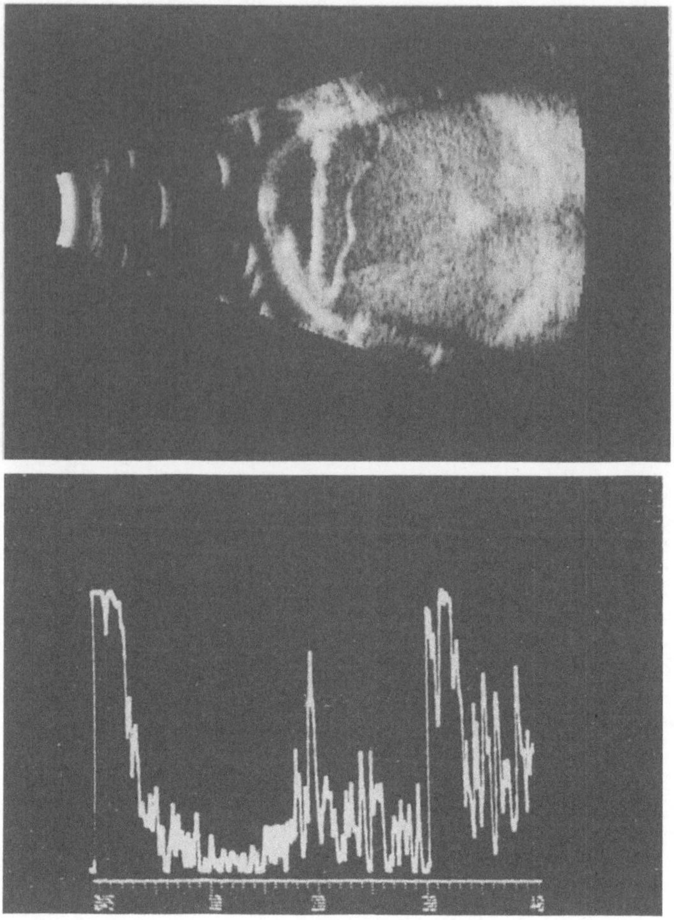

(a)

(b)

Fig. 5. B-scan (a, immersion technique) and standardized A-scan (b, contact method) of the posterior segment

Discussion

This case demonstrates three interesting echographic features. First the lesion in the anterior chamber; this had been correctly diagnosed to be a calcified subluxated lens by echographic characteristics (high reflectivity, irregular internal structure, marked sound attenuation and foreign body signals, indicating calcification).

For the second lesion under the conjunctiva, B-scan gave important topographical information. Because of the intact smooth sclera, scleral staphyloma and tissue prolapse could be ruled out. The most important information concerning the tissue differentiation however was given by standardized A-scan:

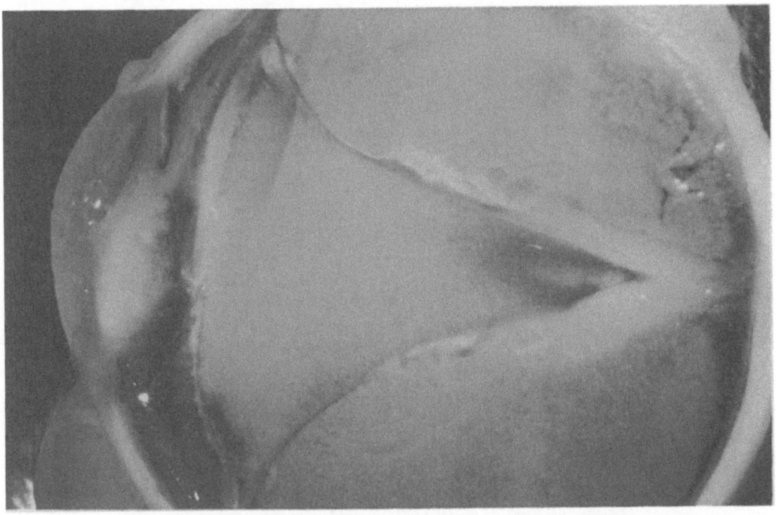

Fig. 6. Macroscopic section of the bulbus with the epibulbar and the anterior chamber lesion and the tent like retinal detachment

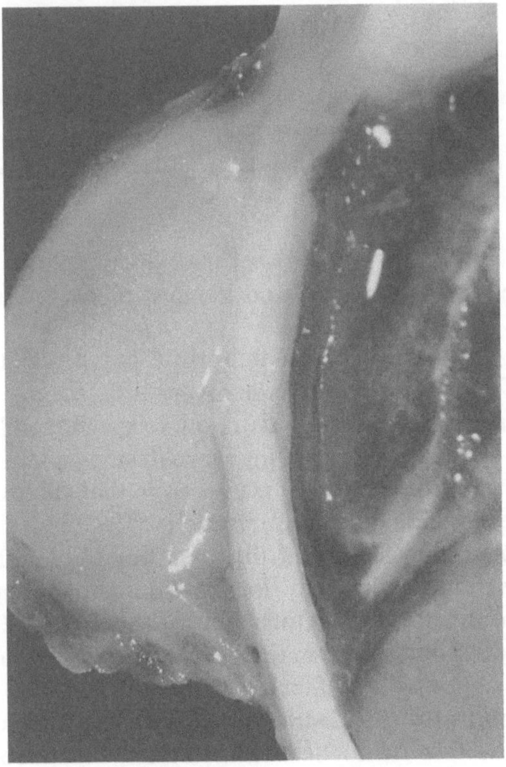

Fig. 7. Macroscopic section of the epibulbar lesion

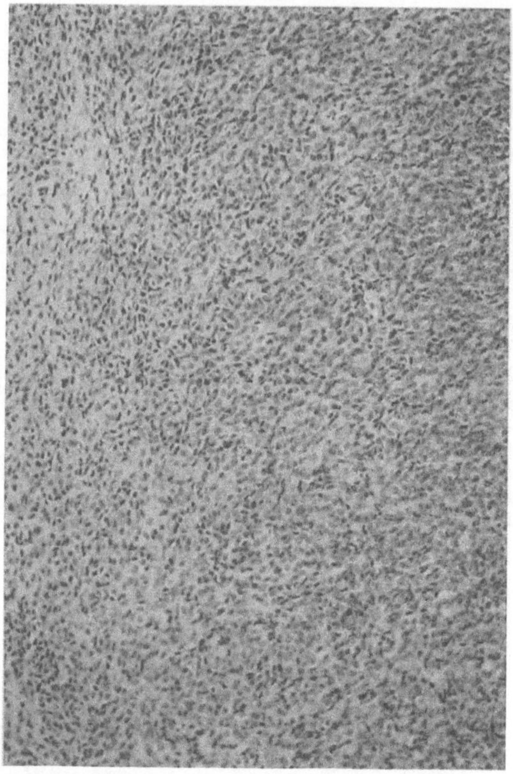

Fig. 8. Histologic specimen of the epibulbar lesion (malignant melanoma)

because of the regular structure and the low internal reflectivity a melanoma was suspected.

The histologic findings of an uniformly composed tumor with regular distribution of monomorphic cells and very little stroma in between seem to account for the ultrasonic picture with low reflectivity and regular structure, a similar picture is usually described for choroidal melanomas [3]. The reason why no vascularity could be detected by A-scan is that the tumor contained only small capillaries but no bigger tumor vessels.

The third interesting feature of this case was the tent-like structure in the blood filled vitreous, which by localisation and configuration had been suspected to be the detached retina. But the lack of a 100% high spike in A-scan, which is described as the major A-scan criteria for the retina by Ossoinig [4], made the diagnosis very difficult.

Histology confirmed the diagnosis and the macroscopic picture might give the clue why the retina did not behave like a retina in ultrasound (Fig. 5). On one hand this could be due to the long standing pathology with an atrophic or fibrotic retina in the posterior vitreous where the fibrosis changed the smooth surface and therefore made it less high reflective. On the other hand, the vitreous cavity was filled with blood cells, which caused a marked sound attenuation for all other intravitreal and retinal structures.

Regarding these three features the immersion technique was very important for diagnosis. It provided an easy to obtain recognizable topographic information with B-scan and helped to differentiate epibulbar structures and tissues which were located directly under or on top of the sclera. In addition, the immersion technique facilitated the examination by aiming the one dimensional A-scan at the right place and in the right direction, so that standardized A-scan echography could be performed, which like in this case, usually provides the most important information concerning the tissue differentiation of a tumor.

References

[1] J.J. Arentsen and W.R. Green. Melanoma of the iris. Ophthal. Surg., 1975;6:23–32.

[2] F.A. Jacobiec. Conjunctival melanoma: Unfinished business. Arch. Ophthalmol. 1980;98:1378–1384.

[3] K.C. Ossoinig. Standardized Echography: Basic principles, clinical application and results. In R.D. Dallox (ed.), Ophthalmic ultrasonography, comparative techniques. Boston: Little, Brown and Company, 1979.

[4] K.C. Ossoinig, G. Islas, G.E. Tamayo and C. Tamburelli. Detached retina versus dense fibrovascular membrane. Standardized A-scan and B-scan criteria. In K.C. Ossoinig (ed.), Ophthalmic Echography. Dordrecht: Junk Publishers, 1987.

Dr. Elisabeth Frieling
Department of Ophthalmology
University of Regensburg
Franz-Josef-Strauß-Allee 11
93042 Regensburg, Germany

19. Ultrasound biomicroscopy and laser treatment

T. AVITABILE, M.G. UVA, V. RUSSO, F. MARANO and A. REIBALDI

(Catania, Italy)

Abstract

We studied 19 patients by means of ultrasound biomicroscopy (UBM). This instrument works with high frequency probes (50 MHz) and it reaches an axial and lateral resolution of about 50 Microns. These patients were affected by anterior segment disorders and received laser therapy. We measured the anterior chamber depth before and after Nd:YAG laser iridectomy to evaluate the consequent changes in depth, and used quantitative gonioscopy to measure the value in degrees of the irido-corneal angle. Changes in cyst structure after Nd:YAG laser treatment were also evaluated. The results of this study confirm that with these instruments it is possible to follow conjunctival blebs after holmium laser treatment in patients affected by open angle glaucoma.

Key words: Ultrabiomicroscopy (UBM), laser therapy, glaucoma, anterior segment

Introduction

Laser procedures can replace surgery in some disorders of the anterior segment of the eye. Thus far, patients affected by these disorders and treated with laser therapy were studied with either optic biomicroscopy or ultrasound biometry. The 10 MHz B-scan equipment was not suitable because of its very low resolution, and because the probe must be placed at a specific distance from the anterior segment because the beam is focused.

In 1990, Pavlin *et al.* [1] developed instruments equipped with a high frequency probe (50–100 MHz), and with an axial and lateral resolution ranging between 20 and 50 μ. Because of the high resolution images obtained with these instruments they were called 'ultrasound biomicroscopes'. These *in vivo* images were comparable to fixed histological specimens.

Using UBM we visualized on an 864 × 432 pixels monitor an image derived from an area of tissue measuring 5 × 5 mm. At a very high frequency, the depth of penetration is approximately 6.5 mm. In particular, cornea, iris, ciliary body, anterior part of the lens can be studied at a very high resolution.

G Cennamo and N. Rosa (eds.), Ultrasonography in Ophthalmology 15, pp. 179–184.

Materials and methods

Beginning in May 1993, we used UBM to study 19 patients affected by diverse disorders before and after different kinds of laser treatment: 1) 7 patients (7 eyes) affected by closed angle glaucoma before and after Nd:YAG laser iridotomy; 2) 5 patients (5 eyes) affected by plateau iris syndrome; 3) 3 patients (3 eyes) affected by open angle glaucoma, in which we performed a holmium laser sclerostomy; 4) 3 patients (3 eyes) affected by pupillary seclusio before and after Nd:YAG laser treatment; and 5) 1 patient (1 eye) affected by a cyst of the anterior layer of the iris, treated with Nd:YAG laser.

1. Patients affected by closed angle glaucoma

In these patients we performed both UBM examination and traditional echography. Using traditional echography we can evaluate [2]:

a) the antero-posterior length of the eye, so obtaining information about the refraction (most of these patients are hypermetropic). In these patients it was 22.08 ± 1.44 mm.

b) lens thickness (5.02 ± 0.36 mm), which was increased in these patients. This also justifies the surgical treatment (ECCE+IOL), even when the lens is transparent [3–11].

c) anterior chamber depth, which is decreased (2.0 ± 0.27 mm) because of the lens thickening and its consequent anterior dislocation.

Ultrasound biomicroscopy provides more information than traditional echography. Indeed, because of the higher resolution of the instrument and the bidimensional images of the anterior segment, UBM leads to more accurate measurements of the anterior chamber. Furthermore, using special software it is possible to perform a quantitative gonioscopy before and after the laser treatment.

This instrument is very important in the study of the ciliary body. In fact, we did not perform laser iridotomy when we found, by means of UBM, that the intraocular hypertension was due to an 'iris plateau syndrome', because in this case the anatomical situation will be unchanged. None of these patients had an acute glaucoma attack before Nd:YAG laser iridotomy, all the eyes were treated with antiglaucomatous drugs. After laser treatment the anterior chamber depth was not changed (2.02 ± 0.24 mm); we also observed a significant peripheral deepening not detectable with traditional echography. Using UBM, we were able to study the profile of the iris convexity caused by the relative pupillary block, without the difficulties of previous optical technique such as the 'Scheimpflug technique' [12–13].

In all the eyes after Nd:YAG laser treatment, we found a decrease of the peripheral convexity of the iris. Using UBM equipped with special software, it is possible to make an approximate measurement of the irido-corneal angle variations. It is not easy to measure the iridocorneal angle because it lacks of reference points, indeed the iris surface is not flat and the inner corneal profile is concave.

Pavlin *et al.* [14,15] measured the distance between two lines drawn through two points separated by 250–500 μ from the scleral spur and perpendicular to the iris surface. Using our software, the angle measurement is performed setting the angle cursor in the iris recess and tracing two tangential lines to the endothelium and to the iris anterior surface. The angle values obtained in our case report were: values before Nd:YAG laser treatment: 11.58 ± 1.55 degrees; values after Nd:YAG laser iridotomy: 19.01 ± 2.38 degrees.

Our values do not coincide with those reported by Pavlin *et al.* [14] either because our instrument is not equipped with software to perform these measurements or because Pavlin used 62 and 80 MHz probes that have a higher resolution than our 50 MHz probe.

We can conclude that UBM is very useful to establish if the angle closure is due to peripheral synechias or to anterior dislocation of the iris root (lens thickening or plateau iris) in patients affected by closed angle glaucoma.

2) Patients with iris plateau syndrome

The plateau iris configuration consists in a normal depth chamber, a flat iris profile and a narrow or closed angle. The 'iris plateau syndrome' is present when the previous situation occurs and spontaneous angle closure is still possible, or after mydriasis when there is also a patent iridotomy [16,17]. Before UBM the anatomical condition of the iris root, which could occlude the angle, was unknown. Many authors tried to explain it by invoking such disorders as peripheral iris anomalies, lens alteration, and anomalous position of the ciliary processes [16–18]. In 1992, Pavlin *et al.* [15] demonstrated that the ciliary bodies play a fundamental role in patients affected by plateau iris. In their study performed on 8 patients, they showed that the angle formed by the iris and the ciliary bodies axis is significantly decreased and that the distance between the zonule and the posterior face of the iris is also decreased.

Because of the anteriorization of the ciliary bodies it is useless to perform an iridotomy in patients with plateau iris, because it is the peripheral iris that causes the angle closure.

We studied five patients with ocular hypertension (the intraocular pressure was high also after iridotomy), normal or slightly decreased (2.42 ± 0.17) anterior chamber depth, flat iris profile (observed with gonioscopy) and normal lens thickness (4.65 ± 0.4 mm). Ultrasound biomicroscopy revealed dislocation of the axis of the ciliary body towards the posterior surface of the iris; consequently, Nd:YAG laser iridotomy was avoided. Indeed, with this instrument the sclerocorneal junction is well demonstrated thanks to the different reflectivity existing between corneal stroma (low reflectivity) and sclera (high reflectivity). The ciliary body is well defined with respect to the sclera because of its low reflectivity. Reflectivity is different depending on whether the ultrasound beam crosses a ciliary process or vallecules.

The scans are very important in ciliary body evaluation. Indeed, using a longitudinal scan the ciliary body appears localized under the iris. This scan allowed us to detect the anteriorization of the ciliary body. We like to use the scleral spur as a reference point because it is easily distinguishable given its high reflectivity.

The ciliary body can be enhanced also with transversal scan. This procedure is best performed with an immersion cup because, with the patient looking in a lateral position, perpendicular scan of the ciliary bodies can be performed, and artifacts can be avoided. With this procedure the processes and valleculas of the ciliary bodies can be studied in detail. Rarely, were we able to visualize the zonular fibers, either because of their low reflectivity or of their peripheral position.

3) Patients with open angle glaucoma

For two years, in our Institute, we treated therapy-resistant open angle glaucomas with holmium laser sclerostomy. After this laser treatment it is important to maintain the bleb open with subconjunctival injections of antimetabolites which delay the scaring processes. We studied, using UBM, three patients who had undergone this treatment. This method can be useful to evaluate the size of the conjunctival bleb and to monitor the scaring processes.

4) Patients with 'pupillary seclusio'

We performed UBM examination in three patients affected by 'pupillary seclusio' before Nd:YAG treatment. This technique reveals a modified iris profile (iris bombé) and synechias between the iris and the anterior surface of the lens. Using a special software program changes in the iridocorneal angle width before and after laser treatment can be measured. It is also possible to show the pupillary synechias close to the iris root. Therefore, the information obtained with this technique allows the surgeon to identify the site where iridotomy should be performed.

5) Patients with iris posterior layer cysts

Finally, using UBM, it is relatively easy to study neoformations of the anterior segment. In particular, differently from traditional echography, UBM distinguishes a solid from a cystic neoformation. Pavlin *et al.* [1,19] attempted to perform a tissue characterization diagnosis of different tumors.

Based on our experience of 14 iris neoformations (11 cystic lesions, 3 solid lesions), a UBM examination should be performed before laser treatment of these tumors, because with UBM one may define exactly the borders of the lesion, the wall thickness, its contents, and the anterior or posterior layer origin. Ultrasound biomicroscopy also shows whether there is a malignant tumor under the lesion.

Among the 14 lesions studied, we treated only one patient with laser (an iris anterior layer cyst located in the iridocorneal angle). The UBM examination before Nd:YAG laser treatment provided information about contents, and in particular we did not find any malignancy under the visible lesion. After laser treatment we found changes in the shape of the irido-corneal angle and reattachment of the anterior layer of the iris to the iris stroma.

References

[1] C.J. Pavlin, M.D. Sherar and F.S. Foster. Subsurface ultrasound microscopic imaging of the intact eye. Ophthalmology 1990;97:244-250.

[2] T. Avitabile, C. Marino, V. Russo and R. Ghirlanda. Ruolo dell'ecografia nella valutazione delle modificazioni di alcuni parametri oculari dopo chirurgia extracapsulare della cataratta in occhi normali e glaucomatosi. Clin. Ocul. e Pat. Ocul. 1992;13(4):173–176.

[3] A. Reibaldi and M.G. Uva. Glaucoma da chiusura d'angolo. In Ghedini (ed.), Trattamento del glaucoma primario. Milan, 1991;299–324.

[4] A. Reibaldi and M.G. Uva. Surgical management of closed angle glaucoma: our experience. Intern. Ophthalmol. 1992;16:405–408.

[5] A. Reibaldi and M.G. Uva. ECCE più IOL in camera posteriore nel glaucoma ad angolo chiuso: ipotesi di protocollo per studio multicentrico. Boll. Ocul. 1993;72(2):257–267.

[6] A. Reibaldi, M.G. Uva, V. Russo, S. Sciacca and S. D'Asero. Il glaucoma 'irritativo' primario: trattamento chirurgico. Clin. Ocul. e Pat. Ocul. 1991;12(6):387–391.

[7] A. Reibaldi, M.G. Uva, G. Giannetto and S. Sciacca. Closed angle glaucoma: a new surgical trend and its rationale. New Trends in Ophthalmol. 1992:7(3):231–235.

[8] A. Reibaldi, M.G. Uva, J.P. Ott and V. Russo. Ein neues chirurgisches Vorgehen beim Winkelblockglaukom. Klin. Mbl., Augenheilk 1992:200;658–661.

[9] M.G. Uva, G. Scalia, G. Panta, F. Valvo and A. Reibaldi. Modificazioni di alcuni parametri oculari dopo chirurgia extracapsulare della cataratta in occhi normali e glaucomatosi. Boll. Ocul. 1991;70(1):289.

[10] M.G. Uva, G. Scalia and F. Valvo. ECCE + IOL in camera posteriore: studio tonografico. Boll. Ocul. 1991;70(2):215–222.

[11] M.G. Uva, G. Panta, F. Cafà, V. Russo and A. Reibaldi. Follow up di occhi con glaucoma ad angolo chiuso operati di sola ECCE con impianto di lente a disco compressible nel sacco. Boll. Ocul. 1992;71(1):101–108.

[12] J.C. Jin and D.R. Anderson. The effect of iridotomy on iris contour. Am. J. Ophthalmol. 1990;110:260.

[13] D.R. Anderson, J.C. Jin and M.M. Wright. The physiologic characteristics of relative pupillary block. Am. J. Ophthalmol. 1991;111:344.

[14] C.J. Pavlin, K. Harasiewicz and F.S. Foster. Ultrasound biomicroscopy of anterior segment structures in normal and glaucomatous eyes. Am. J. Ophthalmol. 1992;113:381-389.

[15] C.J. Pavlin, J.A. McWhae, H.D. McGowan, F. Stuart Foster. Ultrasound biomicroscopy of anterior segment tumors. Ophthalmology 1992;99(8):1220-1228.

[16] R. Tornquist. Angle closure glaucoma in an eye with a plateau type of iris. Acta Ophthalmol. 1958;36:413.

[17] R.F. Lowe and R. Ritch. Angle closure glaucoma. Clinical types. In R. Ritch, M.B. Shield and T. Krupin (eds), The Glaucomas. St. Louis: C.V. Mosby, 1989:845.

[18] R.F. Lowe. Plateau iris. Aust. J. Ophthalmol. 1981;9:71.
[19] C.J. Pavlin, K. Harasiewicz, M.D. Sherar and F.S. Foster. Clinical use of ultrasound biomicroscopy. Ophthalmology 1991;98:287–295.
[20] T. Avitabile, V. Russo and R. Ghirlanda. Primi risultati dell'utilizzo dell'utrabiomicroscopio nello studio delle patologie del segmento anteriore. Clin. Ocul. e Pat. Ocul. 1994;16(3):194–200.
[21] C.J. Pavlin, R. Ritch and F.S. Foster. Ultrasound biomicroscopy in Plateau Iris Syndrome. Am. J. Ophthalmol. 1992;113:390–395.
[22] A. Reibaldi and M.G. Uva. ECCE più IOL in camera posteriore nel glaucoma ad angolo chiuso: oggi. IX AISG Congress, Rapallo, 13–14 March 1993 (in press)
[23] R. Ritch. Plateau iris is caused by abnormally positioned ciliary processes. J. Glaucoma 1992;1:11.
[24] M.D. Sherar and F.S. Foster. Ultrasound backscatter microscopy. IEEE Ultrasonics Symposium Proc. 1988;1:959–966.
[25] M.D. Sherar and F.S. Foster. A 100 Mhz PVDF ultrasound microscope with biological applications. Acoust. Imaging 1988;16:511–520.
[26] M.D. Sherar, B.G. Starkowski, W.B. Taylor and F.S. Foster. A 100 Mhz B-Scan ultrasound backscatter microscope. Ultrasound Imaging 1989;11:95–105.
[27] M.D. Sherar and F.S. Foster. The design and fabrication of high frequency poly (vinylidene fluoride) transducers. Ultrasound Imaging 1989;11:75–94.

T. Avitabile
Institute of Ophthalmology
Catania University
Via Bambino 32
95124 Catania, Italy

20. Ultrasound biomicroscopy in the study of glaucoma

T. AVITABILE, V. RUSSO, M.G. UVA and A. REIBALDI

(Catania, Italy)

Abstract

The high frequency Humphrey UBM System 840 produces bidimensional images of the anterior segment of the eye with a very high resolution (about 50 μ) that are useful to determine the underlying physiopathologic mechanisms in various kinds of glaucoma. With this instrument we studied 20 glaucomatous patients and described the usefulness of quantitative gonioscopy and anterior chamber biometry, in: five eyes with plateau iris syndrome; five eyes with closed angle glaucoma before and after undergoing an ECCE+IOL surgery; seven eyes with closed angle glaucoma before and after Nd:YAG laser treatment; and three eyes affected by pigmentary glaucoma.

Key words: Echography, ultrasound biomicroscopy, glaucoma, iris plateau

Introduction

The physiopathology of some types of glaucoma, e.g., closed angle glaucoma, plateau iris syndrome, pigmentary glaucoma, can account for structural abnormalities of the anterior segment of the globe. A better understanding of particular anatomical features in these eyes yielded the recently proposed innovative therapeutical approaches [1–15].

Although ultrasonography, because of its poor resolution, has always played a secondary role in the study of disorders of the anterior segment in presence of clear media, UBM, which provides high resolution images *in vivo*, is a new means with which to examine the cornea, irido-corneal angle, iris, ciliary body, zonule, posterior chamber by high resolution images [16–20]. With this technique, information not obtainable by other semeiotic means, helped us to select the correct treatment.

We previously described the use of traditional echography in the study of glaucomatous eyes [21–23]. In the present study we describe our experience with ultrasound biomicroscopy (UBM).

G Cennamo and N. Rosa (eds.), Ultrasonography in Ophthalmology 15, pp. 185–190.

Patients and methods

At the Institute of Ophthalmology of the University of Catania we have used the UBM System 840 (Humphrey Instruments, San Leandro, CA) since May 1993.

This system is based on a 50 MHz transducer integrated with a high resolution B-scan imaging device. Axial and lateral resolution is about 50 μ and tissue penetration is approximately 6.5 mm. Therefore, cross sectional images of the anterior globe at microscopic resolution can be obtained. Further information about this device and the investigative technique has been reported elsewhere [24–27]. When necessary, we have combined UBM with traditional echography performed with an Ophthascan S echograph (Biophysic Medical).

Here we report on the following cases: 12 eyes affected by closed angle glaucoma treated with Nd:YAG laser iridectomy (plus ECCE+IOL in five eyes); five eyes affected by plateau iris syndrome; and three eyes affected by pigmentary glaucoma. We have also used UBM to study cases of secondary glaucoma with pupillary seclusio treated with Nd:YAG laser iridectomy; iris cysts treated with Nd:YAG laser ablation; and glaucoma in eyes vitrectomized with silicone oil.

Results

Eyes with closed angle glaucoma

In this group of 12 eyes, the preoperative echobiometric study, performed with the Ophthascan S showed an anterior chamber depth (mean $\pm$ S.D.) of 2.0 ± 0.27 mm; lens thickness (mean $\pm$ S.D.): 5.02 ± 0.36 mm; and axial eye length (mean $\pm$ S.D.): 22.08 ± 1.44 mm.

During the first examination no eye was affected by an acute attack of glaucoma; all eyes were under maximal antiglaucomatous therapy (C.A.I included). These data are comparable with those of our previous papers [3,4,23]. They are quite consistent with the particular anatomo-pathological feature of eyes with closed angle glaucoma which clearly justifies, as surgical approach, the simple ECCE+IOL implantation [2,9–12,28]. Further details about our surgical procedure are provided elsewhere [3,4,9–12,29].

After Nd:YAG laser iridectomy the anterior chamber depth showed no significant variations ($2.0. \pm 0.24$ mm) even if there was an evident peripheral deepening of A.C., not detectable with traditional ultrasound biometry. In the five eyes operated on with ECCE+IOL implantation, the A.C. post-operative depth was 3.6 ± 0.16 mm.

Measurements of anterior chamber depth using the UBM system are very accurate. We were able to measure the axial distance from the internal corneal surface to the lens surface with a finer positioning of end points, and the iris is easily distinguished from the lens surface (which, in the case of myotic pupils, is sometimes difficult using the traditional technique). However, the difference between the sets of measurements obtained with the two methods was not significant.

Bidimensional scanning permits measurements of the anterior chamber at points other than the axial position. The convex contour of the iris, owing to the situation of 'relative pupillary block' typical of these eyes [28] can be analysed over the entire iris length without the difficulties encountered with previous optical techniques, e.g. the Scheimpflug technique [30,31].

After Nd:YAG iridectomy, all the eyes showed a reduction in iris peripheral forward-bowing, and a much straighter configuration was observed, thus reflecting the fall of gradient pressure between the posterior and anterior chambers. These changes in iris profile were even more evident in eyes operated on with ECCE+IOL.

Using the software supplied with the UBM system, we were able to perform a rough measurement of these changes. Thanks to the good resolution imaging of the cross section of the angle structures we were able to assess interactively the angle measurement in degrees by superimposing two lines corresponding to the endothelial and iris surfaces. The angular opening values measured in our case report were: pre-operative values (mean $\pm$ S.D.): 11.58 $\pm$ 1.55 degrees; post-iridectomy values (mean $\pm$ S.D.): 19.01 $\pm$ 2.38 degrees; and post ECCE+IOL values (mean $\pm$ S.D.): 40.1 $\pm$ 4.12 degrees.

Because of the power of resolution of the 50 MHz transducer supplied with our system and the lack of dedicated software for analysis and measurement, we were only able to obtain gross values, that were not reproducible, and not comparable to those obtained by Pavlin *et al.* using higher frequency transducers [15–18].

Regarding the accuracy of UBM to define the state of the angle behind peripheral synechiae or to differentiate an appositional closure from synechial closure in a patient with clear media, because of the resolution of our device, UBM supports but does not substitute dynamic gonioscopy.

Iris plateau syndrome

In this group of five eyes, diagnosis had been made previously in the light of clinical signs (the intraocular pressure behaviour even after iridectomy, visual field, fundus), gonioscopy (extremely narrow/closed angle in the presence of a nearly normal chamber appearance due to a flat iris profile), conventional biometry (nearly normal anterior chamber depth: 2.42 $\pm$ 0.17 mm, normal lens thickness: 4.65 $\pm$ 0.4 mm).

At UBM cross sections these eyes showed an anomalous anterior positioning of the ciliary processes; they were immediately adjacent to the posterior peripheral iris, blocking the ciliary sulcus between the anterior surface of ciliary processes and the posterior iris surface. This picture was remarkably similar in all these cases.

These findings are consistent with Ritch's observation [32], according to which, the position of the ciliary processes provides structural support beneath the peripheral iris, preventing the iris root from moving backward after iridectomy. It is likely that even after cataract extraction, the ciliary processes remain anteriorly positioned and prevent peripheral angle deepening as observed by Pavlin et al. [17,18]. This finding supports our earlier speculation [5] that ECCE+IOL is inadvisable as antiglaucomatous treatment in these type of glaucomas.

Pigmentary glaucoma

In 1979 Campbell presented his theory that mechanical rubbing between anterior packets of zonules and the peripheral iris in predisposed eyes is the cause of the loss of iris pigment in pigmentary glaucoma [33]. At the American Academy meeting held in Chicago on November 1993 he described the new theory that reverse pupillary block in pigmentary glaucoma causes posterior iris movement and increases iris-zonule contact, and reported that this condition could be improved by iridectomy or by flattening of the iris. At the same Congress Pavlin et al. [19] presented a case report of 17 pigmentary glaucomas studied by UBM. Eight eyes showed posterior iris bowing, close iris-zonule relationship and increased iris-lens contact, nine eyes displayed a straight iris outline, separation of the posterior part of the iris from the zonules and reduced iris-lens contact.

We used UBM to study three cases of pigmentary glaucoma. They were being treated with Dapiprazole (T.I.D.), and follow-up was 6, 14 and 18 months, respectively. We examined the eye under passive myotic action and after suspension of the therapy (aimed at obtaining a steady-state test). In all eyes we observed, at the ending of passive myosis, an increase in posterior iris bowing, and with a reduction of the iris-zonule distance, iris lens contact was slightly increased.

Conclusions

Also in the field of glaucomatous disorders, UBM provides valuable information unobtainable with any other technique. With UBM the pathophysiologic mechanism has been clarified and the structural causes elucidated. We have found this device to be very useful and are looking forward to test its potential with higher frequency probes.

References

[1] E.L. Greve. Primary angle closure glaucoma: extracapsular cataract extraction or filtering procedure? Int. Ophthalmol. 1988;12:157.

[2] F. Gunning and E. Greve. Intercapsular cataract extraction with implantation of the Galant disk lens: a retrospective analysis in patients with and without glaucoma. Ophthalm. Surgery 1991;22,(9):531–538.

[3] M.G. Uva, G. Scalia, G. Panta, F. Valvo and A. Reibaldi. Modificazioni di alcuni parametri oculari dopo chirurgia extracapsulare della cataratta in occhi normali e glaucomatosi. Boll. Ocul. 1991;70(1):289–296.

[4] M.G. Uva, G. Scalia and F. Valvo. ECCE+IOL in camera posteriore: studio tonografico. Boll. Ocul. 1991;70(2):215–222

[5] A. Reibaldi and M.G. Uva. Glaucoma da chiusura d'angolo. In Il Trattamento del glaucoma primario, Milano: Ghedini Ed., 1991;299–324.

[6] A. Reibaldi and M.G. Uva. Surgical management of closed angle glaucoma: our experience. Int. Ophthalmol. 1992;16:405–408.

[7] A. Reibaldi and M.G. Uva. ECCE più IOL in camera posteriore nel glaucoma ad angolo chiuso: ipotesi di protocollo per studio multicentrico. Boll. Ocul. 1993;72(2):257–267.

[8] A. Reibaldi and M.G. Uva. ECCE più IOL in camera posteriore nel glaucoma ad angolo chiuso: oggi. IX AISG Congress, Rapallo, 13–14 March 1993. Boll. Ocul. 1994;73(2):271–280.

[9] A. Reibaldi, M.G. Uva, V. Russo, S. Sciacca and S. D'Asero. Il glaucoma "irritativo" primario: trattamento chirurgico. Clin. Ocul. e Pat. Ocul. 1991;12(6):387–391.

[10] A. Reibaldi, M.G. Uva, G. Giannetto and S. Sciacca. Closed angle glaucoma: a new surgical trend and its rationale. New Trends in Ophth. 1992;7(3):231–235.

[11] A. Reibaldi, M.G. Uva, J.P. Ott. and V. Russo. "Ein neues chirurgisches Vorgehen beim Winkelblockglaukom". Klinische Monatsblätter für Augenheilkunde. Klin. Mbl. Augenheilk. 1992;200:658–661.

[12] A. Reibaldi, T. Avitabile and V. Russo. Ecografia del segmento anteriore: da rudimentale visualizzazione a biomicroscopia delle strutture. Proc. XXVII S.O.M. 1994;141–168.

[13] A. Reibaldi, M.G. Uva, V. Russo, G. Panta and J.P. Ott. UBM e glaucoma. Cl. Ocul. e Pat. Ocul. 1994;16(3):201–205.

[14] D.G. Campbell. Pigmentary glaucoma. Another look at mechanism, and possible role of laser iridotomy. Chicago: Am. Acad., November 14–18, 1993.

[15] D.G. Campbell and B. Kurwa. Blinking, reverse pupillary block, iridotomy and pigmentary glaucoma. Scientific poster 53, Chicago: Am. Academy 1993;111.

[16] C.J. Pavlin, M.D. Sherar and F.S. Foster. Subsurface ultrasound microscopic imaging of the intact eye. Ophthalmology 1990;97:244–250.

[17] C.J. Pavlin, K. Harasiewicz, M.D. Sherar and F.S. Foster. Clinical use of ultrasound biomicroscopy. Ophthalmology 1991;98:287-295.

[18] C.J. Pavlin, K. Harasiewicz and F.S. Foster. Ultrasound biomicroscopy of anterior segment structures in normal and glaucomatous eyes. Am. J. Ophthalmol. 1992;113:381–389.

[19] C.J. Pavlin, R. Ritch and F.S. Foster. Ultrasound biomicroscopy in Plateau Iris Syndrome. Am. J. Ophthalmol. 1992;113:390–395.

[20] C.J. Pavlin, G.E. Trope, F. Feldman, K. Harasiewicz and F.S. Foster. High frequency ultrasound biomicroscopic features of pigmentary glaucoma. Abstract Chicago: American Academy, 1993;81.

[21] A. Reibaldi and T. Avitabile. Ecografia e Glaucoma. Boll. Ocul. 1987;Suppl.3:124–127.

[22] A. Reibaldi, T. Avitabile and M.G. Uva. The role of echography in adult glaucoma. In J.M. Thijssen (ed.), Ultrasonography in Ophthalmology. Dordrecht: Kluwer Academic Publisher 1988;235–243.

[23] T. Avitabile, C. Marino, V. Russo and R. Ghirlanda. Ruolo dell'ecografia nella valutazione delle modificazioni di alcuni parametri oculari dopo chirurgia extracapsulare della cataratta in occhi normali e glaucomatosi. Clin. Ocul. e Pat. Ocul. 1992;13(4):173–176.

[24] T. Avitabile, V. Russo and R. Ghirlanda. Primi risultati dell'utilizzo dell'Ultrabiomicroscopio nello studio delle patologie del segmento anteriore. Cl. Ocul. e Pat. Ocul. 1994;16(3):194–200.

[25] T. Avitabile, V. Russo, M.C. Sorce and A. Reibaldi. A new apparatus for the study of anterior segment disorders: ultrasound biomicroscope. XV S.I.D.U.O, Cortina (Italy), January 1994*(in press).

[26] T. Avitabile, M.G. Uva, V. Russo, F. Marano and A. Reibaldi. Ultrasound Biomicroscopy and laser treatment. Proc. X S.I.L.O 1994;239–247.

[27] T. Avitabile, M.G. Uva, V. Russo and A. Reibaldi. Ultrabiomicroscopia e laser. X S.I.L.O. Congr., Cortina (Italy), 1994.

[28] E.L. Greve and M.J. Wagemans. Reduction of intraocular pressure after extracapsular cataract extraction with posterior chamber intraocular lens implantation in patients with narrow angle. In Surgical Management of Coexisting Glaucoma and Cataract, Amsterdam: Ed. E.L. Kupler Publ./Ghedini Ed., 1987.

[29] M.G. Uva, G. Panta, F. Cafà, V. Russo and A. Reibaldi. Follow up di occhi con glaucoma ad angolo chiuso operati di sola ECCE con impianto di lente a disco compressibile nel sacco. Boll. Ocul. 1992;71(1):101–108.

[30] J.C. Jin and D.R. Anderson. The effect of iridotomy on iris contour. Am. J. Ophthalmol. 1990;110:260–269.

[31] D.R. Anderson, J.C. Jin and M.M. Wright. The physiologic characteristics of relative pupillary block. Am. J. Ophthalmol. 1991;111:344.

[32] R. Ritch. Plateau iris is caused by abnormally positioned ciliary processes. J. Glaucoma 1992;1:11.

[33] D.G. Campbell. Pigmentary dispersion and glaucoma, a new theory. Arch. Ophth. 1979;97(9):1667–1672.

T. Avitabile
Institute of Ophthalmology
Catania University
Catania, Italy

21. Preoperative standardized echography in penetrating keratoplasty combined with extracapsular cataract extraction and intraocular lens implantation

A. GALANTUOMO
(Naples, Italy)

Abstract

It is well known that K-readings change as a result of keratoplasty producing either steepening or flattening of the anterior corneal curvature; these changes depend on the preoperative steepness of the host cornea and the extent of donor/recipient graft size disparity. Under these conditions the preoperative calculation of intraocular lens (IOL) power is very difficult to determine and IOL power formulas can predict postoperative refractive error within 2 D of desired power in only 26–62% of cases. Furthermore, in case of unclear media it is crucial to perform a careful examination of anterior and posterior segments with echography, before performing penetrating keratoplasty, especially if combined with extracapsular cataract extraction and IOL implantation. We report our experience in 32 consecutive cases of penetrating keratoplasty combined with ECCE and IOL implantation.

Key words: Standardized echography, triple procedure, intraocular lens, penetrating keratoplasty, keratometry

Introduction

Over the last 15 years, the evolution of cataract surgical techniques, present knowledge regarding corneal physiopathology and the fact that penetrating keratoplasty (PK) brings about, per se, a more rapid evolution of incipient lens opacity have all led to a consensus among ophthalmologists that visual rehabilitation is more successful when, in those cases in which corneal pathologies requiring transplant are associated with corneal opacity, the commonly termed 'triple procedure' (PK, ECCE, IOL implant) is performed [1–3]. Numerous studies have shown that if cataract extraction takes place after corneal transplantation there is the risk of a secondary decompensation of the lemb through progressive loss of endothelial cells following PK [3,4].

The greatest advantage of triple procedure surgery is the quick visual

G Cennamo and N. Rosa (eds.), Ultrasonography in Ophthalmology 15, pp. 191–199.

rehabilitation, which is especially striking in elderly patients. However, it is difficult to calculate the IOL power in the case of a triple procedure. When IOL power is calculated for cataract extraction without keratoplasty, the post-operative corneal power is presumed to be unaffected by the surgical procedure, and can therefore be accurately measured by using the preoperative keratometry reading. However, with the addition of penetrating keratoplasty, the post-operative corneal power can no longer be assumed to remain unchanged from its preoperative state [5].

In the most commonly used IOL power calculation formulas the three most relevant variables are axial eye length, post-operative anterior chamber depth and keratometry. The K value influences the IOL calculation more so in the case of a triple procedure, because there are only small changes in pre- and post-operative AL and ACD measurements [6,7].

Previous studies have shown that K-readings change as a result of kerato-plasty, producing either steepening or flattening of anterior corneal curvature, depending on the preoperative steepness of the host cornea [8] and the extent of donor/ recipient graft size disparity [9–11].

Under these conditions, IOL power formulas can predict postoperative refractive error within 2 D of desired power in only 26 to 62% of the cases [4–7,9]. Furthermore, in the event of unclear media it is very important to perform a complete examination of the globe with standardized echography before a PK [12] so as to evaluate the preoperative state of the anterior segment (anterior synechiae, phakodonesis, lens dislocation, posterior lens capsule rupture and lens shrinkage) and to rule out the presence of vitreoretinal diseases (prolif-erative vitreoretinal membranes, vitreous haemorrhage, retinal detachment, glaucomatous optic nerve damage, age-related macular degeneration, intraocu-lar tumors and bulbar phthisis).

In this study we evaluated the importance of preoperative examinations with standardized echography in 32 cases of triple procedure. We compared the IOL power obtained with preoperative K readings from the receiving or fellow eye with that obtained using the average K readings based on our previous cases. In both instances, we used the SRK formula.

Material and methods

This study was carried out on 32 patients, on whom triple procedure surgery had been performed by the same surgeon. The patients were 17 males and 15 females, whose ages ranged from 24 to 75 (mean 58.4) years. Of these patients, 12 underwent a PK for a keratoconus, 10 for a herpes virus keratitis, 8 for eye injuries and 2 for bullous keratitis. All patients had undergone a complete preoperative slit lamp and echographic examination before the PK was performed in order to rule out the presence of anterior or posterior segment alterations which might have influenced the indications and prognosis of the implantation.

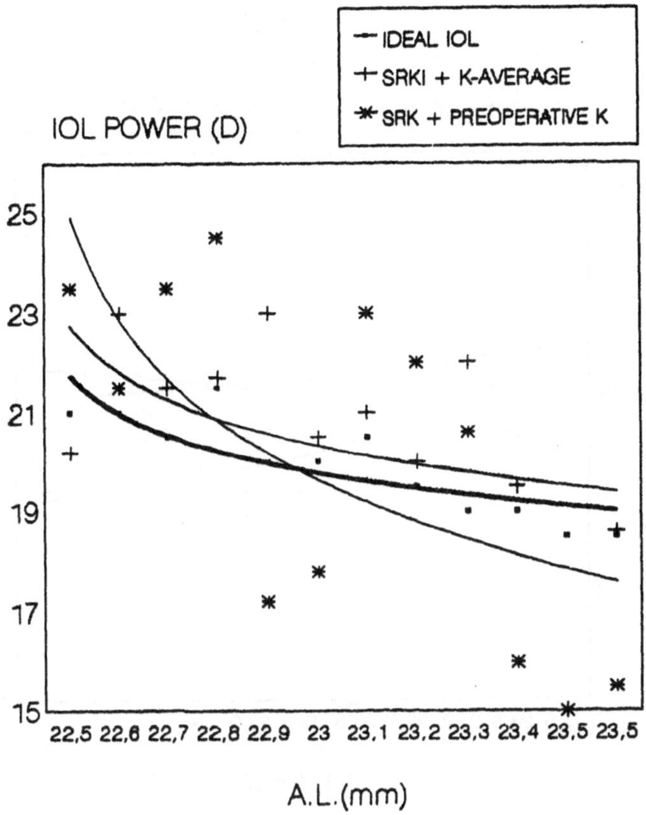

Fig. 1. Group I (12 eyes; 22.5 mm <axial length <23.5 mm)

Open-sky ECCE was performed by using an automated irrigation/aspiration unit for removal of the remaining lens cortex and a posterior chamber IOL was placed in a capsular bag. A peripheral iridotomy was performed and sodium hyaluronate was placed over the implant. The donor corneal button, with the same diameter as the receiving bed, was sutured to the host with double continuous 10/0 monofilament nylon sutures. The 10/0 nylon suture was removed at an average of 5 months after surgery, depending on the amount of astigmatism and on the biomicroscopic condition of the host/donor interface, and glasses were prescribed when the patient's refraction stabilized.

Preoperative keratometry was performed on all operated eyes when possible (45% of the cases). If irregular mires precluded reliable keratometry, an estimate was obtained from the fellow eye. Keratometry readings were taken preoperatively and at every postoperative visit in the steepest and flattest meridians, which were averaged. The mean preoperative K-reading was 43.52 ($\pm$4.23) D. All eyes underwent preoperative A-scan axial length measurement (mean, 23.65 mm), with the immersion technique and T-20 sensitivity.

The IOL power calculation was made by using the SRK formula with an

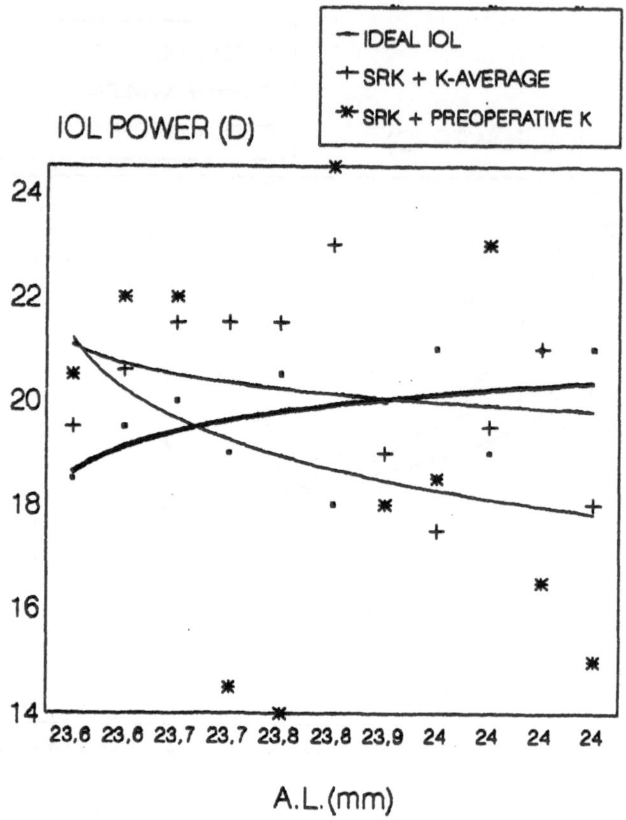

Fig. 2. Group II (11 eyes; 23.6 mm <axial length <24.1 mm)

average postoperative K-reading (44.25 D) based on 60 previous cases of the surgeon, after the removal of a continuous 10/0 nylon suture and at least 12 months after PK.

The refractive outcome obtained with the SRK formula with average K-reading was compared with the result that would have been obtained if the SRK formula had been used with preoperative K-readings of the operated or fellow eye. In order to select an ideal IOL power for the 32 patients, the final refractive outcome was compared with the desired refractive outcome, as determined before surgery, and the IOL power that would have produced the desired outcome was designated the 'ideal IOL power'. The IOL power resulting from application of the SRK formula with preoperative K-readings from the operated or fellow eye and the IOL power resulting from application of the SRK formula with the average K-reading based on the surgeon's previous cases were then compared with the ideal IOL in an attempt to identify the best approach for the estimation of the IOL power in triple procedure surgery.

Student's t-test was used for two-sample comparison and analysis of variance for comparisons of means from more than two samples.

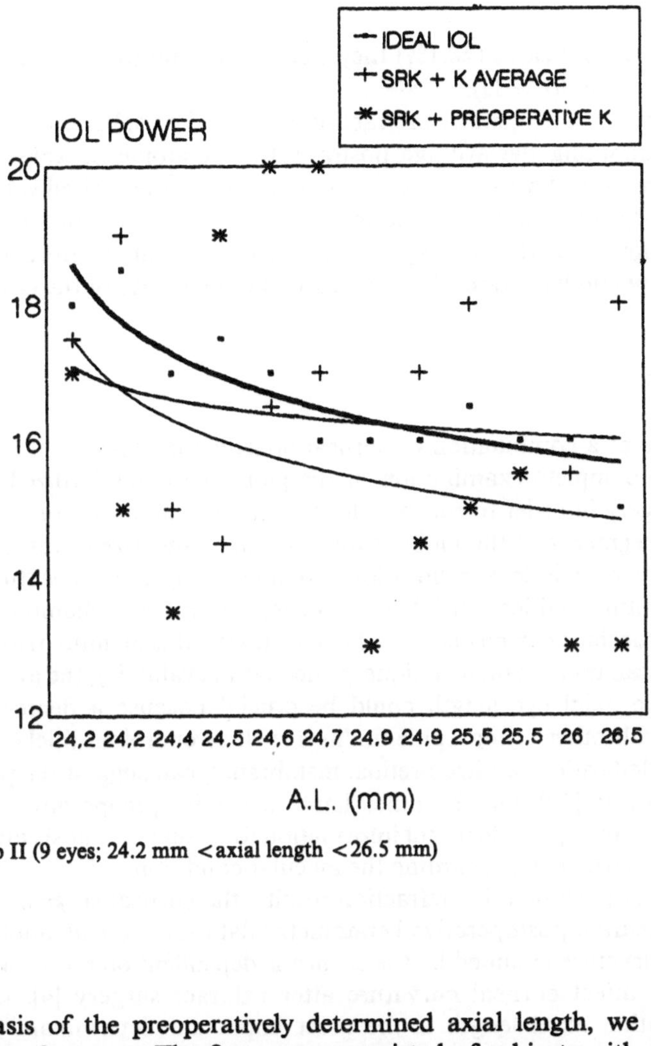

Fig. 3. Group II (9 eyes; 24.2 mm <axial length <26.5 mm)

Results

On the basis of the preoperatively determined axial length, we divided the patients into 3 groups. The first group consisted of subjects with axial length ranging between 22.5 and 23.5 mm (12 cases); the second group of 11 subjects with axial lengths between 23.6 and 24.1 mm range, and the third group of 9 subjects with axial length ranging between 24.2 and 26.5 mm.

All the data we collected were compared with the IOL which ideally would have produced emmetropia in each patient (Figs. 1–3). On the whole, the mean discrepancy between predicted power and ideal power was, by using the SRK formula with postoperative average K-reading, equal to 2.2 (±0.9 D, without relevant differences between the three groups of axial eye length considered. With the SRK formula and preoperative K-readings from the receiving or fellow eye, the mean discrepancy was 2.91 (±1.4) D. These differences were statistically significant ($p < 0.01$).

In 20 cases (62.5%) the average postoperative keratometric values ranged, after suture removal and after at least 10 months postsurgery, between 43.75

and 44.75 D; in 9 cases (28.1%) they were higher (up to 54 D), and in 3 cases (9.4%) lower (up to 37 D).

In summary, postoperative refraction expressed in spheric equivalent, measured by adopting the average postoperative keratometric value in the IOL calculation, ranged between ±2.0 D with respect to the desired value in 75% of the cases. By adopting the preoperative keratometric values of the receiving eye or the fellow eye, the findings would have been much more modest, i.e., refraction would have ranged between 2.0 D only in 54% of the cases.

Discussion

In the case of a combination of corneal opacity and cataract, it is essential to perform a complete examination of the globe with standardized echography before surgery in order to rule out the presence of alterations of the anterior or posterior segments of the globe. Moreover, in traumatized eyes, standardized echography reveals lens dislocation, volume changes, an eventual posterior capsule rupture and lens shrinkage. An irregular anterior chamber depth, with anterior synechiae can be better evaluated with the B-scan immersion technique.

The A-scan immersion technique is effective in evaluating the axial eye length (AEL). The axial eye length could be crucial because a decrease in AEL, together with other echographic findings such as choroidal thickening with or without calcification or vitreo-retinal membranes, can suggest the presence of a bulbar phthisis [12]. On the other hand, a careful preoperative echographic examination may provide useful information for visual prognosis after the triple procedure, particularly regarding the macular condition.

Regarding postoperative refraction results, the corneal surgeon is unable to provide accurate postoperative keratometry data for the lens implant because the final curvature assumed by the cornea is dependent on more variables than those that affect corneal curvature after cataract surgery [4]. Gabel *et al.* suggested that axial length is the most important determinant of the final refractive error [8], in that eyes with preoperative axial length measurements less than 22 mm produced a hyperopic refractive error, whereas eyes with an axial length greater than 24 mm produced myopic refractive errors. However, our finding of the lack of marked differences in the final refraction in the three groups of axial lengths considered, did not confirm their results, possibly due to a difference in lens calculation formulas and surgical techniques.

Corneal graft, cataract extraction and lens implantation were first combined by Taylor [13] in an implanted IOL of one standard power. Subsequently, several methods have been proposed to predict the post-operative corneal power: some surgeons used the preoperative K of the operated or fellow eye in their formulas [14]; but recently Katz and Foster [7] and Crawford *et al.* [6] demonstrated that recipient or fellow eye keratometry readings do not provide predictable refractive results after a triple procedure and the results emerging from our study seem to confirm such observations.

It has been suggested that certain eyes with marked preoperative deviation from normal in keratometry and axial lengths values would benefit more from two separate surgical procedures, namely penetrating keratoplasty and ECCE, followed later by posterior chamber IOL implantation, when post-operative K values have been stabilized [15,16]. However, the major disadvantage of a two-stage procedure is the fact that patients would be subjected to two separate operations and, of course, there would be an increased risk of graft failure at the time of secondary implant. Binder *et al.* found that a significant number of corneas failed after secondary intraocular lens implantation even with the use of viscoelastic substances [17].

Other surgeons use average K values derived from their own previous series on the assumption that there is no correlation between pre- and post-operative K values. However, Gabel *et al.* [8] found that preoperative recipient eye K-readings had an effect on the final refractive error and therefore separate regression equations may be necessary for patients with preoperative K-readings which are flat (<42 D), average (42–45 D), or steep (>45 D). Although the amount of change in corneal curvature between the preoperative and post-operative condition differs in these three categories, Gabel and coworkers found that the average post-operative K-readings at 12 months were similar, regardless of the preoperative K-readings; this was also true when using disparate sizes between the recipient opening and donor graft tissue.

Musch *et al.* [5] developed a regression equation resulting from the analysis of a previous consecutive series of triple procedure cases, in which IOL power = 56.95–1.62 × axial eye length. Using this formula prospectively in 52 consecutive patients undergoing triple procedure surgery, 67% of eyes were within 2 D of the desired refraction. However, when the regression formula was compared with the SRK and Binkhorst formulas (using K-values based on the surgeon's previous average 12-month postoperative K-readings), the results were not significantly different with the three methods of calculation. The authors conclude that even though a surgeon-specific regression formula relying on preoperative axial length performed as well as either the SRK or Binkhorst formula, the choice of which formula to apply remains entirely in the surgeon's discretion.

Our results suggest, in the case of a triple procedure, that the use of a K value of 44.25 D in the calculation of IOL power yields refractive values ranging between ±2.0 D of the preoperatively desired value in 75% of the cases. In our case study the IOL calculation was less precise when recourse was made to the preoperative keratometric values of the receiving or the fellow eye. The results of this study once again clearly demonstrate that the most important determinant of the postoperative refraction in patients undergoing the triple procedure are the postoperative K-readings. If one assumes that for each diopter of kerato-metry change, the refractive error changes by 1.5 D [18], then one can assume that for every 0.50 D of keratometry change, there will be a refractive error of 0.75 D.

In the current study, 20 of the 32 eyes had a mean postoperative reading within 0.50 D of the assumed mean preoperative reading and 75% of the patients achieved refractive errors within 2.0 D of desired refraction: Only in 25% of the cases did we have a superior myopia or mild hyperopia.

In conclusion, we are unable to derive a single formula to predict IOL power because of the wide variation in postoperative corneal curvature that occurred after penetrating keratoplasty. Among individual surgeons, and even in the hands of the same surgeon, there may be a variation in the recipient bed configuration, the donor button shape, the pattern of suturing, the depth of suture placement, the tightness of the sutures, and the ratio of donor to host diameters [6].

At present, therefore, we are still far from reaching a common criterion for IOL calculation in the event of a triple procedure, and the best results will be obtained by a careful re-examination of the average postoperative keratometric results recorded by each surgeon in a fairly large sample of patients.

References

[1] J.D. Hunkeler and L.L. Hyde. The triple procedure: Combined penetrating keratoplasty, extracapsular cataract extraction and lens implantation. An expanded experience. Am. Intraocular Implant. Soc. J. 1983;9:20–24.

[2] S.G. Kramer. Penetrating keratoplasty combined with extracapsular cataract extraction. Am. J. Ophthalmol. 1985;100:129–133.

[3] G. Rama and P. Rama. Cataratta e cheratoplastica. In Buratto (ed.), Chirurgia della cataratta nei casi complicati. 1991;285–315.

[4] P.S. Binder. Intraocular lens powers used in the triple procedure; effect on visual acuity and refractive error. Ophthalmology 1985;92:1561–1566.

[5] D.C. Musch and R.F. Meyer. Prospective evaluation of a regression-determined formula for use in triple procedure surgery. Ophthalmology 1988;95:79–85.

[6] G.J. Crawford, R.D. Stulting, G.O. Waring, W.S. van Meter and L.A. Wilson. The triple procedure. Analysis of outcome, refraction, and intraocular lens power calculation. Ophthalmology 1986;93:817–824.

[7] H.R. Katz and R.K. Foster. Intraocular lens calculation in combined penetrating keratoplasty, cataract extraction and intraocular lens implantation. Ophthalmology 1985;92:1203–1207.

[8] M.G. Gabel, R.F. Meyer and D.C. Musch. Intraocular lens power. In F.S. Brightbill (ed.), Corneal surgery: Theory, technique, and tissue. St. Louis: The C.V. Mosby Co., 1986;250–257.

[9] P.S. Binder. The triple procedure. Refractive results. 1985 Update. Ophthalmology 1986;93:1482–1488.

[10] W.M. Bourne, J.A. Davison and W.M. O'Fallon. The effects of oversize donor buttons on postoperative ocular pressure and corneal curvature in aphakic penetrating keratoplasty. Ophthalmology 1982;89:242–246.

[11] D.G. Heidemann, A. Sugar, R.F. Meyer and D.C. Musch. Oversized donor grafts in penetrating keratoplasty: A randomized trial. Arch. Ophthalmol. 1985;103:1807–1811.

[12] G. Cennamo, A. Loffredo, N. Rosa, A. Pezone and E. Guida. Standardized echography and triple procedure. In P. Till (ed.), Ophthalmic Echography. Kluwer Academic Publishers, 1993;13:415–420.

[13] D.M. Taylor. Keratoplasty and intraocular lenses. Ophthalmic Surg. 1976;7(1):31–42.

[14] D.M. Taylor, A.L. Starn and P.L. McDonald. Long-term observations. In F.S. Brightbill (ed.), Corneal surgery: Theory, technique, and tissue. St. Louis: The C.V. Mosby Co., 1986;250–257.
[15] S.C. Richards, R.J. Olson, and W.L. Richards. Factors associated with poor predictability by intraocular lens calculation formulas. Arch. Ophthalmol. 1985;103:515–518.
[16] W.J. Stark and A.E. Maumenee. Cataract extraction after successful penetrating keratoplasty. Am. J. Ophthalmol. 1973;75:751–754.
[17] P.S. Binder. Secondary intraocular lens implantation during or after corneal transplantation. Am. J. Ophthalmol. 1985;99:515–520.
[18] J.I. McNeill and H.E. Kaufman. A double running suture technique for keratoplasty: Earlier visual rehabilitation. Ophthalmic Surg. 1977;8(4):58–61.

A. Galantuomo
II University of Naples
Institute of Ophthalmology
Naples, Italy

22. The usefulness of echography before and after Osteo-Odonto-Kerato-Prosthesis

G.C. FALCINELLI, T. AVITABILE,[1] P. COLLIARDO, V. RUSSO[1] and R. GHIRLANDA[1]

(Rome and [1]Catania, Italy)

Abstract

The Osteo-Odonto-Kerato-Prosthesis (OOKP) is a particular biological prosthesis whose implant is performed in two steps: in the first, the cornea is covered with mouth mucous and an acrylic cylinder, fixed on an osteo-odonto layer, is implanted in the eyelid. Three months later, the cornea, iris and lens are removed and the OOKP is implanted. The role of echography before OOKP is very important because it allows us to evaluate such aspects of the ocular conditions as: the different corneal layers, the anterior chamber with the depth and content alterations; the pupillar diameter and the condition of the iris, the irido-corneal, irido-lenticular synechias, the lens anomalies, and the vitreo-retinal conditions that could make OOKP surgery useless. Because of the acrylic cylinder, only the posterior pole can be visualized with ophthalmoscopy. Consequently, the echographic examination provides information on the conditions of the peripheral posterior segment.

Because these eyes are often affected by high intraocular pressure, which is not detectable by tonometry, echography should be used to evaluate the optic disk excavation and, after OOKP implantation, any previous antiglaucomatous surgery. Here, we report our experience with traditional equipment, new generation B-scan and with high frequency equipment (ultrasound biomicrosopy; UBM), which is particularly useful in the study of the anterior segment of these injured eyes.

Key words: Osteo-odonto-kerato-prosthesis, echography, ultrasound biomicroscope

Introduction

The Osteo-Odonto-Kerato-Prosthesis (OOKP) is a biological prosthesis limited to patients affected by severe corneal injuries. This implant is performed in two steps: in the first, the cornea is covered with mouth mucous and an acrylic cylinder, fixed to an osteo-odonto layer, is implanted in the eyelid. Three months

G Cennamo and N. Rosa (eds.), Ultrasonography in Ophthalmology 15, pp. 201–205.

later, the cornea, iris and lens are removed and an OOKP is implanted.

In ophthalmology the echographic examination is essential in the presence of opaque media. It plays a very important role in patients who require OOKP surgery. Indeed, echography allows us to evaluate both the posterior and the anterior segment of the eye, which cannot be examined because of the corneal opacity or a symblepharon. Echography is useful both before surgery, as an aid to planning surgery, and after surgery to explore the retinal periphery. Indeed, the size of the acrylic cylinder implanted allows us to visualize only 30°–40° of the retina using ophthalmoscopy [1–5].

Materials and methods

To perform this study we used standardized A- and B-scan techniques. We used the following equipment: the Kretztechnick 7200 MA; Ophthascan S Biophysic Medical and Ultrascan System II Cooper Vision, equipped with an 8 MHz A-scan not focused probe and a 10 MHz B-scan focused probe; the Sonovision STT-100 equipped with a 10 MHz B-scan focused probe which can visualize digital images in grey scale and in pseudo-colour; the Humphrey UBM System 840, last generation ultrasound biomicroscope, which using a 50 MHz probe, gives bidimensional images with an axial and lateral resolution of almost 50 μ. The anterior segment examination was performed with a B-scan probe and immersion technique. The UBM equipment is very useful in this case because of the detailed visualization of the anterior segment structures. Indeed, it allows us to examine the different corneal layers, the anterior chamber and its alterations (flattening of the anterior chamber, atalamia, hyphema, etc.). Consequently, we can make very accurate measurements. We can also evaluate of the pupillary diameter, the iris conditions, the possible presence of irido-corneal or irido-lens synechias, and the anterior part of the lens. All these data obtained by means of echography assist the surgeon in planning this particular kind of surgery on the anterior segment.

We performed this study in collaboration with the Department of Ophthalmology of St. Camillo's Hospital in Rome; we examined 123 patients, 76 male and 47 female, ranging from 21 to 83 years of age (average: 53.8 years), from 1980 to 1993. All the patients were examined echographically either before undergoing OOKP surgery, to evaluate the anatomical conditions of the eye, or in the post-surgical follow-up, to examine the retinal periphery. Echographically, the acrylic cylinder reacts like a foreign body, causing a sound attenuation with shadowing of the posterior structures. With UBM, the cylinder ringing decreases because of the very high frequency and in this case, it is possible to perform an accurate examination of this eye.

It is more complex to perform an echographical examination in an eye that has undergone OOKP surgery than in a normal eye, because of the acrylic cylinder, which must be avoided during the examination [6–9].

Results

Using the above-mentioned techniques, we evaluated the various ocular structures. We evaluated anomalies in the shape and dimensions of the cornea, in particular we measured the corneal thickness using the ultrasound DGH 2000 pachymeter. The data obtained with pachymeter are useful to choose the acrylic cylinder; indeed, the posterior part of the prosthesis will be either in the corneal stroma or in the anterior chamber. The corneal thickness measurements are easier using the UBM equipped with a 50 MHz probe, with an axial and lateral resolution of 20 μ. The normal shape of the anterior chamber can be modified by anterior or posterior synechias, which, in particular cases, can resemble large membranes on the anterior surface of the iris and the lens, and the irido-corneal angle. Using the UBM equipment it is possible to measure exactly the anterior chamber depth, setting one gate on the inner corneal layer and the other on the lens anterior surface. The iris can be examined easily using the B-scan technique.

It is more difficult to perform an echographic examination of the pupil, although it is easier if the pupil is mydriatic; B-scan is possible using tangential ultrasound beam to the iris surface. The anterior chamber depth can decrease to atalamia, or can increase because of aphakia or lens luxation in the vitreous chamber. The angle structures can be visualized using UBM; thus it is possible to perform a quantitative gonioscopy and to detect the presence of synechias.

The lens shape and dimensions must be carefully studied to decide the best surgical procedure for its extraction – lens extraction being necessary in this kind of surgery. If the patient is pseudophakic we can visualize the presence of the IOL in the anterior or posterior chamber echographically. The echographical examination of the posterior segment is important to detect any vitreal or retino-choroidal disorder such as inflammatory vitreous alterations, recent or old vitreous haemorrhage, vitreous detachment, and age-related macular degeneration. In the case of traumatized eyes, it will be necessary to detect an endocular foreign body, a choroidal thickening, a choroidal or retinal detachment.

Furthermore we can detect previous surgery for retinal detachment and we can identify the type of surgical procedure performed (e.g., with internal tamponade substances like gas, silicon oil or PFCL).

In the glaucomatous patients we perform an examination of the optic nerve head to show an eventual optic disk excavation.

Strampelli's original surgical technique has been improved. In particular, the acrylic cylinder can now be customized. Indeed, on the basis of the axial length, obtained with ocular biometry, and of personal formula calculated to obtain the acrylic cylinder optical power, 'personalized' optical cylinders are prepared. The biometry is performed with the immersion A-scan technique. If there is a symblepharon which hinders the echography execution, the biometry is performed during the first part of surgery.

The role of echography is fundamental also in the post-surgical follow-up because of the limited part of the retina that can be examined by ophthalmoscopy. The most common pathologies that can be found immediately after surgery are vitreous haemorrhage and choroidal detachment. Vitreous haemorrhage can be studied with topographic, kinetic and quantitative criteria to evaluate both the progressive reabsorption and the membrane neoformation.

The choroidal detachment, in particular if localized in the pre-equatorial sector, can be diagnosed only with echography; with this technique the extension and evolution of the detachment can be evaluated.

An echographic examination of a patient who has undergone glaucoma surgery associated to OOKP shows unusual patterns. For instance, in cyclodiastasis there is a sovrachoroideal space extending from the limbus to the lateral rectus muscle insertion and communicating with anterior chamber: the iris root and ciliary body are separated from the sclerocorneal trabeculate and sclera using Supramid or Prolene 5/0.

The B-scan technique can detect diastasis because of an anechogenic sector localized between the iris root, ciliary body and choroids and scleral wall, caused by the aqueous humour infiltration.

Another kind of surgery consists in the insertion into the anterior chamber of a silicon tube 0.3 mm in diameter (length of 30–35 mm) whose posterior part is left free in the orbit.

In such cases, the B-scan technique reveals an unechogenic space due to aqueous humour accumulation in I and II Benedict spaces, behind the scleral wall.

Conclusions

Echography has rarely been used to examine patients who have undergone OOKP surgery, and there are no data in the literature on this topic. The echographical examination undoubtedly plays an essential role in these cases, both before and after surgery: before surgery because of opaque media and the structural alterations; after surgery to observe the posterior segment and retinal periphery, a procedure that is not possible with ophthalmoscopy because of the presence of the acrylic cylinder, which allows us to visualize only 30°–40° around the posterior pole.

It is difficult to interpret the echographical patterns arising from cases of OOKP surgery, because there are no previous reports and because structural alterations before surgery caused by the severe anatomical damage, and the presence of cylinder materials (bone, acrylic cylinder) after surgery cause various artifacts.

References

[1] F. Iannetti, and M. Liberali. Cataract and glaucoma in osteo-odonto-kerato-prosthesis. Ann. Oftalmol. Clin. Ocul. 1986;112(10):905–909.

[2] V. Marchi, F. Fiormonte and A. De Martiis. Osteo-odonto-kerato-prosthesis (the basic and the additional procedure). Part II: the cataract extraction procedure the retroprosthesis membrane treatment. Ann. Ottalmol. Clin. Ocul. 1989;115(4):349–354.

[3] V. Marchi. Osteo-odonto-kerato-prosthesis (the basic and the additional procedure). Part I: osteo-kerato-prosthesis operation. Ann. Ottalmol. Clin. Ocul. 1989;115(4):325–338.

[4] V. Marchi, F. Fiormonte, G.L. Manni and A. De Martiis. Osteo-odonto-kerato-prosthesis (the basic and the additional procedure). Part III: t-he surgical treatment of glaucoma. Ann. Ottalmol. Clin. Ocul. 1989;115(4):403-421.

[5] R. Ricci, I. Pecorella, A. Ciardi, C. Della Rocca, U. Di Tondo e V. Marchi. Strampelli's osteo-odonto-kerato-prosthesis. Clinical and histological long-term features of three prosthesis. Br. J. Ophthalmol. 1992;76(4):232–234.

[6] G. Falcinelli, A. Missiroli, V. Pettiti and C. Pinna. Osteo-odonto-kerato-prosthesis up to date. In F. Blodi (ed.), Acta: XXVth Int. Congr. Ophthalmol., Rome, Italy, May 4–10, 1986. Berkeley: Kugler, Milan: Ghedini, 1988;2:2772–2776.

[7] K. Hruby. Were keratoprosthetics a progress or failure? Fortschr. Ophthalmol. 1987;84(2): 142–143.

[8] F. Iannetti. Twenty years follow-up of osteo-odonto-kerato-prosthesis. In F. Blodi (ed.), Acta: XXVth Int. Congr. Ophthalmol., Rome, Italy, May 4–10, 1986. Berkeley: Kugler, Milan: Ghedini, 1988;1:1165–1168.

[9] V. Marchi. Results of 62 osteo-odonto-kerato-prosthesis. In F. Blodi (ed.), Acta: XXVth Int. Congr. Ophthalmol., Rome, Italy, May 4–10, 1986. Berkeley: Kugler, Milan: Ghedini, 1988;1:1244–1249.

T. Avitabile
Institute of Ophthalmology
Catania University
Catania, Italy

[1]Department of Ophthalmology
St. Camillo's Hospital
Rome, Italy

23. Corneal topography pachymetry

U. FRIES, C. OHRLOFF and R. MAKABE
(Frankfurt am Main, Germany)

Abstract

For refractive surgical procedures and medical therapy a correct assessment of corneal thickness is crucial. We conducted corneal ultrasound pachymetry in 200 eyes, and found that the peripheral thickness was significantly greater than central thickness (0.669 versus 0.54 mm). The thinnest point was below the center. The more distant from the centre the corneal thickness, the greater the upper thickness (0.689 mm) with respect to the lower thickness (0.627 mm).

Key words: Corneal pachymetry, ultrasound, corneal thickness.

Introduction

The importance of the clinical parameter corneal thickness is largely underestimated. The count of endothelial cell numbers and the evaluation of their shapes are well established methods; consequently, alterations in corneal thickness give a good indication of endothelial cell function. Correct evaluation of corneal thickness is an important parameter in cases of dystrophy, degeneration and treatment, and it is crucial for a good outcome of refractive surgery.

To obtain safe and accurate results the equipment must have a minimum standard such as the IEC-standard or German KV-Norm [1,2], with at least 20 MHz, a lowest axial resolution of 0.1 mm and a maximum tolerance in precision of 0.05 mm. Some early devices have much lower frequencies and are not sufficiently accurate for the needs of predictable refractive surgery, which might account for the rare spreading of corneal pachymeters.

To measure the low reflective corneal endothelium using high frequencies, the 'gain' must be increased, a procedure which might cause untoward bioeffects. This is very important because A-mode, which is used in corneal pachymeters, aims at the target that is more affected by ultrasound than it would be in the short strike by the B-mode measurement. If standard values of corneal mapping are obtained in a large population, the amount of ultrasound energy used in routine patients can be limited because it will be necessary to measure only the corneal region of interest.

In clear corneas, optical [3–5] and ultrasound [6–8] measurements can be

G Cennamo and N. Rosa (eds.), Ultrasonography in Ophthalmology 15, pp. 207–211.

performed. The optical measurement might be more accurate because of its shorter wave length, but the parameter-dependent calculation of thickness may be a source of error.

Method

We performed corneal pachymetry in 200 eyes of 100 Caucasian Central Europeans (50 females and 50 males). We used a system equipped with a 20 MHz contact probe with an integrated laminary introduction. The measurement was done quickly to avoid artifacts caused by drying on the anesthesized cornea (1 drop of 5% proximetacainhydrochloride) without using artificial tears or lubricating agents. Pachymetry was performed at 25 points, the center, and on three peripheral rings (2 mm, 4 mm, 6 mm from center); six measurements were made at each point (one point every 1.5 hours). The measurement was standardized in all eyes starting in the center going peripheral clockwise. Measurements were performed perpendicular to the endothelium/Descemet's membrane. The probe was applied very delicately without applanating the center of the eye. Slight applanation was necessary when applying the probe to the periphery because of the difference in the inner and outer curvature of the cornea, which looks like a small trapezium (Figs. 1 and 2). Slight applanation of the periphery is essential in order that the ultrasound is reflected to the probe. This is also crucial when measuring with lubricants to avoid the fluid meniscus being counted as part of cornea thickness.

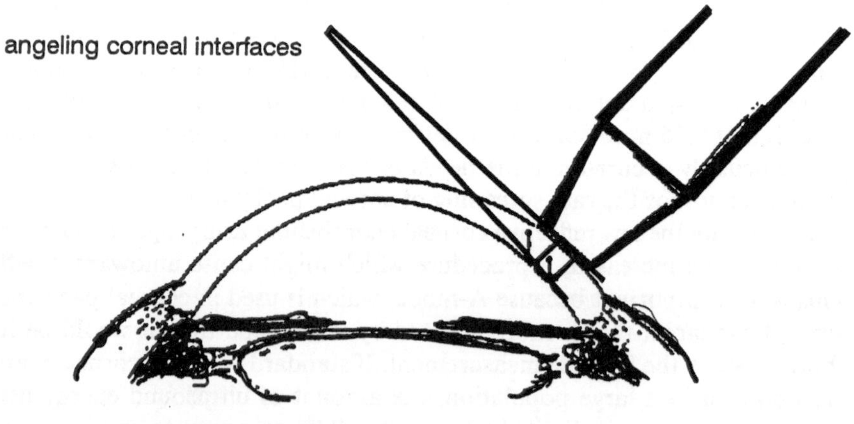

Fig. 1. Peripheral pachymetry measurement without applanation-angle between epithelial and endothelial tangent. Ultrasound beam will not be reflected to probe

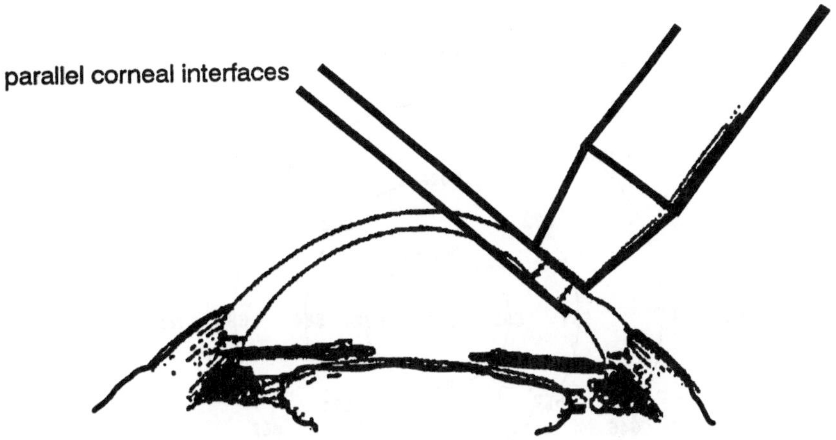

Fig. 2. Parallel tangents of corneal interfaces. Ultrasound beam will be reflected towards probe

Result

In all eyes the center was thinner than at the periphery of the cornea (Fig. 3). Central corneal thickness was about 0.54 mm. Cornea was thickest in the upper periphery (about 0.69 mm); the lower periphery was relatively thinner (about 0.64 mm; average: 0.05 mm). The thinnest point measured in our population sample was between 1 and 2 mm below center. The difference between right and left eyes was not significant. The average thickness of the concentric rings was 0.551 mm in ring 1, 0.585 mm in ring 2 and 0.669 mm in ring 3 (going from the center to the periphery).

Discussion

In early studies peripheral corneal measurements were made in post mortem eyes [9], however, those studies did not take account of *post mortem* swelling of the cornea, and thus, the results reported are not reliable for clinical examinations or for therapeutical or surgical purposes [10]. In clear corneas, an optical measurement can be performed, whereas in cases of opaque corneas caused by edema or scars the ultrasound examination is the only way to measure corneal thickness.

A study of corneal compressibility caused by applanation in corneal pachymetry demonstrated a lack of significant differences at applanation pressures from 0 to 80 mmHg [11], with an accuracy 2.5 microns. To use a similar technique with soft applanation causes no artifacts by compression, as the cornea has a non detectable compressibility during measurements.

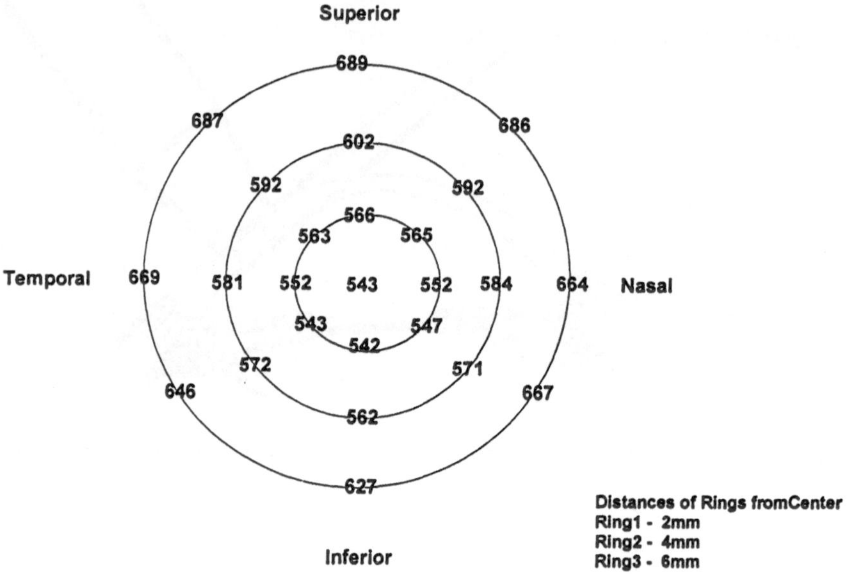

Fig. 3. Map of corneal thickness in pachymetry

The central corneal thickness in our population sample is in accordance with previous studies [8,12]. Ultrasound and optical measurements have been shown to be comparable [6,13], whereas corneal thickness was greater in cadaver eyes measured with ultrasound than with optical measurements [8]. However, the latter finding may depend on the device used; on the whole, indeed, the early pachymeters used lower frequencies with respect to modern equipment.

A difference has been found in thickness between the centre and periphery, even though it was not statistically significant [7]. On the contrary, the difference found by us was big. Moreover, we did not detect a decrease of peripheral thickness in our population sample in relation to age [12]. Even in elderly subjects (aged over 70 years) we did not detect any statistical or clinical difference with respect to the younger age group. This lack of difference might be due to a difference in the examination technique [11] or the probe used. The difference in corneal thickness that we found in this study corresponds to the changes in shape [14] (flattening towards the periphery of the cornea) found in photokeratography in normal eyes.

References

[1] Ultraschallvereinbarung. Dt. Ärztebl. 1993;90(8):390–403.

[2] IEC 1157, Genève, 1992.

[3] D. Green, B.R. Frueh and J. Sharpio. Corneal thickness measured by interferometry. J. Opt. Soc. Am. 1975;65:119–1213.

[4] D.M. Maurice and A.A. Giardini. A simple optical apparatus for measuring the corneal thickness and the average thickness of the human cornea. Br. J. Ophthalmol. 1951;35:169–177.

[5] S. Mishima and B.O. Hedbys. Measurement of corneal thickness with the Haag-Streit pachometer. Arch. Ophthalmol. 1968;80:710–713.

[6] P.S. Binder, J.A. Kohler and D.A. Rorabaugh. Evaluation of an electronic corneal pachometer. Invest. Oph. & Vis. Sci. 1977;16:855–858.

[7] N.K. Hiryi and J.R. Larke. Thickness of human cornea measured by topographic pachometry. Am. J. Optom. Physiol. Opt. 1978;55:97–100.

[8] J.J. Salz, T. Lee, J.V. Jester *et al.* Analysis of incision depth following experimental radial keratotomy. Ophthalmology 1983;90:655–659.

[9] M. Salzmann. The anatomy and histology of the human eyeball in the normal state. Chicago: The University of Chicago Press, 1912;26.

[10] J. Sobanski. Die Hornhautdicke in vivo und ihre Bestimmung. Zbl. Ophthal. 1934;32:354–355.

[11] A. Dybbs A. and O.D. Solomon. Is the cornea compressible. Invest. Ophthalmol. & Sci. 1993;34(4):1249.

[12] E.L. Martola and J.L. Baum. Central and peripheral corneal thickness. Arch. Ophthalmol. 1968;79:28–30.

[13] R.D. Lepper and H.G. Trier. Neuartige Ultraschallbiometrie. Klin. Mbl. Augenheilkd. 1983:177;101–106.

[14] S.A. Dingeldein and S.D. Klyce. The topography of normal cornea. Arch. Ophthalmol. 1989;107:512–518.

Dr. med. U. Fries
Universitäts-Augenklinik
Theodor-Stern-Kai 7, H8b
D-60590 Frankfurt/Main
Germany

24. Echographic evaluation of the Ahmed valves

E. MORAGREGA, C. VELASCO-BARONA, V. SÁNCHEZ and F. GIL
(México City, México)

Abstract

The Ahmed valves are one of the aqueous drainage devices used for glaucoma treatment. It has a venturi type valve that permits the drainage of the aqueous to the equatorial orbital space across a limbal shunt. The echographic characteristics of other valves have been described. We studied 24 patients with this implant, and describe the echographic characteristics at 4 weeks after surgery. We found that 33% had a large filtering bleb, 45% had a moderate filtering bleb and 12.5% had a small filtering bleb. The echographic characteristics are similar to those described previously.

Key words: Ahmed valves, glaucoma shunt devices, echographic characteristics, bleb, intraocular pressure

Introduction

Of the modern aqueous drainage devices used for the treatment of glaucoma, translimbal equatorial shunts are the most effective. Molteno, Shocket, Krupin, Baerveldt implants are the most widely used. These devices have in common an anterior chamber shunt to an episcleral, equatorial, bleb-promoting device or plate. A fibrous reservoir develops over the plate and accommodates aqueous humor drainage post-operatively. The surface area of this reservoir may be one of the key factors in long-term post-surgery control of intraocular pressure [1–3].

These four devices are similarly designed glaucoma implants that allow aqueous to drain through the tubes (which are placed through the limbus) into encapsulated spaces surrounding the equatorially positioned plates. Intraocular pressure is lowered as aqueous then passively diffuses through the bleb walls [4–6]. Because these aqueous drainage devices are positioned relatively posteriorly on the globe, the associated blebs are often difficult to detect clinically. In this context, Lloyd *et al.* have described the characteristic echographic appearance of the plates and the presence or not of the blebs [7].

G Cennamo and N. Rosa (eds.), Ultrasonography in Ophthalmology 15, pp. 213–218.

Material and methods

At the Association to Prevent Blindness in the Mexico Hospital 'Dr. Luis Sánchez Bulnes' we use the Ahmed glaucoma shunt device, because it has a venturi type valve. This means that when the pressure in the tube increases, the valve opens and the aqueous drains to the plate and to the episcleral space forming the bleb. There are several descriptions of the echographic findings related to the Molteno and Baerveldt glaucoma implants [7], but to our knowledge there are no reports about the echographic findings of Ahmed glaucoma implants. Consequently, we performed echographic examinations in 24 patients who underwent surgery with Ahmed valve implants. The examinations were performed using the Digital IV A–B Scan (Alcon).

Results

When the bleb was not present, it was difficult to distinguish the plate from the scleral wall. The plate however cast a shadow on the orbital tissue, and the shadow was more evident at the edges of the plate. Furthermore, when the bleb was absent, a thin echolucent line adjacent to the echogenic plate was frequently observed. In this case the line represented a small amount of fluid (Fig. 1). When a bleb was present, an area of echolucency underlying and/or overlying the plate was typically present (Fig. 2). The following very simple classification of the bleb sizes was used in this study:

No fluid	<2 mm in height
Small	2 mm to 4 mm
Moderate	4 mm to 6 mm
Large	>6 mm

When the echographic exams were performed 24 hours after surgery, most of the patients showed no evidence of a bleb formation (20 patients: 83.33%); but we did see a thin echolucent line adjacent to the plate, as described above, representing a small amount of fluid. One week after surgery, most of the patients showed evidence of bleb formation. The blebs were small in 10 patients (41.66%); moderate in 9 patients (37.5%) and large in 3 patients (12.5%). We re-examined the 24 patients at 4 weeks post-surgery and we noted that the bleb had increased in size in 22 patients as compared with previous evaluations. In this third measurement, the blebs were: small in 3 patients (12.5%), moderate in 11 (45.83%), and large in 8 patients (33.33%). In only 2 patients (8.33%) was there no evidence of bleb formation. When the bleb was moderate to large; it was related to applanation of the scleral wall (Fig. 3).

The plate is best located with B-scan using both transversal and longitudinal views.

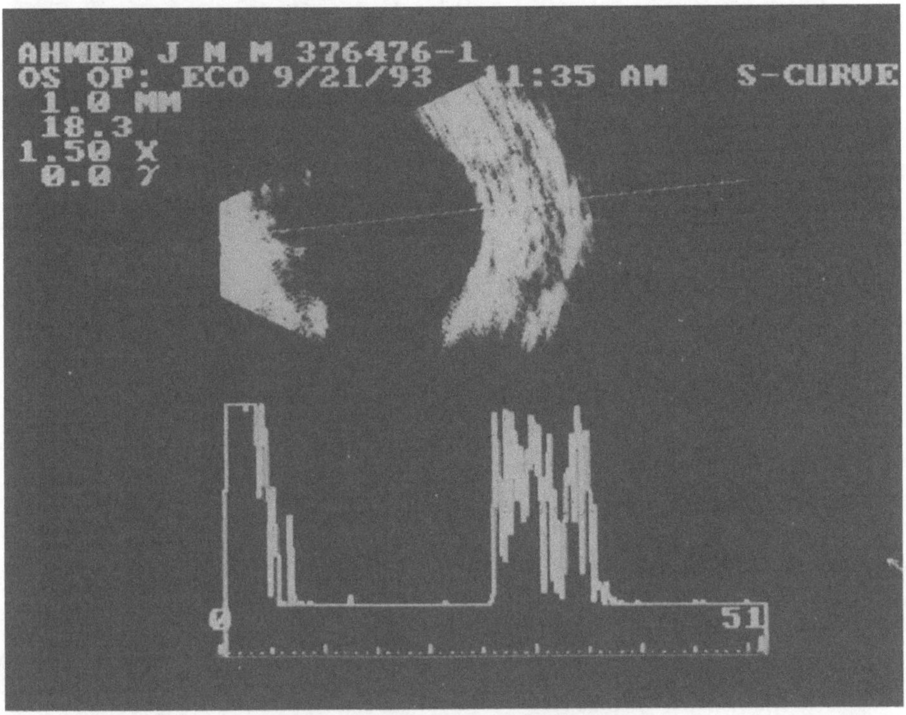

Fig. 1. Transverse A–B scan of the Ahmed plate. (P) plate, (S) shadowing and (E) episcleral fluid (thin line)

Conclusion

In summary, B-scan echography is useful in demonstrating the sizes, locations and characteristics of blebs associated with Ahmed valves. Echography is therefore useful in the postoperative management of patients with hypotony or elevated intraocular pressure who have undergone these glaucoma shunting procedures and in whom bleb existence cannot be determined on slit-lamp examination. The echographic characteristics found in this study are similar to those previously described by Lloyd *et al.* [7].

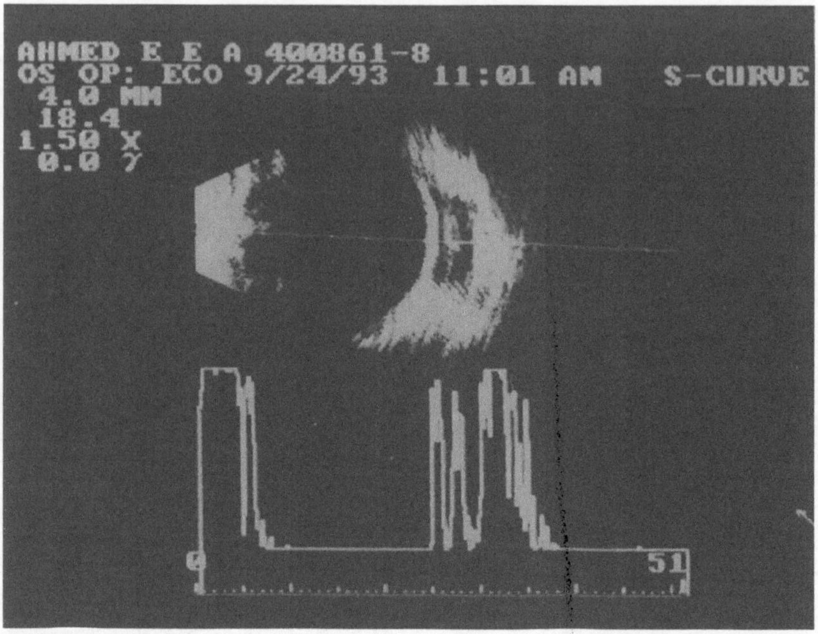

(a)

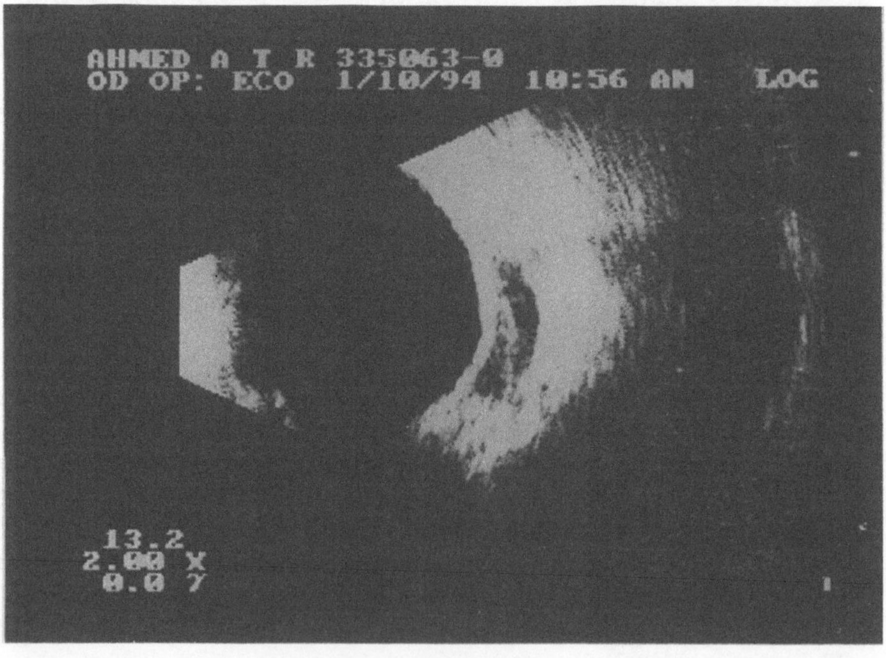

(b)

Fig. 2. a) Transverse A–B scan of the Ahmed plate with overlying and underlying bleb. b) Transverse B-scan of the Ahmed plate with overlying and underlying bleb. c) A-scan of the Ahmed plate with associated underlying and overlying bleb. The plate is represented by one spike

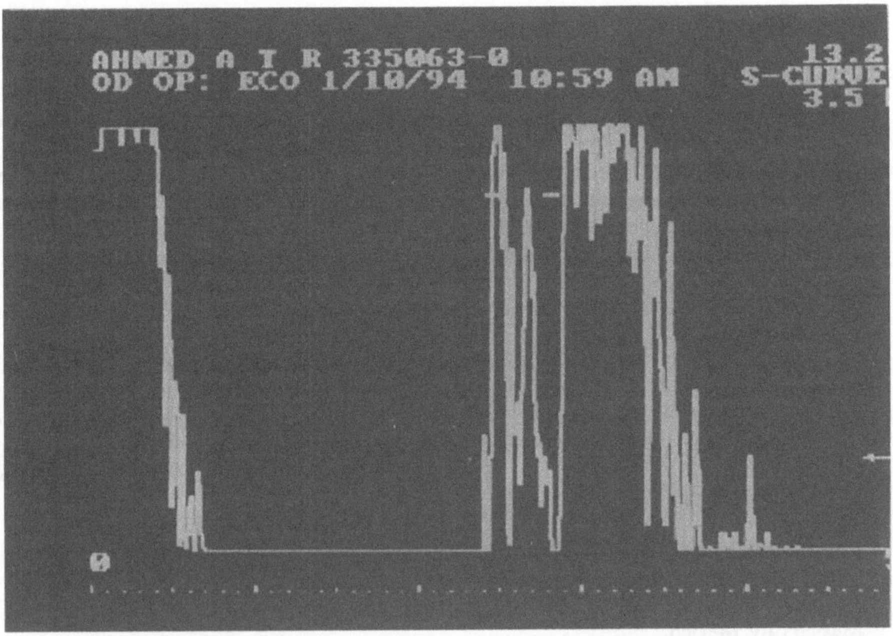

(c)

Fig. 2 (cont.) (see opposite page)

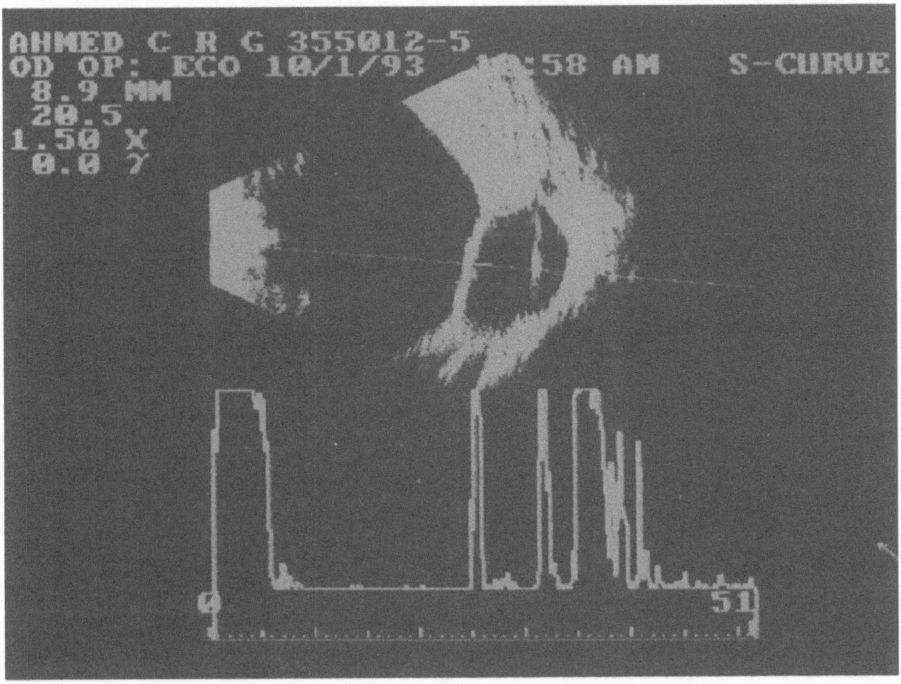

Fig. 3. Transverse A–B scan of the Ahmed plate with overlying and underlying bleb and scleral flattening

References

[1] M.A. Lloyd, T. Sedlack, D.K. Heuer *et al.* Clinical experience with the single-plate Molteno implant in complicated glaucomas. Update of a pilot study. Ophthalmology 1992;99:679–687.

[2] D.K. Heuer, M.A. Lloyd, D.A. Abrams *et al.* Which is better? One or two? A randomized clinical trial of single-plate versus double-plate Molteno implantation for glaucomas in aphakia and pseudophakia. Ophthalmology 1992;99:1512–1519.

[3] K.U. Loeffler and J.L. Jay. Tissue response to aqueous drainage in a functioning Molteno implant. Br. J. Ophthalmol. 1988;72:29–35.

[4] A.C.B. Molteno. New implant for drainage in glaucoma: clinical trial. Br. J. Ophthalmol. 1969;53:606–615.

[5] D.S. Minkler, D.K. Heuer, B. Hasty *et al.* Clinical experience with the single plate Molteno implant in complicated glaucomas. Ophthalmology 1988;95:1181–1188.

[6] D.S. Minkler, A. Shammas, M. Wilcox and T.E. Ogden. Experimental studies of aqueous filtration using the Molteno implant. Trans. Am. Ophthalmol. Soc. 1987;85:368–392.

[7] M.A. Lloyd, D.S. Minkler, R.L. Green *et al.* Echographic evaluation of glaucoma shunts. Ophthalmology 1993;100:919–927.

Eduardo Moragrega
Asociación para Evitar la Ceguera en México
Hospital "Dr. Luis Sánchez Bulnes"
México City, México

25. Echographic and tomographic evaluation of Molteno and Baerveldt implants in three children

S.M. PANARELLO, A. DOLCI, P. TORTORI DONATI,[1] A. POLIZZI,[2]
C.E. TRAVERSO[2] and P. VITTONE
(Genoa, Italy)

Abstract

The authors describe and discuss the peculiar echographic and tomographic features of Baerveldt and Molteno implants in three children with refractory glaucomas who had undergone goniotomy and trabeculectomy.

Key words: Baeverveldt implant, Molteno implant, refractory juvenile glaucoma

Introduction

Most infants and young children with glaucoma respond satisfactorily to treatment with goniotomy or trabeculectomy. The postoperative use of anti-metabolites such as 5-fluorouracil and mitomycin have improved the results of filtering surgery for those who have difficult forms of glaucoma or who have not benefitted from previous, filtering operations, because sub-conjunctival injections are difficult in young children. The encouraging results obtained with the Molteno implant in adults have led us to apply this surgical procedure in children [1–3]. However, clinical examination alone may not be sufficient to evaluate the efficiency of the filtering bleb of the Molteno implant. In these cases ultrasound is very helpful [4,5].

Material and methods

In 1991–92 three children out of a group of 34 with congenital glaucoma received Molteno and Baerveldt implants at the Department of Ophthalmology of the G. Gaslini Institute.

Case I, C.V., a five-day-old female with bilateral buphthalmos: corneal oedema in both eyes, corneal diameter 13.5 mm in right eye, 13 mm in left eye, axial length 21.5 mm in right eye, 20 mm in left eye; intraocular pressure 37 mmHg in right eye, 30 mmHg in left; optic nerve was slightly faded. The patient under-

G Cennamo and N. Rosa (eds.), Ultrasonography in Ophthalmology 15, pp. 219–223.

went four bilateral goniotomies and a trabeculectomy in the left eye without improvement. At six months she underwent trabeculectomy with mitomycin in the right eye and received a one-stage Molteno implant in the left eye.

Case II, R.V., a seven-year-old female who had previously undergone five goniotomies and one trabeculotomy in the right eye and 4 goniotomies in the left. Corneal diameter was 13 mm in the right eye and 14 mm in the left; axial length 22.20 mm in the right eye and 26.60 in the left. Intraocular pressure was 27 mmHg in the right eye and 17 mmHg in the left; optic nerve was slightly faded in both eyes; visual acuity: 0.6 Snellen in the right eye, 0.1 Snellen in the left eye with correction. She received a Baerveldt implant in the right eye.

Case III, F.J., a seven-day-old female with corneal oedema in both eyes; corneal diameter 10 mm in the right eye, 10.5 mm in the left eye; axial length 17.60 mm in the right eye and 17.32 mm in the left eye; Intraocular pressure 48 mmHg in the right eye and 40 mmHg in the left. After trabeculectomy and goniotomy, she underwent trabeculectomy with mitomycin in the right eye and received a Molteno implant in the left eye at two months. In all three cases the drainage tube was closed with a nylon suture and reopened by Argon laser after 15 days.

Results

Case I. The ophthalmological examination 24 months after surgery showed: no conjunctival reaction, drainage tube in anterior chamber; corneal diameter 14.2 mm in the right eye 14.4 mm in the left; axial length 22.80 mm in the right eye 21.30 mm in the left; intraocular pressure 20 mmHg in both eyes.

Case II. The ophthalmological examination 24 months after surgery showed: no conjunctival reaction; drainage tube in the anterior chamber, intraocular pressure 19 mmHg in both eyes; visual acuity unchanged.

Case III. Ophthalmological examination 10 months after surgery showed: cornea slightly oedematous in both eyes; corneal diameter 11 mm in both eyes; axial length 19.80 mm in the right eye 18.50 mm in the left; intraocular pressure 24 mmHg in the right eye and 22 mmHg in the left.

Discussion

Experimental studies [6,7] have shown that aqueous flow passes from the outer sclera along the thin tube to the compartment created by the plate from which it can filter into the surrounding tissues. A and B-scan ultrasound showed the presence of surrounding fluid and scleral flattening adjacent to the plate in all three cases (Figs. 1 and 2).

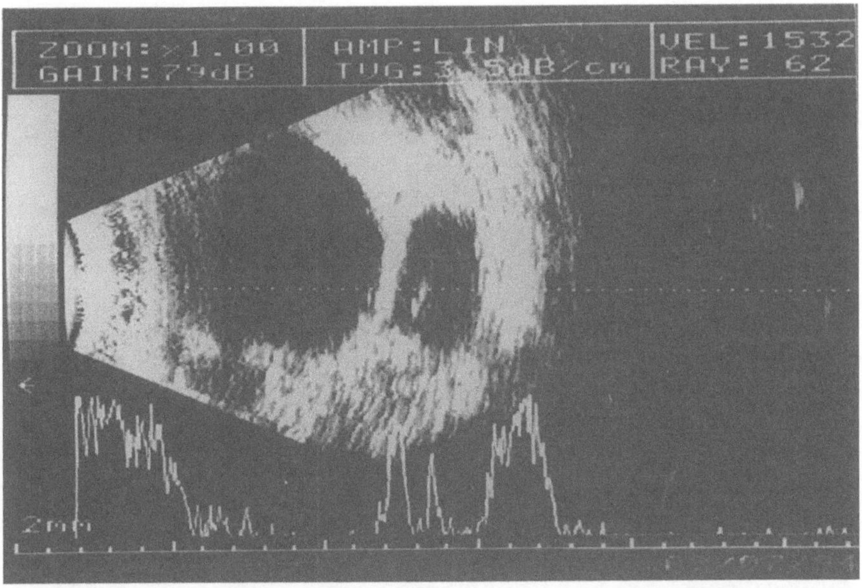

Fig. 1. Ultrasound of Molteno implant

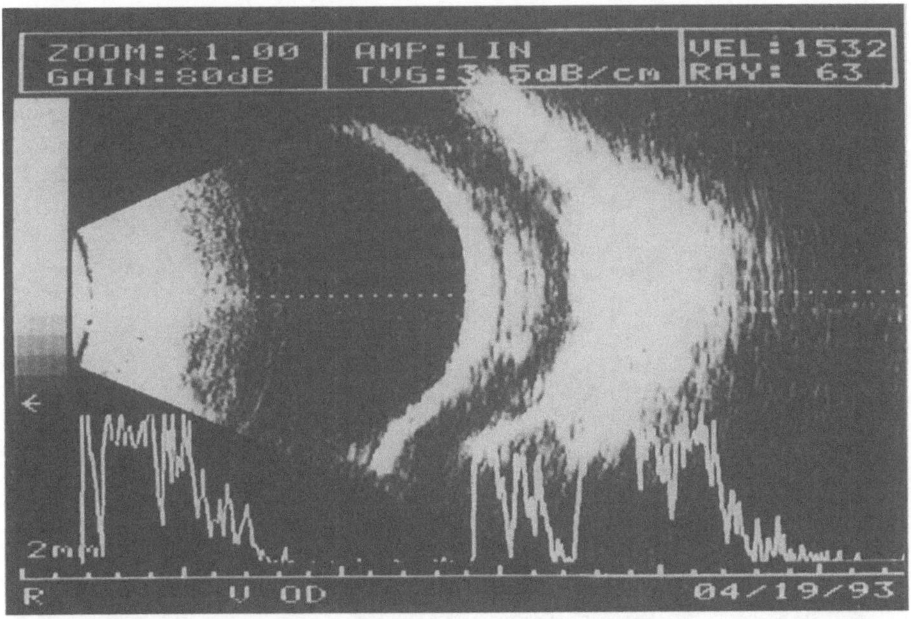

Fig. 2. Ultrasound of Baerveldt implant

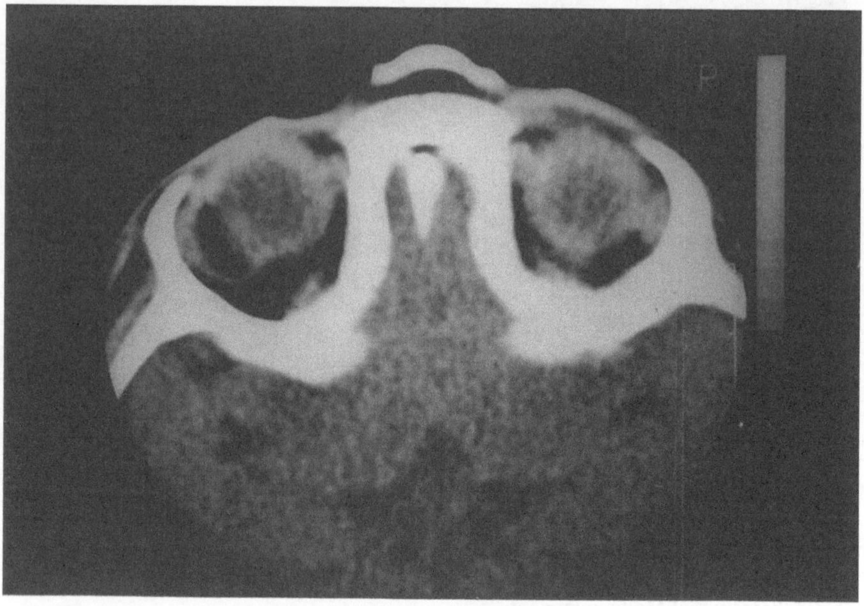

Fig. 3. CT-scan of Molteno implant shows low reflective area

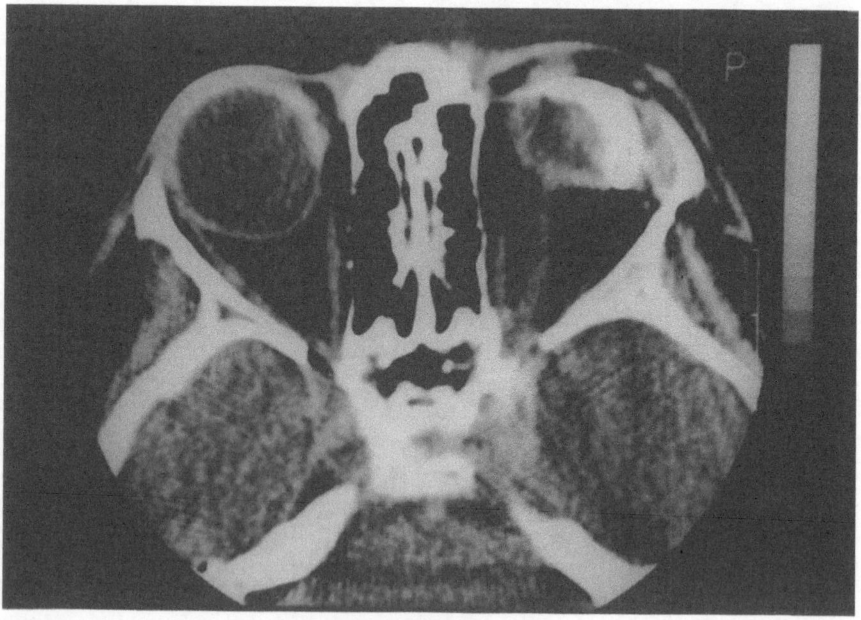

Fig. 4. CT-scan of Baerveldt implant shows high reflective area

There were differences in the echographic images of the various materials constituting the implants: the Molteno implant consisting of a silicone tube attached to polypropylene plate; the Baerveldt implant consisting of a silicone tube attached to a silicone plate embedded in radio-opaque barium. Ultrasound showed a more highly reflective membrane in the Baerveldt implant than in the Molteno implant in which a low reflective fluid surrounded a highly reflective plate (Figs. 1 and 2). CT-scan confirmed this information (Figs. 3 and 4).

Ultrasound has proved to be extremely helpful in monitoring and documenting the cyst-like blebs that form around the plates. Ultrasound B-scan measurements demonstrated the presence of persisting filtration blebs around the Molteno plate even when the latter could not be reliably detected at clinical examination.

References

[1] P. Vittone, S.M. Panarello, A. Dolci, E. Priolo and C.E. Traverso. Applicazione di impianto drenante nella terapia del glaucoma congenito refrattario: presentazione di due casi. Boll. Ocul. 1993;6 suppl.:413–416.

[2] A.C.B. Molteno, E. Anckler and G. Van Biljon. Surgical technique for advanced juvenile glaucoma. Arch. Ophthalmol. 1984;102:51–57.

[3] C.E. Traverso, K.F. Tomey and A. Al-Kaff. La protesi drenante di Molteno per il trattamento dei glaucomi congeniti refrattari alla chirurgia antiglaucomatosa convenzionale. Boll. Ocul. 1989;68:385–395.

[4] M. Munoz, K.F. Tomey, C.E. Traverso, S.H. Day and S.H. Senft. Clinical experience with the Molteno implant advanced infantile glaucoma. J. Pediatr. Ophthalmol. Strabismus 1991;28:68–72.

[5] R.L. Green, M.A. Lloyd, D.S. Minckler *et al.* Echographic evaluation of Molteno implants. In Arvo Abstracts, Invest Ophthalmic Ecography. Dordrecht: Dr. W. Junk., 1987.

[6] J. Hughes and S.F. Byrne. Detection of posterior ruptures in opaque media. In Ossoinig K.C., Ophthalmic Ecography, Dordrecht: D.R. W. Junk, 1987.

[7] D.S. Minckler, A. Shammas, M. Wilcox *et al.* Experimental studies of acqueous filtration using the Molteno implant. Trans. Am. Ophthalmol. Soc. 1987;84:368.

S.M. Panarello
Department of Ophthalmology
G. Caslini Institute
Genoa, Italy

[1]Department of Neuroradiology
G. Gaslini Institute
Genoa, Italy

[2]Eye Clinic
University of Genoa
Genoa, Italy

26. Reliability of ultrasound biomicroscopic measurements of the anterior segment

G. MARCHINI, R. TOSI, A. PAGLIARUSCO, P. MONTI and L. BONOMI

(Verona, Italy)

Abstract

We determined the precision of the measurement obtained by ultrasound biomicroscopy (UBM) of the anterior segment of the eye. In 10 subjects (10 eyes) we evaluated the reproducibility of two measurements on the same UBM image and on two images obtained at different times, calculating the coefficient of correlation (*r*). In 10 other subjects (10 eyes) we assessed the variability of 5 measurements taken during 5 successive examinations, calculating the mean coefficient of variation (CV) for each parameter.

On the same UBM image, the within-observer agreement was high for all parameters (*r* values ranging between 0.95 and 0.99), whereas the between-observer agreement was less satisfactory for the angle-opening distances and for iris thickness 1 (*r* ranging from 0.74 to 0.79). On images of the same ocular section obtained at two different times the within- and between-observer agreement was unacceptable for 5 parameters (angle-opening distance 250 and 500 μm, iris thicknesses 1 and 2, iris-lens angle) and for 6 parameters (same measurements plus scleral-ciliary process angle), respectively, with *r* values ranging between 0.21 and 0.76.

Analysis of the CV of 5 measurements showed good reproducibility (CV <10%) for the determination of anterior chamber depth, scleral thickness, trabecular-ciliary process distance, iris thicknesses 2 and 3, iris-zonule distance, scleral-iris angle and scleral-ciliary process angle. Less satisfactory CV values, ranging from 10.5 to 19.8%, were obtained for trabecular-iris angle in degrees, angle-opening distance 250 and 500 μm, iris-ciliary process distance, iris thickness 1, iris-lens contact distance and iris-lens angle.

In conclusion, the precision of UBM is insufficient for many parameters. The reproducibility of the technique may be increased by more strictly standardized examination conditions and by better training of the observers.

Key words: Ultrasound biomicroscopy (UBM), reliability, reproducibility

G Cennamo and N. Rosa (eds.), Ultrasonography in Ophthalmology 15, pp. 225–231.

Introduction

Ultrasound biomicroscopy (UBM) is a new ultrasonographic diagnostic procedure that provides images of the anterior segment of the eye with a resolution of 40–50 μm [1,2]. UBM enables us to examine structural details of the angle region and, for the first time, permits direct visualization of the retro-iridial anatomical formations. This has led to a new approach, in both qualitative and quantitative terms, to the study of glaucoma and may contribute towards clarifying the mechanisms of some forms of the disease [3–6]. In particular, UBM enables us to measure a series of linear and angular parameters capable of defining the characteristics of normal and glaucomatous eyes [7]. These parameters may prove invaluable for an understanding of angle closure mechanisms and for the evaluation of the effects of therapy in angle-closure glaucoma. It is therefore important to know the precision of the measurements obtained with UBM. To this aim, we have evaluated the reproducibility of the measurements of 15 UBM parameters in a series of 20 normal subjects.

Materials and methods

The examinations were performed using a UBM 840 instrument (Humphrey-Zeiss, San Leandro, California) with a 50 MHz transducer that gives a resolution of 40–50 μm and 5 mm tissue penetration. The examination technique is very similar to the normal B-scan ultrasonographic immersion procedure and has previously been described in detail elsewhere [2].

Only one eye was examined in each subject. Each eye was studied in its axial section, exploring the transverse diameter passing through the apex of the cornea from 3 o'clock to 9 o'clock, in constant ambient lighting conditions. Images centered on the pupil, angular region and ciliary process were obtained and recorded for each eye. The 15 parameters defined by Pavlin *et al.* [7] and listed below, were measured on these images using a special caliper issued with the instrument software package:

- anterior chamber depth (ACD)
- trabecular-iris angle in degrees Θ1 (AW)
- angle-opening distance 250 μm (AOD 250)
- angle-opening distance 500 μm (AOD 500)
- iris thickness 1 (ID I)
- iris thickness 2 (ID 2)
- iris thickness 3 (ID 3)
- scleral thickness (SD)
- trabecular-ciliary process distance (TCPD)
- iris-ciliary process distance (ICPD)
- iris-zonule distance (IZD)

- iris-lens contact distance (ILCD)
- iris-lens angle in degrees Θ2 (ILA)
- scleral-iris angle in degrees Θ3 (SIA)
- scleral-ciliary process angle in degrees Θ4 (SCPA)

Measurements of linear parameters are expressed in thousandths of a millimetre, whereas angular measurements are expressed in degrees.

Two types of study were conducted. In an initial group of 10 subjects we evaluated, for each parameter, two measurements, both within and between observers, on the same image and on two different images obtained at different times. First, the same observer measured the parameters twice on the same image. Secondly, the parameters were measured on the same image by two different observers. The same observer then measured the various parameters on two images of the same ocular section obtained in two successive examinations on the same day. Lastly, the parameters on these images were measured by two different observers. In each of the 4 combinations, the degree of agreement between the two measurements was assessed using regression analysis and calculating the coefficient of correlation *r* for each parameter.

In a second group of 10 subjects we determined the variability of 5 measurements on images of the same ocular section obtained in 5 successive examinations in the course of 3 days. In this case, the data analysis was done using the coefficient of variation (CV = standard deviation/mean × 100). For each parameter, the CV value was first determined in each eye, and the mean CV value was then calculated for all eyes.

Results

When the same observer took the two measurements on the same image, the within-observer agreement was very good for all parameters, with *r* values ranging from 0.95 to 0.99 (Table 1). When two observers measured the parameters on the same image the *r* values ranged from 0.93 to 0.99 for 13 parameters; between-observer agreement was lower for the angle-opening distances (AOD 250, AOD 500) and for iris thickness 1 (ID1) with *r* values of 0.74, 0.79, respectively (Table 2).

The measurements taken by the same observer on two images of the same ocular section obtained in two successive examinations were characterized by *r* values ranging from 0.81 to 0.98 for 10 parameters. By contrast, for the angle-opening distances (AOD 250, AOD 500), the iris thicknesses 1 and 2 (ID1 and ID2) and the iris-lens angle (Θ2), the within-observer agreement was characterized by *r* values ranging from 0.38 to 0.76 (Table 3).

The measurements by two different observers on images of the same ocular section obtained on two successive occasions yielded good between-observer agreement for 9 parameters with *r* values ranging from 0.80 to 0.99, whereas for the measurements of AOD 250, AOD 500, ID1, ID2, the iris-lens angle (Θ2)

Table 1. Within-observer agreement for two measurements of 15 UBM parameters obtained on the same image

Parameter	r	p	Parameter	r	p
ACD	0.99	0.000	ID 3	0.99	0.000
Θ 1 (AW)	0.99	0.000	ILCD	0.99	0.000
AOD 250	0.99	0.000	ID 1	0.98	0.000
AOD 500	0.99	0.000	IZD	0.98	0.000
ST	0.99	0.000	Θ 3 (SIA)	0.97	0.000
TCPD	0.99	0.000	Θ 4 (SCPA)	0.95	0.000
ICPD	0.99	0.000			
ID 2	0.99	0.000			

Table 2. Between-observer agreement for two measurements of 15 UBM parameters obtained on the same image

Parameter	r	p	Parameter	r	p
ACD	0.99	0.000	ICPD	0.95	0.000
IZD	0.99	0.000	ID 2	0.94	0.000
ILCD	0.99	0.000	Θ 4 (SCPA)	0.94	0.000
ID 3	0.99	0.000	TCPD	0.93	0.000
Θ 3 (SIA)	0.99	0.000			
SD	0.97	0.000	ID 1	0.79	0.006
Θ 2 (ILA)	0.97	0.000	AOD 500	0.75	0.013
Θ 1 (AW)	0.96	0.000	AOD 250	0.74	0.015

Table 3. Within-observer agreement for two measurements of 15 UBM parameters obtained on images of the same ocular section at two successive observation times

Parameter	r	p	Parameter	r	p
ACD	0.98	0.000	ILCD	0.83	0.003
ICPD	0.95	0.000	SD	0.81	0.004
Θ 3 (SIA)	0.93	0.000			
TCPD	0.92	0.000	ID 1	0.76	0.011
IZD	0.89	0.000	AOD 250	0.62	0.057
Θ 4 (SCPA)	0.89	0.000	Θ 2 (ILA)	0.56	0.091
ID 3	0.86	0.001	ID 2	0.46	0.181
Θ 1 (AW)	0.84	0.002	AOD 500	0.38	0.274

Table 4. Between-observer agreement for two measurements of 15 UBM parameters obtained on images of the same ocular section at two successive observation times

Parameter	*r*	*p*	Parameter	*r*	*p*
ACD	0.99	0.000	SD	0.80	0.007
Θ 3 (SIA)	0.93	0.000			
ICPD	0.92	0.000	Θ 4 (SCPA)	0.64	0.045
Θ 1 (AW)	0.88	0.000	AOD 500	0.48	0.165
IZD	0.86	0.001	ID 1	0.45	0.194
ILCD	0.84	0.002	Θ 2 (ILA)	0.43	0.125
TCPD	0.83	0.003	AOD 250	0.27	0.456
ID 3	0.81	0.005	ID 2	0.21	0.557

Table 5. Mean values, 95% confidence intervals (95% CI) and coefficients of variation (CV) for 15 UBM parameters

Parameter		Mean	C.I. 95% (±)	C.V. %
ACD	μm	2.427	0.214	1.4
SD	μm	1.014	0.072	3.9
TCPD	μm	0.928	0.113	5.9
ID 2	μm	0.411	0.035	9.7
ID 3	μm	0.522	0.051	4.4
IZD	μm	0.495	0.068	6.6
Θ 3 (SIA)	degrees	26.251	4.266	7.5
Θ 4 (SCPA)	degrees	33.518	2.980	8.6
Θ 1 (AW)	degrees	18.618	5.263	12.4
AOD 250	μm	0.194	0.046	19.8
AOD 500	μm	0.283	0.062	18.0
ICPD	μm	0.271	0.077	15.6
ID 1	μm	0.401	0.052	10.5
ILCD	μm	0.707	0.176	14.2
Θ 2 (ILA)	degrees	16.607	1.750	12.5

and the scleral-ciliary process angle (Θ4) the degree of between-observer agreement was unacceptable with *r* values ranging from 0.21 to 0.64 (Table 4).

The results of analysis of variability of 5 measurements obtained on UBM images of the same ocular section obtained in 5 successive examinations are reported in Table 5, which shows the mean values, 95% confidence intervals and coefficients of variation (CV) for the 15 parameters studied. Coefficients of variation ranging from 1.4 to 9.7% were obtained for anterior chamber depth, scleral thickness, trabecular-ciliary process distance, iris thicknesses 2 and 3, iris-zonule distance, scleral-iris angle and scleral-ciliary process angle. Trabecular-iris angle in degrees, angle opening distances 250 and 500 μm, iris-ciliary process distance, iris thickness 1, iris-lens contact distance and iris-lens angle were characterized by CV values ranging from 10.5 to 19.8%.

Discussion

Ultrasound biomicroscopy constitutes a new diagnostic imaging method which has substantially modified the approach to the study of the anterior segment in both qualitative and quantitative terms. In the overall assessment of UBM three distinct aspects should be considered, namely, its clinical significance, its accuracy and its precision.

Undoubtedly, the clinical value of UBM is considerable. To mention but a few examples, UBM allows visualization of the retro-iridial structures, formerly not possible *in vivo*; it provides precise information in filtering [3,7] and in cataract surgery [8]; it can be used to visualize and study tumours of the anterior and intermediate segments [9] and has already contributed towards clarifying the pathogenetic mechanisms of some forms of glaucoma [4–6].

To-date no data are available as to the accuracy of UMB. Little is known about the correct speed of sound in ocular tissues when using frequencies of the order of 50–100 MHz [7], and thus, at present, we do not know exactly what the effective correspondence is between the UBM image and the 'actual' anatomical size. Further studies may be expected to shed light on this issue.

As regards the precision of UBM, a prime concern is the reproducibility of UBM measurements. The term 'precision' is a synonym for reproducibility and expresses the degree of agreement between repeated measurements of the same phenomenon. The precision is usually greater when the measurements are made on the same section and by the same observer and decreases when measurements are taken by different observers and at different times. From this standpoint, the data obtained in our study show that the variability of the measurements obtained on the *same image* is low and results in a good, or at any rate an acceptable degree of both within- and between-observer agreement for all the parameters measured. However, the precision of the UBM method was much less satisfactory when measurements made on images referring to the same ocular section but obtained at different times. In this case, the within- and between-observer reproducibility of the examination proved unacceptable for 5 and 6 of the 15 parameters considered, respectively. While the within- and between-observer agreement on different images was still very good for such linear measurements as anterior chamber depth, scleral thickness and trabecular-ciliary process distance, UMB measurements were less precise in estimating of the trabecular-iris angle and, at least partly, in evaluating the iris thickness. These conclusions are confirmed by CV analysis of the measurements.

Many of the UBM parameters processed for quantitative determinations of the anterior segment [7] are thus not sufficiently reproducible and the best method of evaluating them has yet to be defined. The precision of the measurements might be improved by more strictly standardized examination conditions and by better training of the observers.

References

[1] C.J. Pavlin, M.D. Sherar and F.S. Foster. Subsurface ultrasound microscopic imaging of the intact eye. Ophthalmology 1990;97:244.

[2] C.J. Pavlin, K. Harasiewicz, M.D. Sherar and F.S. Foster. Clinical use of ultrasound biomicroscopy. Ophthalmology 1991;98:287.

[3] C.J. Pavlin and F.S. Foster. Ultrasound biomicroscopy in glaucoma. Acta Ophthalmol. 1992;204 suppl.:7.

[4] C.J. Pavlin, K. Harasiewicz and F.S. Foster. Ultrasound biomicroscopy in plateau iris syndrome. Am. J. Ophthalmol. 1992;113:390.

[5] C.J. Pavlin, M. Easterbrook, K. Harasiewicz and F.S. Foster. An ultrasound biomicroscopic analysis of angleclosure glaucoma secondary to ciliochoroidal effusion in IgA nephropathy. Am. J. Ophthalmol. 1993;116:341.

[6] S.D. Potash, C. Tello, J. Liebmann and R. Ritch. Ultrasound biomicroscopy in pigment dispersion syndrome. Ophthalmology 1994;101:332.

[7] C.J. Pavlin, K. Harasiewicz, F.S. Foster. Ultrasound biomicroscopy of anterior segment structures in normal and glaucomatous eyes. Am. J. Ophthalmol. 1992;113:381.

[8] C.J. Pavlin, D. Rootman, S. Arshinoff, K. Harasiewicz and F.S. Foster. Determination of haptic position of transsclerally fixated posterior chamber intraocular lenses by ultrasound biomicroscopy. J. Cataract Refract. Surg. 1993;19:573.

[9] C.J. Pavlin, J.A. McWhae, H.D. McGown and F.S. Foster. Ultrasound biomicroscopy of anterior segment tumors. Ophthalmology 1992;99:1220.

G. Marchini
Istituto di Clinica Oculistica,
Università di Verona
Verona, Italy

27. A dynamic study of accommodation using ultrasound biomicroscopy

J.A. McWHAE, A.C.S. CRICHTON and J. REIMER

(Calgary, Alberta, Canada)

Abstract

Accommodation is fundamental to vision, yet our understanding of the process remains limited. Highly detailed images of the iris and ciliary body region can be obtained through the use of ultrasound biomicroscopy. This technique utilizes high frequency transducers to produce B-scan images with axial and lateral resolution approaching 20 microns.

We performed a dynamic study of accommodation using ultrasound biomicroscopy and video recording. A 50 MHz transducer was used. Seven patients, ranging in age from 18 to 64 years, were examined. The anterior segment of one eye was imaged while the patient alternated between near and distance fixation with the other eye. The most remarkable changes were noted in the region of the posterior chamber. A posterior bowing of the iris occurred during accommodation, resulting in marked shallowing of the posterior chamber. This phenomena was most prominent in the younger patients of the group.

The use of ultrasound biomicroscopy provides a dynamic view of the anterior segment showing a characteristic posterior bowing of the iris during accommodation. This observation increases our understanding of ocular changes during accommodation.

Key words: Accommodation, iris bowing, ultrasound biomicroscopy

Introduction

The process of accommodation has been of interest to ophthalmologists for at least two centuries. In 1970, Coleman [1] presented a unified model for the accommodative mechanism which combined previous theories and emphasized the importance of the vitreous body in accommodation. Coleman's theory of accommodation proposes that contraction of the ciliary muscle relaxes tension on the zonules allowing the lens to assume a more spherical shape. The anterior portion of the vitreous body moves forward supporting the back of the lens. The lens protrudes anteriorly shallowing the anterior chamber. Opening of the trabecular meshwork allows reduced outflow resistance to produce a gradual

G Cennamo and N. Rosa (eds.), Ultrasonography in Ophthalmology 15, pp. 233–240.

lowering of intraocular pressure and maintain the vitreo-lens-aqueous pressure gradient to favour the accommodated lens position. Studies using ultrasound [1–6] have generally confirmed that the central anterior chamber shallows in the accommodated state. These studies also confirm an increase in lens thickness. In a recent paper, Shum *et al.* [6] concluded that axial length increases during accommodation, although some authors found conflicting results [4,5].

Pupillary constriction is another known component of accommodation. Changes in the peripheral iris have not been described to the best of our knowledge. We are not aware of any previous methods that could provide a dynamic cross-sectional view of the iris during accommodation.

Ultrasound biomicroscopy is a recent development in high resolution ocular ultrasound. It was developed by Drs. Pavlin, Sherar and Foster [7,8] and allows for very detailed imaging of the anterior segment. Using high frequency transducers of 50–100 MHz, a B-scan view of the anterior segment with resolution approaching 20 microns can be obtained [8]. Humphrey Research Division, Carl Zeiss Inc., has developed a clinical prototype of this machine which we have had in use at Foothills Hospital. We proposed a dynamic study of accommodation in order to increase our understanding of the accommodative process.

Patients and methods

Seven patients participated in our study (ages 18, 23, 24, 28, 37, 41, 64, alternating male/female). Detailed informed consent was obtained from each patient to participate in the study, which had been approved by Foothills Hospital Bioethics Committee. Each patient had a spherical equivalent refractive error of between –0.75 and +0.50 in each eye with cylinder less than 1.00 diopter. Each patient had at least 6/7.5 corrected vision in each eye. With the exception of the pseudophakic 64-year-old patient, none had significant past ocular problems. The 64-year-old patient had developed unilateral cataract, for which surgery was performed six months prior. The left eye had had a phacoemulsification procedure with placement of a 5.5 mm round posterior chamber intraocular lens and the posterior capsule was clear. Refractive error was +0.25 OD and plano OS. As this study was intended to be a qualitative study, it was performed without correction, but with a considerable accommodative stimulus.

A Humphrey Instruments Ultrasound Biomicroscope Prototype (Humphrey Research Division, Carl Zeiss Inc., San Leandro, CA) was used. It was operating at 50 MHz for the study. With the patient in the supine position, topical tetracaine 0.5% drops were applied to the study eye. An appropriate sized plastic eye cup (Humphrey Instruments Inc.) was placed within the palpebral fissure and filled with 2% methylcellulose solution. The ultrasound transducer, which had been previously immersed in sterile water, was then placed in the methycellulose solution and radial scanning was performed in the iris and ciliary body region. A non-accommodative target was placed two metres above the patient for fixation of the fellow eye. An accommodative target was located at 20 cm and the patient was instructed to alternately view the distance and near target. This would provide a 4.5 diopter accommodative stimulus for the emmetropic patient. Presbyopic patients who were unable to focus on the 20 cm target were instructed to focus on it to the best of their ability. The targets were aligned in such a fashion that the convergence movement of the eye examined with ultrasound was neutralized. The image was recorded directly from the monitor into a ¾-inch U-matic video recorder. Using the ultrasound biomicroscope, images could also be frozen and stored. Both a distance and near image of the iris/ciliary body region was stored for each patient, as well as a profile of the central anterior chamber for distance and near fixation.

Results

Ultrasound biomicroscopy with continuous video recording provided a dramatic view of anterior segment changes during accommodation. It was initially intended to concentrate on changes in the ciliary body region. Ciliary processes could be seen to move centrally, however, striking and unexpected changes were noted in the profile of the iris. Following this observation, the radial scanning was performed so as to best image the iris and the region of the posterior chamber.

Good quality studies were obtained in six of the seven patients. Two patients experienced some discomfort from the eye cup. One patient had difficulty accomplishing the accommodative task, resulting in a poor quality study. The other patient complained of some residual eye discomfort following the study and a small amount of central corneal punctate staining was noted. This patient's cornea returned to normal by the following day.

During distance fixation, the profile of the iris was either flat or slightly convex in all patients. With near fixation, there was an immediate posterior bowing of the peripheral iris with resultant shallowing of the posterior chamber. This phenomenon was most prominent in the youngest patients in the study and though it was progressively less apparent with increasing age, this movement was still present to some extent even in the older patients of the group.

The difference in the iris profile between the unaccommodated state and the accommodated state is shown in Figs. 1–3. It was noted in the four youngest patients in the study that the iris posterior pigment epithelium came to within a short distance of the zonules but in no case did it appear to make contact. Also of note, the changes in iris profile were sustained during prolonged near fixation (up to at least 20 seconds in the younger patients who were able to maintain near fixation).

Studies on the pseudophakic 64-year-old patient were particularly interesting. Initially, the patient's left pseudophakic eye was studied while the patient

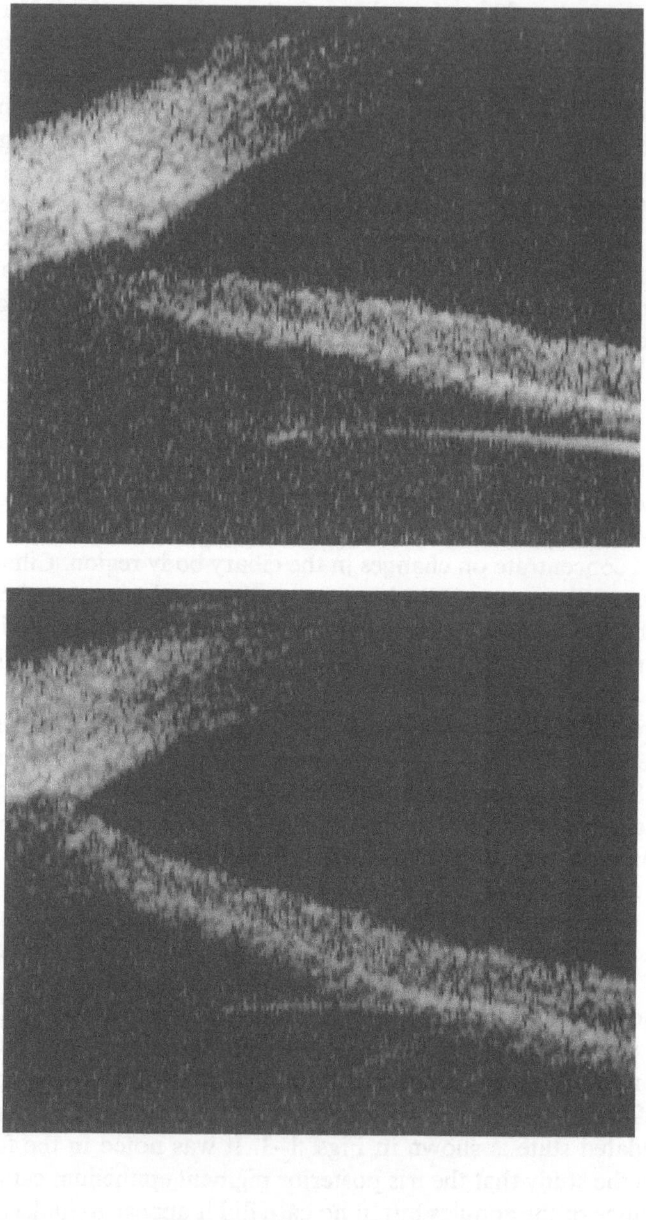

(a)

(b)

Fig. 1.
(A) Radial scan of angle region in an 18-year-old man during distance fixation. note slightly convex iris profile. Highly reflective line at the bottom of the picture represents the lens capsule
(B) Same patient during near fixation. Iris profile is now concave, posterior chamber has shallowed

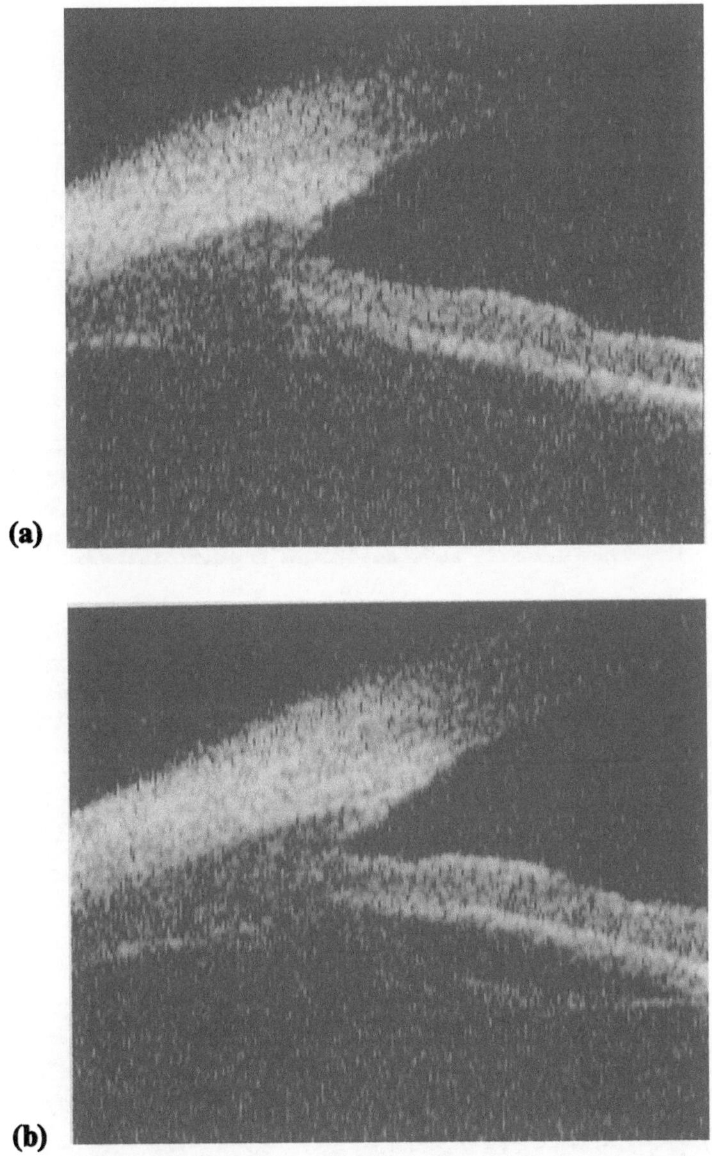

Fig. 2.
(A) Radial scan of angle regione in a 24-year-old man during distance fixation. Iris profile is convex
(B) Same patient during near fixation, iris profile now concave

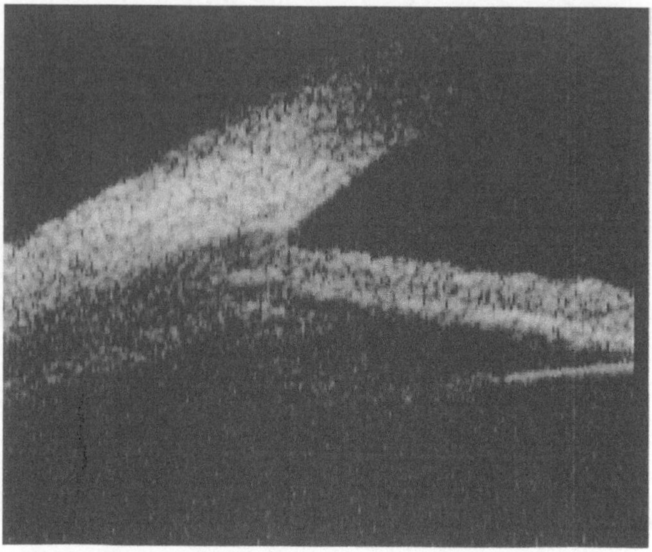

(a)

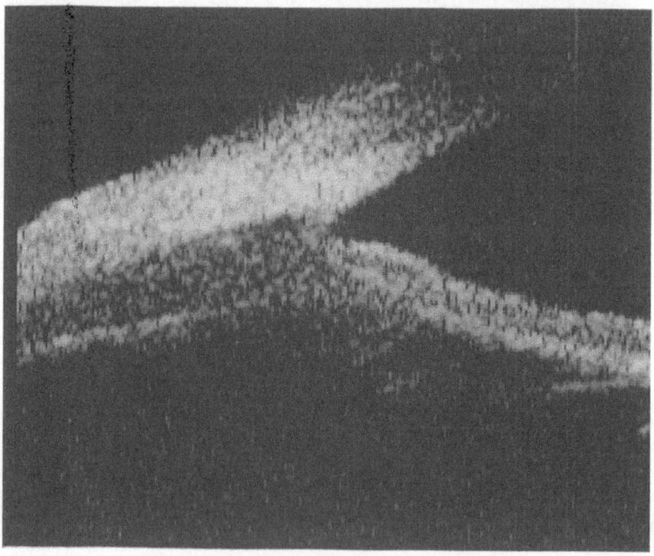

(b)

Fig. 3.
(A) Radial scan of angle region in a 28-year-old woman during distance fixation. Iris profile is straight
(B) Same patient during near fixation, iris profile now concave

alternated fixation with the right eye. In the resting state, the intraocular lens could be clearly demonstrated on the ultrasound and was seen to be placed within the capsular bag. With the lens implant in this position, there was ample space between the iris and optic with no potential for pupillary block. During accommodative effort, there was no change in the iris profile. With central scanning involving the pupil, there was a small amount of pupillary constriction. The study was then repeated while scanning the phakic right eye and using the left eye for fixation. The patient was unable to focus to any extent on the near target, but he was instructed to make an effort. Interestingly, a small but observable posterior bowing of the iris of the phakic eye did occur with accommodative effort.

Shallowing of the central anterior chamber was observed in our study. By freezing images centered over the pupil during distance and near fixation, we could then measure the central anterior chamber depth using an electronic caliper. The shallowing of the anterior chamber was relatively small, varying from 0.02 mm to 0.08 mm.

Discussion

Studies using ultrasound have increased our knowledge of ocular changes during accommodation. Ultrasound biomicroscopy, which can provide a dynamic high resolution view of anterior segment structures, is ideal for studying the accommodative process. This technique allowed us to make a video recording of the profile of the iris during the act of accommodation.

It would appear that the iris is much more active during accommodation than previously understood. The central iris moves forward with the lens while the peripheral iris bows posterior, shallowing the posterior chamber. This effect is age dependent. Further, this effect still occurs in the presbyopic eye as noted by our 64-year-old patient. The findings were absent in the pseudophakic eye, however.

Ideally our study would have been performed with the patient in the upright position. Logistically this would be very difficult. The fact that the iris was initially flat or convex and that the changes varied with age suggest gravity was not a significant factor in our observations.

Studies using ocular ultrasound have tended to confirm the Coleman theory of accommodation. Studies [2–6] support the idea that ciliary muscle contraction allows the lens to assume a more spherical shape. The anterior surface of the lens moves forward towards the cornea. It is likely [6] that total axial length increases slightly in the accommodative state.

Our study suggests there may be a further component to the accommodative mechanism. We propose that with the forward movement of the lens during accommodation, reverse pupillary block may occur. Due to the reduction of volume centrally in the anterior chamber, there is a movement of aqueous not only out of the trabecular meshwork [1] but also towards the periphery of the chamber resulting in the iris being bowed posteriorly. This movement would allow for total anterior chamber volume to remain relatively constant. Further, it would tend to distribute pressure more evenly between the anterior chamber and the posterior chamber. This provides further support for the peripheral lens, encouraging and helping to maintain changes in the shape of the lens for near fixation. The observation that iris profile changes did not occur in a pseudophakic eye which did not have the potential for pupillary block tends to support this theory. The fact that posterior bowing of the iris continued during prolonged near fixation would suggest these iris changes may have a role in maintaining the accommodated state, rather than being incidental movements.

We observed a characteristic posterior bowing of the iris during near fixation. The iris is thus more dynamic than previously felt during accommodation. This observation furthers our understanding of the accommodative process and will likely have implications in pathological states. Studies in this area may be able to confirm or deny the proposed pathophysiology of pigmentary glaucoma, namely rubbing of the zonules on the posterior iris surface.

References

[1] D.J. Coleman. Unified model for accommodative mechanism. Am. J. Ophthalmol. 1970;69:1063–1079.

[2] D.J. Coleman and R. Weininger. Ultrasonic M-mode technique in ophthalmology. Arch. Ophthalmol. 1969;82:475–479.

[3] J.K. Storey and E.P. Rabie. Ultrasound – A research tool in the study of accommodation. Ophthalmic Physiol. Opt. 1983;3:315–320.

[4] H.M. Soriano. Echographic findings in accommodation. In K.C. Ossoinig (ed.), Doc. Ophthalmol., Proc., Series 48, Ophthalmic Echography, Dordrecht: Martinus Nijhoff/Dr. W. Junk Publishers, 1987;163–169.

[5] R.D. Lepper and H.G. Trier. Measurement of accommodative changes in human eyes by means of a high-resolution ultrasonic system. In K.C. Ossoinig (ed.), Doc. Ophthalmol., Proc. Series 48, Ophthalmic Echography, Dordrecht: Martinus Nijhoff/Dr. W. Junk Publishers. 1987;157–162.

[6] P.J. Shum, L.S. Ko, C.L. Ng. and S.L. Lin. A biometric study of ocular changes during accommodation. Am. J. Ophthalmol. 1993;115:76–81.

[7] C.J. Pavlin, M.D. Sherar and F.S. Foster. Subsurface ultrasound microscopic imaging of the intact eye. Ophthalmology 1990;97:244–250.

[8] C.J. Pavlin, K. Harasiewicz, M.D. Sherar and F.S. Foster. Clinical use of ultrasound biomicroscopy. Ophthalmology 1991;98:287–295.

Dr. John McWhae
University of Calgary
Faculty of Medicine
Calgary, Alberta T2N 4N1
Canada

Vitreoretinal disorders

28. Detached retina vs. dense fibrovascular membrane: A-scan and B-scan signs for the differential diagnosis with standardized echography

K.C. OSSOINIG
(Iowa City, USA)

Introduction

In eyes with opaque ocular media, especially in those with dense vitreous and subvitreal hemorrhages forming membraneous structures with the vitreous cavity the differentiation between a detached retina and a dense fibrovascular membrane is often a difficult challenge to the echographer. Yet the (early and reliable) diagnosis of retinal detachment in eyes with opaque media is of paramount importance, especially in eyes that have suffered severe trauma as well as in eyes with severe proliferative vitreoretinopathy, i.e., in eyes where timely vitrectomy and retinal re-attachment surgery often decide the outcome and are the only way for recovery of useful vision.

When real-time contact B-scan echography became popular in the 1970's, and more so, when B-scan resolution improved dramatically in the 1980's it was thought that B-scan would readily solve the challenge of correctly differentiating fibrovascular membranes from retinal detachments. Kinetic B-scan, in particular, was expected to help in this differentiating process simply on the basis that posterior vitreous detachments most closely resembling retinal detachments morphologically are, in contrast to retinal detachments, very mobile and show incomparably more extensive aftermovement than the typically limited, undulating aftermovement known from large rhegmatogenous retinal detachments.

However, this clear-cut kinetic difference holds true only for large surfaces separated widely from the fundus and not complicated by any fibrotic changes. But in cases with opaque ocular media (with the exception of plain cataracts), i.e., vitreous hemorrhages, such fibrotic changes occur rather regularly often rendering the kinetic B-scan information worthless. The denser a vitreous membrane is, the more sluggish becomes its aftermovement which then may not be detected by B-scan any longer. Conversely, detached retinas also become less mobile with progressing fibrotic changes so that both detached retinas and fibrovascular membranes become similar (if not immobile) as far as B-scan kinetic evaluation is concerned. In contrast, A-scan kinetic evaluation still shows typical aftermovement in retinal detachments regardless how severe the proliferative changes are.

G Cennamo and N. Rosa (eds.), Ultrasonography in Ophthalmology 15, pp. 243–262.

The custom of calling a membraneous structure which is 360° continuous with surrounding attached retina or which inserts in a more or less funnel-shaped fashion into the optic disc (as evidenced by B-scan) automatically a 'detached retina' and of calling a membraneous structure automatically a 'membrane' when it seems to by-pass the optic disc on B-scan or when B-scan fails to easily demonstrate a 360° continuity of its signals with those from surrounding fundus is a wide-spread and popular simplification which leads to misdiagnoses and is therefore diagnostically unacceptable. Especially in eyes with severe proliferative vitreoretinal changes caused by diabetes or trauma vitreous membranes easily mimic detached retina. At times retinal detachments cannot be recognized as such as they mimic membranes. When considering all types of retinal detachments and vitreous fibrovascular membrane formations the B-scan effectiveness in differentiating between the two does not look good. Thirty-six percent of retinal detachments in this study were not positively diagnosed by the combined effort of using all four B-scan criteria (see Table 3 and Figure 9). Almost as often false-positive diagnoses of retinal detachment resulted from such illicit simplification as has been shown in our study even if sophisticated B-scan techniques are applied. One can imagine what happens when overly simplified B-scan techniques (e.g., 'free-style' B-scanning applied through closed lids) are applied. In contrast, Standardized Echography (using combined standardized A-scan and B-scan instrumentation and techniques) allows more than 99% of the cases to be reliably and clearly differentiated using a number of A-scan and B-scan criteria to arrive at a 'hard' differential diagnosis (see Table 3 and Figure 9).

Since the 1960's, specific A-scan and B-scan criteria for retinal detachment vs. dense fibrovascular membranes were incorporated into Standardized Echography. Since about 1980 a fixed set of 4 A-scan and 4 B-scan criteria was successfully used by us to achieve a differential diagnosis between retinal detachments and vitreous membranes (or other strongly reflecting surfaces mimicking retinal detachments such as the surfaces of posterior hyphemas or of pools of Fluorocarbon liquids) close to a 100% sensitivity and specificity [1,2]. In an 18-month period between January 1987 and June 1988 we performed a study to test each of these echographic criteria for their sensitivity, specificity, and positive as well as negative predictive values, and graded them according to their availability and to the ease as well as quickness of their application.

A-scan and B-scan criteria

Four A-scan and four B-scan criteria are useful in the diagnosis of retinal detachment and its differentiation from simulating surfaces such as the surfaces of fibrovascular membranes, of posterior vitreous detachment enhanced by hemorrhage, of posterior hyphemas, etc.

A₁ *(Fig. 1)*

This A-scan sign is positive for retinal detachment when the maximized surface spike is 100% high at Tissue Sensitivity of the instrument showing a sharply rising left limb with very few (less than 3) high-frequency nodules between base and peak ('Quantitative Echography I' [3]).

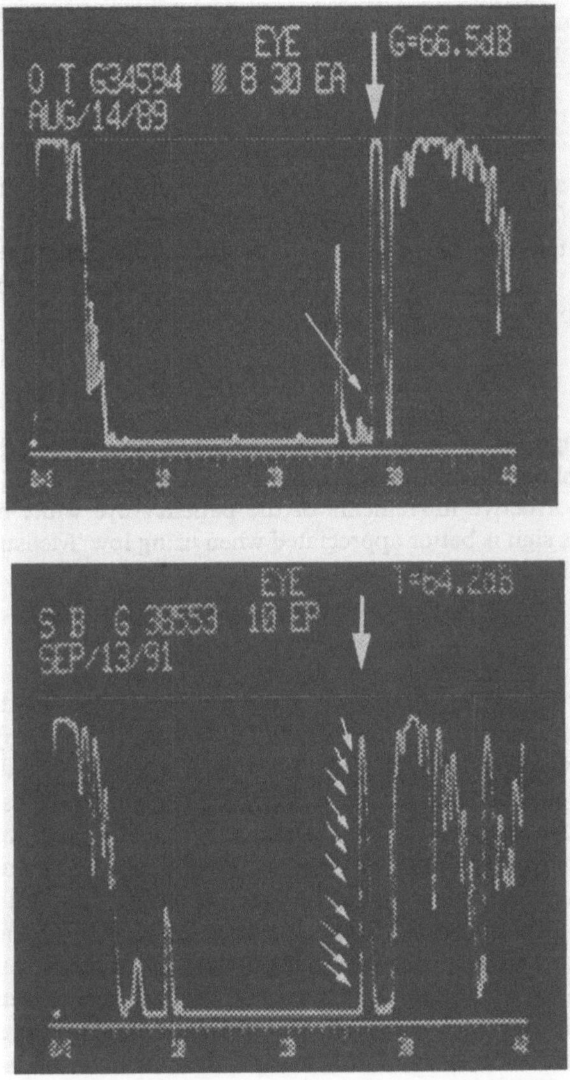

Fig. 1. A. Positive A_1 sign (retinal detachment–large arrow). B. Negative A_1 sign (membrane–large arrow). Small arrows point out high-frequency nodules on left limb of retinal and membrane spikes

The A_1 sign is negative for retinal detachment, when the left limb shows more than 4 high-frequency nodules or the height is less than 97% (when maximized!). This sign is equivocal, when 3 high-frequency nodules are seen along the left limb or the spike height is about 99%. It is also considered equivocal, when a typical retinal signal can only be obtained in one single beam direction although the surface is very large.

In order to be able to use this highly sensitive and specific sign the A-scan instrument must be standardized. To date, the B-scan S, the Mini A-scan, the Ophthascan S, the Sonokretz, and the Kretztechnik 7200 MA are the only instruments offering standardized A-scan; no other instrument can be used for this A_1 evaluation.

A_2

This A-scan sign is positive for retinal detachment when the surface spike remains high (at least 95% display height) or becomes that high when the beam is shifted anteriorly toward the ora serrata. This phenomenon was first described by Freyler [4]. Again, a standardized A-scan instrument is required for a useful application of this sign (see above).

A_3

This A-scan sign is positive for retinal detachment when the surface spike shows minimal, trembling, vertical, brief aftermovement following each of the minimal inadvertant corrective movements of the patient's eye while fixating a stable target [5]. This sign is better appreciated when using low 'Measuring Sensitivity' of a Standardized A-scan instrument.

A_4 *(Fig. 2)*

This A-scan sign results from a quantitative measurement of the reflectivity of the surface in question ('Quantitative Echography II' [3,6]). During this evaluation, the maximal signal from the surface is displayed and compared with the maximal signal from the sclera of the same eye being used as reference [7]. A difference between the maximal surface and scleral signals of 15 db or less indicates retinal detachment whereas a difference of 17 db and above proves membrane. A difference of 16 db is borderline and can still be resolved by including the maximal signal from the prescleral surface. In the case of retinal detachment, this surface is pigment epithelium and reflects less strongly than when the retina is attached and the prescleral surface is retinal surface. A difference of 12 db or less between the maximal scleral and prescleral surfaces indicates attached retina while a difference of 14 db or more is consistent with retinal detachment.

This acoustic criterion too requires the use of a Standardized A-scan instrument to be reliable and useful (see above). The latest model of a

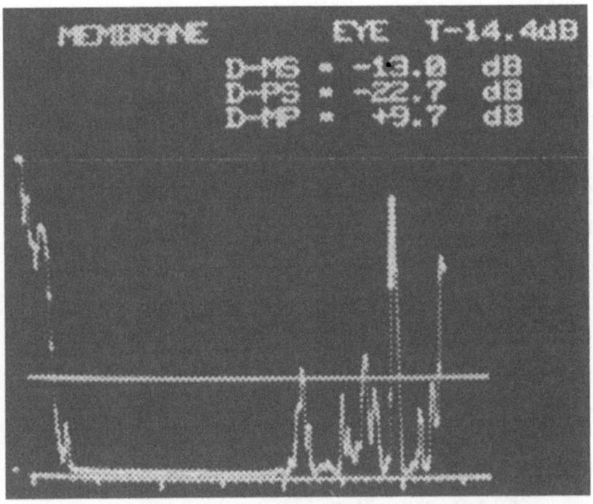

A

Fig. 2. Maximal signals from detached retina (A), sclera (B), and 'presclera' (C) as memorized by the instrument (B-scan S – BVI) are highlighted by electronic gates. The difference in decibels between the maximal signals from 'membrane' (detached retina in this case) and sclera (D-MS = –13.0 dB), between 'presclera' and sclera (D-PS = –22.7 dB), and between 'membrane' and 'presclera' (D-MP = +9.7 dB) are displayed: Positive A_4

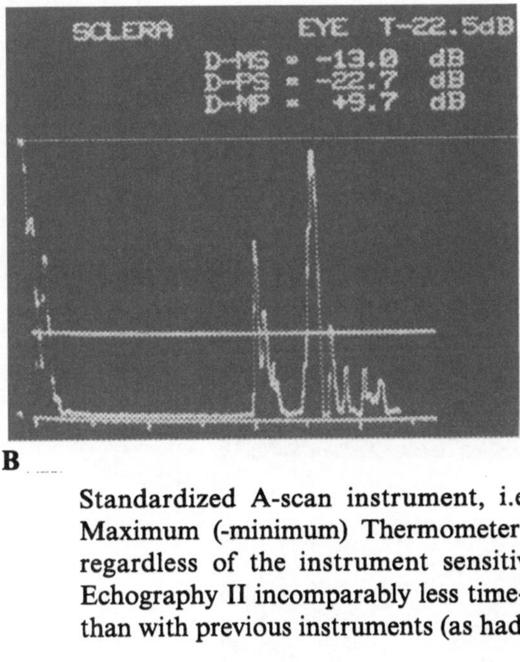

B

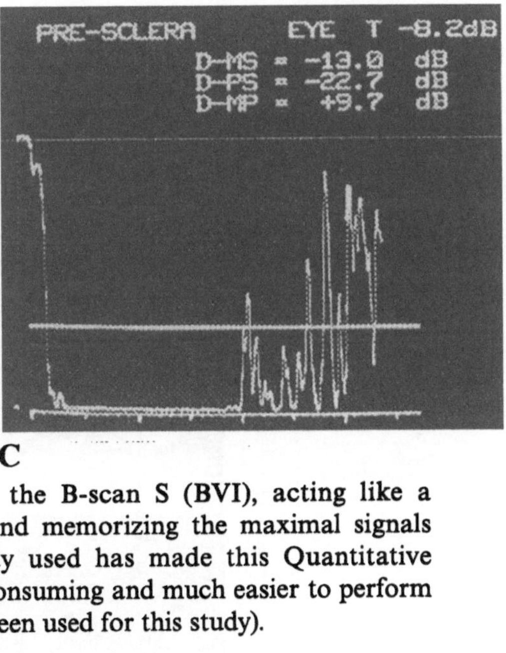

C

Standardized A-scan instrument, i.e., the B-scan S (BVI), acting like a Maximum (-minimum) Thermometer and memorizing the maximal signals regardless of the instrument sensitivity used has made this Quantitative Echography II incomparably less time-consuming and much easier to perform than with previous instruments (as had been used for this study).

B_1 *(Fig. 3)*

This B-scan sign represents shapes of surface signals that are specific for retinal detachment and not produced by fibrovascular membranes or other surfaces that may mimic retinal detachment. The most commonly seen typical shape is an 'angled' surface line representing detached retina which is subjected to traction. Figure 3A illustrates such angling (arrows) in a total funnel-shaped retinal detachment ('triangular' detachment; Fuller [8]) and Figure 3B shows it in localized, tent-like tractional detachments.

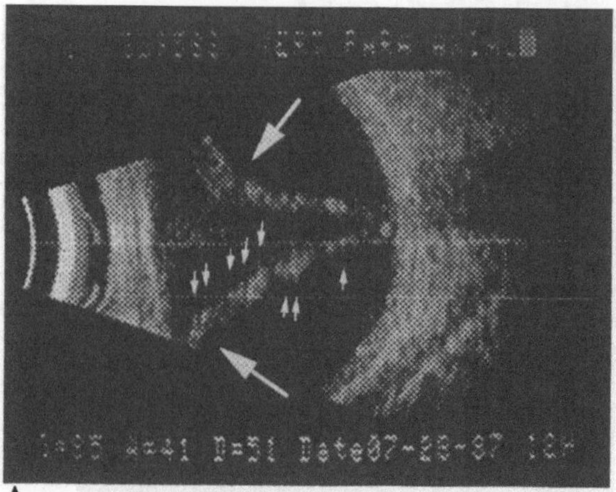
A=41 D=51

A

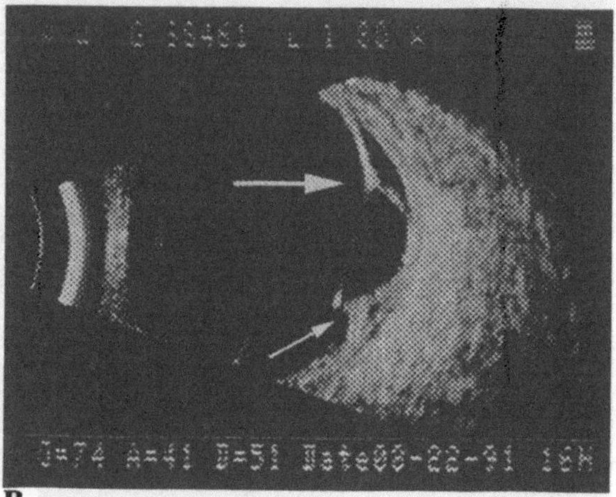
G=74 A=41 D=51 Date08-22-91 16H

B

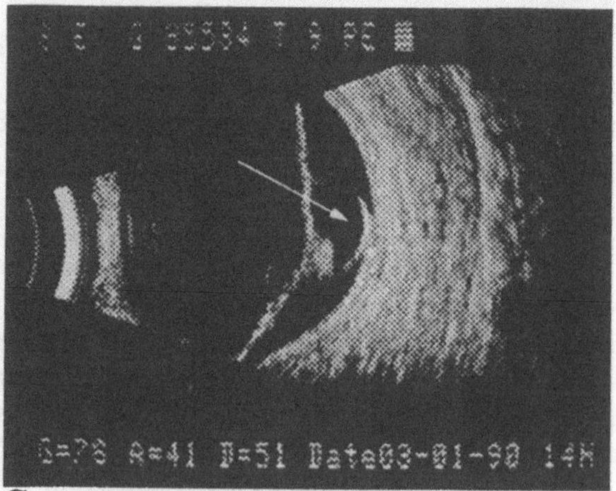
G=76 A=41 D=51 Date03-01-90 14H

C

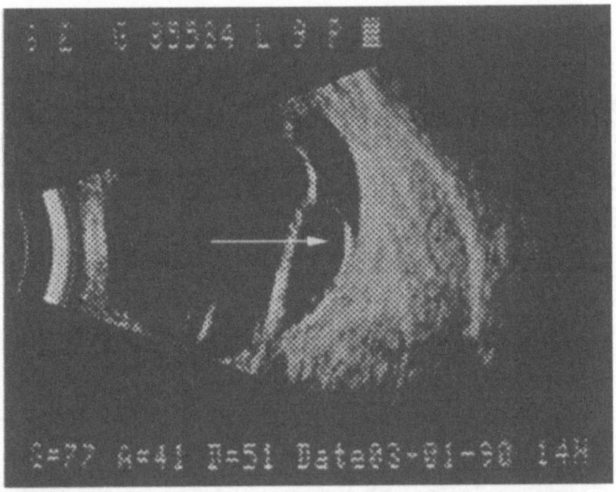

D

Fig. 3. Total funnel-shaped retinal detachment (A) and tractional retinal detachments (B) showing phenomenon of 'angling' (large arrows). Smooth macrofolds are also present (small arrows). Transverse (C) and longitudinal (D) scans of retinal cyst (arrows point at signals from posterior cyst wall)

Another typical shape is caused by cyst formation which too is specific for retina. In order to safely differentiate a retinal cyst from a large retinal fold, the cyst pattern must be shown in two echographic planes that are perpendicular to each other and thus reveal the 3-dimensional character of a cyst and dispel the possibility that a 2-dimensional fold is the cause for the pattern. Figures 3C and 3D show a tranverse and a longitudinal section from such a retinal cyst proving its 3-dimensional character.

B_2

This B-scan sign is caused by smooth 'macro-folds' of a large surface. Only those portions of the surface reached by an approximately perpendicular sound beam produce echoes while those portions reached by an oblique beam reflect all the energy away from the probe and thus remain 'anechoic' (mirror-like reflection on large smooth interface). This results in an interrupted echo line. The individual short echo lines originate only at the tiny point-like portions of the smooth surface, which are reached by a perpendicular beam. These lines are longer or shorter depending on the echo intensity. Moreover, these lines are oriented perpendicular to the direction of the sound beam and not according to the course of the large surface (Fig. 3A, small arrows).

B₃ *(Fig. 4)*

This B-scan sign is positive for retinal detachment when a funnel-shaped surface structure inserts into the optic disc with clear separation of its two leaves in the B-scan section. One often has to search for an optimal scanning approach to clearly display the B_3 sign. In Figure 4A this was achieved through a transverse scan of the optic disc area.

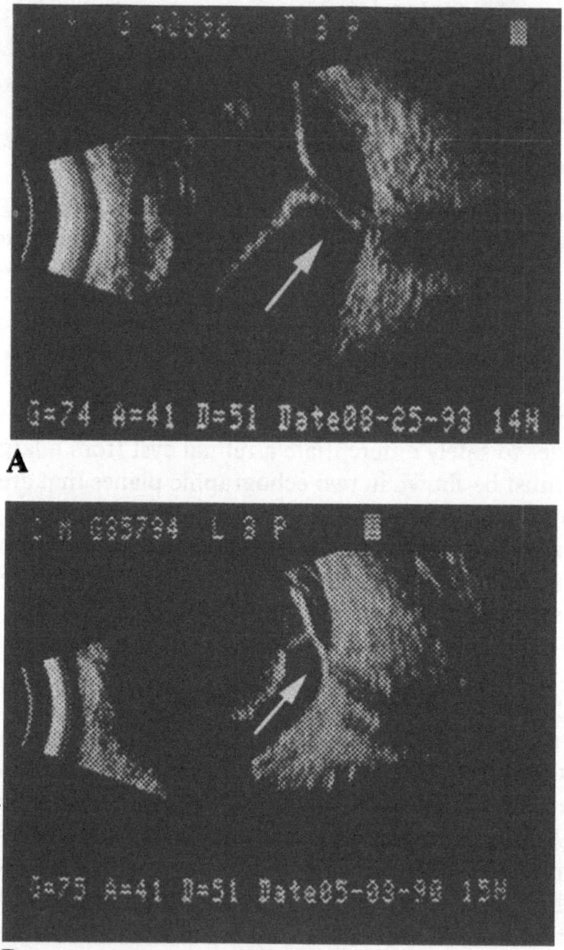

Fig. 4. A. Total funnel-shaped retinal detachment showing separate insertion (arrow) of the two retinal leaves into the disc (positive B_3). B. Funnel-shaped fibrovascular vitreous membrane inserting into disc with common stalk (arrow) (negative B_3)

A retinal detachment is unlikely when the two leaves of the funnel-shaped surface structure are seen to insert into the disc with one common stalk (Fig. 4B). Only a clear-cut separation or a distinct common stalk of the two leaves at their optic disc insertion allow a useful application of the B_3 sign. Often the insertion of a detached retina or a funnel-shaped membrane show neither clear-cut type of insertion into the disc and thus offer no unequivocal B_3 sign that would be useful for the differential diagnosis.

B_4

This sign may be applicable in partial retinal detachments. When the echo line obtained from the detached portion can be followed clearly into the attached area and thus both the detached and attached portions of the echo line are clearly continuous the B_4 sign is positive for retinal detachment. While inserting membranes usually do not show this sign, a partially detached vitreous with its posterior surface being enhanced by hemorrhage may simulate retina in this regard. However, such non-membraneous positive vitreous surface behaves very differently from detached retina in quantitative and kinetic terms. Also, the direction in which the fusion occurs in large surfaces is clearly opposite in detached retina vs. vitreous: the attached portion is seen only peripherally in detached vitreous whereas it is located either both peripherally and posteriorly or only posteriorly (when the retina is detached to the ora). Since the posterior surface of a detached vitreous (even if it is acoustically enhanced by dense vitreous hemorrhage) reflects clearly less than a detached retina the B_4 sign should be recruited as additional help for the diagnosis of detached retina only after a positive A_1 sign has been established first.

The study

In a clinical study we tested the usefulness of the four A-scan and four B-scan criteria by determining their availability, (general and particular) sensitivity, (general and particular) specificity, and their (general and particular) positive as well as negative predictive values. We also determined the ease (vs. difficulty) of applying each of the acoustic criteria, and the time required for their application (quickness vs. slowness of procedure).

The study originally involved all patients seen consecutively in our Echography Service between January 1987 and June 1988 because of densely opaque ocular media. All those patients who had only a plain cataract with or without a rhegmatogenous retinal detachment, or only a simple vitreous or subvitreal hemorrhage without proliferative complications were excluded from the study. Furthermore, all those patients were excluded from the study, in whom a verification of the real status of the retina could not be obtained within 10 days of the echographic examination. After the exclusion of these cases the study included a total of 61 eyes in 58 patients (55% male, 45% female). All of these eyes had densely opaque ocular media and strongly reflective 'membraneous' structures within the vitreous cavity (most of them as a consequence of severe proliferative diabetic retinopathy or severe ocular trauma).

In all but two of the eyes verification of the echographic diagnosis was obtained through a vitrectomy. In one case a vitreous hemorrhage cleared enough in time to allow ophthalmoscopic verification. In another case histologic verification was obtained following enucleation. In 48 (79%) of the eyes included in the study the 'membraneous structure' which had been evaluated with the acoustic criteria for retinal detachment, was confirmed to be detached retina. Conversely, fibrovascular membranes were confirmed in the remaining eyes.

Availability

The availability of an acoustic criterion is the percentage of all eyes studied, in which a particular criterion could be applied whether the result was unequivocal for the diagnosis of retinal detachment and its differentiation from a dense fibrovascular membrane, or not. If the availability, for instance, was 98%, the criterion was available in all but one of the 61 cases.

The A-scan and B-scan criteria basically fall into two categories.

Category 1

This includes those criteria (i.e., A_1, B_1, and B_2), which by nature are always available, though not always diagnostic. The maximal height of a surface spike at Tissue Sensitivity and the smoothness of its left ascending limb (A_1), for instance, can always be evaluated. Typical shapes (B_1) such as angling of an echo line and cyst pattern may or may not be present but can always be looked for, in a B-scan. These typical shapes may also be present but be equivocal and misleading. The same holds true for smooth macrofolds (B_2).

Category 2

This includes those criteria (i.e., A_2, A_3, B_3 and B_4) which if available may be either positive, negative or equivocal. On the other hand these criteria may not be available for reasons extrinsic to the study. They then are useless for the diagnosis but at least cannot be misleading as the equivocal criteria are. A_2, for instance, is only available to begin with if a large surface extends to the ora (or vitreous base). It cannot be used when the large surface is limited to a more posterior fundus area. The A_3 sign may be impossible to evaluate in a patient who continuously moves the eyes as those movements may be subtle. An A_4 may not be available if an eye is extremely soft for lack of standard scleral signals. The B_3 sign may be out of order because the surface structure is neither funnel-shaped nor inserting into the disc. The B_4 sign finally cannot be included when a retinal detachment or simulating surface structure is total. In all these instances, these particular criteria cannot be used but also cannot mislead the diagnostician. For this reason particular (not only general) sensitivities etc. were determined for the category 2 criteria (see below).

Sensitivity

The sensitivity of a criterion indicates how reliable it is in determining retinal detachment. It is the probability or percentage of true positives. This is the rate that a true detached retina will be identified as such. Any misinterpretation in this regard is a false-negative diagnosis. If, for instance, the sensitivity of the A_1 criterion in the study was 98%, then it was positive in all cases of retinal detachment but one.

Specificity

The specificity of a criterion is the probability (or percentage) of true negatives. This is the rate that a normal (not detached) retina will be identified. Any misinterpretation in this regard is a false-positive diagnosis. If, for instance, the specificity of the A_1 criterion in the study was 100%, then it was not positive for retinal detachment when there was no retinal detachment. It never indicated detached retina when the retina was attached.

There are two ways to look at the sensitivity and specificity of an acoustic criterion for the diagnosis of a retinal detachment vs. a dense fibrovascular membrane. In a general sense, the sensitivity is the percentage of correct cells in the total group of retinal detachments (i.e., 48 cases in the study). Any such diagnosis not indicated by the criterion is a false-negative regardless of whether the criterion was negative for retinal detachment or was not even available for use. In this report such a sensitivity is called 'general' sensitivity. In the same way, the specificity is called general, when all the true negatives are counted against the criterion being negative for retinal detachment regardless of whether the criterion was indeed negative or was not even used for the diagnosis because it was not available. This general consideration of a criterion's sensitivity and specificity is important to evaluate the value of the criterion in the differential diagnosis of retinal detachment vs. dense fibrovascular membrane.

For the clinician in clinical practice this general sensitivity and specificity of a criterion, however, are much less important than what – in a narrower definition – is called 'particular' sensitivity and 'particular' specificity: it is the percentage of correctly diagnosed true positives and true negatives, respectively among those cases for which the criterion was available. If, for instance, the A_3 sign was available only in 92% of all 48 cases of true retinal detachment but correctly indicated retinal detachment in all these cases, the particular sensitivity of the A_3 sign is 100% whereas its general sensitivity is only 92%. For the clinician, however, it is important to know that this criterion is available in 92% of all cases and that it is 100% reliable in detecting retinal detachment in the cases where it is available.

Positive predictive value

The positive predictive value of a criterion is the probability (or percentage) that a positive outcome of the test will actually be a detached retina.

Negative predictive value

The negative predictive value of a criterion is the probability (or percentage) that a negative outcome of the test will actually be an attached retina.

To both the positive and negative predictive values the definition of a general and a particular kind were applied as outlined for the sensitivity and specificity above. Again, the particular values are more interesting to the echographer than the general ones since the echographer does know when a test cannot be applied and therefore a conclusion is not possible. On the other hand the echographer needs to know how reliable a criterion is once it is available.

Ease

Another important factor in choosing and weighing various criteria for the differentiation between detached retina and dense fibrovascular membranes are the skill and effort the echographer needs to apply to get a useful result. Usually the easier and faster techniques are applied first and the more difficult procedures are left for later if needed. For the evaluation in this study, the easier techniques were given a ++ and the more difficult tests were rated as - -.

Time

Similarly, the value of a criterion was also judged by the length of time needed to get a useful result. Again the speediest procedures were rated with a ++, whereas the more time-consuming evaluations were given a - -.

Results

The results of the study are presentetd in Tables 1–3 and Figures 5–9. Table 1 tabulates the percentages of the availability of each of the eight acoustic criteria (both for the entire group of patients [bold numbers] and for the 48 eyes with subsequently proven retinal detachment [numbers in parenthesis]). The particular sensitivities and specificities as well as positive and negative predictive values are highlighted in bold type to stress their greater importance for the clinician. The general and particular indicators are illustrated side by side in the bar charts (Figs. 5–8).

Table 2 lists the ranking of the four A-scan and four B-scan criteria in regard to the various indicators listed in Table 1. As can be seen, the A-scan criteria (especially the A_1 sign) clearly lead the B-scan criteria in all indictors. Among

Table 1. Results of the four A-scan and four B-scan criteria used in the diagnosis of retinal detachment and its differentiation from dense fibrovascular vitreous membranes according to their availability (**AV**), general sensitivity (S_G), particular sensitivity (S_P), general specificity (SP_G), particular specificity (SP_P), general positive predictive value ($+Pred_G$), particular positive predictive value ($+Pred_P$), general negative predictive value ($-Pred_G$), particular negative predictive value ($-Pred_P$), ease vs. difficulty of application (**Ease**), and quickness vs. slowness of procedure (**Time**)

%of	AV (av)	S_G	S_P	SP_G	SP_P	$+Pred_G$	$+Pred_P$	$-Pred_G$	$-Pred_P$	East	Time
A_1	**100** (100)	98	**98**	100	**100**	100	**100**	93	**93**	++	++
A_2	**69** (67)	67	**100**	62	**89**	86	**97**	33	**100**	+	+
A_3	**92** (92)	92	**100**	92	**100**	98	**100**	75	**100**	±	++
A_4	**77** (71)	65	**91**	92	**92**	97	**97**	41	**80**	--	--
B_1	**100** (100)	44	**44**	85	**85**	91	**91**	29	**29**	+	++
B_2	**100** (100)	75	**75**	38	**38**	82	**82**	29	**29**	±	++
B_3	**44** (42)	25	**60**	31	**67**	57	**86**	10	**33**	--	±
B_4	**57** (60)	40	**66**	15	**33**	63	**83**	6	**17**	--	--

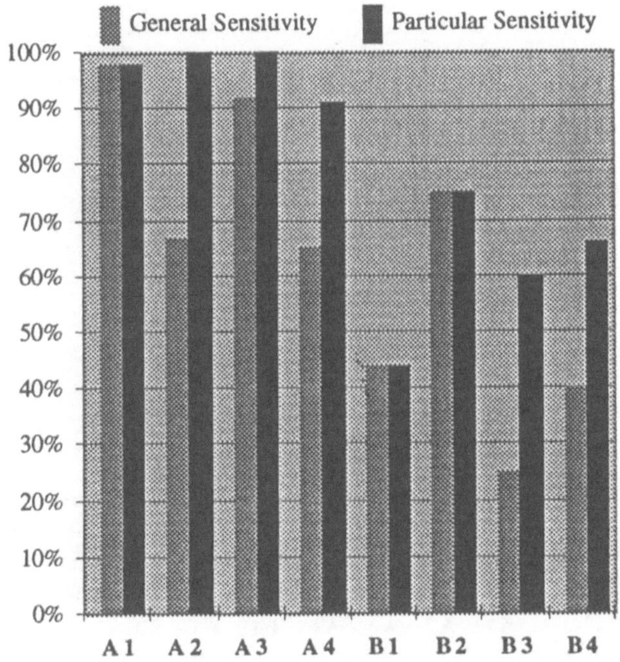

Fig. 5. Illustration of the (general and particular) sensitivities of the four A-scan and the four B-scan criteria used in the study for the diagnosis of retinal detachment

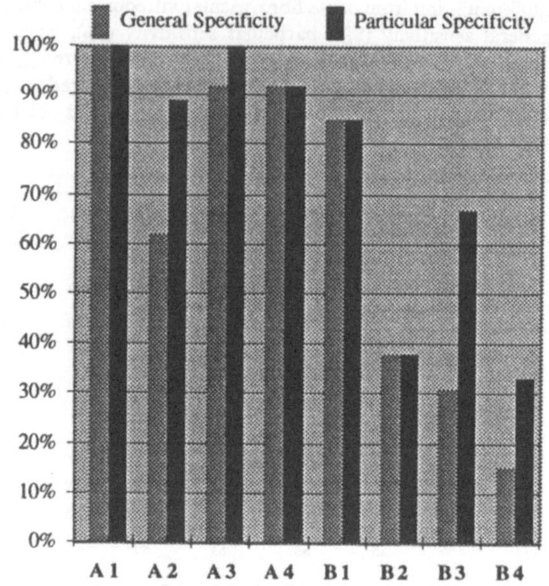

Fig. 6. Illustration of the (general and particular) specificities of the four A-scan and the four B-scan criteria used in the study for the diagnosis of retinal detachment

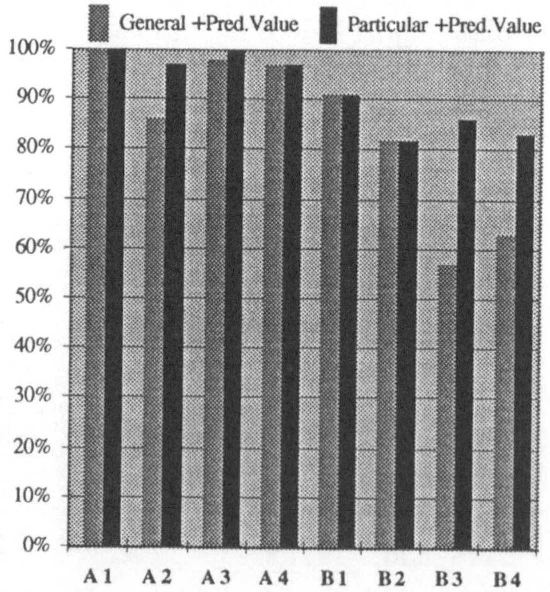

Fig. 7. Illustration of the (general and particular) positive predictive values of the four A-scan and the four B-scan criteria used in the study for the diagnosis of retinal detachment

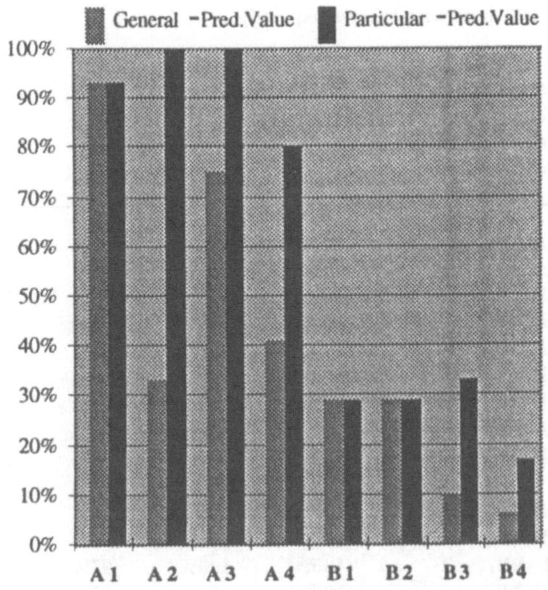

Fig. 8. Illustration of the (general and particular) negative predictive values of the four A-scan and the four B-scan criteria used in the study for the diagnosis of retinal detachment

Table 2. Ranking of differential criteria (from left to right) according to left indicators

Availability	A_1&B_1&B_2, A_3, A_4, A_2, B_4, B_3
Sensitivity (general)	A_1, A_3, B_2, A_2, A_4, B_1, B_4, B_3
Sensitivity (particular)	A_2&A_3, A_1, A_4, B_2, B_4, B_3, B_1
Specificity (general)	A_1, A_3&A_4, B_1, A_2, B_2&B_3, B_4
Specificity (particular)	A_1&A_3, A_4, A_2, B_1, B_3, B_2, B_4
Positive predictive value (general)	A_1, A_3, A_4, B_1, A_2, B_2, B_4, B_3
Positive predictive value (particular)	A_1&A_3, A_2&A_4, B_1, B_4, B_2, B_3
Negative predictive value (general)	A_1, A_3, A_4, A_2, B_1&B_2, B_3, B_4
Negative predictive value (particular)	A_2&A_3, A_1, A_4, B_3, B_1&B_2, B_4
Ease of operation	A_1, A_2&B_1, A_3&B_2, B_3&B_4, A_4
Swiftness of operation	A_1&A_3&B_1&B_2, A_2, B_3, B_4, A_4

The clinically most important parameters and the percentages which are $\geqslant 90$ are printed in **bold type**

Table 3. Effectiveness of various combinations of diagnostic criteria in positively diagnosing retinal detachment (at least two positive criteria required)

Among the 48 proven cases of retinal detachment were at least acoustic criteria positive for retinal detachment	1	2	3	4	5
$A_1\&A_2\&A_3\&A_4\&B_1\&B_2\&B_3\&B_4$	(100%)	**100%**	100%	83%	65%
$A_1\&A_2\&A_3\&B_1\&B_2\&B_3\&B_4$	(100%)	**100%**	98%	79%	42%
$A_1\&A_2\&A_3\&A_4\&B_1\&B_3\&B_4$	(100%)	**100%**	98%	71%	48%
$A_1\&A_2\&A_3\&A_4\&B_1\&B_2\&B_4$	(100%)	**100%**	98%	85%	65%
$A_1\&A_2\&A_3\&A_4\&B_1\&B_2\&B_3$	(100%)	**100%**	98%	79%	60%
$A_1\&A_2\&A_3\&A_4\&B_2\&B_3\&B_4$	(100%)	**100%**	96%	77%	56%
$A_1\&A_3\&A_4\&B_1\&B_2\&B_3\&B_4$	(100%)	**100%**	96%	77%	48%
$A_2\&A_3\&A_4\&B_1\&B_2\&B_3\&B_4$	(100%)	**100%**	90%	60%	40%
$A_1\&A_2\&A_3\&A_4\&B_1\&B_2$	(100%)	**100%**	96%	77%	56%
$A_1\&A_2\&A_4\&B_1\&B_3\&B_4$	(100%)	**100%**	96%	73%	48%
$A_1\&A_3\&B_1\&B_2\&B_3\&B_4$	(100%)	**100%**	92%	58%	19%
$A_1\&A_2\&B_1\&B_2\&B_3\&B_4$	(100%)	98%	89%	40%	17%
$A_2\&A_3\&B_1\&B_2\&B_3\&B_4$	(100%)	98%	81%	44%	17%
$A_2\&A_4\&B_1\&B_2\&B_3\&B_4$	(100%)	90%	71%	42%	10%
$A_1\&A_2\&A_3\&B_1\&B_2$	(100%)	**100%**	92%	63%	19%
$A_1\&A_2\&A_3\&A_4\&B_1$	(100%)	**100%**	85%	65%	15%
$A_1\&B_1\&B_2\&B_3\&B_4$	(100%)	96%	62%	21%	–
$A_2B_1\&B_2\&B_3\&B_4$	(98%)	90%	44%	19%	2%
$A_2\&A_4\&B_1\&B_3\&B_4$	(100%)	77%	50%	13%	–
$A_1\&A_2\&A_4\&B_1$	(100%)	**100%**	85%	65%	15%
$A_1\&A_3\&B_1\&B_2$	(100%)	**100%**	83%	25%	–
$A_1\&A_2\&A_3\&A_4$	(100%)	96%	79%	46%	–
$A_1\&A_4\&B_1\&B_3$	(100%)	83%	46%	2%	–
$B_1\&B_2\&B_3\&B_4$	(96%)	62%	25%	2%	–
$A_1\&A_3\&A_4$	(100%)	96%	60%	–	–
$A_1\&A_2\&A_3$	(100%)	94%	60%	–	–
$A_1\&A_4\&B_1$	(100%)	81%	25%	–	–
$A_1\&A_2\&A_4$	(98%)	83%	48%	–	–
$A_1\&A_3$	(100%)	90%	–	–	–
$A_1\&A_4$	(98%)	65%	–	–	–
$B_1\&B_2$	(92%)	29%	–	–	–
$B_1\&B_3$	(58%)	10%	–	–	–

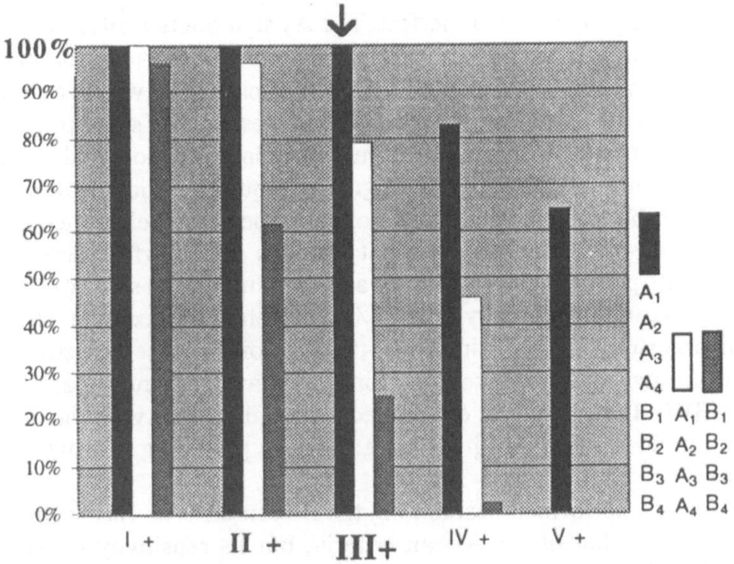

Fig. 9. Comparison of results (in %) when using A_1&A_2&A_3&A_4+B_1&B_2&B_3&B_4, A_1&A_2&A_3&A_4, and B_1&B_2&B_3&B_4 echographic criteria and harvesting at least one (I+), at least two (II+), at least three (III+), four (IV+) and five (V+) criteria positive for retinal detachment in the 47 cases (100%) of proven retinal detachment in the study

the B-scan signs the B_1&B_2 signs rank first. Those criteria which ranked higher than 90% are highlighted in Table 2; so are the indicators of greater importance.

Table 3 lists the diagnostic effectiveness of various combinations of A-scan and B-scan criteria in terms of their overall sensitivities. Figure 9 shows a bar chart illustrating the differences in this group effectiveness between a diagnostic pool of all eight criteria and a combined effort of all A-scan and all B-scan criteria, respectively. While the combined pool of all eight criteria harvested at least 3 positive criteria in each single case of retinal detachment and thus provided a 'hard' correct diagnosis in 100% of the proven cases of retinal detachment, the success rate of the combined effort of all A-scan criteria was only 79% in achieving at least 3 positive criteria, and that of all B-scan criteria was only 25%.

Discussion

When scrutinizing the performance of each of the acoustic differential criteria as indicated in Table 1 and Figures 5–8, it becomes evident that no single acoustic criterion can give an entirely satisfying result. Each of the criteria has its strengths and weaknesses though to quite different degrees.

The A_1 sign offers a perfect specificity and positive predictive value, but its sensitivity is slightly less than perfect. The A_2 sign offers a 100% sensitivity and negative predictive value, at least regarding the 69% of the true retinal detachments where it was available. Its specificity, however, is only 89% and, besides, it was not available in a third of the cases. The A_3 sign appears to be the best of all with a 100% record for all the particular indicators and an availability of 92%. It is, however, a subjective sign and requires a good deal of experience before it can be trusted completely. For the experienced examiner it is a pearl. The A_4 sign shows another excellent but less than perfect performance. In particular, its poor time performance and demand on the skills of the examiner hampered its use (availability only 77%) in severely injured eyes. However, this A-scan criterion has been improved tremendously since the study was performed through the use of software programs available nowadays with the *B-scan S* (BVI). It now may be considered an equal partner with the other A-scan criteria. It does offer the great advantage of providing a truly quantitative measure.

The B_1 sign performed best among the B-scan criteria. Its specificity of 85% comes close to that of the A-scan criteria, but its sensitivity is very low. The reason for this is the relative rarety of typical shapes occurring in retinal detachments across the board. The B_2 sign, by contrast, offers a much higher though still not ideal sensitivity while being not at all specific. The characteristics of the B_2 sign, however, are better understood today than at the time of the study, so that clearly better results can be expected from its use. The same holds true of the B_3 sign: when accepting only clear-cut cases of separate insertion of the two leaves of a funnel-shaped surface structure into the disc, the rate of false-positives is likely to drop further; at the same time, however, false-negatives are likely to increase as a consequence of more equivocal outcomes. A major weakness of both the B_3 and the B_4 signs has been and continues to be their low availability rates (44% and 57%, respectively).

As this study clearly shows, none of the acoustic criteria is always available and sensitive enough to diagnose each case of retinal detachment. Moreover, the specificities of some of the criteria are so poor that one cannot trust them even though their sensitivity may be high. The solution is to use a pool of several criteria and attempt to harvest at least 2 positive ones to make the diagnosis of retinal detachment a safe one. If one of the two successful criteria has a poor specificity record a third positive criterion has to be added to make the diagnosis 'hard'. As the study shows, only the utilization of the entire pool of A-scan and B-scan criteria has a chance to achieve this goal in all cases (see Table 3 and Fig. 9). Combinations of only seven, and in some instances even of fewer than seven A-scan and B-scan criteria may be successful to get at least 2 positive hits, and in the majority of cases even 3 positive answers (Table 3). But such a limited approach risks misdiagnoses and does not offer a significant shortening of the examination times needed. It is definitely better to always use the entire pool of eight acoustic differential criteria. The question remains of how to apply the various A-scan and B-scan criteria successively in order to save time and effort and still obtain the hard diagnosis desired.

Experience has shown that the B_1 sign, followed by the B_2 and B_3 signs, and then by the A_1&A_2&A_3 group leads to hard diagnoses quickly. Since the B-scan basic examination usually detects a large surface suspicious of being a retinal detachment, it is quite natural to first look at the presence of smooth macro-folds and typical shapes. If the surface structure inserts into disc in a funnel-shaped fashion, this insertion would be scrutinized next (B_3). Since none of these B-scan signs has a good specificity record, they are not sufficient to safely diagnose retinal detachment even if 2 of them should be positive. It is always an easy and very safe approach to quickly add the A_1&A_2&A_3 signs to secure the diagnosis of retinal detachment. Should the absolutely required number of two positive signs or the always preferable minimal score of three clearly positive answers still not be achieved by this approach, one will add the somewhat more time-consuming and difficult A_4 and B_4 evaluations. Ever since the software program for Quantitative Echography II has become available with the *B-scan S* instrument (BVI), the A_4 sign can be mastered in a very short time. We use the A_4 sign regularly in many cases of retinal detachment, simply because it is next to the A_1 sign, the only objective quantitative measurement available and gives the diagnosis the extra security.

Conclusion

The safe diagnosis of retinal detachment in eyes with dense vitreous and/or subvitreal hemorrhages and with proliferative complications requires the use of all eight A-scan and B-scan criteria of Standardized Echography. Any shortcuts trying to use fewer acoustic criteria softens the diagnosis considerably and fails to come up with a solid diagnosis in every single case. The use of B-scan signs alone misses on a large scale and the exclusive use of A-scan signs is also insufficient.

When utilizing the entire pool of all eight A-scan and B-scan criteria the echographer is guaranteed to safely diagnose retinal detachment even under the most adverse circumstances as found in severe cases of trauma and vitreoretinal proliferative disease. However, not all criteria need to be applied in all cases. To economize their usage time- and effort-wise, the examiner is recommended to apply them in a certain order until at least 2 clearly positive criteria are obtained. If one or the other of these positive criteria has a poor specificity record it will be wise to safeguard the diagnosis with one of the two quantitative criteria (i.e., A_1 and A_2).

The recommended order of application (as far as available) is this: B_1, B_2, B_3, A_1, A_2, A_3, B_4 and A_4. Even if it should be necessary to apply all eight criteria in a rare case, the total evaluation time should not exceed 10 minutes in the hand of an experienced echographer. The reward for utilizing this approach well will be a nearly 100% diagnostic record.

References

1. K.C. Ossoinig, G. Islas, G.E. Tamayo and C. Tamburrelli. Detached retina versus dense fibrovascular membrane (standardized A-scan and B-scan criteria). In K.C. Ossoinig (ed.), Ophthalmic echography (SIDUO 1984). Dordrecht/Boston/London: Kluwer Academic Publishers, Docum. Ophthal. Proc. Series.Docum Ophthal Proc Series, 1987;48:275–284.
2. K.C. Ossoinig. Standardized ophthalmic echography of the eye, orbit and periorbital region. A comprehensive slide set and study guide, 3rd edn. Iowa City: Goodfellow Co., 1985:44.
3. K.C. Ossoinig. Quantitative echography – the basis of tissue differentiation. J. Clin. Ultrasound. 1974;2(1):33.
4. H. Freyler. Echography – an important auxillary examination in the surgical management of retinal detachment (German). Klin. Monatsbl. Augenheilk. 1970;157:617–633.
5. K.C. Ossoinig. Standardized echography. Basic principles, clinical applications, and results. In Int. Ophthalmol. Clin. Boston: Little Brown and Co., 1979;19(4):127–210.
6. A. Sawada, M. Inahara, Y. Masuyama and Y. Baba. Significance of quantitative echography in membrane-like structures in the vitreous. Acta. Soc. Ophthal. Japonicae. 1979;83(8):1434–1444.
7. P. Till and A. Neumann. Reliability of biological standards (German). In K.C. Ossoinig (ed.), Ultrasonographia media (Proc 1st World Congress on Ultrasonic Diagnostics in Medicine and SIDUO III). Verlag Wien Med. Akad. 1971;II:119–124.
8. D.F. Fuller. Triangular retinal detachment – ultrasonic identification of massive periretinal proliferation in eyes with opaque media. Mod Prob Ophthalmol. 1977;18:68.

Karl C. Ossoinig
Department of Ophthalmology
UI Hospitals and Clinics
Iowa City
U.S.A.

29. A-B scan echographic imaging in a case of Terson's syndrome

P. LIZZI, S. DA POZZO, L. BORZAGHINI and P. PERISSUTTI

(Trieste, Italy)

Abstract

A 35-year-old male patient, after suffering a subarachnoid hemorrhage (SAH), complained of severe bilateral visual impairment, due to a vitreous hemorrhage (VH). Five months after receiving surgery for SAH, visual acuity had not improved and A-B scan echography revealed that a dense and widespread VH, associated with bilateral posterior vitreous detachment (PVD), was still detectable in both eyes. Furthermore, echography revealed the presence of a preretinal image, visible by both A and B scan, lying upon the posterior pole of the left eye; this image suggested the presence of a dome-shaped preretinal membrane. Then, in order to accelerate visual acuity improvement, the patient underwent a pars plana vitrectomy (PPV) in the left eye, and the excision of a preretinal membrane. One month after PPV, visual acuity in the left eye was 9/10. The case described emphasizes the usefulness of standardized A-B scan echography when VH precludes ophthalmoscopic examination of fundus oculi. The combination of these techniques allows a complete and reliable assessment of vitreoretinal conditions both in the diagnostic phase and in the planning of vitreoretinal surgery.

Key words: A-B scan echography, Terson syndrome, vitreous hemorrhage, pars plana vitrectomy

Introduction

The vitreous hemorrhage (VH) occurring as the direct result of subarachnoid hemorrhage (SAH) was first described in 1900 by Terson. At present, Terson's syndrome includes all cases of intraocular hemorrhage (IH) associated to all forms of intracranial bleeding. Intraocular hemorrhage, usually confined to the retina, is observed in 20–40% of adult patients with SAH [1–3], while vitreous hemorrhage appears in 3–5% patients presenting with SAH [4]. When the vitreous is penetrated by blood, the syndrome is very severe and the death rate is substantially higher. In most patients there is a slow progressive improvement of visual acuity because of spontaneous clearing of vitreous hemorrhage and the

G Cennamo and N. Rosa (eds.), Ultrasonography in Ophthalmology 15, pp. 263–268.

short-term visual outcome is generally good both in patients treated conservatively and in those treated surgically [5].

Here we describe the case of a young male who was affected by SAH at the age of 35, and who subsequently developed Terson's syndrome with bilateral vitreous hemorrhage. Five months later, he came to our observation because visual acuity had not improved at the predicted rate. Echography revealed a bilateral vitreous hemorrhage, with a total posterior vitreous detachment (PVD); these echographic findings suggested a pars plana vitrectomy (PPV) be performed.

Case report

On December 27, 1992, a 35-year-old male, complaining of a sudden frontal headache, was admitted to a medical centre (different from ours); the patient had a history of a mild treated hypertension. Computed tomography and cerebral angiography revealed the presence of a SAH caused by the rupture of a single aneurysm of the anterior communicating artery. Visual acuity was count fingers in both eyes; the ophthalmoscopic examination was impossible because of the presence of a massive bilateral vitreous hemorrhage. A few days later, the aneurysm was surgically clipped and, from the neurological point of view, the patient recovered well enough to be discharged, but visual acuity did not show significant signs of subjective or objective improvement. Three months later, the patient was examined by an ophthalmologist who suggested to perform a PPV to accelerate the visual acuity improvement.

At that point, he came to our observation on May 15, 1993 to undergo a complete eye examination and an A–B-scan echographic assessment. The best corrected visual acuity was 20/200 in the right eye and 20/400 in the left eye; the anterior segment was normal, while vitreous hemorrhage precluded the ophthalmoscopic examination. Intraocular pressure was 15 mmHg in both eyes.

A–B scan echography revealed a bilateral, widespread, dense and partially condensed vitreous hemorrhage (Figs. 1, 2A and B) in the right eye; there was a total PVD in both eyes. No echographic signals were recorded from the space between the collapsed vitreous and the retinal surface: no echographic image resembling a retinal detachment was found, while a preretinal echogenic image upon the posterior pole of the left eye and visible with both A and B-scan techniques suggested the presence of a dome-shaped preretinal membrane (Fig. 2B).

On September 17, 1993, the patient underwent a PPV in the right eye and less than one month later, the best-corrected visual acuity was 9/10 (Fig. 3). At present, the patient is waiting for vitreous surgery on his left eye (Fig. 4).

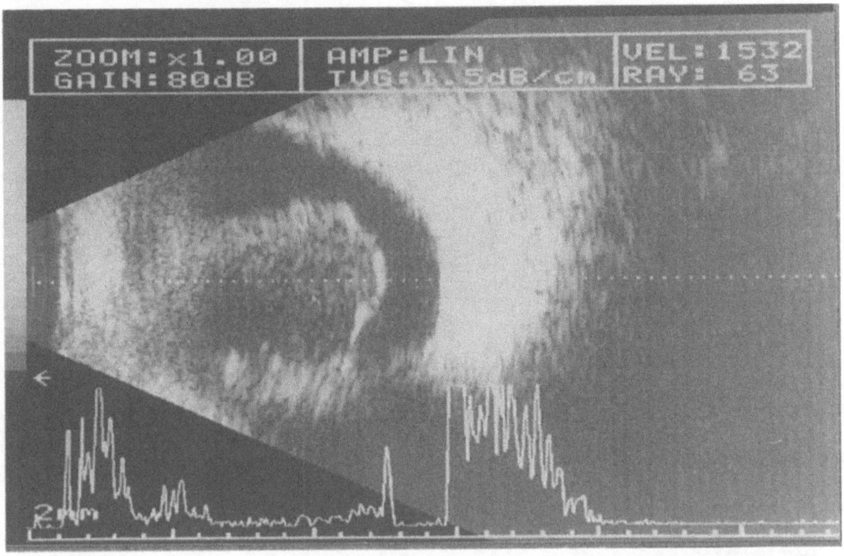

Fig. 1. A–B scan image of the right eye. Note the vitreous detachment with a posterior cortical high-reflectivity spike. There is an empty preretinal space

Discussion

A severe loss of visual acuity and its effects on daily life may be a serious problem for patients who survive SAH. A conservative treatment is represented by a 12-month waiting period, during which vitreous hemorrhage can sometimes clear spontaneously. After this period has elapsed, the alternative is to perform a PPV, which is technically facilitated by the presence of PVD. This surgical technique is considered the treatment of choice [3]; only visual immature children or adults with bilateral vitreous hemorrhage that are unlikely to resolve, must undergo early vitrectomy [6]. Schultz et al. [5] reported that in 25 of 30 considered eyes (83%), 12 treated conservatively and 13 with vitrectomy, visual acuity improved to 20/50 or better of best-corrected visual acuity, after an average follow-up of 48 months from SAH onset. However, the average time to best visual acuity is significantly shorter for eyes treated with vitrectomy than for those treated conservatively; 4.5 vs. 15 months, as reported by Schultz et al [5].

The case report described here confirms that in all cases of Terson's syndrome, therapeutic choices must always be preceded by an A–B scan echographic assessment of vitreoretinal conditions. In fact, echography overcame the vitreous opacity, and visualized the vitreous condition (total posterior detachment and condensation) and the retinal attachment.

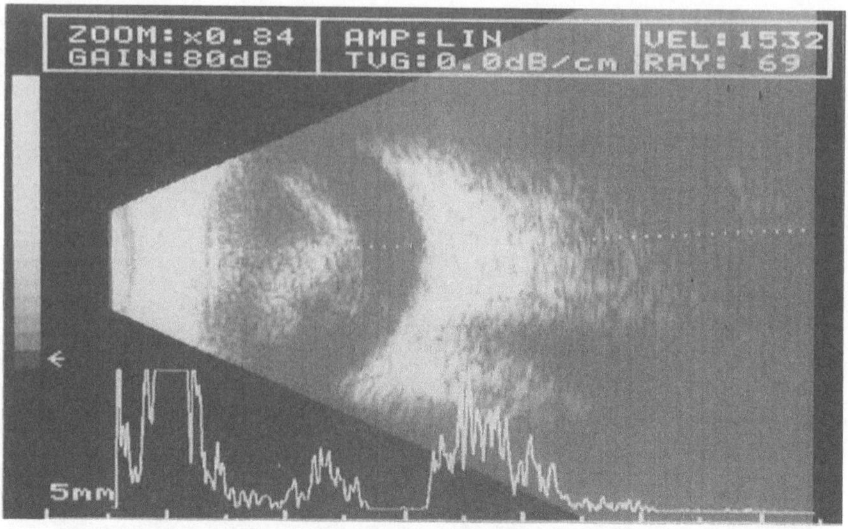

(A)

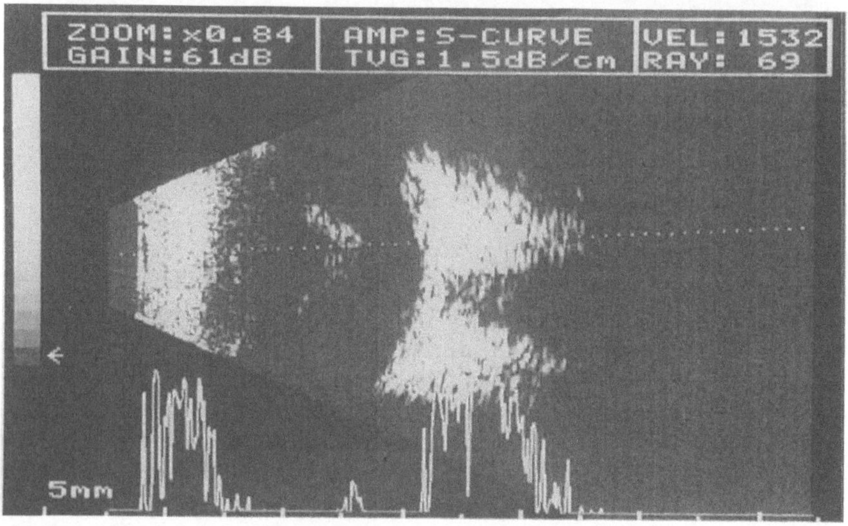

(B)

Fig. 2. (A) A–B scan image of the left eye. Note the vitreous detachment. (B) scan image of the left eye. The lower reflectivity of the preretinal A-scan spike suggests the presence of a preretinal membrane

Furthermore, A–B scan echography is an effective diagnostic tool for the visualization of preretinal membranes. Also in our patient we obtained an image that suggested the presence of a left preretinal, dome-shaped membrane (Fig. 2B). As reported by Weingeist et al. [6], the presence of these membranes can represent an obstacle to the recovery of good visual acuity, because they often lie

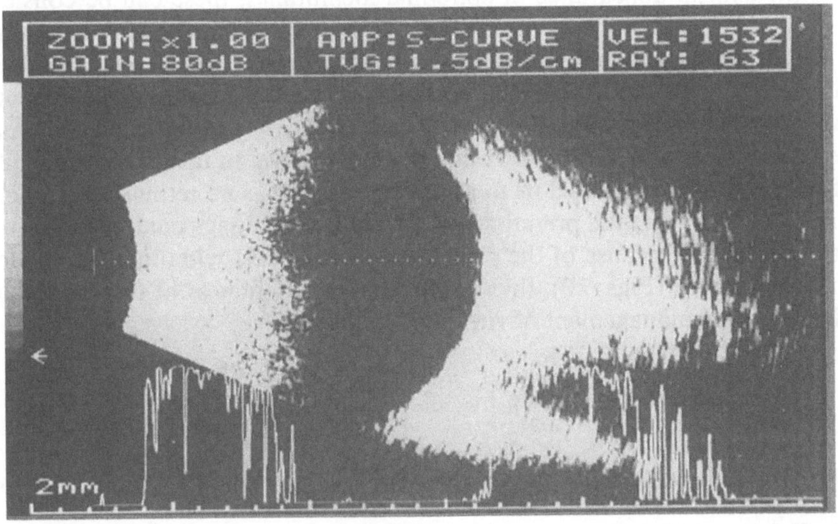

Fig. 3. ***A–B*** **scan post-surgical image of the right eye; a pars plana vitrectomy has been performed and actual best-corrected visual acuity is 20/25**

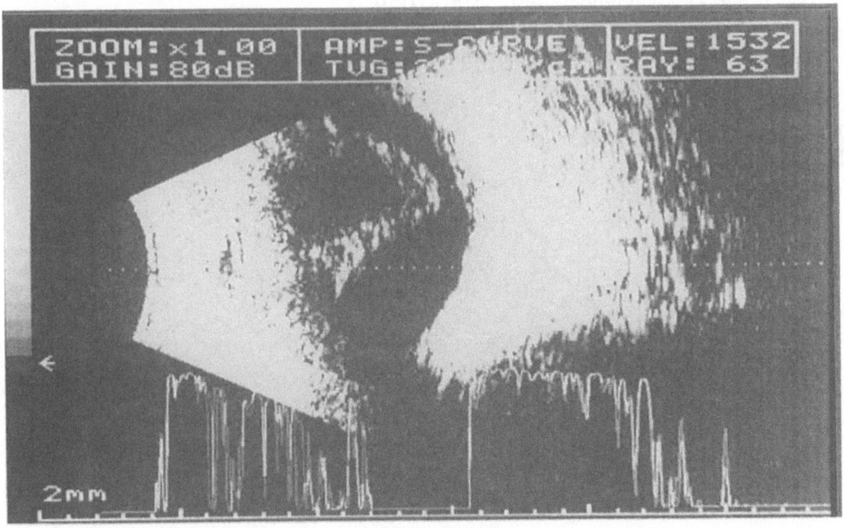

Fig. 4. ***A–B*** **scan image of the left eye (four months later after the scan shown in Figure 2B and 9 months after the onset of SAH): the persistence of vitreous hemorrhage can be clearly seen**

over the macular area. In 19 of 30 eyes (63%) observed by Schultz et al. [5], there was the clinical appearance of epiretinal membranes; these can be considered real sequelae of Terson's syndrome and they rarely recur even after excision.

These membranes are not easily visualized echographically: with B-scan alone, they can be misinterpreted as the expression of a retinal detachment [6]; but, with A- and B-scan combined they can be clearly differentiated from retina, because they appear thinner and much less reflective. In fact, the combined use of both techniques allowed us to assess that there was no retinal detachment in the left eye and that the preretinal echogenic B-scan image could be interpreted as a membrane because of the preretinal A-scan peak, with a reflectivity lower than retinal one (Figs. 2B), thus confirming the usefulness of this technique in diagnosis and management of vitreoretinal diseases.

References

[1] F.B. Walsh and W.F. Hoyt. Clinical neuro-ophthalmology, 3rd ed. Baltimore: Williams and Wilkins Co., 1969;176.

[2] H.E. Shaw, M.B. Landers and C.F. Sydnor. The significance of intraocular hemorrhages due to subarachnoid hemorrhage. Ann. Ophthalmol. 1977;9:1403–1405.

[3] J.G. Clarkson and H.W. Flynn. Vitrectomy in Terson's syndrome. Am. J. Ophthalmol. 1980;90:549–552.

[4] A.M. Garfinkle, I.R. Danys, D.A. Nicolle, A.R.T. Colohan and S. Brem. Terson's syndrome: a reversible cause of blindness following subarachnoid hemorrhage. J. Neurosurg. 1992;76:766–771.

[5] P.N. Schultz, W.M. Sobol and T.A. Weingeist, Long-term visual outcome in Terson syndrome. Ophthalmology 1991;98:1814–1819.

[6] T.A. Weingeist, E.J. Goldman, J.C. Folk, A.J. Packer and K.C. Ossoinig. Terson's syndrome: clinicopathologic correlations. Ophthalmology 1986;11:1435–1442.

Lucio Borzaghini
Department of Ophthalmology
Children's Hospital – I.R.C.C.S.
Trieste, Italy

30. Echographic findings in 'brawny' scleritis. A ten-year follow-up

V. MAZZEO, P. PERRI, P. MONARI and G. DEGLI INNOCENTI

(Ferrara, Italy)

Abstract

A case of nodular ('brawny') scleritis is reported together with its echographic findings. Data on a ten-year echographic follow-up are described; this case was first described by us in 1988, and the duration of its clinical history is 25 years. Whatever apparatus was used over the years, the B-scan images showed a fusiform enlargement of the ocular wall; the anterior aspect bulged towards the vitreous cavity like a tumor, while the posterior aspect bulged towards the orbital space giving rise to a staphyloma-like appearance. This appearance and the very strong acoustic shadowing behind the lesion helps to differentiate this condition from choroidal melanomas. The A-scan internal reflectivity of posterior scleritis is still much debated. The different A-scan patterns might be explained by the diverse pathological changes that occur in the various types of sleritis

Key words: A- and B-scan, follow-up, differential diagnosis, malignant melanoma, nodular ('brawny') scleritis

Introduction

Scleritis is an uncommon disease characterized by oedema and inflammatory cell infiltration of the sclera and episclera. Several forms exist thereby presenting problems for differentiation and for clinical classification [1–3]. Our case shows some peculiar clinical features, namely: a 25-year-duration and different clinical manifestations over time. The early clinical history of this patient is reported in the Proceedings of the SIDUO Congress held in Iguazù [4]. The first nodular manifestation decreased when therapy was discontinued. Ten years later the former pathological area is still echographically visible, while other inflammatory phenomena are present in other scleral areas [5]. We therefore believe that this echographic follow-up may help clarify the acoustic behaviour of this lesion.

G Cennamo and N. Rosa (eds.), Ultrasonography in Ophthalmology 15, pp. 269–275.

Case history

From 1985 to 1990 the patient was followed-up with several controls, the situation being stable without therapy. Best corrected visual acuity (BCVA) decreased due to a subcapsular and nuclear cataract. A visual field examination was performed before the cataract was complete.

In April 1991 intraocular pressure suddenly increased to 26 mmHg (applanation tonometry; AT) it immediately returned to normal levels with two daily drops of a beta-blocker agent. In November 1991 the patient underwent ECCE with IOL implantation in the capsular bag. Post-operative BCVA was 20/30 and reached 1 in October 1992. On ophthalmoscopy a degenerate vitreous and very pale disc were seen. At the retinal periphery very old pigment dispersion was also present. After surgery intraocular pressure was normal without local or general therapy. In spite of these findings several visual fields revealed progressive damage.

In February 1993 BCVA dropped to 20/70. Ophthalmoscopy and fluorescein angiography revealed vitreous opacities and vitreoretinal interface pathology, i.e., 'cellophane maculopathy'. In the meantime, several episodes of deep purple redness occurred particularly in the lower temporal sclera that looked swollen. In May deflazacort therapy was begun (90 mg per day) and tapered over two months.

In August 1993, at a 15-day interval, two peribulbar injections of methyl prednisolone plus ialuronic acid were administered with good results. The injections were repeated in October but no benefit was observed after the second one. In the meantime intraocular pressure increased again to 22 mmHg (AT) and beta-blocker eye drops are still in use.

In December 1993, the clinical examination showed a deep purple scleral bulge with dilated episcleral vessels in the lower temporal area. The anterior segment was within normal limits; the best corrected visual acuity was 20/25. The Ophthalmoscopic examination showed no change.

Because the eye was painful, a systemic non steroidal antinflammatory therapy was begun (Ibuprofen, 1600 mg per day) together with indomethacin eye-drops. Visual field did not worsen and the pain disappeared.

Echographic findings

All the echograms taken from 1983 to-date were reviewed to evaluate the changes over time. A detailed description of the first images has been published elsewhere [4]. Various techniques, representing the most commonly used procedures at the time, have been used over these years (Figs. 1 and 2).

Until October 1988 no changes occurred in the lesion. Whatever the machine used, the B-scan echograms showed a fusiform enlargement of the ocular wall; the anterior aspect of this area bulged towards the vitreous cavity like a tumor, while the posterior one bulged towards the orbital space giving rise to a

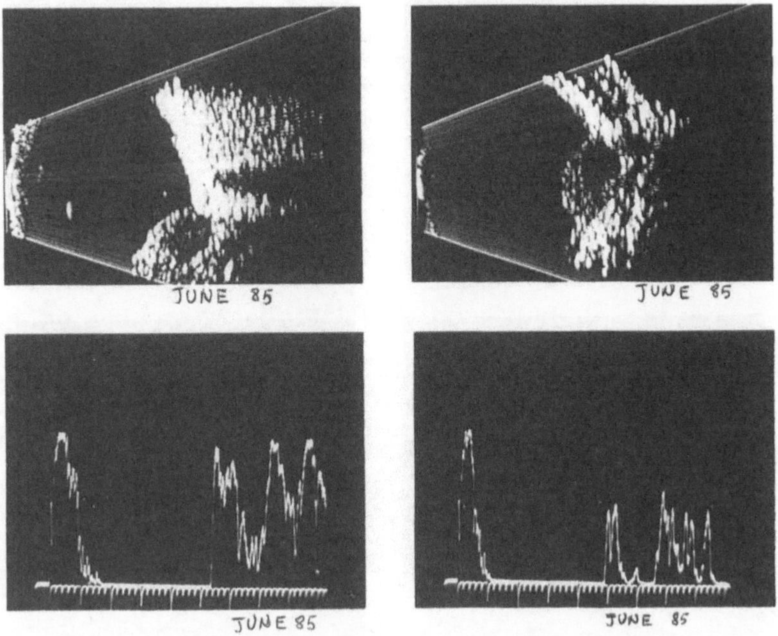

Fig. 1. Nodular scleritis. Row 1. Xenotech equipment. On the left: tumour-like lesion, the anterior aspect is highly reflective. A pseudochoroidal excavation reveals the acoustic shadowing behind the lesion. On the right: the same lesion scanned transversely. The sensitivity is lowered by 18 dB. An almost empty fusiform enlargement bulges towards the vitreous cavity and towards the orbital space. A staphylomatous deformation of the external ocular wall is clearly visible, while the acoustic shadowing simulates an extrascleral extension. Row 2. Kretztecknik 7200 MA. On the left, the anterior group of high spikes is interpreted as representing the thickened retino-choroidal layer. The low echospikes are interpreted as representing the swollen sclera; on the left Rs-24 dB

staphyloma-like appearance. Acoustic shadowing was present behind the lesion particularly in the early images. This acoustic shadowing was, in our opinion, higher than that produced by malignant melanoma of the same thickness.

Images taken in 1988 and subsequently (Figs. 3–5) when the lesion began to shrink, resembled the images published by Guthoff in 1991 [6] and Byrne and Green in 1992 [7]: the fusiform enlargement was still visible, the bulging towards the vitreous space was reduced, while the space towards the orbit was more evident.

In the newly involved temporal area, the echographic findings revealed a slight thickening of the sclera with some oedema in the Tenon space (Fig. 6).

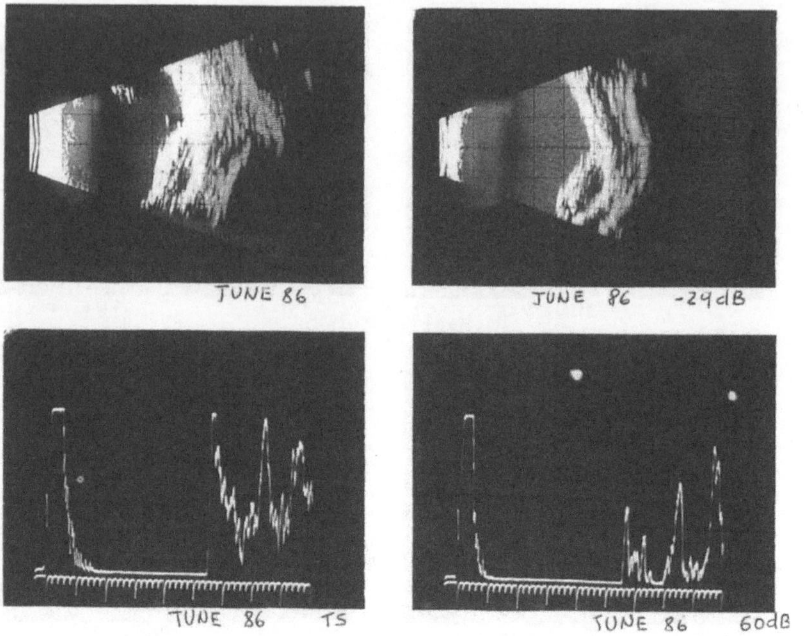

Fig. 2. Nodular scleritis. Row 1. Ocuscan 200. The fusiform enlargement of the sclera is still present. The anterior part of the lesion bulging towards the vitreous space resembles a thick layer. On the left: by lowering the sensitivity of the equipment the staphylomatous deformation of the ocular wall is more clearly visible. Row 2. A-scan echotraces at Ts and at 60 dB

Discussion

In 1988 we reported that A-scan of scleritis was characterized by a series of low spikes. In the discussion of the paper, Karl Ossoinig stated that the scleritis was characterized by high internal reflectivity. These diverse points of view are still present in Guthoff's book [6] and in Byrne and Green's book [7]. This is most likely a question of personal experience of the various examiners. Five years ago we suggested that the A- and B-scan echograms of the anterior aspect of our lesion were due to the retino-choroidal layer characterized by a thickened choroid as occurs in scleritis [1,2]. The almost empty middle or low reflective area was believed to be produced by the swollen sclera; the more posterior brilliant line with B-scan and the high reflective echo-spike in the A-scan were thought to be the sclera/Tenon interface. The different pathological events that can take place in a scleritis [1] may lead to a lowering of the internal reflectivity of the sclera. Most of the pathological specimens published, also by Guthoff [6], show a fusiform enlargement of the sclera that bulges both towards the vitreous

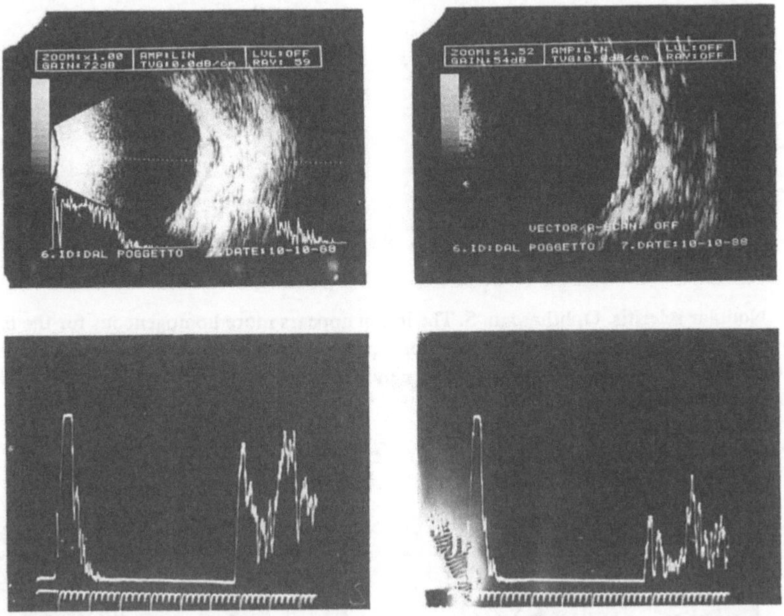

Fig. 3. **Nodular scleritis. Row 1: Sonomed 3000. The lesion shows a reduced thickness; the bulging towards the vitreous space is greatly reduced, while the staphylomatous deformation appears at lower amplification. Row 2. Kretzteknik 7200 MA**

space and the orbit. The low reflective area has instead been interpreted by Ossoinig and Harrie [8] and by Byrne and Green [7] as an infiltration in the Tenon's space.

Guthoff [6] reported that the infiltration of Tenon's space could be documented over several months, but in our case one infiltration lasted ten years. We tend to the opinion that some pathological changes occurring in the more superficial scleral tissue together with some infiltration in Tenon's space may lead to a low reflective area. The temporal area involved by the disease since early 1993 shows different acoustic characteristics: the sclera shows only a slight diffuse thickening with some infiltration of Tenon's space. The differential diagnosis with choroidal melanoma occurs only in the highly localized forms where the intravitreal bulging of the lesion simulates an intraocular tumour. In case of malignant melanoma, even if sound attenuation due to the lesion thickness is present, the anterior aspect of the lesion itself never resembles an irregular layer. Furthermore, in nodular forms the orbital bulging assumes a staphylomatous appearance that has never been reported in extrascleral extension of choroidal melanomas.

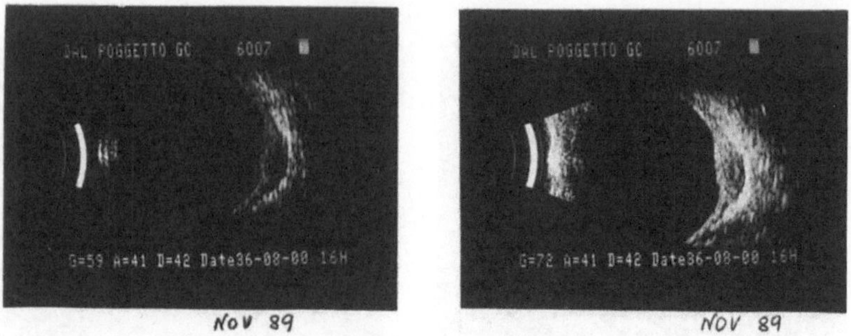

Fig. 4. **Nodular scleritis. Ophthascan. S. The lesion appears more homogeneous for the first time. By lowering the sensitivity setting, the anterior aspect assumes the appearance of a thick layer, the fusiform enlargement looks 'empty', while the enhancement of the line we believe represents the sclera/Tenon interface**

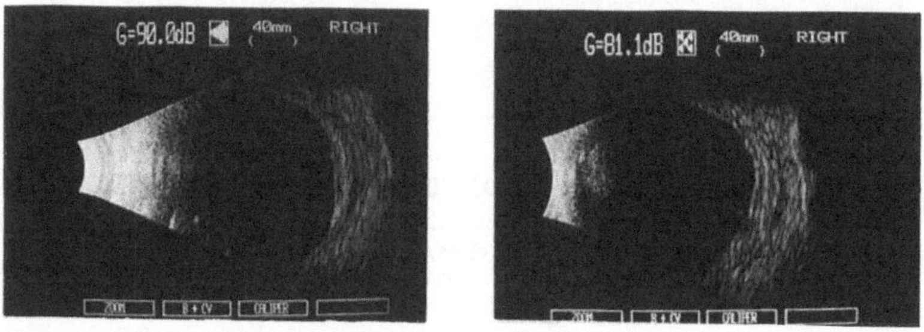

Fig. 5. **Nodular scleritis – Biovision. A highly reflective zone is seen behind the group of very high echospikes that represents either the retinochoroidal layer or the ocular wall followed by some infiltration in the Tenon's space**

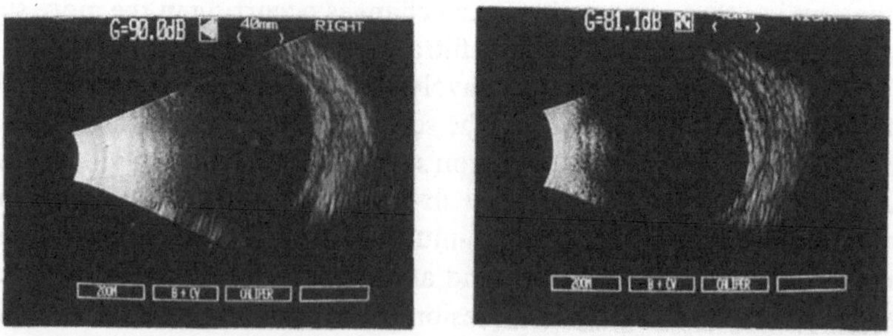

Fig. 6. **Diffuse anterior scleritis. Biovision. A flattening of the normal concavity of the ocular wall is present which is due to an enlargement of the choroidal scleral layer. There is some diffuse oedema and/or infiltration in Tenon's space**

References

[1] W.H. Spencer. Sclera. In W.H. Spencer, Ophthalmic pathology. An Atlas and Textbook. 3rd Edition. AAO 1985;389–411.

[2] P. Watson. Disease of the sclera and episclera. In W. Tasman and E.A. Jaeger (eds), Duane's Clinical Ophthalmology, Vol. 4. Philadelphia: Lippincott Co., 1992;18–22.

[3] P.G. Watson. The diagnosis and management of scleritis. Ophthalmology 1980;716–720.

[4] V. Mazzeo, P. Perri and P. Monari. Ultrasound findings in brawny scleritis. Dordrecht: Kluwer Academic Publishers. Doc. Ophthalmol. Proc. Series 1988;53:411–417.

[5] M. Sainz de la Maza, N.S. Jabbour and C.S. Foster. An analysis of therapeutic decision for scleritis. Ophthalmology 1992;100:1372–1376.

[6] R. Guthoff. Ultrasound in ophthalmologic diagnosis. A practical guide. Stuttgart: Georg Thieme Pub., 1991.

[7] S.F. Byrne and R.L. Green. Ultrasound of the eye and orbit. St. Louis: Mosby Year Book, 1992.

[8] K.C. Ossoinig and R.P. Harrie. Diagnosis of intraocular tumors with standardized echography. In P.K. Lommatzsch and F.C. Blodi (eds). Intraocular tumors. Berlin: Springer Verlag, 1983;154–182.

[9] G. Singh, R. Guthoff and C.S. Foster. Observations on long term follow-up of posterior scleritis. Am. J. Ophthalmol. 1986;101:570–575.

Prof. Vincenzina Mazzeo
via Polonia 79
44100 Ferrara, Italy

31. Echographic diagnosis of acute retinal necrosis

W.A.J. VAN HEUVEN and J. MCADAM
(San Antonio, Texas, USA)

Abstract

Two cases of acute retinal necrosis (ARN) and severe vitritis in immunologically compromised patients, one monocular and one binocular, were found to have similar echographic characteristics. The response to appropriate medication and vitreous and retinal biopsy confirmed the diagnoses. Subsequently, a third case in an immunologically competent patient was found to have identical echographic findings, suggesting a diagnosis of herpetic ARN, which permitted appropriate treatment to be given. The typical echographic picture consists of vitreous opacities, vitreous schisis and loculation (cyst-like), vitreo–retinal traction, retinal detachment, subretinal opacities and choroidal thickening.

Key words: Herpes, acute retinal necrosis

Case reports

Case 1

C.T.F.: In January, 1992, a 38-year-old black male was admitted to the hospital from the Immunosuppression Clinic with fatigue, influenza-like symptoms, a productive cough with white sputum and decreasing vision. In July, 1991, he had a bout of herpes zoster of the scalp and right ear. In October, 1991, he was diagnosed with optic neuritis OU with severe visual loss, treated with prednisone, and septic arthritis of the hip with a positive salmonella culture, treated with ciprofloxacin. A few days later he also developed a herpes simplex type II infection of the buttocks. Because of a low T-helper cell count of 23, he was also treated with AZT 100 mgm p.o. q.i.d. The vision improved slightly with treatment and the hip became asymptomatic. In December, the vision decreased again. The eye examination showed an absence of light perception OD and only light perception OS. Intraocular pressure was zero in each eye. Pupils were irregular with posterior senechiae. Anterior chambers had 2+ flare and some cells. The vitreous was very cloudy with many whitish cells, through which the fundus could be seen vaguely, indicating pallor of the discs and white patches of the retina throughout, each patch roughly round and 3–4 mm in diameter. No hemorrhages were seen.

G Cennamo and N. Rosa (eds.), Ultrasonography in Ophthalmology 15, pp. 277–283.

The ultrasound examination showed similar findings in both eyes: moderate vitreous opacities; multiple vitreous membranes, some of which were parallel and suggested vitreous schisis (Fig. 1), while others showed a loculated pattern; vitreous traction with tenting of the retina and areas of retinal detachment with subretinal opacities.

At our recommendation, with the tentative diagnosis of herpes retinitis and vitritis, intravenous acyclovir was started, which changed later to Gancyclovir, because CMV retinitis could not be ruled out. During the next two weeks, the vitritis improved but the vision did not. Gancyclovir was then discontinued because there was no hope of improving the vision further because of severe optic atrophy.

Case 2

R.G.: In March, 1992, a 58-year-old white male hospital patient was referred by the Transplant Service three days after admission because of right eye pain, redness and watering for two days. He had been admitted to the hospital because of left chest pain, a productive cough, mild fever and chills two months

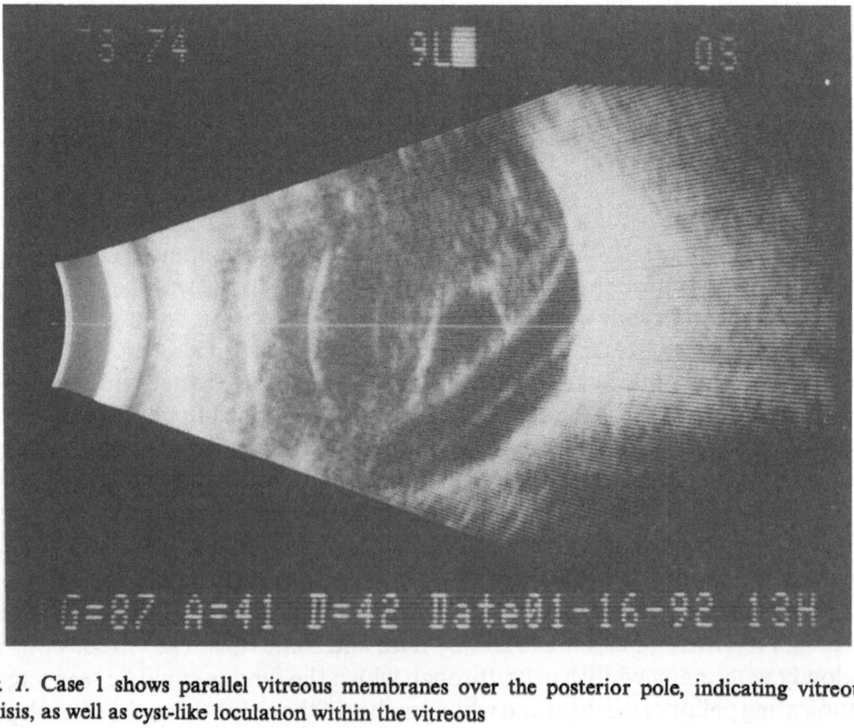

Fig. 1. Case 1 shows parallel vitreous membranes over the posterior pole, indicating vitreous schisis, as well as cyst-like loculation within the vitreous

following a left single lung transplant for idiopathic pulmonary fibrosis. His medications were imuran 100 mgm/day, cyclosporin 150 mgm b.i.d., and prednisone 45 mgm/day. He had been immediately started on antibiotics, but bronchoscopy showed no transplant rejection and no bacteria, but it did show candida, aspergillus and mucor. He was thus started on amphotericin, which he tolerated poorly, so that only a low dose could be given. The eye examination showed 20/200 OD and 20/30 OS. The left eye was essentially normal. Abnormal findings in the right eye included a small hypopyon, severe vitritis and hemorrhagic retinitis which was difficult to visualize. A diagnostic paracentesis was done, the culture results of which were negative. Because of the possible diagnosis of CMV retinitis, gancyclovir was started. During the next week, the hypopyon cleared and the eye pain decreased, although the vision and the vitritis did not improve.

The ultrasound examination showed moderately vitreous opacities, multiple vitreous membranes with some loculation, vitreous attachment to an area of retinal detachment peripherally, subretinal opacities and possible detachment or thickening (Figs. 2 and 3).

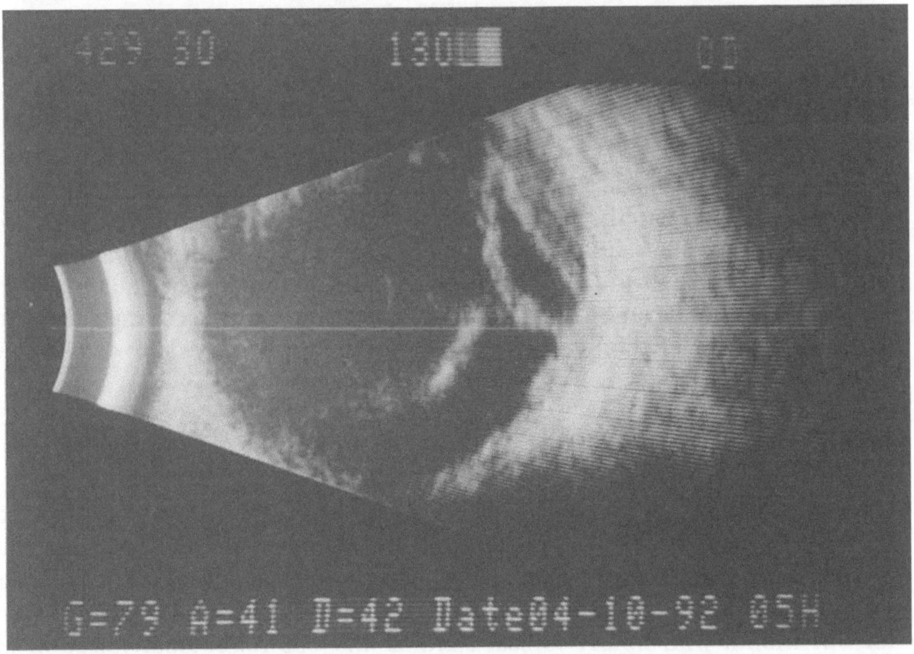

Fig. 2. Case 2 shows a vitreous membrane inserting into a bullous retinal detachment with a layered accumulation of debris (confirmed at surgery) under the retina

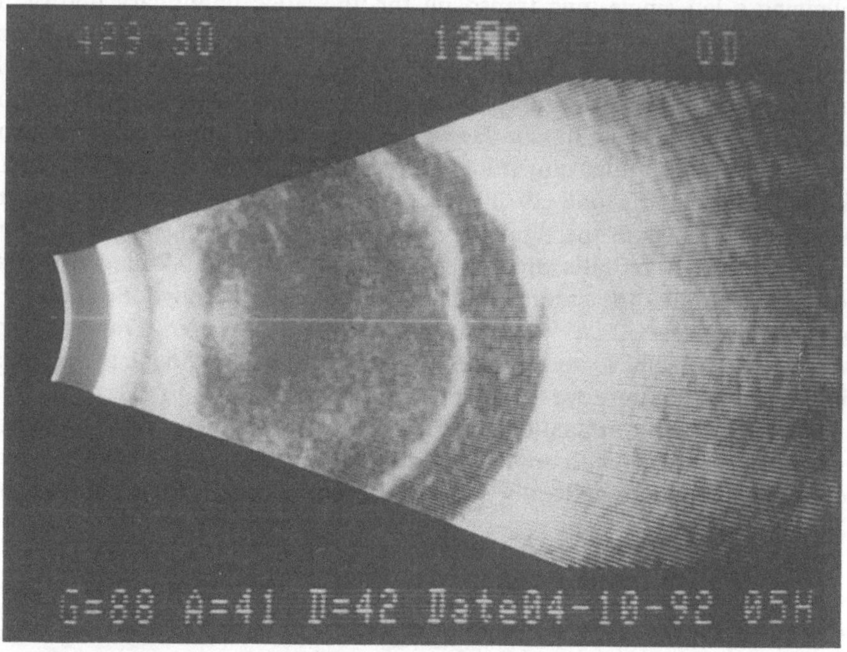

Fig. 3. Case 2 shows a retinal detachment near the equator with many subretinal opacities and an irregularly thickened choroid

The decision was made to do a vitreo-retinal biopsy so that an etiology could be found. At surgery, the vitreous had multiple membranes and pockets of liquefaction, and the retinal detachment was necrotic with a large amount of subretinal white debris (Fig. 3). Biopsies and cultures were taken which demonstrated mucor and aspergillus. An enucleation was recommended and performed 3 days later, following which the patient died 4 days later of systemic mucormycosis.

Case 3

S.L.M.: In June, 1993, a 42-year-old Latin-American male was examined because of photophobia and progressively decreasing vision OS since December, 1992 and increasing ocular pain not related to eye movement since January, 1993. He had been treated for anterior uveitis by the referring ophthalmologist for one month with hourly topical steroids and one retrobulbar injection of Kenalog (depo-steroid) without improvement. Other past social, medical and ocular history was negative, except for a 2-week loss of appetite. The eye examination showed light reception only OD and 20/25 OS. The right conjunctiva was intensely injected and had a deep red-violet color with little discharge. The cornea had mild microcystic epithelial edema with no staining and no keratic precipitates or flare. The vitreous, however, was densely packed with whitish cells, so that no view of the retina was possible. The iris had posterior senechiae temporally, but no nodules. The lens had mild nuclear sclerosis, similar in degree to the left eye. However, otherwise the left eye was entirely normal. Pressures were 32 mmHg OD and 22 mmHg OS. Laboratory tests already done were all normal and included chest x-ray, brain and orbital MRI, complete blood count, RPR, sedimentation rate and toxoplasmosis, toxocara, cytomegalovirus, herpes I and II and HIV titres.

The ultrasound examination showed moderate vitreous opacities with evidence of vitreous schisis and loculation (Figs. 4 and 5). Vitreous traction was present over low-lying retinal detachments. There were also subretinal opacities and thickening of the choroid.

Although the original clinical diagnosis had been posterior scleritis and uveitis, the echographic characteristics suggested ARN, so that lymphocyte studies and anti-HSV and VSN ELISA and IgM studies were repeated. Lymphocyte studies showed no evidence of cellular immunologic abnormality, but the anti-VZV IgM and ELISA, as well as the anti-HSV IgM were all sero positive. The patient was started on oral acyclovir and prednisone and the uveitis gradually improved, although the vision never recovered.

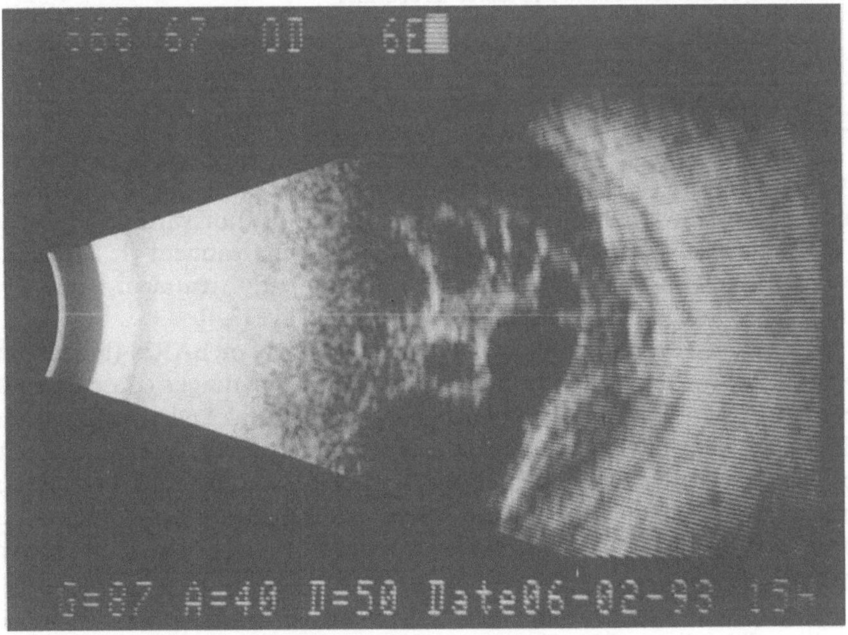

Fig. 4. Case 3 shows vitreous loculation and retina-choroid thickening

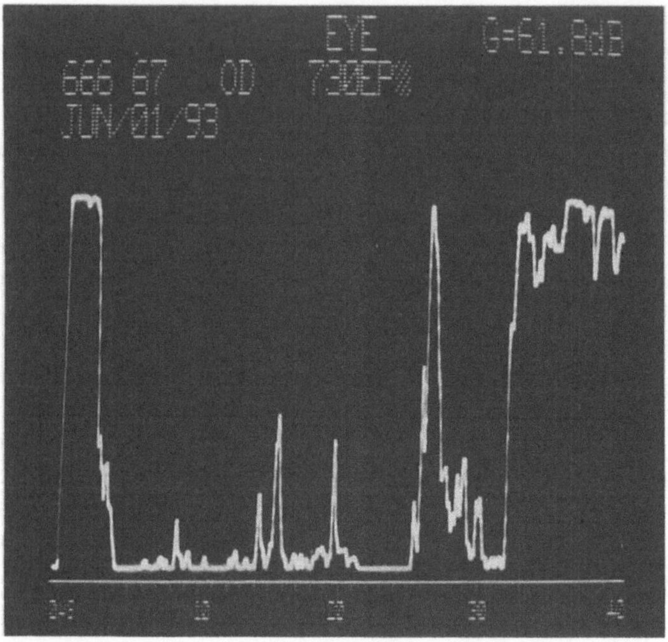

Fig. 5. **Using standardized A-scan, Case 3 shows multiple vitreous opcities throughout, vitreous membranes, retinal detachment and subretinal opacities**

Discussion

Acute retinal necrosis syndrome in immune competent patients can usually be assumed to be caused by herpes simplex virus (HSV) or varicella zoster virus (VZV), both of which are susceptible to acyclovir treatment [1, 2]. Thus, the early recognition of this condition can lead to early treatment (Case 3) and possible prevention of involvement of the second eye [3,4].

In immune compromised patients, however, ARN or BARN (bilateral) may be caused by a variety of infectious agents, including fungus (Case 2). In these cases, biopsy of the choroid, pigment epithelium, retina and vitreous should be done early [5,6], so that appropriate specific therapy can be started. In addition, because the vitritis may be very severe, a vitrectomy to visualize the fundus may uncover hints about the etiology before cultures are positive, such as optic neuritis (possible VZV) or hemorrhagic retinitis (possible CMV) or perivenous retinal sparing (CMV or resistant HSV and VZV) [7,8].

Thus, in any case with severe vitreous involvement, where the fundus is not easily visible, diagnostic ultrasound can be an invaluable aid to make or to rule out the diagnosis of ARN, so that appropriate action, which is often invasive (toxic drugs or ocular biopsy), can be started or else avoided. The ARN-related echographic characteristics in the three cases presented here showed moderate vitreous opacities, vitreous schisis and loculation, vitreous traction, secondary retinal detachment, subretinal opacities and choroidal thickening.

Supported by a Research Development Award from Research to Prevent Blindness, Inc., New York.

References

[1] J.S. Duker and M.S. Blumenkranz. Diagnosis and management of the acute retinal necrosis (ARN) syndrome. Surv. Ophthalmol. 1991;35:327–343.

[2] D.S. Gartry, D.J. Spalton, A. Tilzey and P.G. Hykin. Acute retinal necrosis syndrome. Br. J. Ophthalmol. 1991;75:292–297.

[3] A. Palay, P. Sternberg Jr., J. Davis, H. Lewis, G.N. Holland, W.F. Mieler, D.A. Jabs and C. Drews. Decrease in the risk of bilateral acute retinal necrosis by acyclovir therapy. Am. J. Ophthalmol. 1991;112:250–255.

[4] J. Martinez, H.M. Lambert, A. Capone, P. Sternberg Jr., T.M. Aaberg, P.F. Lopez and C. Davidson. Delayed bilateral involvement in the acute retinal necrosis syndrome. Am. J. Ophthalmol. 1992;113:103–104.

[5] R.B. Nussenblatt and A.G. Palestine. Editorials: Human immunodeficiency virus, herpes zoster, and the retina. Am. J. Ophthalmol. 1991;112:206–207.

[6] W.S. Foulds. The uses and limitations of intraocular biopsy. Eye 1992;6:11–27.

[7] D.J. Forster, P.U. Dugel, G.T. Grangieh, P.E. Liggett and N.A. Rao. Rapidly progressive outer retinal necrosis in the acquired immuno-deficiency syndrome. Am. J. Ophthalmol. 1990;110:341.

[8] J.S. Duker and E.P. Shakin. Letter to Editor – Correspondence. Am. J. Ophthalmol. 1991;111:255–256.

W. A. J. van Heuven
University of Texas Health Science Center
Department of Ophthalmology
7703 Floyd Curl Drive
San Antonio, TX 78284-6230
U.S.A.

Orbital and periorbital tumors

32. Orbit lymphoma: echographic findings – our experience

P. PERRI, V. MAZZEO, L. RAVALLI, D. BRIENZA, P. DE PALMA and A. ROSSI

(Ferrara, Italy)

Abstract

Sixteen patients, eight men and eight women, with mono- or bilateral exophthalmos caused by lymphoma, were observed at the University Eye Clinic of Ferrara, between 1982 and 1993. We describe in detail the echographic characteristics and the essential features for the diagnosis. We also discuss the role of the ultrasonography in the differential diagnosis and in the follow-up.

Key words: Lymphoma, A and B-scan echography

Introduction

Lymphomas represent a group of tumors which mainly originate in the lymph nodes and in the regions containing lymphoid tissue. Orbital involvement is an exception because the orbit does not usually contain lymphoid tissue [1,2]. Lymphoid orbital tumors are classified as follows: Hodgkin's lymphomas, non-Hodgkin's lymphomas, Burkitt's lymphoma, reticulum cell sarcoma and fungoid mycosis [2].

Both in its primary and in its secondary form with systematic diffusion, lymphoma is rarely found in the orbit [1–3]; the most frequent histologic forms are represented by non-Hodgkin's lymphomas. The site of orbital lesions varies: the frequency with which it involves the upper quadrants is similar to that of other tumors and cysts but the frequency with which it involves the lower quadrants is certainly higher than that of other tumors [4].

The mass can be either intraconic or extraconic, multiple masses are often present and they can rarely affect both orbits. The mass often has a 'shell' configuration, with infiltration in Tenon's capsule, concentrical to the eyeball [5].

Symptomatology is often misleading: blepharoedema is the first symptom; the exophthalmos appears subsequently. Exophthalmos can be either direct or indirect, depending on the mass location. Sometimes, a hard and not reducible mass can be palpated. It is often associated with diplopia, but the most characteristic sign is a pinkish mass which moves from the conjunctival fornix toward the limbus [6]. Bilateral location is a sign of marked malignancy [1].

G Cennamo and N. Rosa (eds.), Ultrasonography in Ophthalmology 15, pp. 287–292.

Case reports

Between 1982 and 1993, at the University Eye Clinic of Ferrara, 43 patients, aged between 19 and 96 who were affected by mono- or bilateral exophthalmos, were observed (Table 1). These patients underwent A- and B-scan echography: they showed the echographic findings of the lymphoma-sarcoma-pseudotumor group. Seventeen of them were excluded because the diagnosis had no clinical support these patients being lost during follow-up.

For 10 of the 43 patients the final diagnosis was pseudotumor orbitae. Five of them were men and 5 were women. The women were aged between 25 and 35, the men between 45 and 78, with a median age of 40 years. Three cases of the five women were previously presented during the 5th Congress of the Italian Society of Echophthalmology [7].

The remaining 16 patients represent the lymphoma cases that we observed during the last 11 years; eight are men and eight are women. Thirteen patients were affected by monolateral exophthalmos (seven in the right orbit and six in the left orbit) while the remaining three patients suffered from bilateral exophthalmos. In 15 patients the orbital manifestation was primary, while in one patient it was a systematic form.

As shown in Table 2, the mean age was 51.5 with a minimum of nine years and a maximum of 88 years, with no significant differences between men and women. However, it should be noted that the difference in the mean of pseudotumors is lower in our case study.

Fifteen patients underwent incisional biopsy which supported the diagnosis of lymphoma (Table 3). The exact histologic report is missing in one case. In another case the diagnosis was made on the basis of hematochemical findings. All the lymphomas we observed were classified as non-Hodgkin's lymphomas: 10 had a low degree of malignancy and belong to the immunocytoma, monocytoid, centrocyte and lymphocyte type, three had a high degree of malignancy, one of which B-T lymphocyte, one T-lymphocyte and one immunoblast, finally one was classified as Castleman's disease, which is a particular angiofollicular hyperplasia, a form with an inevitable lymphomatosis clinical development [8].

Table 1.

	Pseudotumors	Lymphomas	Lost to follow-up	Total
Male	5	8	8	21
Female	5	8	9	22
Total	10	16	17	43
Age min.	25	19	28	
Age max.	78	88	96	
Median	40	51.5	54	

Table 2.

Patient		Sex	Age	Situs	Onset	Cell-type
1.	B.M.	M	19	Orbit sx	Primary	Castleman's disease
2.	R.N	F	29	Orbit dx	Primary	B-cell monocytoid
3.	T.G.	F	30	Bilateral	Primary	B-cell monocytoid
4.	M.U.	M	35	Orbit dx	Primary	T-cell malignant
5.	A.G.	M	40	Orbit sx	Primary	B-cell immunoblastic
6.	S.V.	F	42	Orbit sx	Primary	B-cell centrocytic
7.	R.C.	F	44	Orbit dx	Primary	Unknown
8.	N.G.	M	51	Orbit dx	Primary	Hematochemistry
9.	D.F.	F	52	Bilateral	Primary	B-cell centrocytic
10.	F.F.	F	55	Orbit dx	Primary	B-cell monocytoid
11.	A.M.	M	62	Bilateral	Primary	B-cell centrocytic
12.	N.M.	M	72	Orbit dx	Primary	B-cell lymphocytic
13.	R.C.	F	81	Orbit dx	Primary	B-T cell malignant
14.	P.P.	M	82	Orbit sx	Primary	B-cell immunocytoma
15.	F.A.	M	87	Orbit sx	Primary	B-cell immunocytoma
16.	G.V.	F	88	Orbit sx	Secondary	B-cell immunocytoma

Table 3.

A-scan and B-scan ultrasound characteristics of lymphomas	
Localization	Various, intra or extraconic, sometimes multiple lesions, often localized in both orbits, typical 'shell' arrangement
Shape	Irregular
Borders	Various, sometimes well-outlined, often irregular
Relations	Optical nerve, muscles, orbit walls
Reflectivity (A-scan)	Low
Structure (B-scan)	Homogeneous
Sound at tenuation (A-scan)	Small K angle
Sound transmission (B-scan)	Moderate
Compressibility	None
Vascularity	None

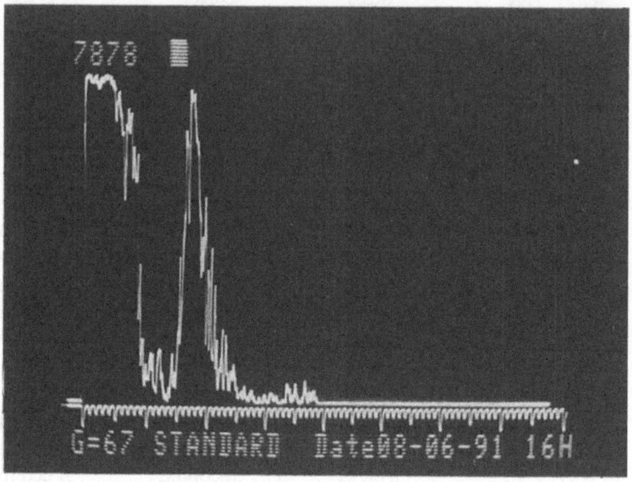

Fig. 1. **Parabulbar A-scan (Ophthascan S). Well out-lined lesion with low internal reflectivity**

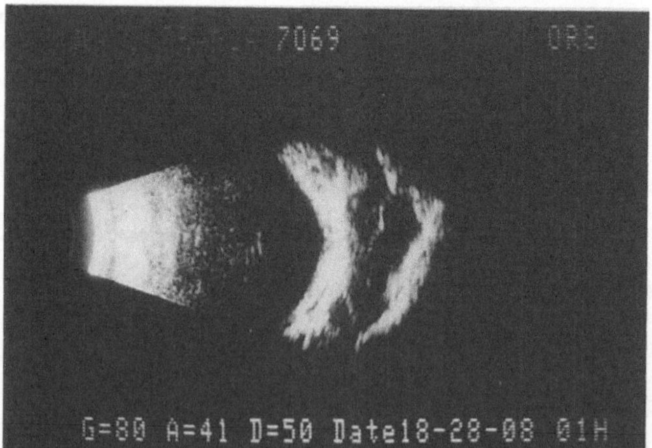

Fig. 2. **B-scan (Ophthascan S). Solid lesion with irregular borders, low internal reflectivity with septa**

Discussion

In the echographic diagnosis of orbital disorders the lymphoma-sarcoma-pseudotumors are notoriously classified under a single group, which causes numerous problems for the differential diagnosis [9]. This difficulty, as we will see, is due to the fact that the echographic findings of these diseases are very similar. This similarity reflects the pathology of such lesions. Both lymphomas and pseudotumors are, in fact, characterized by an accumulation of lymphocytes that are thickly packed together with only small interfaces between the cellular groups and the intercellular substance [10]. Whatever site they occupy, lymphomas are invariably irregular in shape and, usually well-defined, but at times the borders may be blurred.

The echographic criteria of lymphomas in A- and B-scan have been well codified [1,4,9,11] (Table 3): the study of the shape and of the relationship to the other structures of the orbit is much easier with B-scan. Therefore, it is possible to study the relationships between the lymphoma and the optic nerve, the muscles and the eyeball profile. B-scan will reveal whether the muscles are an integral part of the pathological process or whether they are only shifted; whether there is dilatation of the ophthalmic veins or alterations of the bone walls as happens in the most penetrating forms [10].

The most important characteristics of lymphomas in A-scan (Fig. 1) are the low reflectivity (5–40%) and the small angle 'K' which expresses a poor sound attenuation [12,13]; this peculiarity is due, as previously mentioned, to the typical pathological appearance [10]. When the lesion is well-defined, maximal opening and closing spikes are present in A-scan; the closing spike is difficult to maximize in the penetrating and widespread forms. In these cases the neoplastic process, separating orbital structures with different reflectivity, can therefore determine the formation of irregular echoes in the tracing [4]. It should be noted that a lymphoma is not a compressible lesion and never shows any sign of vascularization in its internal part [14].

The main B-scan characteristics (Fig. 2) are those of a solid and infiltrating lesion with an irregular outline but a fairly good demarcation of the adjacent structures. The internal echogenicity is low and internal echoes are absent or infrequent [15]. Furthermore, in our experience and in that of others [16,17], the sound transmission in B-scan is good. On the contrary, Coleman *et al.* [15] found that lymphomas show poor sound transmission, and that therefore the borders and the orbital wall cannot be observed.

Finally it should also be noted that by penetrating Tenon's capsule, the lymphoma can simulate a tenonitis with its characteristic 'T' sign [18].

Conclusion

Echography is only one of the tools in the pseudotumor-lymphoma-sarcoma differential diagnosis. Other diagnostic examinations (computerized tomography and nuclear magnetic resonance) should be performed to obtain as much information as possible. Echography is also important in monitoring the efficacy of therapy during follow-up thus avoiding further computerized tomographical examinations. In the case of inflammatory idiopathic pseudotumor, mainly involving the fat tissue, besides the instrumental diagnostic criteria, clinical evolution and prompt therapeutic response to cortisone treatment are important in the differential diagnosis.

References

[1] A.F. Jakobiec and R.L. Font. Orbit. In W.H. Spencer, Ophthalmic pathology. Philadelphia: Saunders Co., 1986.
[2] J.A. Shields. Diagnosis and Management of Orbital Tumours. Philadelphia: Saunders Co., 1989.
[3] R. Frezzotti. Patologia, clinica e terapia della malattie dell'orbita 65 Congresso SOI, Siena, 1985.
[4] V. Mazzeo, L. Ravalli and R. Scorrano. L'ecografia nei tumori dell'orbita. Ferrara: A. Rossi-Clinica dei tumori dell'occhio e dell'orbita. S.A.T.E. 1981;453–504.
[5] W. Schroeder. Zur Topographie lymphome. Klin. Mbl. Augenheilk. 1979;174:157–165.
[6] G. Pirazzoli and P.E. Gallenga. I tumori dell'orbita. Clinica dei tumori dell'occhio e dell'orbita – A. Rossi, Ferrara, S.A.T.E. 1981;505–581.
[7] V. Mazzeo, P. Perri, P. Monari, M. Chiarelli and F. Franco. Pseudotumor dell'orbita in gravidanza. Clin. Ocul. e Pat. Ocul. 1991;4:290–292.
[8] G. Castoldi and V. Liso. Malattie del sangue e degli organi ematopoietici. McGraw-Hill Ed., 1993;289.
[9] V. Mazzeo. Ecografia dell'apparato oculare. Testo-Atlante. Fogliazza ed., 1987.
[10] K.C. Ossoinig and P. Till. Ten year study on clinical echography in orbital disease. In J. Frañois and F. Goes, Ultrasonography in Ophthalmology. Basle: Karger, 1975;200–216.
[11] R. Guthoff. Ultrasound in ophthalmologic diagnosis – A practical guide. Stuttgart: Georg Thieme, 1991.
[12] K.C. Ossoinig. A-Scan echography and orbital disease. 'Orbital disorders'. Bleeker G.M. *et al.* Mod. Probl. Ophtal. 14. Basle: Karger. 1975;203–235.
[13] K.C. Ossoinig. The role of clinical echography in modern diagnosis of periorbital and orbital lesions. III International Symposium on Orbital Disorders. The Hague: Junk, 1978;469–540.
[14] S.F. Byrne and R.L. Green. Ultrasound of the Eye and Orbit. St. Louis: The Mosby Year Book, 1992.
[15] D.J. Coleman, R.L. Jack and L.A. Franzen. High resolution B-scan ultrasonography of the orbit. III. Lymphomas of the orbit. Arch. Ophthalmol. 1972;88:375–379.
[16] M. Restori. Ultrasound in orbital diagnosis. Trans. Ophthal. Soc. U.K. 1979;99:223–225.
[17] M.J. Dadd, G. Kossoff and H.L. Hughes. Application of grey scale echography in retrobulbar examination. In Investigative Ultrasonology 2. Clinical. Advances. Bath: Pitman Press, 1981;287–294.
[18] D.J. Coleman, F.C. Lizzi and R.L. Jack. Ultrasonography of the Eye and Orbit. Philadelphia: Lea & Febiger, 1977.

Paolo Perri, M.D.
University Eye Clinic of Ferrara
Via A. Cassoli 30
44100 Ferrara, Italy

33. Merkel cell carcinoma: an echographic study

F. GENOVESI-EBERT, F. TRANFA, N. ROSA,[1] G. BONAVOLONTÁ[1] and G. CENNAMO[1]

(Pisa and [1]Naples, Italy)

Abstract

Merkel cell neuroendocrine carcinoma is a cutaneous neoplasm rarely affecting the eyelids and periocular tissue. Merkel cells, which are probably of epithelial origin, are clear oval cells in the epidermis and outer root sheaths of hair follicles. They share ultrastructural features with neuroendocrine cells and have been reported to be associated with touch receptors.

This is an aggressive tumor with high rates of local recurrence and metastases. Because of its rarity, diagnosis can be difficult and treatment is thus often delayed. Standardized echography may be a useful tool with which to diagnose orbital recurrence because Merkel cell carcinoma often mimics lymphoma or undifferentiated carcinoma, both clinically and histopathologically.

Here we describe a patient with an orbital recurrence of Merkel cell carcinoma. To the author's knowledge, this is the first such case examined with echography. Therefore, the echographic findings of this lesion are compared with the histopathological features. Moreover, this experience indicates that an aggressive approach be used in the management of this tumor to avoid recurrence and metastasis.

Key words: Merkel cell carcinoma, echography, orbital lesion

Introduction

Merkel cells are clear oval cells in the epidermis and in the outer root sheaths of hair follicles, probably of epithelial origin, which resemble the neuroendocrine cells ultrastructure [1]. First described by Friedrich Merkel in 1875 in the basal layer of the epidermis of birds [2], they were suggested to be tactile sensory cells (*Tastzellen*) being in continuity with dermal nerve endings. This hypothesis has been substantiated recently by electron microscopy in human skin [3]: in fact they are often associated with touch receptors.

In the eyelid, Merkel cells occur singly in the epidermis, in the external root sheaths of hairs and eyelashes, and in specialized touch spots alternating with

G Cennamo and N. Rosa (eds.), Ultrasonography in Ophthalmology 15, pp. 293–302.

eyelashes. The typical electron microscopic feature is the presence of dense-core granules, intranuclear rodlets and spinous processes.

Merkel carcinoma (neuroendocrine carcinoma, trabecular carcinoma) is a rare primary tumor of the skin with peculiar ultrastructural and immunohistochemical characteristics. It probably develops from precursor cells which give rise to keratinocytes and Merkel cells. This tumor, first described in 1972 by Toker [4], was thought to derive from sweat glands; however, the ultrastructural similarity to normal Merkel cells, demonstrated only in 1978 by Tang and Toker [5], suggested the neoplasia arose from these cells.

Merkel cell carcinoma is more common in the elderly, with a male/female ratio of 2/3 [6]. The prevalence of this tumor is unclear, because many patients have been reported more than once by different groups of authors. The typical clinical appearance is a non-tender red nodule with intact overlaying skin. The tumor affects more frequently the lids, the eyebrows, the orbital rim, and the cantus [1]. The eyelid and periocular Merkel cell carcinoma has the potential for local recurrence and metastatic spread. Its recurrence rate is 33%; almost two-thirds give rise to regional lymph node metastases, and up to 50% metastasize widely and result in death. Given the histological and clinical features of this tumor, a lifetime follow-up is recommended.

The rarity of eyelid Merkel cell carcinoma may lead to difficulty in its diagnosis and delay in the treatment of this highly malignant, potentially lethal tumor. Immunohistochemical studies on tumor cells showed the presence of both neuron-specific enolase, and cytokeratin [7]. The ultrastructural study demonstrated dense-core granules within the tumor cells [5], whose identification is the only means of confirming the diagnosis.

Standardized echography provides data about location, extent and type of tissue differentiation of orbital tumors [8]. Moreover, standardized echography [9] is the method of choice for the examination, evaluation, diagnosis and follow-up of patients with suspected or proven orbital and periorbital disease. However, to the best of our knowledge, the echographic features of the orbital localization of Merkel tumors have never been described.

Case Report

A 74-year-old white woman was referred to our Department for the treatment of an orbital mass in November 1993. In April 1993 a red nodule appeared under the left eyebrow arch, and a wide excision of the tumor was performed. Histopathology lead to the diagnosis of Merkel cell carcinoma.

In August 1993 another nodule was excised and histological examination confirmed the diagnosis of Merkel cell tumor recurrence. In November 1993 the patient had another orbital recurrence, and consequently, she was referred to our Department. Physical examination showed severe left exophthalmus with displacement of the eyeball, and a third degree ptosis. The right eye was normal. An orbital lump with hard-elastic consistency and a diameter of about 2.5 cm was detected under the outer third of the eyebrow arch. The best corrected visual acuity in the left eye was 20/200. The left eye slit lamp examination showed diffuse corneal disepithelization and marked sclerosis of the lens, ophthalmoscopy revealed angiosclerotic retinal vessels and normal optic disc; and the intraocular pressure was 18 mmHg.

A computerized tomographic scan examination with contrast enhancement showed a solid mass lesion in the superotemporal left orbit. This involved the superior rectus and lateral rectus muscle, and induced a downward and forward displacement of the eyeball, without affecting the contiguous bony structure.

An orbital echographic examination was performed [9], with Mini A and Ophthascan S (Biophysic Medical). Standardized echography showed a regularly structured, hard, vascularized and well-defined lesion with a medium-low reflectivity and medium angle kappa. A total orbital exenteration was performed.

Quantitative echography showed a regular internal structure, with a medium-low reflectivity (Fig. 1), and a medium sound attenuation with medium angle kappa (Fig. 2). Kinetic echography showed a vascularized hard lesion (Figs 3 and 4). Topographic echography (Figs. 5 and 6) showed that this solid, oval mass lesion was located in the superotemporal mid posterior orbit. The lesion was well outlined (Fig. 7), and measured 24.1 mm × 18 mm (Figs. 8 and 9). The pathologist's report confirmed the diagnosis of Merkel cell tumor.

The immunohistochemistry examination showed a positive reaction to cytokeratin and a positive reaction to chromogranin and the electron microscopy examination showed typical dense-core granules.

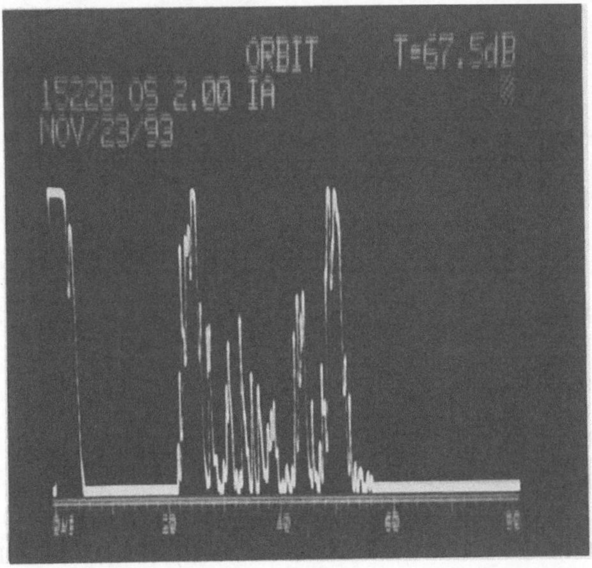

Fig. 1. **Standardized A-scan at T sensitivity showing a low-medium reflective lesion**

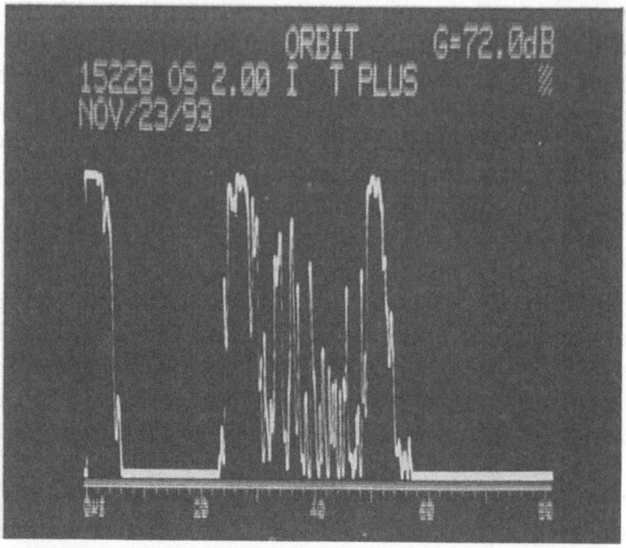

Fig. 2. Standardized A-scan at T plus sensitivity showing a medium angle K

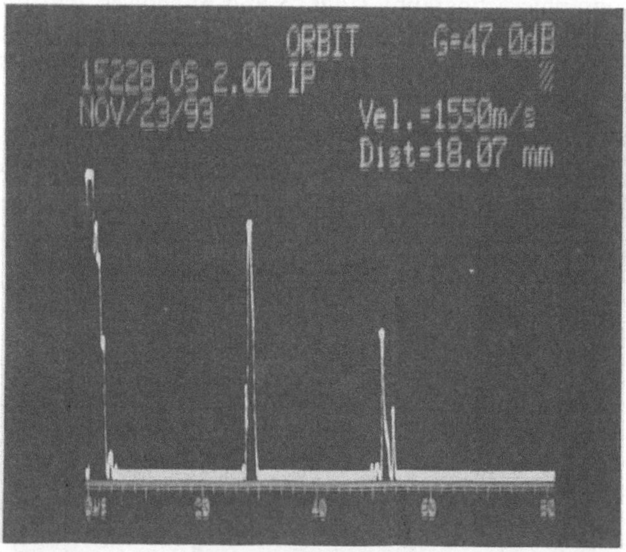

Fig. 3. Standardized A-scan at T minus sensitivity showing the size of the lesion without compression

Discussion

Merkel cell carcinoma has been established as an important and highly malignant primary neoplasm of the skin. It is difficult to give a precise number of the published cases; however, Hitchcock [10] reviewed 400 cases of overall cutaneous tumor, while Kivela and Tarkkanen [1] estimated that about 600

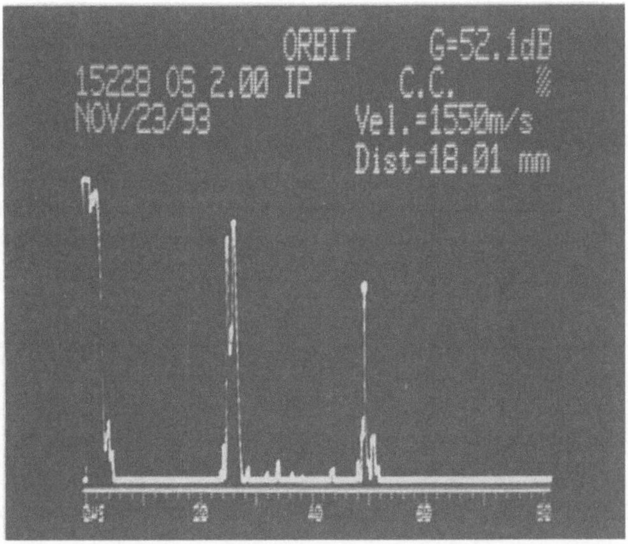

Fig. 4. Standardized A-scan at T minus sensitivity showing the size of the lesion during compression

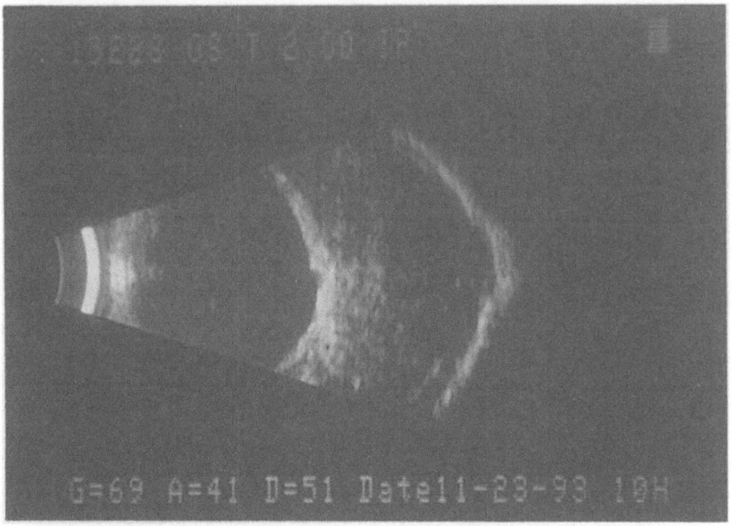

Fig. 5. Contact B-scan showing the lesion in a transversal section

cases of cutaneous carcinoma had been described between 1982 and 1990. This tumor rarely occurs in the eyelid or in the periocular region: Kivela [1] reported 50 cases, Rubsamen [11] in a review of the literature found 34 cases, while Furuno [6] found 22 cases. Eyelids have been reported to be involved in 31 patients, whereas four tumors affected the cantus, nine were localized to the eyebrows, and six have been removed from the orbital rim [1]. Thus far, only

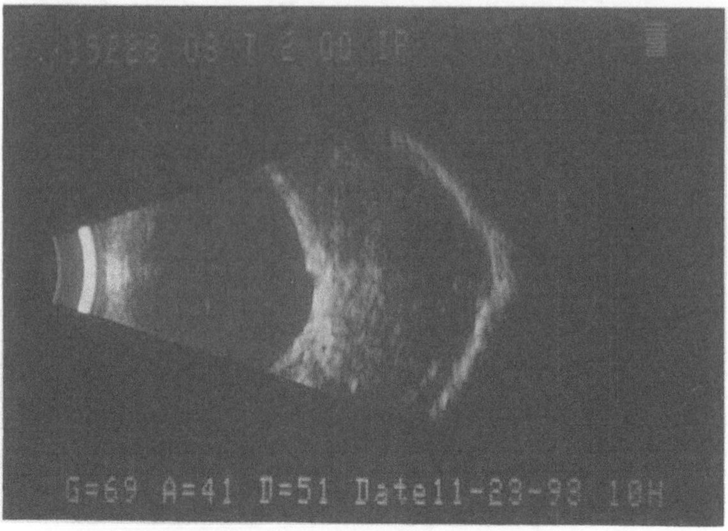

Fig. 6. **Contact B-scan showing the lesion in a longitudinal section**

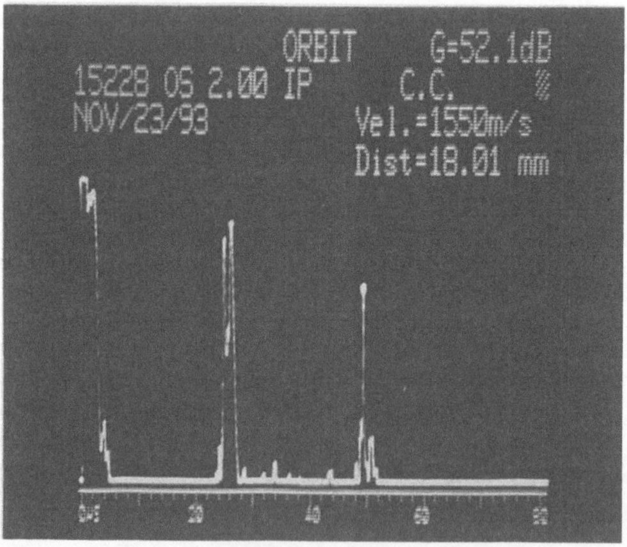

Fig. 7. **Standardized A-scan in a paraocular approach showing the lesion to be well outlined**

four cases of orbital recurrence have been reported [1,12,13].

The typical clinical appearance is a non-tender red nodule with intact overlaying skin; superficial telangiectases may be present. In the eyelid, it arises near the lid margin and may cause partial loss of the eyelashes. Several eyelid tumors have been pedunculated or mimic a chalazion. Because of the high rate of local recurrence and spread, the recommended treatment for Merkel cell

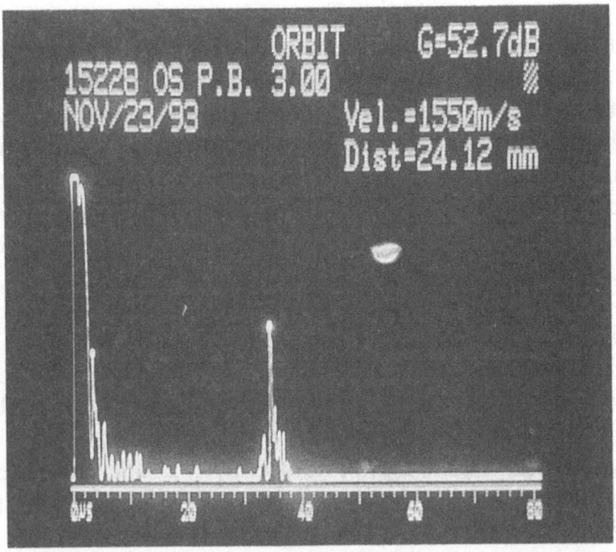

Fig. 8. Standardized A-scan at T minus sensitivity showing the size of the lesion in a paraocular approach

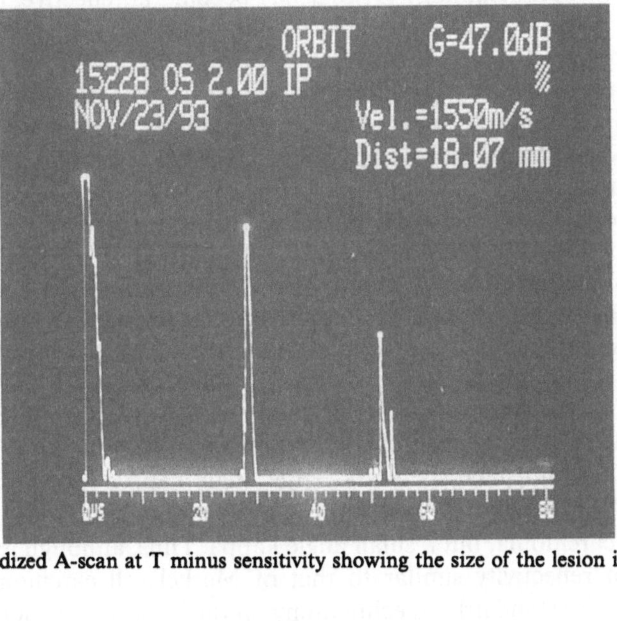

Fig. 9. Standardized A-scan at T minus sensitivity showing the size of the lesion in a transocular approach

carcinoma is a wide surgical excision; the infiltrative pattern of this lesion can be difficult to identify on frozen-section slides, therefore a wide surgical margin of excision is required to compensate for the potential microscopic spread of the tumor beyond the boundary of the main lesion [11]. The tumor, at least in an early stage, responds to local radiotherapy, which has been used in primary [10,14] and recurrence [11] treatment and in cases of lymphatic spread. The examination for regional spread to lymph nodes should be directed toward the submandibular, superficial preauricular and cervical lymph nodes. The most common sites of distant spread are liver, lungs, brain and bones [10,14].

Immunohistochemical studies have been conducted on tumor cells expressing both neuron-specific enolase and cytokeratin. Less commonly chromogenin and neurofilament can be detected [6]. The tumor cells seem thus to possess neuronal and epithelial features. Therefore the origin of the tumor remains enigmatic and controversial.

On light microscopy examination, the monotonous nature of the dermal round cell infiltrate is responsible for the frequent misdiagnosis as malignant lymphoma [15] and immunohistochemistry is needed: in our case report the cells showed a positive reaction to cytokeratin, which is an epithelial marker, and to chromogranin, which is a neuroendocrine marker.

Clinical appearance and light microscopy are not always characteristic. Therefore, a non invasive method that can assist the physician to distinguish among different masses and to plan surgical treatment would be of great help. Standardized echography is a non invasive, advanced method of diagnostic ultrasound in ophthalmology [9] that has become an effective, clinically very useful and sometimes indispensable diagnostic aid in the evaluation of the orbital lesion.

This paper focuses on the differential diagnosis with the following tumoral lesions: mixed tumors, adenoid cystic carcinoma, metastatic tumors and lymphoma. The standardized echography of the Merkel cell carcinoma showed a low reflectivity and a medium angle kappa: the low reflectivity is related to the histopathologic features of the tumor, which is homogeneous, poor in connective tissue and rich in cells.

At low magnification the light microscopy appearance is of the typical round uniform cells of Merkel cell carcinoma (Fig. 10). There is a diffuse cellular proliferation. At higher magnification there was a pale nucleus without nucleolus and scanty cytoplasm. A high rate of mitosis was also observed, as was the muscle infiltration, indicating an aggressive lesion.

Mixed tumor has high reflectivity and medium angle kappa; adenoid cystic carcinoma has high reflectivity and large angle kappa; metastatic tumor has irregular reflectivity and a V pattern; lymphoma has low reflectivity, as does Merkel cell carcinoma, but a small angle kappa. Thus, although lymphoma has a pattern of reflectivity similar to that of Merkel cell carcinoma, it can be differentiated by standardized echography on the basis of the angle kappa.

Quantitative echography of Merkel cell carcinoma and in particular the study of the sound attenuation (angle kappa) was of great importance in the differential diagnosis of these disorders. Complementary information on the consistency of the lesion is obtained by kinetic echography, which moreover shows that Merkel cell carcinoma is vascularized while all the other tumors have no detectable blood flow.

Standardized echography is thus a useful tool with which to distinguish the orbital recurrence of Merkel cell carcinoma from other disorders that can affect

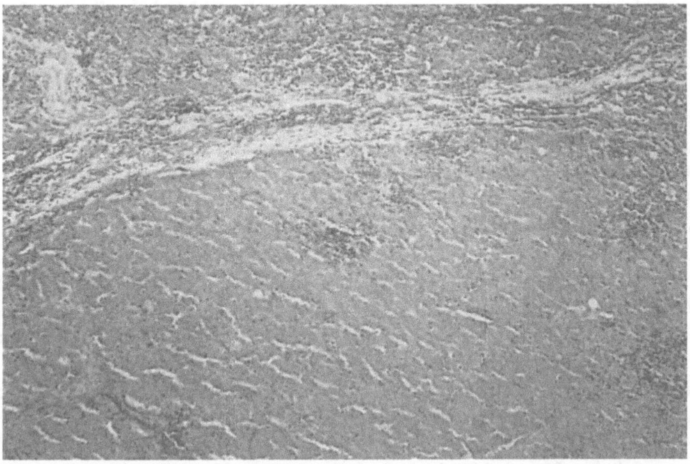

Fig. 10. Histologic appearance of Merkel cell carcinoma. Note the diffuse cellular proliferation of round uniform cells. Hematoxylin and eosin. 4 ×

the orbit. In particular, in the case reported in this paper, which showed a superotemporal localization, this technique helped to exclude the most common orbital lesions that can involve the lacrimal fossa as described by Cennamo *et al.* [16], i.e., lacrimal gland lesions (dacryops, dacryoadenitis, lymphoma, pseudolymphoma, benign mixed tumor, adenoid cystic carcinoma) and other diseases (dermoid cysts, cavernous hemangioma and swannoma in atypical location).

In conclusion, standardized echography provides new insights into the diagnosis of orbital masses and in particular, presents typical characteristics even in case of Merkel cell carcinoma. A standardized echographic pattern suggestive of Merkel cell carcinoma should be followed by immunohistochemical and electron microscopy to confirm diagnosis of this aggressive tumor.

References

[1] T. Kivela and A. Tarkkanen. The Merkel cell and associated neoplasms in the eyelids and periocular region. Surv. Ophthalmol. 1990;35:171–187.

[2] F. Merkel. Tastzellen und Tastkörperchen bei den Hausthieren und beim Menschen. Arch. Mikrosc. Anat. 1875:11:636–652.

[3] M. Mihara, K. Hashimoto, K. Veda *et al.* The specialized junction between Merkel cell and neurite: an electron microscopy study. J. Invest. Dermatol. 1979;73:325–334.

[4] C. Toker. Trabecular carcinoma of the skin. Arch. Dermatol. 1972;105:107–110.

[5] C.K. Tang and C. Toker. Trabecular carcinoma of the skin. An ultrastructural study. Cancer 1978;42:2311–2321.

[6] K. Furuno, M. Wakakura, K. Shimizu, K. Iwabuchi and T. Kameya. Immunohistochemical studies of Merkel cell carcinoma of the eyelid. Jpn. J. Ophthalmol. 1992;36:348–355.

[7] Y. Merot. Is the neuroendocrine carcinoma of the skin a Merkel cell tumor? What we can learn from immunohistochemical and ultrastructural studies. Int. J. Dermatol. 1990;29:102–104.
[8] P. Till and W. Hauff. Differential diagnostic results of clinical echography in orbital tumors. In J.M. Thijssen and A.M. Veerbeek (eds), Ultrasonography in ophthalmology. The Hague: W. Junk, Doc. Ophthalmol. Proc. Ser. 1981;29:277–282.
[9] K.C. Ossoinig. Standardized echography: basic principles, clinical applications, and results. In R.L. Dallow (ed.), Ophthalmic ultrasonography: comparative techniques. Boston: Little, Brown & Co., Int. Ophthal. Clin. 1979;19(IV):127–210.
[10] C.L. Hitchcock, K.I. Bland, R.G. Laney, D. Franzini, B. Harris and E.M. Copeland. Neuroendocrine (Merkel cell) carcinoma of the skin. Its natural history, diagnosis and treatment. Ann. Surg. 1988;207:201.
[11] P.E. Rubsamen, M. Tannenbaum, A.S. Grove and E. Gould. Merkel cell carcinoma of the eyelid and periocular tissues. Am. J. Ophthalmol. 1992;113:674–680.
[12] H. Offret, N. Badarani, J. Quillard, E. Bloch-Michel. Envahissement orbitaire d'une tumeur à cellules de Merkel palpebrale. J. Fr. Ophtalmol. 1992;15:605–609.
[13] R.K. Sibley, J. Rosai, E. Foucar, L.P. Dehner and G. Bosl. Neuroendocrine (Merkel cell) carcinoma of the skin. A histologic and ultrastructural study of two cases. Am. J. Surg. Pathol. 1980;4:211–221.
[14] J.H. Raaf, C. Urmacher, W.K. Knapper, M.H. Shiu and E. Cheng. Trabecular (Merkel cell) carcinoma of the skin. Treatment of primary, recurrent and metastatic disease. Cancer 1986;57:178.
[15] J. Rosai. Ackerman's Surgical Pathology. VIII edition, St. Louis: The C.V.Mosby Co., 1994;166–168.
[16] G. Cennamo, F. Tranfa and G. Bonavolontà. Lesions of the lacrimal fossa: a retrospective echographic study. Proceedings of 12th SIDUO Congress. Doc. Ophthalm. Proc. 1988;53:63,78.

F. Genovesi-Ebert
Pisa
Italy

34. Neurilemmoma (neuroma) of the infraorbital nerve

A. STANOWSKY, F. MORASCH, T. WAGNER and R. WERTHEIMER[1]
(Augsburg and [1]München, Germany)

Abstract

A neurilemmoma located at the infraorbital nerve showed an untypically high reflectivity by standardized A-scan. Moreover, in the same obit we detected enlarged extraocular muscles resembling Graves' disease.

Key words: Neurilemmoma, neurinoma, infraorbital nerve, ultrasound, echography

Introduction

The name neurinoma was introduced by Verocay [1] in 1910. Since Verocay's publication, many other names, e.g., peridural fibroma, Schwannoma, have been proposed for this disease. These names indicate that the tumor is of a mesodermal or neuroektodermal rather than neurogenic origin [2]. Stout [3] clarified in 1935 that the term 'neurinoma' should apply only to a tumor of the nerve fibres, and not to this kind of tumor that is arising in nerve sheaths (neurilemma). He therefore proposed the term 'neurilemmoma'.

A neurilemmoma can appear in all peripheral and cranial nerves. The acoustic nerve is the most frequently affected one. Among the peripheral nerves, the brachial plexus, the flexor surfaces of extremities, the nerves within the mediastinum and the spinal chord are the most frequent sites of neurilemmoma. Within the orbit, a neurilemmoma is found mainly in the area of the oculomotor nerve, but it can also occur after enucleation [4].

Among 877 orbital tumors, Reese [5] found 13 neurilemmomas, a percentage of 1.5%.

We had the opportunity to examine a neurilemmoma of the infraorbital nerve.

Case description

The female patient, R.M., born in 1947 had a known unilateral right-sided exophthalmos since childhood. In February 1991, the patient first noticed a

G Cennamo and N. Rosa (eds.), Ultrasonography in Ophthalmology 15, pp. 303–307.

pressure sensation as well as paresthesia in the area of her right eye and cheek and increased rhinorrhoea and epiphora. Computerized tomography indicated an inflammatory process in the area of the infraorbital foramen with a simultaneous broadening of the horizontal and inferior eye muscles.

Within these muscles standardized A-scan showed a high reflectivity and Graves' disease was suspected. The endocrinological examination showed a small right-sided grade 1 struma with normal thyroid blood parameters and a normal thyroid regulatory circuit.

After high dose steroid therapy, the patient initially felt some subjective improvement of the symptoms. However, a steroid-induced diabetes mellitus was diagnosed, and the steroid therapy therefore was discontinued.

In June 1991 (see Fig. 1) we found a right-sided exophthalmos of 3 mm. Vision was 20/20 bilaterally with a regular visual field, normal fundus appearance and unimpaired ocular motility. In the area of the right lower lid there was a defined tumorous thickening with a mild inflammatory reaction.

Standardized A-scan revealed a thickening of the medial, lateral and inferior muscle with high reflectivity. In the area of the infraorbital foramen a 6 to 7 mm sized, barely compressible, non vascularized structure with low to intermediate reflectivity was found. The internal structure was heterogeneous (see Fig. 2). Magnetic resonance imaging showed a bony defect in the area of the infraorbital foramen. The consulted otolaryngologists and neuro-surgeons did not see any indication for surgery.

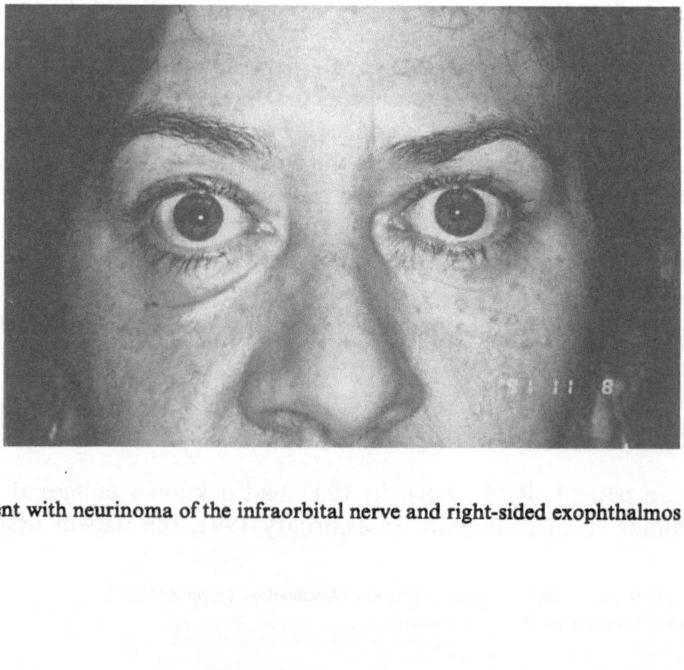

Fig. 1. Patient with neurinoma of the infraorbital nerve and right-sided exophthalmos

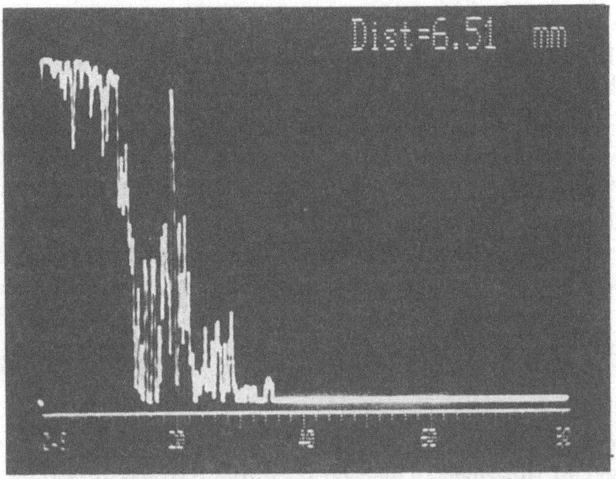

Fig. 2. **Standardized A-scan, showing a non-vascularized tumor with low to medium reflectivity and a heterogeneously regular internal structure. The neurilemmoma had not yet penetrated the infraorbital floor**

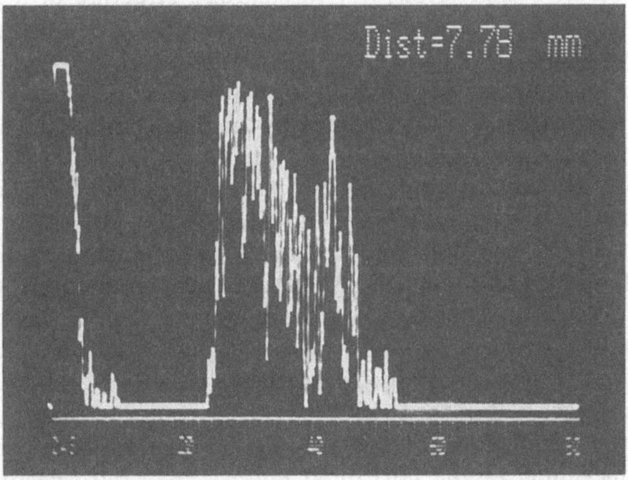

Fig. 3. **After penetration of the infraorbital floor, the internal reflectivity (standardized A-scan) of the neurilemmoma had clearly increased**

During an echographical control examination in August 1991, for the first time a tumorous structure was detected within the orbit. The transocular A-scan examination showed, at 6 o'clock, within the anterior orbit a medium to highly reflective heterogeneously structured tumor showing medium absorption (see Fig. 3).

The tumor was well-defined, barely compressible and showed no signs of vascularisation. It could be assumed that the process that had originated within the infraorbital foramen, had now penetrated the orbital floor and thereby had invaded the orbit itself.

Examination of the right maxillary sinus by the otolaryngologists revealed a mucosal indentation, but no bony or mucosal defect in the area of the superior maxillary sinus wall. We prepared a bony lamella of the upper sinus wall, and a histological sample was removed from the suspected area. The histological examination showed a neurilemmoma. The tumor was excised in a second operation.

Discussion

The diagnosis of this disease was rather difficult, particularly because it is very rare [6,7]. In addition, the thickening of the horizontal eye muscles was misleading.

Our first echographical examination showed in the area of the infraorbital foramen a barely compressible, not vascularized structure of low to medium reflectivity; this had a heterogeneous internal structure and low sound attenuation with well outlined borders.

Because this process was initially located outside the orbit, the existing exophthalmos was thought to be caused by the thickening of the horizontal eye muscles. After the neurilemmoma had penetrated the orbital floor the tumor could be demonstrated echographically within the orbit. By standardized A-scan a somewhat higher reflectivity and sound attenuation was detected. We assume that this change in reflectivity and attenuation may be explained by the fact that after perforation of the bony channel the neurilemmoma could expand to its normal size. In particular, the smaller cystic and vascular components of the tumor may have been affected by this mechanism. In our case, we did not detect the typical echographical characteristics described by Byrne [8], i.e., the vast cystic changes within the tumor. Perhaps we failed to detect these changes because of the specific location and a somewhat different histological composition. The thickening of the horizontal muscles may retrospectively be interpreted as a chronic inflammatory reaction within the orbit caused by the presence of the neurilemmoma.

References

[1] J. Verocay. Zur Kenntnis der Neurofibrome. Beitr. Pathol. Anat. 1910;48:1–69.

[2] J.W. Henderson. Orbital tumors. Philadelphia, London, Toronto: W.B. Saunders Company, 1973;307–312.

[3] A.P. Stout. The peripheral manifestations of the specific nerve sheath tumor (neurilemoma). Am. J. Cancer 1935;24:751–796.

[4] F.C. Blodi. Amputation neuroma in the orbit. Am. J. Ophthalmol. 1949;32:929.

[5] A.B. Reese. Expanding lesions of the orbit. Soc. UK, Trans. Ophthalmol. 1971;63:85–104.
[6] L.A. Pereira and Y.B. Choo. Schwannoma of the infraorbital nerve. Ear, Nose and Throat Journal 1979; 58(6):236–239.
[7] R.I. Kahl. Ein Neurinom des Nervus infraorbitalis. Zeitschrift für Neurologie 1973;204 (2):155–158.
[8] B.W. Byrne, W.A. van Heuven and A.W. Lawton. Echographic characteristics of benign orbital schwannomas (neurilemomas). Am. J. Ophthalmol. 1988;106(2):194–198.

Alexamder Stanowsky
Augenklinik am Zentralklinikum Augsburg
Augsburg, Germany

[1]Augenklinik rechts der Isar
München, Germany

35. Early diagnosis of orbital rhabdomyosarcoma by ultrasonography

K. SÉNYI and J. NÉMETH
(Budapest, Hungary)

Abstract

A case of orbital rhabdomyosarcoma with diplopia as the presenting sign is reported. A four-year-old girl complained of diplopia two weeks after an eyelid puncture by a pine tree needle. She was referred to our department for evaluation after a detailed pediatric and neurological examination. Routine ophthalmological examination and Lancaster projection test revealed a slight disturbance of ocular motility, but no other disorder was found

Ultrasound examination was performed using an Ultrascan Digital B 2000 equipped with a 10 MHz A/B-scan probe, according to routine orbital scanning procedure. The orbital B-scan examination showed that the right rectus inferior muscle was enlarged by a sharply delineated mass, measuring about 16–18 mm in width. A striking feature of the mass was an internal movement mimicking muscle contraction synchronous with rectus muscle contraction noticed when the patient was asked to look in different directions. The finding raised the possibility of a rhabdomyosarcoma involving the inferior rectus muscle.

The patient underwent an inferior orbitotomy and biopsy of the mass. As the intraoperative frozen section confirmed the diagnosis of rhabdomyosarcoma, the tumor was excised. Postoperatively the patient received chemotherapy. One year later she was reoperated because of recurrence of the tumor. Then she was given radiation therapy and cystostatic treatment again. Three years after the last operation, she is doing well without evidence of further tumor recurrence.

In case of unexplained ocular motility disturbance, an ultrasound screening of the orbit should be considered as a diagnostic procedure.

Key words: Orbital embryonal and alveolar type tumor, rhabdomyosarcoma, immunocytochemistry, CWS-86 protocol, VACA-II chemotherapy

Introduction

Rhabdomyosarcoma is rare but is the most frequent primary malignant tumor of the orbit in children [1]. Its presenting signs are progressive proptosis and displacement of the eyeball, diplopia, and sometimes inflammatory signs

G Cennamo and N. Rosa (eds.), Ultrasonography in Ophthalmology 15, pp. 309–314.

mimicking orbital inflammation [2]. Baron and colleagues [3] described the case of a 5-month-old boy where rhabdomyosarcoma manifested as acquired nasolacrimal duct obstruction.

The diagnosis of rhabdomyosarcoma is based principally on orbital biopsy [2]. Of eight orbital fine needle aspiration biopsies in children reported by O'Hara *et al.* [4], three patients had rhabdomyosarcoma. As Gloor and Kalman emphasized, the diagnosis of rhabdomyosarcoma was often made rather late despite the use of such modern diagnostic procedures as ultrasound, CT, MRI and angiography [1]. The most common misleading anamnestic data are a history of trauma, or inflammation and a haemangioma-like angiographic result [1]. Here we describe a case where the presentation sign of orbital rhabdomyosarcoma was diplopia following orbital injury.

Case report

A four-year-old girl was referred to our pediatric outpatient department by a pediatric neurologist because of a two-week-long history of diplopia.

The girl suffered an eyelid puncture by a pine tree needle four weeks earlier. After the injury, the right eye became slightly red and it was treated with antibiotic drops. The conjunctival redness resolved quickly but two weeks after the injury, the patient complained of intermittent diplopia and mild lower eyelid pain. Because of the diplopia, a neurologic examination was performed. The neurological status of the patient was negative, and she was referred to our department for a Lancaster red-green projection test.

The routine ophthalmologic examination revealed slight redness and oedema on the right side: a narrower lid fissure, eyelid involvement, and palpable enlargement of the lower rectus muscle. No proptosis was found. The anterior and posterior segments of the eye were normal. The ocular motility of the right eye was reduced in the downward gaze; this was associated with diplopia.

Ultrasound examination was performed as a routine orbital scanning procedure with an Ultrascan Digital B 2000 A- and B-scan instrument equipped with 10 MHz probes. The echography showed the right side rectus inferior muscle enlarged by a sharply delineated mass, measuring about $10 \times 12 \times 18$ mm. A striking feature of the mass was an internal movement mimicking muscle contraction synchronous with rectus inferior muscle contraction noticed when patient was asked to look in different directions. The internal reflectivity was medium high and angle kappa was 30°. The ultrasound findings raised the possibility of rhabdomyosarcoma involving the lower rectus muscle (Figs. 1 and 2).

Computed tomography of the orbit revealed no anomalies on the left side. On the right side, in the postero-inferior part of the orbit there was a mass of about 25×20 mm that was as dense as the soft part which, breaking through the lower wall of the orbit, reached the right maxillary sinus. The bulbus in the right side was sound.

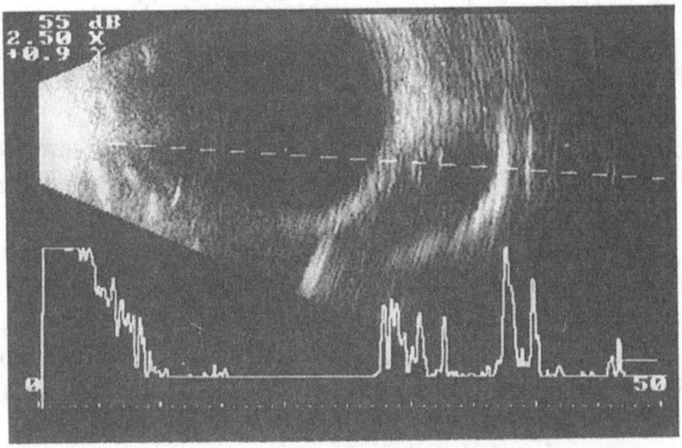

Fig. 1. The right side rectus inferior muscle measuring about 10 × 12 × 18 mm

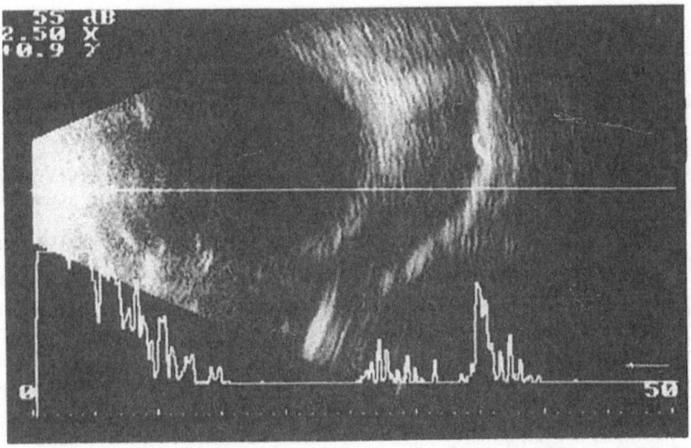

Fig. 2. The internal reflectivity was medium high

The patient underwent an inferior orbitotomy and biopsy of the mass. The intraoperative frozen section confirmed the diagnosis of embryonal rhabdomyosarcoma. The tumor was totally excised. Postoperatively she received cytostatic drugs, namely intravenous Vincristin 1.0 mg daily for 3 weeks and according to the 'CWS-86 protocol' 3 × VACA II. cyclus: vincristin 1.5 mg/m^2

intravenous bolus injection daily and actinomycin D 0.5 mg/m^2 and cyclophosphamide 1200 mg/m^2 and adriamycin 20 mg/m^2.

Bone scintigraphy showed no pathognostic activity. There was reflective mass of $6 \times 12 \times 17$ mms at the site of the rectus inferior muscle under the bulb. Eighteen months after the first operation, she was reoperated because of tumor recurrence and was again given cytostatic treatment.

Histology showed a malignant neoplasm that had the features of alveolar rhabdomyosarcoma. The sections showed fragments consisting almost entirely of tumor without normal structures. The tumor was arranged in layers of polygonal cells essentially without intervening stroma. The tumor was penetrated by numerous small blood vessels that formed partial fine fibrovascular septa. Focally, there was a poorly formed alveolar pattern characterized by a cluster of tumor cells around the periphery of the fibrovascular septa that became less dense towards the middle of the cluster. There was no confluent necrosis, but numerous single tumor cells were necrotic. The tumor cells contained large round to slightly irregular hyperchromatic nuclei with a stippled chromatin pattern, no nucleoli and numerous mitotic figures. The tumor cells contained slight to moderate amounts of eosinophilic cytoplasm either around the nucleus or eccentrically. The neuron-specific enolase stain showed diffuse cytoplasmic reactivity throughout the tumor. The pathologic diagnosis was: Orbit right excision: Rhabdomyosarcoma, recurrent, unfavorable histology (alveolar).

Discussion

The ultrasound diagnostic features of rhabdomyosarcoma have been described by Ossoinig [5], Boparai [6], Guthoff [7] and S.F. Byrne, R.L. Green [8]. Rhabdomyosarcoma is the most common primary orbital malignancy of childhood and frequently presents with a rapidly developing exophthalmos. In general, rhabdomyosarcomas are highly cellular, vascularized lesions that echographically may resemble a pseudotumor or lymphomas. However, the echographic features of this tumor usually differentiate it from the other more common tumors in children, i.e., capillary haemangioma, lymphangioma with hemorrhage and dermoid cyst.

Rhabdomyosarcoma does not affect preferentially any part of the orbit. On the basis of three other cases, it can be affirmed that these neoplasms extend into the anterior orbital areas and are characterized by a homogeneous echographic pattern. The tumor is distinct from the adipose tissue and can be imaged echographically without any difficulty. We occasionally also see areas of medium or low reflectivity, especially when the growing tumor infiltrates and destroys normal orbital structures.

According to Ossoinig, rhabdomyosarcoma together with lymphoma and pseudotumor of the orbit are among the so-called 'low-reflective orbital lesions' [5,9].

The echogram alone does not provide unequivocal information and, in suspected cases, a biopsy is necessary for diagnosis. During recent years, the treatment of these lesions has shifted from radical operation to a combined radio- and chemotherapy. Echography can be useful for follow-up examinations in order to avoid unnecessary radiation exposure by repeated CT scans [10,11]. Opinions still differ concerning the therapy of rhabdomyosarcoma. The treatment possibilities are: surgery [2], irradiation [2,12] chemotherapy [1] and the combination of these three procedures [1,2,6,12].

Conclusion

In case of unexplained ocular motility disturbance, ultrasound screening of the orbit should be considered as a diagnostic method. A 4-year-old white female patient developed orbital rhabdomyosarcoma in the area of the right inferior rectus muscle, and was treated with local excision and chemotherapy. There was no evidence of metastatic disease. Excisional biopsy in February 1992 showed recurrent rhabdomyosarcoma. Further examinations showed no apparent extraorbital disease or metastases. She was subsequently treated with chemotherapy and radiotherapy.

Acknowledgements

Thanks are due to: Dr. Imre Rényi and his colleagues, who completed the cytostatic therapy at the 1st Department of Children, Semmelweis Medical University Budapest, Hungary. Dr. Márta Hajda and her team, who performed the operation at the Neurosurgical Institute, Budapest, Hungary. Professor Barnhill and his colleagues, who performed the second operation and cytostatic therapy at the Hospital for Children, Department of Pathology, Division of Pediatric Pathology, Indianapolis, USA.

References

[1] B. Gloor and A. Kalman. Neoplastische Raumveränderung in der Orbita. I. Klin. Mbl. Augenheilk. 1992;201:291–301.

[2] W.P. Boger and R.A. Petersen. Pediatric Ophthalmology. In D. Pavan-Langston (ed.), Manual of Ocular Diagnosis and Therapy. Boston: Little, Brown and Co., 1980.

[3] E.M. Baron, R.C. Kersten and D.R. Kulwin. Rhabdomyosarcoma manifesting as acquired nasolacrimal duct obstruction. Am. J. Ophthalmol. 1993;115:239–242.

[4] B.J. O'Hara, H. Ehya, L.A. Shields, J.J. Augsburger, C.L. Shields and R.C. Eagle. Fine needle aspiration biopsy in pediatric ophthalmic tumors and pseudotumors. Acta Cytol. 1993;37:125–130.

[5] K. Ossoinig. Quantitative echography – the basis of tissue differentiation. J. Clin. Ultrasound. Vol. 2. 1974;1:33–46.

[6] M.S. Boparai. Clinical ultrasonographic and CT evaluation of orbital rhabdomycosarcoma with management. Indian J. Ophthamol. 1991;35:125–131.
[7] R. Guthoff. Ultrasound in Ophthalmologic Diagnosis. Rhabdomycosarcoma 1991;124–125.
[8] S.F. Byrne and R.L. Green. Ultrasound of the eye and orbit. St. Louis: Mosby Year Book, 1992;288–289.
[9] K. Ossoinig. Standardized echography: basic principles, clinical applications and result. In R.D. Dallow (ed.), Ophthalmic ultrasonography comparative techniques, 1979;172–173.
[10] R. Rochels and G. Reis. Echographic bei orbitalen Rabdomycosarcoma in Kindesalter. Ophthalmologica 1980;180:274.
[11] K. Bluth and J. Planitzer. Comparison of echographic and computer-tomographic examinations in orbital diseases. Doc. Ophthalmol. Proc. Ser. 1981;29:293.
[12] D.H. Abramson, R.M. Ellsworth, P. Tretter, J.A. Wolff and F.D. Kitchin. The treatment of orbital rhabdomyosarcoma with irradiation and chemotherapy. Ophthalmology 1979;86: 1330–1335.

K. Sényi
1st Department of Ophthalmology
Semmelweis University Medical School
Budapest, Hungary

36. Echographic patterns of neurofibromatosis – 1

L. COLLAÇO, P. CANDELÁRIA, C. BATALHA and P. ABRANTES
(Lisbon, Portugal)

Abstract

Four cases of neurofibromatosis-1 were studied with B-scan and standardized A-scan echography. We describe the echographic pattern of plexiform neurofibroma, Lisch nodules, retinal hamartoma and optic nerve glioma.

Key words: Neurofibromatosis-1, plexiform neurofibroma, Lisch nodule, retinal hamartoma, optic nerve glioma

Introduction

The most frequent neurofibromatosis, neurofibromatosis-1 (NF-1), has diverse ophthalmic manifestations [1,5]. The major lesions are Lisch nodules, neurofibromas, optic nerve gliomas and various architectural abnormalities [7,8]. Retinal hamartomas are a rare finding in this condition.

The complications of NF-1, mainly the neurogenic tumours, may require a neurosurgical approach for complete removal and, thus, differentiation from other orbital tumours is important. Standardized A- and B-scan ultrasonography is very useful in the differential diagnosis of several orbital tumours [2,3,6]. We describe the echographic findings in our four NF-1 cases and discuss their value in the diagnosis.

Case reports

Case 1

A nine-year-old black boy presented with unilateral exophthalmos. The ophthalmic examination revealed a vascularized plexiform neurofibroma of soft consistency involving the right anterior orbit and the temporal fossa (Fig. 1). The other orbital and systemic findings ("café-au-lait" spots and larger wing sphenoid bone hypoplasia at computed tomography) led to the diagnosis of NF-1.

G Cennamo and N. Rosa (eds.), Ultrasonography in Ophthalmology 15, pp. 315–322.

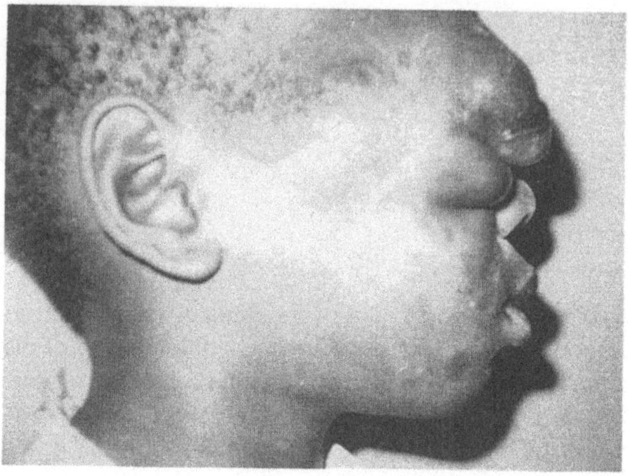

Fig. 1. Plexiform neurofibroma of the right anterior and superior orbit with involvement of the temporal fossa. Case one

A-scan sonography was performed using a 10 MHz probe. An irregularly structured mass lesion with medium to high internal reflectivity was found. There were signs of vascularity and delayed compressibility. B-scan sonography was performed with the echo scan US-3300 equipped with a 10 MHz probe and showed an infiltrative non encapsulated tumour (Fig. 2).

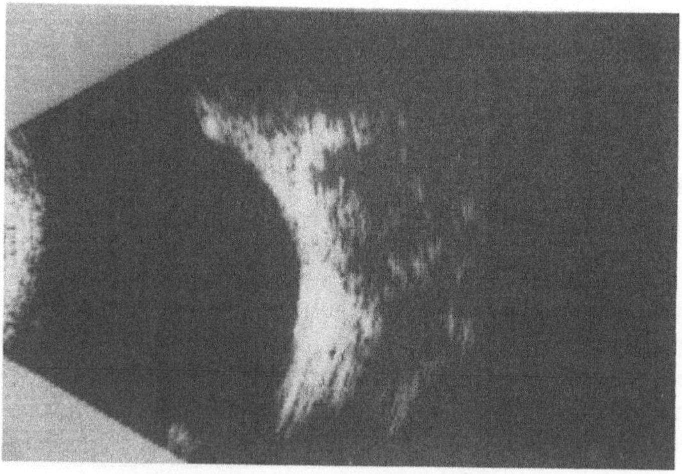

Fig. 2. B-scan showing irregularly shaped and poorly outlined lesion. Case one

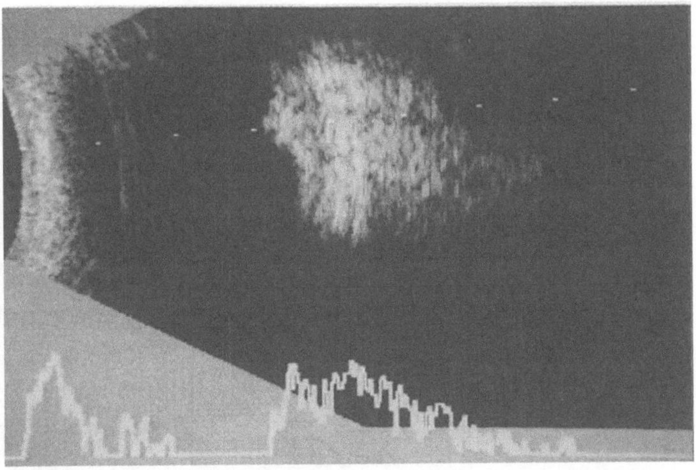

Fig. 3. B- and A-scans. Case two. The trace suggests a solid pattern throughout a retinal hamartoma with a dome-shaped configuration and medium to high reflectivity

Case 2

A five-year-old black girl with multiple subcutaneous neurofibromas and hyperpigmentated areas on the trunk and gluteal region was referred to our Department for further examination. Ophthalmoscopy and fluorescein angiography showed retinal hamartoma near the posterior pole and glial tissue overlying the optic disc.

On B- and A-scan we noted solid neoplastic lesions with medium to high reflectivity in the posterior pole and in the anterior optic nerve (Fig. 3).

Case 3

A 35-year-old white woman had noticed blurred vision in her right eye and displacement of her right globe one year before examination. There was a 16-mm Hertel difference.

A- and B-mode sonograms revealed an enlargement of the optic nerve shadow showing a sonolucent roundish tumour (Fig. 4). On the axial computerized tomographic scan, we observed a unilateral marked widening of the optic nerve (Fig. 5). Systemic examination revealed kyphoscoliosis, multiple 'caf³ au lait' maculas and a pileous cutaneous naevus.

Case 4

A two-year-old white girl was first seen because of a progressive unilateral exophthalmos. Ophthalmic examination revealed a strabismus with limited

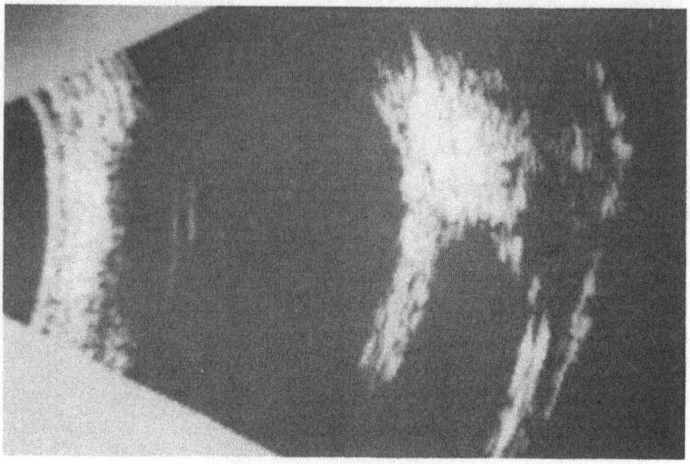

Fig. 4. B-mode sonogram. Case three. The optic nerve tumour appears sonolucent thereby indicating homogeneity

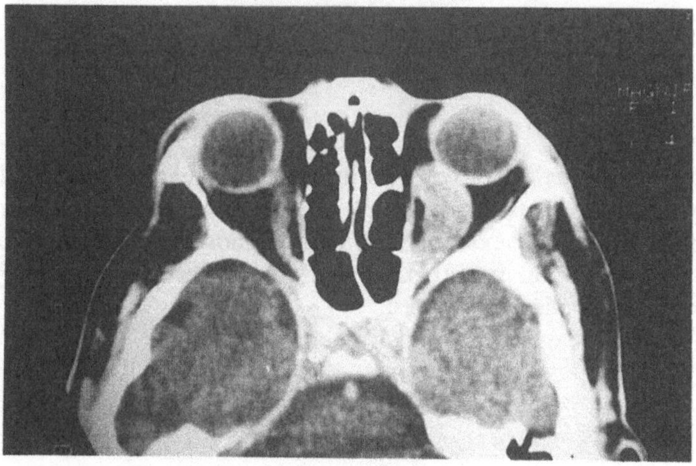

Fig. 5. Axial CT scan, case three. Unilateral marked enlargement of the optic nerve

adduction and elevation. Three millimeter proptosis of the right eye with orbital resistance was also detected. Biomicroscopy of the dark iris of both eyes showed well-defined brown wart-like lesions, features typical of Lisch nodules and ophthalmoscopic findings of pale disks pointed to an optic nerve lesion.

On ultrasonography, an A-scan through the Lisch nodules at a reduced gain setting showed a high lesion spike (Fig. 6). Multiple internal echoes in the optic nerves with medium to high reflectivity were also detected. B-mode sonogram was performed with the Humphrey 835 using a 12 MHz probe; this showed high spikes in the iris hamartomas and spindle-shaped widening of the optic nerves (Fig. 7).

Computed tomography showed a uniform thickening of the entire optic nerve

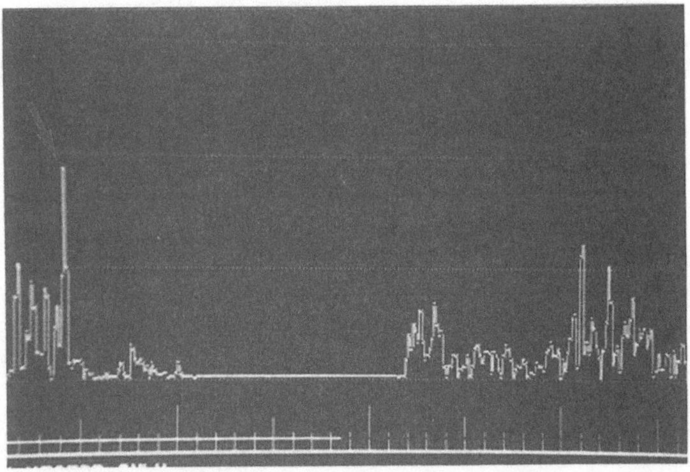

Fig. 6. A-scan through the Lisch nodule at reduced gain setting, left eye, case four. Note the high spike (arrow) corresponding to the iris lesion

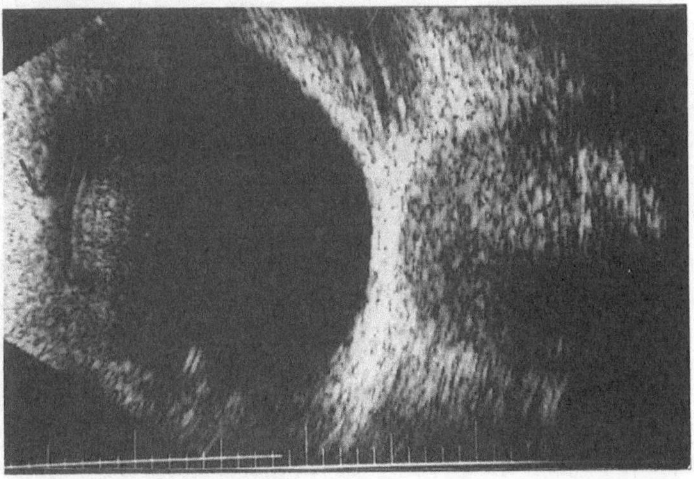

Fig. 7. B-mode sonogram, left eye, case four. Note the high echoes in one iris hamartoma (arrow) and the widening of the optic nerve

(Fig. 8). The T1-weighted images obtained with magnetic resonance imaging showed fusiform sharply delineated optic nerves extending posteriorly into the chiasma. Bright lesions, on T2-weighted images were seen in globus pallidus, brainstem and cerebral peduncles (Fig. 9). An optic nerve incisional biopsy revealed a grade 2 pilocytic astrocytoma (Fig. 10).

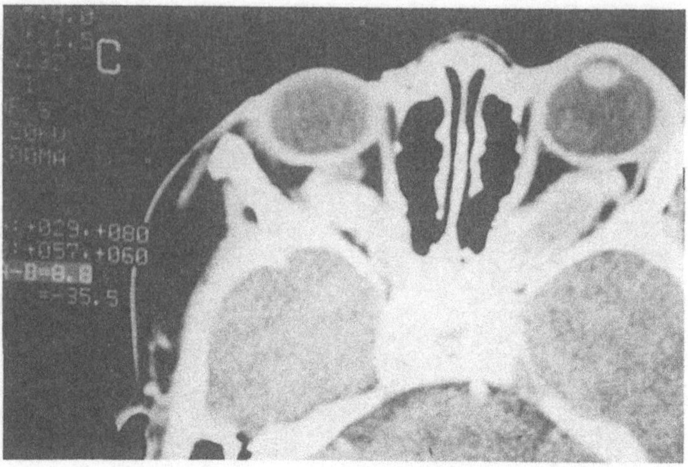

Fig. 8. Axial CT scan showing a uniform thickening of the entire convoluted optic nerves, case four

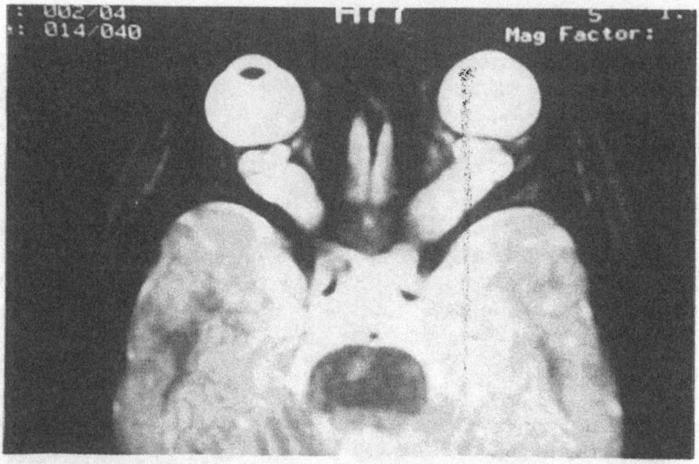

Fig. 9. Axial MRI scan (T2) shows bilateral large optic nerve gliomas with intracanalicular and chiasmal involvement, case four

Discussion

Lisch nodules which are iris melanocytic hamartomas, are the commonest feature of NF-1 echographic pattern that we have found in our cases and are similar to iris naevus.

The ultrasonic patterns of peripheral nerve tumours differ significantly from those of tumours that involve the optic nerve. They are often poorly or not encapsulated [4]. The plexiform neurofibroma that we have studied was an infiltrative non encapsulated lesion, irregularly-shaped and poorly outlined with

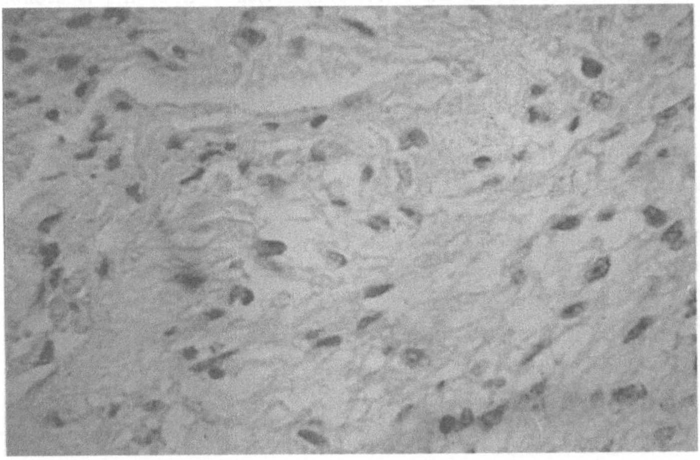

Fig. 10. Histologic section shows a pilocytic astrocytoma (Van Gieson 1000 ×), case four

an irregular internal structure; it had a predominantly high reflectivity and minimal sound attenuation.

Gliomas may involve the optic nerves, the chiasm and hypothalamic area. The echography shows only the orbital tumour with sharply defined anterior borders relatively well-demarcated from the surrounding orbital fat. The posterior extent of the tumour cannot be acoustically evaluated. Low amplitude echoes within the internal structure of the glioma indicate minor tissues interfaces (homogeneous solid lesion); occasional acoustic discontinuities are seen like in case 4, and may represent collagenous connective tissue septae.

Conclusion

Standardized A- and B-scan echography allows us to detect NF-1 orbital and ocular lesions and to differentiate them from other tumours.

References

[1] D.J. Bergin and V. Parmley. Orbital neurilemoma. Arch. Ophthalmol. 1988;106:414.

[2] B.M. Byrne, W.A. Van Heuven and A.W. Lawton. Echographic characteristics of benign orbital schwannomas (neurilemmomas). Am. J. Ophthalmol. 1988;106:195.

[3] S.F. Byrne and B.M. Byrne. Differential diagnosis of orbital neurilemmoma (schwannoma) with standardized echography. In K.C. Ossoinig (ed.), Ophthalmic Echography. Dordrecht: Dr. W. Junk, 1987;491.

[4] D.J. Coleman, F.C. Lizzi and R.L. Jack. Ultrasonography of the Eye and Orbit. Philadelphia: Lea and Febiger, 1977.

[5] J.J. Mulvihill. Neurofibromatosis I (Recklinghausen disease) and Neurofibromatosis II (bilateral acoustic neurofibromatosis): An update. Ann. Inter. Med. 1990;113:39–52.
[6] K.C. Ossoinig. A-scan echography and orbit disease. Mode Probl. Ophthalmol. 1975;14:203–231.
[7] V.M. Riccardi. von Recklinghausen neurofibromatosis. N. Engl. J. Med. 1981;305:1617–1627.
[8] J. Rootman and W. Robertson. Neurogenic tumours. In J. Rootman, Diseases of the Orbit. Philadelphia: J.B. Lippincott & Co., 1988;319.

Dr. Luis Collaço
Department of Ophthalmology
Hospital de S. José
Lisbon, Portugal

37. Standardized echography in Recklinghausen's neurofibromatosis with congenital glaucoma

H. MAIER and G. HASENFRATZ
(Würzburg, Germany)

Abstract

In December 1989 we first saw a three-year-old girl with a congenital glaucoma diagnosed when the child was four weeks of age, together with high intraocular pressure (IOP) of the right eye (40 mmHg). Goniotomy was performed twice in the right eye, but the IOP remained elevated. She presented an asymmetry of the face with displacement of the right eye downwards and nasally, and signs of congenital glaucoma in the right eye, i.e., a large excavation of the optic disc, a corneal enlargement and an IOP of as much as 28 mmHg. The axial eye length was 27.0 mm in the right eye and 21.7 mm in the left eye. In standardized echography a parabulbar lesion was found in the superotemporal right orbit. The anamnestic data and the diagnostic ultrasound suggested a neurofibroma. This was supported by nuclear magnetic resonance and computerized tomography. Thus, an orbitotomy was performed. Histopathology confirmed a neurofibroma.

In 1990 and 1991 café au lait patches and other neurofibromas developed elsewhere, and the diagnosis of Recklinghausen's neurofibromatosis was made. We found that for more than three years the congenital glaucoma and the retrobulbar lesion of the right eye had been the only signs of this disease.

Key words: Congenital glaucoma, Recklinhausen's neurofibromatosis, standardized echography

Introduction

The differential diagnosis of exophthalmos in childhood may cause difficulties. An exact diagnosis can only be established by several examination techniques and a complete clinical examination, such as clinical echography with A-scan and B-scan and radiologic findings obtained by computerized tomography and nuclear magnetic resonance. In this study the clinical data and the echographic findings obtained with standardized echography in an unusual case of Recklinghausen's neurofibromatosis with congenital glaucoma in a child are described.

G Cennamo and N. Rosa (eds.), Ultrasonography in Ophthalmology 15, pp. 323–329.

Case report

In December 1989 we first saw this three-year-old girl. A congenital glaucoma had been diagnosed when the patient was four weeks old, together with the intraocular pressure of 40 mmHg in the right eye. Goniotomy of the right eye was performed when the patient was two months old. A second operation was necessary one month later. After a period of medically well regulated intraocular pressure, the intraocular pressure was 36 mmHg six months later.

The visual acuity in December 1989 was 1/25 in the right eye and 0.9 in the left eye. The anterior segment was within normal limits on both sides. She presented an asymmetry of the face with displacement of the right globe downwards and nasally, and signs of congenital glaucoma in the right eye, i.e., large excavation of the optic disc and corneal enlargement [1].

The intraocular pressure in the right eye was 28 mmHg and normal in the left eye (15 mmHg). The corneal diameter (13.5 mm) was slightly enlarged in the right eye. In the left eye the corneal diameter was normal with 11 mmHg, the optic disc had a glaucomatous excavation with a cup disc ratio of 0.8.

The asymmetry of the face was not typical for congenital glaucoma. The right orbit seemed to be greater than the left one. Furthermore, there was an exophthalmos of the right eye of 9 mm. The globe was displaced nasally and downwards. The parents recorded that globe displacement appeared a long time ago and had developed very slowly.

Echographic findings obtained with standardized echography

The echographic examination was performed using standardized echography [2–5]. The devices used were a standardized A-scan (Mini A-Scan, Alcon, 8 MHz NF) and a contact B-Scan (Mini-B, Alcon, 10 MHz NF); biometry was performed with the biometric system (GBS) or with the standardized A-scan.

Biometry showed that the axial eye length of the right eye was clearly above the normal range with 27.0 mm compared to 21.7 on the left eye (Fig. 1). Since the difference did not explain the asymmetry of the face, diagnostic ultrasound was performed and a lesion in the superotemporal orbit was detected (Fig. 2).

In contact B-scan we saw a parabulbar lesion in the superotemporal anterior orbit, extending to the middle orbit. The lesion was clearly separated from the extraocular muscles (musculus rectus superior and musculus rectus lateralis). We found no indentation of the globe. The lesion was oval-roundish in shape.

Standardized A-scan examination showed a well-outlined lesion with low reflectivity, regular internal structure and moderate sound attenuation. The consistency was hard, and vascularity poor (Fig. 3).

According to Byrne [3] several differential diagnoses were possible. The main criteria for the differential diagnosis were the internal structure, the sound attenuation, the vascularity and the consistency.

Lymphomas and pseudotumors of the orbit also present a regular internal structure, a firm consistency and a poor vascularity, but their sound attenuation

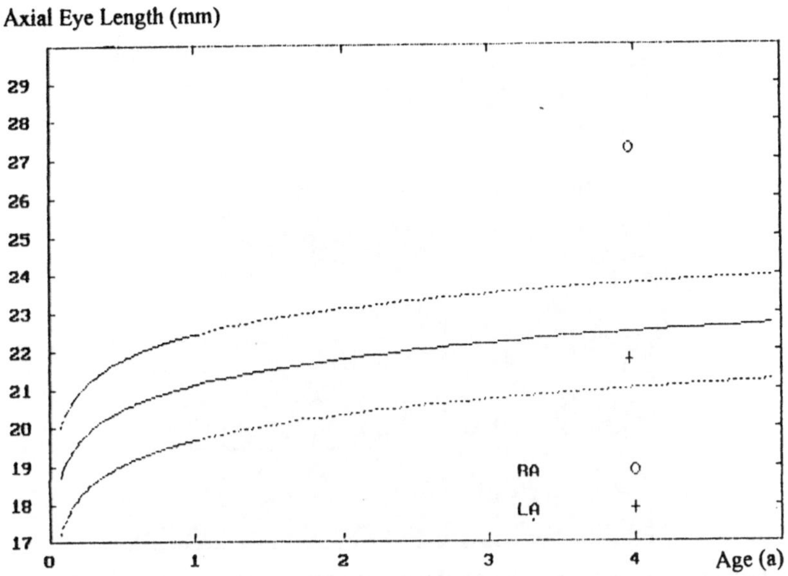

Fig. 1. Axial eye length (mm) in relation to age (a): Axial eye length, determined with the immersion-technique. Biometry showed that the axial length of the right globe was clearly above the normal range, which is determined as the area between the scattered lines of the normal axial eye length growth

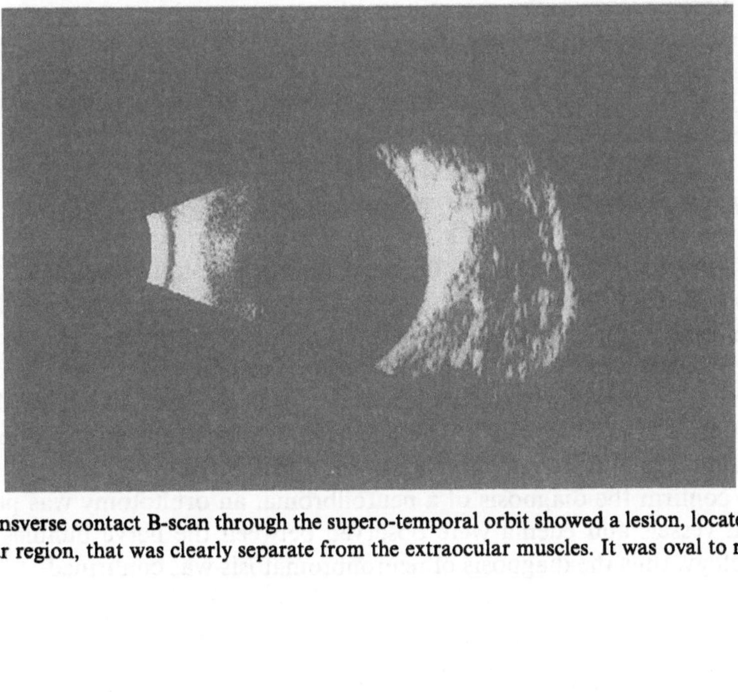

Fig. 2. Transverse contact B-scan through the supero-temporal orbit showed a lesion, located in the parabulbar region, that was clearly separate from the extraocular muscles. It was oval to roundish in shape

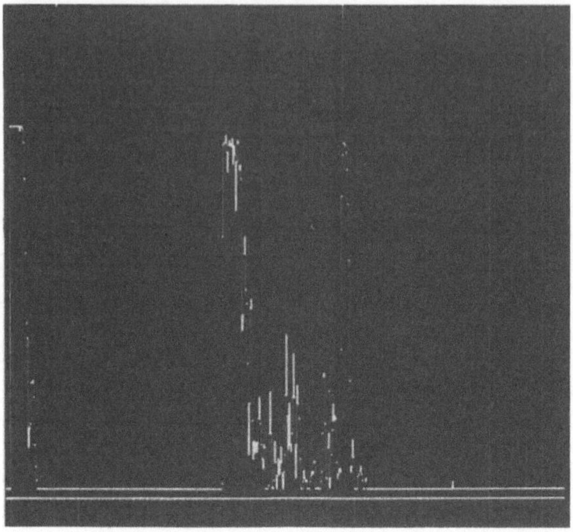

Fig. 3. Transocular standardized A-scan through the superotemporal orbit. The lesion was well outlined with low reflectivity, a regular internal structure and a moderate sound attenuation. The consistency was hard and the vascularity poor

is very weak. Rhabdomyosarcomas have an irregular structure and a strong vascularity, not a regular structure and a poor vascularity as presented in our case. Schwannomas have a strong vascularity and thus were unlikely. We found the echographic findings consistent with a solitary neurofibroma, a fibrous histiocytoma was suspected as differential diagnosis. This coincided with the clinical findings and the congenital glaucoma [2–4,6–8].

Computerized tomography and nuclear magnetic resonance imaging

Computerized tomography of the head showed a lesion in the superotemporal orbit consistent with a neurofibroma (Fig. 4). There was no thickening or enhancement of the choroid, sclera, posterior ciliary nerves or small intraconal nerves as can occur when these structures are involved [9].

Nuclear magnetic resonance showed a well-outlined lesion in the superotemporal orbit on coronar and axial section. Particularly in the latter section, the tumor could be separated from the muscles (Fig. 5).

To confirm the diagnosis of a neurofibroma, an orbitotomy was performed. Blood vessels and edema were observed between the nerve bundles in histopathology, thus the diagnosis of neurofibromatosis was confirmed.

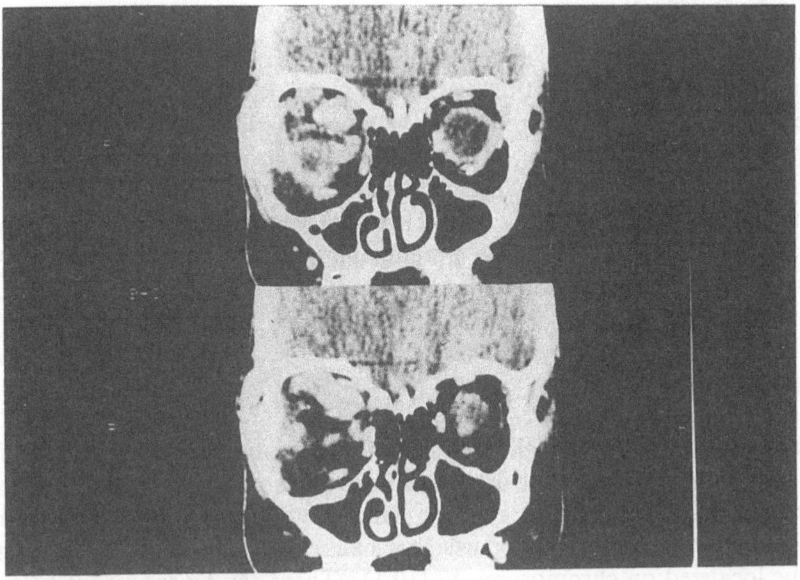

Fig. 4. Computerized tomography of the head in coronar sections. The lesion in the superotemporal orbit was in the parabulbar region. The right orbit is enlarged compared with the left one. The maxillary sinus is smaller than the left one. There is no indentation of the brain

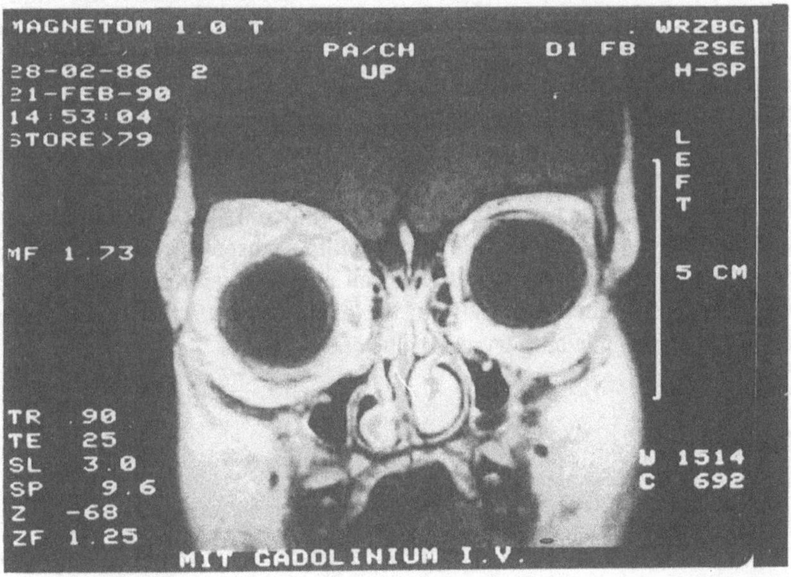

Fig. 5. Nuclear magnetic resonance imaging in coronar sections showed the lesion in the superotemporal orbit

Clinical course

Until March 1990, the neurofibroma of the orbit was the first and only neurofibroma found in this patient. Together with congenital glaucoma, Recklinghausen's neurofibromatosis was suspected. In June 1990 the girl had a spontaneous fracture of the left tibia, caused by an intraosseal lipoma.

In November 1990 café-au-lait patches and other neurofibromatomas were detected, thus the diagnosis of Recklinghausen's neurofibromatosis was confirmed. In August 1991, the parents had begun to recognize neurologic symptoms, e.g., speech difficulties.

Discussion

Manifestation of Recklinghausen's neurofibromatosis (neurofibromatosis type 1) can be systemic with localisation of neurofibromas in the brain, gliomas or meningiomas and in the viscera. There can be skeletal deformities and phenochromocytomas. The genes that cause neurofibromatosis are suspected to be localized on chromosome 17 [10,11]. There can be cutaneous café au lait patches, plexiform neurofibromas or pedunculated skin lesions [10,11].

Ocular lesions of the neurofibromatosis are neurofibromas of the eyelids, optic nerve gliomas, hamartomas of the iris (Lisch nodules), underdevelopment of the sphenoid, and retinal lesions [10]. A secondary glaucoma can develop by infiltration of the anterior chamber angle by a neurofibroma of the ciliary body, or abnormalities of the anterior chamber angle such as a fibrovascular membrane [1]. In case of glaucoma an ectropion uvea is common [12–14]. Therapy of the glaucoma is topic medication or a goniotomy, as was performed in this child. Filtration surgery is not as a rule successful [1].

The elevation of the intraocular pressure may be high with painful buphthalmos. In these cases enucleation is necessary [15,16].

For more than three years the congenital glaucoma and the retrobulbar lesion in the right eye were the only signs of Recklinghausen's neurofibromatosis. The shape of the neurofibroma and the visual acuity have been constant for three years. Thus, no further surgery than the orbitotomy 1990 was performed. The girl will have cosmetic surgery when she starts school.

References

[1] Shields and G.K. Kriegelstein. Glaukom-Grundlagen, Differentialdiagnose, Therapie. Berlin, Heidelberg, New York: Springerverlag, 1993;335.

[2] S.F. Byrne. Standardized echography in the differentiation of orbital lesions. Surv. Ophthalmol. 1984;29:226

[3] S.F. Byrne and R.L. Green. Ultrasound of the Eye and Orbit. St. Louis: Mosby Year Book, 1992;243–312.

[4] G. Hasenfratz and U. Lewan. Results of standardized echography in orbital diseases. A review of 311 cases. In P. Till (ed.), Ophthalmic echography 13. Dordrecht: Kluwer Academic Publishers, 1990;135–144
[5] K.C. Ossoinig. Standardized echography: basic principles, clinical applications and results. Int. Ophthalmol. Clin. 1979;19(4):127.
[6] D.J. Bergin and V. Parmely. Orbital neurilemoma. Arch. Ophthalmol. 1988;106:414.
[7] S.F. Byrne and B.M. Byrne. Differential diagnosis of orbital neurilemoma (Schwannoma) with standardized echography. In K.C. Ossoinig (ed.), Ophthalmic Echography, Dordrecht: Dr. W. Junk, 1987;491.
[8] S.F. Byrne, W.A. van Heuven and A.W. Lawton. Echographic characteristics of benign orbital Schwannomas (Neurilemonas). Am. J. Ophthalmol. 1988;106:195.
[9] D. Reed, W.D. Robertson, J. Rootman and G. Douglas. Plexiform neurofibromatosis of the orbit: CT evaluation. Am. Jour. of Neuroradiology 1986;7(2):259–263.
[10] W.P. Boger and R.A. Petersen. Pediatric ophthalmology. In D. Paran-Langston (ed.), Manual of ocular diagnosis and therapy. 3 rd ed. Boston: Little Brown and Company, 1991;274–275.
[11] J.A. Mitchell, J. Wray and K. Michalski. Neurofibromatosis and fragile – X syndrome in the same patient. Am. J. Med. Genetics 1985;22(3):571–575.
[12] A. Bechetoille, J.M. Ebran and J. Bigorgne. Ectropion congenital de l'epithelium iridien et glaucome. Journal Français d'Ophthalmologie 1985;8(8–9):529–534.
[13] R. Herzberg. Congenital ectropion uvease and glaucoma. Australian and New Zealand Journal of Ophthalmology 1985;13(1):45–48.
[14] R. Rich, M. Forbes, J. J.R. Hetherington, R. Harrison and S.M. Podos. Congenital ectropion uvea with glaucoma. Ophthalmology 1984;91(4):326–331.
[15] S. Brownstein and J.M. Little. Ocular neurofibromatosis. Ophthalmology 1983;90(12):1595–1599.
[16] J.P. Burke, R.J. Leicht, J.F. Talbot and M.A. Parsons. Choroidal Neurofibromatosis with congenital iris ectropion and buphthalmos: relationship and significance. Journal of Pediatric Ophthalmology and Strabismus 1991;28(5):265–267.

G. Hasenfratz, M.D.
University Eye Clinic
Josef-Schneider Str. 11
97080 Würzburg
Germany

38. Standardized echography in diagnosing orbital tumors: our experience with cases verified with echo-assisted fine needle aspiration

D. DORO, E. MIDENA and E. MANTOVANI
(Padua, Italy)

Abstract

We checked the standardized echographic diagnosis by fine needle aspiration (FNA) performed under ultrasonic guidance in 31 patients with orbital mostly low reflective tumors. Optimal B-scan visualization of the aspirating needle was achieved when a specifically designed needle-obturator with a highly reflective tip was used. Echo-assisted FNA was useful in differentiating orbital lymphoma from idiopathic orbital inflammation and lymphoid hyperplasia, and consequently the most appropriate radiation and/or systemic therapy could be planned. Echographic prediction of an orbital lymphoproliferative disorder was very good: lymphoma involving the lateral rectus muscle was correctly identified in one out of two cases. Because of the low amount of material aspirated from hard compact lesions, we were unable to make a cytologic diagnosis (obtained after surgery) in patients with sclerosing pseudotumor, recurrent rhabdomyosarcoma, recurrent orbital melanoma, high reflective metastatic carcinoma and glomangioma. Fine needle aspiration confirmed the echographic diagnosis in single cases of low reflective metastatic carcinoma, dermoid cyst and mucocele.

Key words: Standardized echography, fine needle aspiration, orbital tumor, orbital lymphoma, orbital idiopathic inflammation, orbital lymphoid hyperplasia

Introduction

We agree with Hasenfratz [1] that clinical information on patients, time dedicated to echographic examinations and the experience of examiners are all factors influencing the accuracy of standardized echography in diagnosing and differentiating orbital masses. Moreover, the accuracy of the diagnosis varies according to the type of the examined tumor [2]. Whereas, for instance, the accuracy of the echographic diagnosis of orbital cavernous hemangioma has

G Cennamo and N. Rosa (eds.), Ultrasonography in Ophthalmology 15, pp. 331–342.

been reported to be around 90%, idiopathic orbital inflammation, lymphoid hyperplasia and lymphoma, which are lymphoproliferative disorders probably representing a continuous spectrum of disease [3], cannot be reliably differentiated on the basis of echographic patterns.

Fine needle aspiration (FNA) of orbital disorders under ultrasonic guidance has been reported to be a useful technique to establish the diagnosis made with the combined use of standardized echography, computerized tomography (CT) or magnetic resonance imaging (MRI) and to plan the proper therapy [4–7]. Here we report the results of standardized echography and echo-assisted FNA performed in patients with lymphoproliferative orbital disorders, and in selected patients with non lymphoproliferative orbital masses.

Patients and methods

We conducted a standardized echographic examination (Coopervision ultrascan Digital B® and Biophysic Ophthascan S mini-A) on 31 patients (age range 14–76 years) with unilateral or bilateral proptosis due to an orbital mass. Fine needle aspiration of the orbital mass was carried out under B-scan guidance after local anesthesia. The tip of the 20 gauge needle, equipped with an obturator to avoid contamination during insertion, was usually easily identified on longitudinal B-scan sections at a low system sensitivity setting when the inserted needle was gently tilted. In some recent cases, we used a specifically designed needle obturator with a highly reflective spiral tip (Echojekt®) for optimal visualisation of echo-assisted FNA (Fig. 1). After removing the

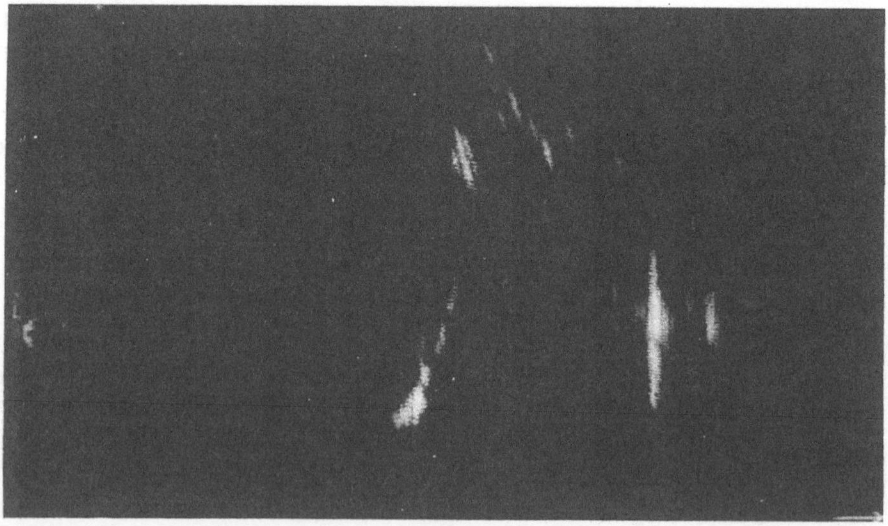

Fig. 1. Lymphoid hyperplasia of the left lateral rectus. At low system sensitivity setting the Echojekt® needle with its very high reflective obturator-tip can be displayed within the orbital lesion on B-scan

obturator, the aspiration is aided by a pistol grip connected to a syringe, as described elsewhere [4,6]. The cytological specimen stained with Giemsa was promptly examined by a cytopathologist; in some cases immunocytochemical techniques were used. When the amount of material was insufficient, a second FNA biopsy was taken.

Results

By means of standardized echographic examination we were able to identify 12 patients with low or very low reflective regularly structured lymphoproliferative orbital disorders (Fig. 2). Evaluation of FNA material revealed a lymphoma in a patient with a low reflective thick lateral rectus muscle, echographically consistent with a metastatic origin (Figs. 3 and 4). As shown in Table 1, FNA results enabled us to distinguish among lymphoma (13 cases), lymphoid hyperplasia (4 cases) and orbital idiopathic inflammation (3 cases). There were no remarkable differences among the three groups concerning age range, sex, typical supero-temporal location and motility impairment. Periocular inflammation was the rule in orbital idiopathic inflammation; it was distinctly rare in lymphoma and frequent (50% of cases) in lymphoid hyperplasia. The T sign was not observed in any case of orbital idiopathic inflammation (Figs. 5 and 6). Visual loss was due to compressive optic neuropathy in two cases of lymphoma and orbital idiopathic inflammation and to associated exudative retinal detachment in a case of orbital lymphoid hyperplasia involving the choroid [8]. Bilaterality and multiple mass lesions were uncommon in lymphoma patients. The width of lymphoproliferative orbital lesions exceeded 10 mm except in lymphoid hyperplasia cases.

Echo-assisted FNA confirmed the echographic diagnosis in six patients with very low or low reflective orbital masses (Table 2) including orbital extension of choroidal melanoma, mucocele and dermoid cyst. A patient with an orbital low reflective metastatic carcinoma from the rectum was correctly diagnosed after FNA (Fig. 7). No material could be obtained from single cases of recurrent orbital melanoma and rhabdomyosarcoma.

In four out of five selected cases of medium-high reflective orbital masses the results of standardized echography were dubious or inconclusive (Table 3); FNA failed to obtain adequate material in a case of glomangioma and metastatic carcinoma but was helpful in differentiating single cases of adenoid cystic carcinoma, cavernous hemangioma and a rare orbital wall meningioma (Fig. 8).

Discussion

In our experience, standardized echography identified 19 out of 20 patients with lymphoproliferative orbital disorders; a false negative diagnosis of metastasis due to a low reflective lateral rectus muscle was made in one case. From the

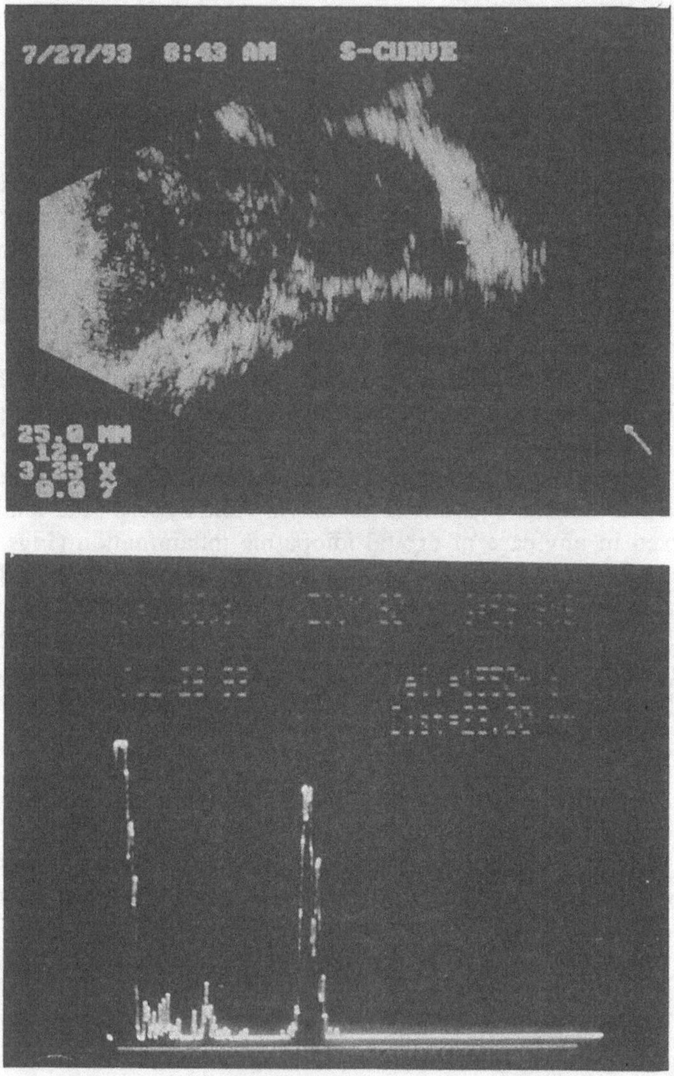

Fig. 2. **Orbital lymphoma. B-scan; single poorly echogenic mass in the superotemporal orbit (top). Standardized A-scan: the lesion shows very low reflectivity, regular structure and defined borders (bottom)**

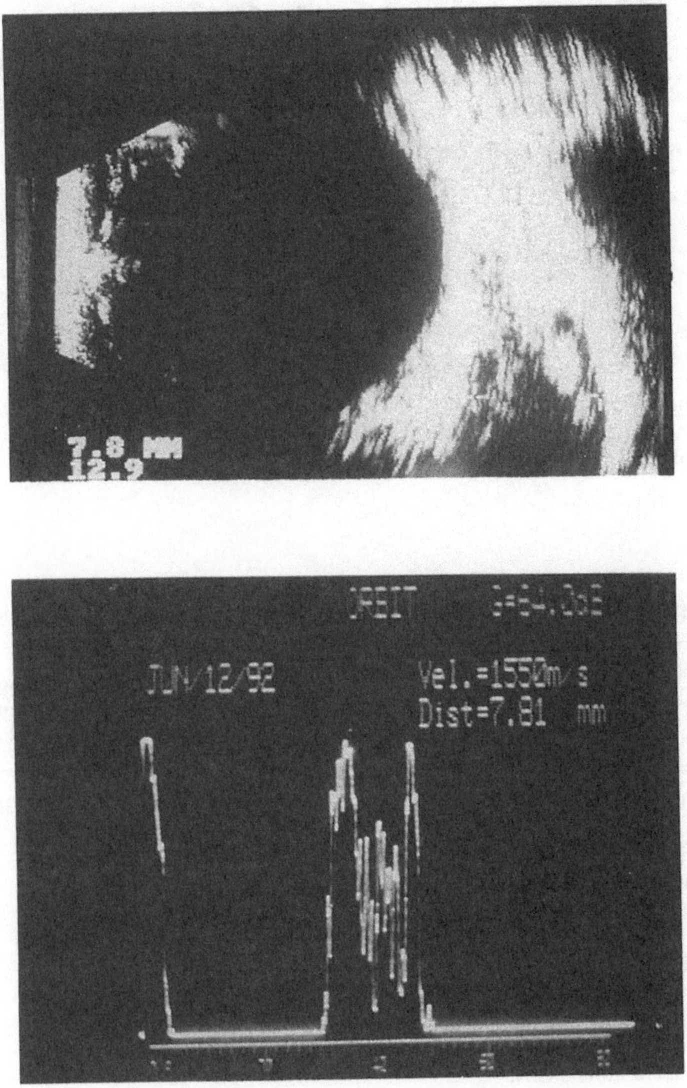

Fig. 3. Lymphoma involving the lateral rectus, B-scan imaging: enlarged belly of the lateral rectus (top). Standardized A-scan: the reflectivity of the muscle appears medium with irregular structure (bottom)

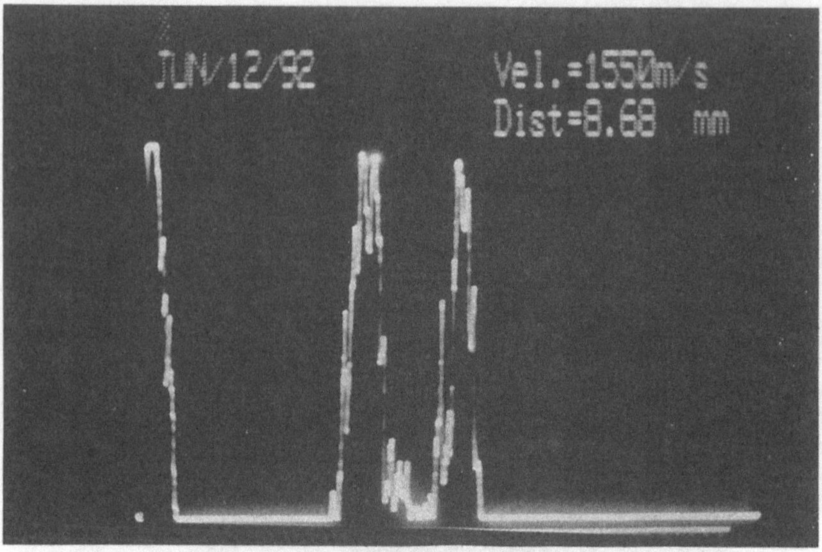

Fig. 4. Same patient as in Fig. 3. Very low reflectivity and regular structure in another A-scan echogram of the lateral rectus muscle. An identical scan was obtained in a patient with lateral rectus lymphoid hyperplasia

Table 1. Types of lymphoproliferative orbital disorders after echo-assisted FNA: clinical features

	Lymphoma (13 cases)	Lymphoid hyperplasia (4 cases)	Idiopathic inflammation (3 cases)
Age (range)	49–73	50–78	35–75
Sex M/F	7/6	2/2	1/2
Periocular inflammation	1	2	3
Motility impairment	5	1	2
Visual loss	1	1	1
Bilaterality	1	–	1
Main location (22 orbits)			
– superior or superotemporal	10	2	2
– lateral rectus	1	1	–
– nasal	2	–	–
– intraconal or around O.N.	1	2	–
– extraconal diffuse	1	–	–
Maximal width (mm)	10÷20	2÷10	12÷15
Multiple mass lesion	2	1	2

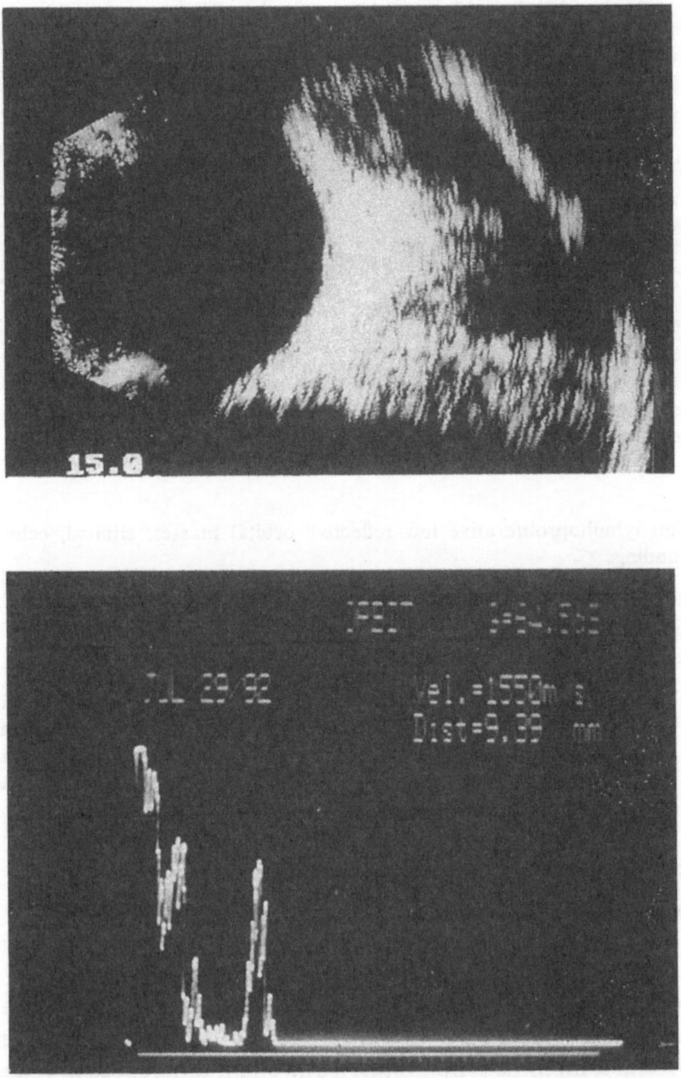

Fig. 5. **Orbital idiopathic inflammation. Contact B-scan showing a large mass involving the superotemporal orbit (top). Paraocular standardized A-scan showing very low reflectivity and regular structure of the orbital lesion**

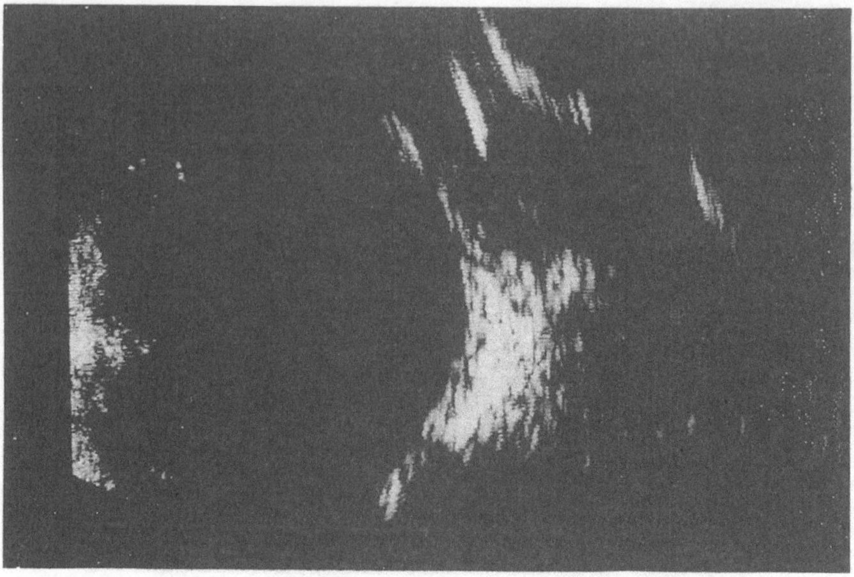

Fig. 6. Same patient as in Fig. 5. The highly reflective needle tip, with 'normal' obturator, inserted in the orbital mass is clearly displayed on B-scan

Table 2. Non lymphoproliferative low reflective orbital masses: clinical, echographic and cytological findings

Pat.	Age	Reflectivity	Strucrture	FNA	Final diagnosis
1.	54	Low	Irregular	Adenocarcinoma	Metastatic carcinoma (rectum)
2.	62	Very low	Regular	Epithelioid melanoma	Orbital extension of choroidal melanoma*
3.	65	Low	Regular	No material	Recurrent melanoma (anophthalmia)*
4.	14	Low	Regular	No material	Recurrent rhabdomyosarcoma*
5.	76	Absent	–	Mucus	Mucocele*
6.	23	Low	Irregular	Sebaceous material	Dermoid cyst*

* Correct echographic diagnosis

echographic examination we could not distinguish among the various types of lymphoproliferative disorders, moreover, the 'T' sign was absent in all three cases of orbital idiopathic inflammation and slight differences in reflectivity and structure between lymphoma and orbital idiopathic inflammation [1] could not be detected.

We found echo-assisted FNA useful in differentiating orbital lymphoma from lymphoid hyperplasia and orbital idiopathic inflammation ('pseudotumor orbitae'); in all patients, but one with histologically-diagnosed sclerosing pseudotumor, the amount of material aspirated was sufficient for cytological

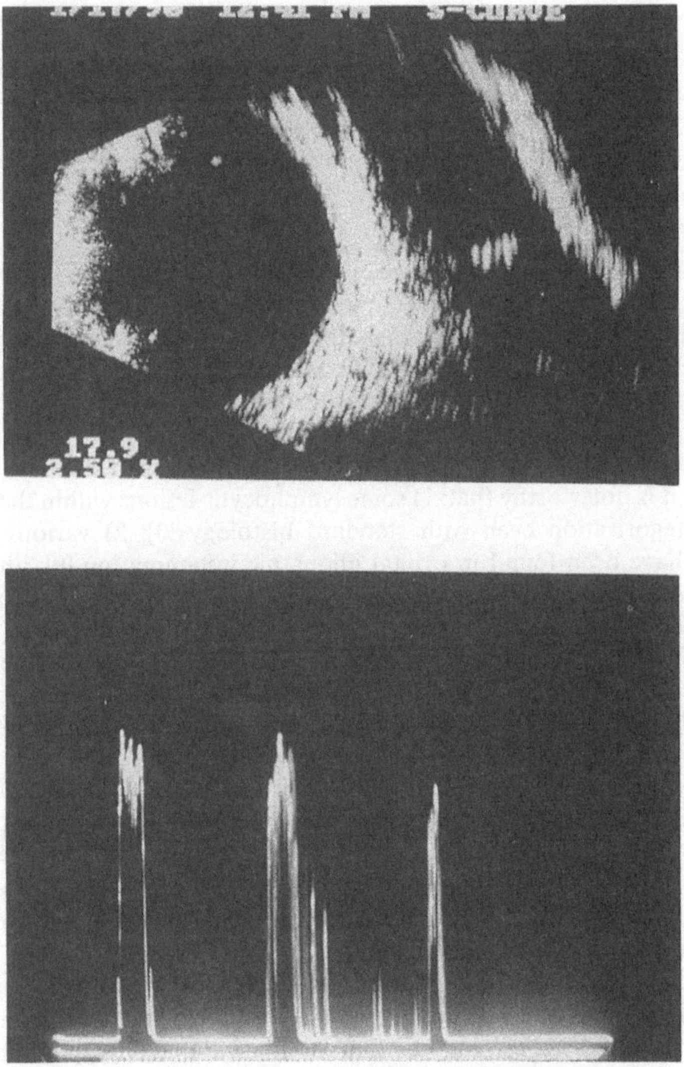

Fig. 7. **Low reflective orbital metastasis from rectum carcinoma. Transverse B-scan section of the needle tip into the orbital mass (top). Low reflectivity and regular heterogeneous structure are evident on standardized A-scan (bottom)**

Table 3. Medium-high reflective orbital masses: clinical, echographic and cytological findings

Pat.	Age	Reflectivity	Structure	FNA	Final diagnosis
1.	73	Mid-high	Irregular	No material	Metastatic carcinoma (bladder)
2.	46	Mid-high	Irregular	Malignant epithelial cells	Adenoid cystic carcinoma*
3.	42	Mid-high	Irregular	Blood	Cavernous hemangioma*
4.	71	High	Regular heterogeneous	Meningothelial cells	Orbital wall meningioma*
5.	41	Mid	Regular heterogeneous	No material	Glomangioma*

* Inconclusive echographic diagnosis..

evaluation. We are aware that the conventional but more invasive open biopsy is preferred by many orbital surgeons. However, Char and Miller [9] found CT-guided FNA useful in differentiate lymphomas from pseudotumors [9]. They had no false positive results but negative results were observed in 10% of FNA samples.

Our FNA results have not been routinely compared with standard histology; however, it is noteworthy that: 1) some lymphocytic lesions within the orbit defy ready categorisation even with standard histology [3]; 2) various histologic patterns have been found in orbital idiopathic inflammation [9]; and 3) long-term follow-up has shown that extraorbital lymphoma develops in more than 25% of patients with histologically 'benign' orbital lymphoid lesions [10].

A competent cytopathologist is essential for FNA of an orbital mass. We did not use sophisticated analytical techniques such as flow cytology or Southern blot analysis, but only standard (Giemsa) staining; monoclonal antibodies for kappa and lambda chains were used in a few cases.

Obviously fibrotic lesions represent a limit of FNA. In our series of patients the material aspirated from histologically verified fibrotic acoustically low reflective tumors (single cases of sclerosing pseudotumor, recurrent orbital melanoma and recurrent rhabdomyosarcoma) was insufficient for analysis. A correct echographic diagnosis was made in five out of six non lymphoproliferative low reflective orbital masses with poor or well defined borders; FNA was contributory only in a case of metastatic adenocarcinoma. Probably echo-assisted FNA should be limited to selected cases of medium-high reflective orbital masses where cytology can substantiate the echographic and clinical diagnosis or is requested prior to surgery, radiation or systemic therapy. Even though standardized echographic examination can reveal differences between adenoid cystic carcinoma and cavernous hemangioma [11], sometimes only experienced examiners can appreciate them; in such cases we found FNA useful for the pre-surgical diagnosis. Fine needle aspiration did not help in single cases of high reflective metastatic carcinoma and glomangioma, both of which were histologically verified [12].

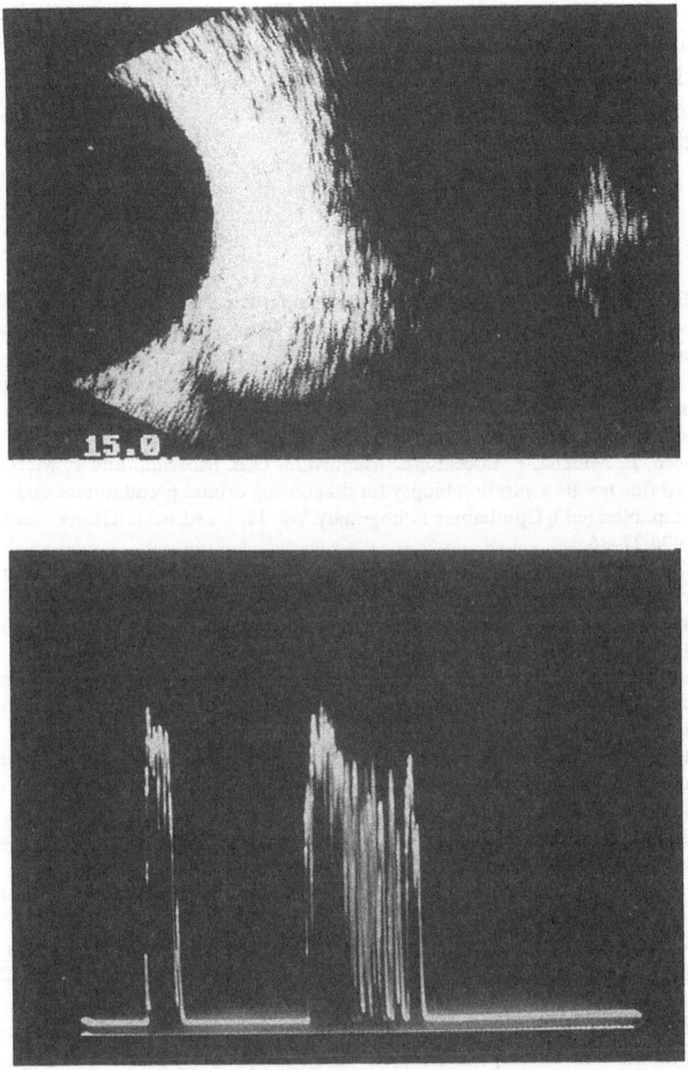

Fig. 8. **Orbital wall meningioma. B-scan: echogenic mass with strong sound attenuation (top). Transocular standardized A-scan: high reflective lesion with a regular heterogeneous structure (bottom)**

No complications, such as orbital hematoma or inflammation, optic nerve injury or globe perforation occurred in our series of patients; however, in other patients with tumors located in the posterior orbit echographic visualisation was poor and CT-guided FNA had to be performed.

We are not advocating echo-assisted FNA as a constant alternative to incisional or excisional surgical biopsy; however, in lymphoproliferative or metastatic orbital disorders FNA can provide useful diagnostic information in outpatients, rapidly and at low cost, provided that cytopathological specimen are correctly interpreted.

References

[1] G. Hasenfratz and V. Lewan. Results of standardized echography in orbital diseases. A review of 311 cases. In P. Till (ed.), Ophthalmic Echography. Dordrecht: Kluwer Academic Publishers, 1993;13:135–144.

[2] K.C. Ossoinig. Standardized echography: basic principles, clinical applications and results. Intern. Ophthalmol. Clinics 1979;19:107–210.

[3] A. Garner. Orbital lymphoproliferative disorders. Br. J. Ophthalmol. 1992;76:47–48.

[4] D. Doro, E. Midena, P. Boccato, E. Mantovani, G.B. Moschini and F. Moro. Echography assisted fine needle aspiration biopsy for diagnosing orbital pseudotumor and lymphoma. In R. Sampaolesi (ed.), Ophthalmic Echography. Vol. 12. Dordrecht: Kluwer Academic Publishers, 1990;27–36.

[5] J.S. Kennerdell, A. Dekker, B.L. Johnson and P.J. Dubois. Fine needle aspiration biopsy; a report of its use in orbital tumors. Arch. Ophthalmol. 1979;97:1315–1317.

[6] E. Midena, T. Segato, S. Piermarocchi and P. Boccato. Fine needle aspiration biopsy in ophthalmology. Surv. Ophthalmol. 1985;29(6):410–422.

[7] C. Tamburrelli, F. Focosi and A. Fabiano. Echodriven fine needle aspiration biopsy in orbital tumor diagnosis. In R. Sampaolesi (ed.), Ophthalmic Echography. Dordrecht: Kluwer Academic Publishers, 1990;12:15–25.

[8] V. Mazzeo, L. Ravalli and P. Perri. Echographic findings in lymphoid hyperplasia of the choroid. In R. Sampaolesi (ed.), Ophthalmic Echography. Vol. 12. Dordrecht: Kluwer Academic Publishers, 1990;419–425.

[9] D. Char and T. Miller. Orbital pseudotumor. Fine needle aspiration biopsy and response to therapy. Ophthalmology 1993;100:1702–1710.

[10] F.A. Jakobiec and D.M. Knowles. An overview of ocular adnexal lymphoid tumors. Trans. Am. Ophthal. Soc. 1989;87:420–444.

[11] G. Cennamo, F. Tranfa and G. Bonavolontà. Lesions of the lacrimal fossa: a retrospective echographic study. In R. Sampaolesi (ed.), Ophthalmic Echography. Vol. 12. Dordrecht: Kluwer Academic Publishers, 1990;63–72.

[12] D. Doro, E. Mantovani and L. Bergamo. Glomus tumor of the eyelid and anterior orbit: echographic and histological features. In P. Till (ed.), Ophthalmic Echography. Vol. 13. Dordrecht: Kluwer Academic Publishers, 1993;233–237.

Daniele Doro
Clinica Oculistica
Università di Padova
Via Giustiniani, 2
I-35128 Padua, Italy

39. Preliminary report of echographic findings in a case believed to be a meningocele of the right orbit, examined with standardized echography

J. SCHUTTERMAN
(Stockholm, Sweden)

An 18-year-old man with right-side ptosis since birth, longstanding depression of the right globe and more than half a year's history of marked proptosis was examined with both magnetic resonance imaging and standardized echography of the orbit. Magnetic resonance showed cerebral dysplasia of the right frontal lobe and, in the superior part of the right orbit, a 3 × 2 × 6-cm process, with two stalks connecting to the superior orbital fissure and the pterygopalatine fossa. Standardized echography showed an encapsulated, soft lesion, connected to the orbital wall by two thin processes. Most of the lesion showed a low reflectivity. Both magnetic resonance and echography findings were consistent with meningocele of the right orbit.

A more detailed history revealed a strabismus operation for extropia before school age, and medical treatment for epilepsy when the patient was between the ages of 9 and 17. During this period repeated EEG examinations showed an asymmetric pattern suggesting a lesion of the right hemisphere.

Jan Schutterman
Dept. of Ophthalmology
Södersjukhuset Hospital
11883 Stockholm, Sweden

G Cennamo and N. Rosa (eds.), Ultrasonography in Ophthalmology 15, p. 343.

Extraocular muscles and orbital disorders

40. Basedowian ophthalmopathy: diagnostic criteria and new therapeutical prospectives

L. SABETTI, M.G. SERRA, N. FURCESE, I. BASCHIERI[1] and E. BALESTRAZZI

(L'Aquila, Italy)

Abstract

Basedowian ophthalmopathy is an autoimmune disorder that occurs in 5% of patients affected by thyroid disease. These ocular and palpebral alterations cause severe aesthetic and functional damage. We studied five patients (age range: 54–65 years) who had undergone a new therapeutical protocol with immunoglobulin in high doses. The protocol foresaw the administration of intravenous Ig for two days every 21 days for seven courses. The drug used was human monomeric Ig, structurally unmodified. The control group consisted of 24 patients aged between 51 and 64 years treated with thyreostatics. The haematochemical requirements of the thyroid function, necessary to start the treatment, were the normalization of the following tests: TT3, TT4, FT3, FT4 and THS. If supported by other studies, on larger populations, treatment with intravenous Ig may be an important step forward in the cure of Basedowian ophthalmopathy, particularly as it does not cause the serious side effects that occur with steroid therapy. In fact, no relevant side effects were recorded in our study which included a follow-up of 2 years from the beginning of the treatment. However, because these therapeutical cycles are costly, we have not been able to treat a large number of patients (at present only patients with high ATA index have been given this treatment). Studies on larger populations may help to establish the most favourable time to begin therapy.

Key words: Basedowian ophthalmology, immunoglobulin, exophthalmus, echobiometry

Introduction

Basedowian ophthalmopathy is an autoimmune disorder that occurs in 5% of patients affected by thyroid disease [1]. The characteristic signs of this condition are: spastic retraction of the upper eyelid, corneal disease, orbital oedema, optic nerve compression, exophthalmus, increased thickness of extraocular muscles, and an increase in intraocular pressure.

G Cennamo and N. Rosa (eds.), Ultrasonography in Ophthalmology 15, pp. 347–353.

These ocular and palpebral alterations cause severe aesthetic and functional damage. In fact, frequent findings are extraocular motility disorders with initial alterations of adduction and elevation, and consequent dyplopia. In addition, the involvement of the corneal epithelium can lead to initial dystrophy with the possibility of evolution toward corneal ulceration, while the involvement of the optic nerve can lead to irreversible damage of visual function [2–4]. Given the complexity and severity of these alterations timely treatment is important. The therapeutical approach is often difficult, because the pathogenetic mechanism of this disease is not well known [5–8].

The exophthalmos can appear several years before the clinical signs of the thyroid disease. In these cases a correct echography can help to obtain the diagnosis [9–11]. In our experience, A–B scan echography is essential during the follow-up of Basedowian ophthalmopathy because it allows the physician to monitor the increase in the size of the extraocular muscles, and evaluate the different tissutal reflectivity [12].

Material and methods

We studied five patients (4 females and 1 male; age range: 54–65 years, mean 59.8 ± 3.6), who had undergone a new therapeutical protocol with immunoglobulin (Ig) in high doses (two of these patients had previously been treated with systemic corticosteroids for 6 months with poor results). The therapeutical protocol foresaw the administration of intravenous Ig (IVIG): 1 gr/pro kilo/die for two days every 21 days for seven courses, as used in other autoimmune diseases. The drug used was human monomeric Ig, structurally unmodified [13,14]. The control group consisted of 24 patients aged between 51 and 64 years treated only with thyreostatics.

The inclusion criteria for therapy with IVIG were: informed consent from the patients, age between 20 and 65 years, bilateral ophthalmopathy, index of ophthalmopathy above 4 according to Donaldson-ATA. We excluded from this treatment patients who did not respond to the inclusion criteria and who, furthermore, had an IgA deficit, neutropenia, a high rheumatic factor, allergy or intolerance to the administration of serum derivatives, cardiac decompensation, or kidney insufficiency.

The haematochemical requirements of the thyroid function, necessary to start the treatment, were the normalization of the following tests: TT3, TT4, FT3, FT4 and THS. The ophthalmologic follow-up, carried out every 3 months for 24 months from the beginning of treatment, consisted of an examination of the anterior segment, analysis of the Break Up Time (BUT), evaluation of visual acuity, applanation tonometry, fundus oculi, exophthalmometry according to Hertel, evaluation of ocular motility, orthoptic examination, Hess frame, Ishiara test, computerized visual field, electrofunctional examinations, echobiometry of extra-ocular muscles and of the optic nerve. For the latter examinations we used a standardized A-scan instrument (Ophthascan S mini A).

Results

Our data refer to a check-up carried out 3, 12 and 24 months from the start of the treatment. Visual acuity progressively improved in the patients treated with IVIG, while there was no variation in the patients of the control group (Table 1).

The echobiometric follow-up of the extra-bulbar muscles showed that in patients treated with IVIG there was gradual and progressive reduction of the thickness (Fig. 1). In the control group, on the contrary, muscle thickness remained stable and in some cases even increased (Fig. 2).

Also the exophthalmometric control revealed improvements of the proptosis, a natural consequence of a minor perorbital oedema and of a minor muscular thickness, in the study group versus the control group (Figs. 3 and 4).

Table 1. Visual acuity

	Patient's eyes treated with IVIG 1st control	Patient's eyes treated with IVIG after 2 years	Control group eyes I control	Control group eyes after 2 years
8–10/	4 (40%)	6 (60%)	48 (100%)	48 (100%)
6–7/10	4 (40%)	3 (30%)	–	–
3–5/10	–	1 (10%)	–	–
<2/10	2 (20%)	–	–	–
I–III	6 (60%)	8 (80%)	48 (100%)	48 (100%)
IV–VI	3 (30%)	2 (20%)	–	–
VII–IX	1(10%)	–	–	–

5 patients treated with IVIG

24 patients treated with thyreostics

Conclusions

To date, patients affected by this condition were treated with steroids, which did not cure the thyroid ophthalmopathy, although in some cases it helped control and reduce the progression of the disease. However, it resulted such serious side effects as diabetes, high blood pressure, Cushingoid's syndrome, osteoporosis, and damage to the gastrointestinal tract. Therefore, alternative therapeutic approaches, which cause less serious side effects, have been proposed: cyclosporin, radiant therapy, plasmapheresis and somatostatin.

Our experience with high doses of Ig is encouraging. The most important

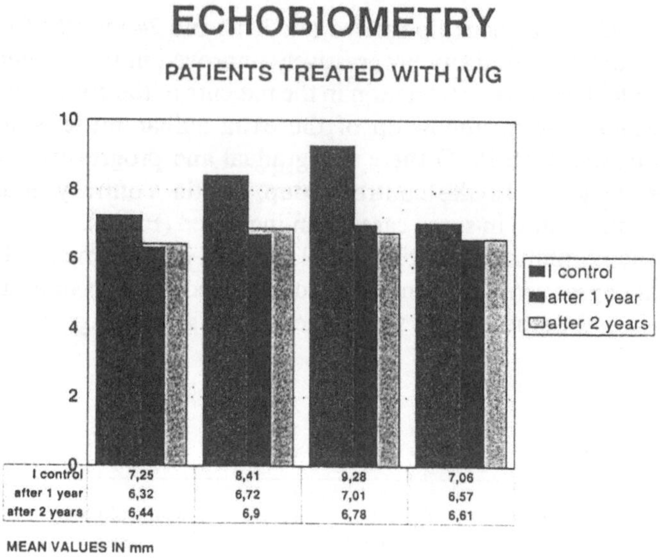

Fig. 1. There was a progressive reduction of muscle thickness during follow-up

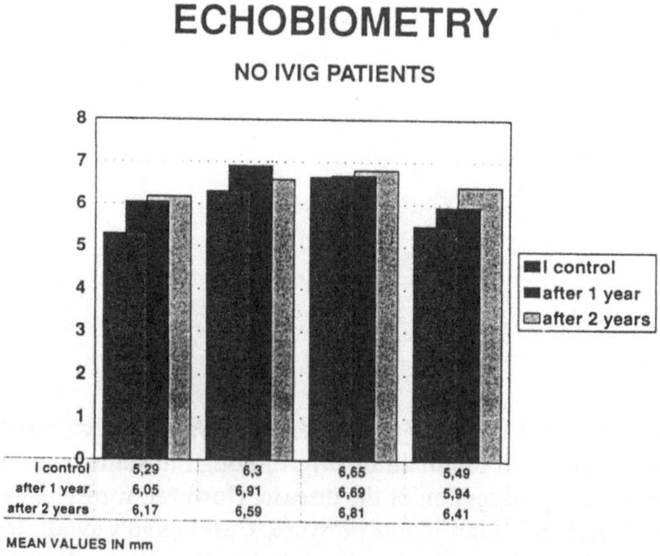

Fig. 2. The muscle thickness remains stable or increases after two years

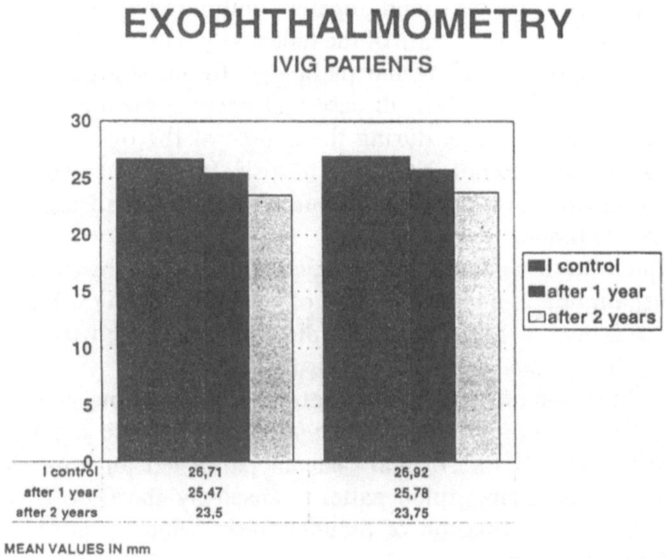

Fig. 3. There was a reduction of the proptosis during follow-up

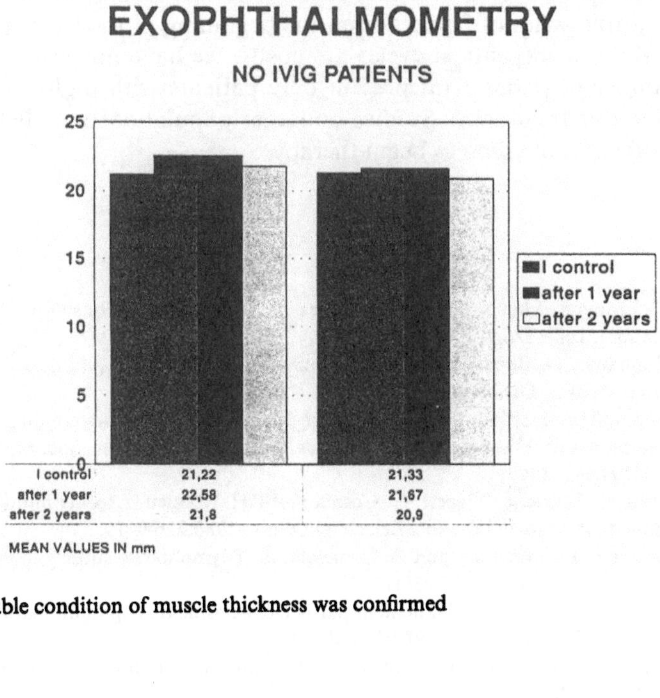

Fig. 4. The stable condition of muscle thickness was confirmed

result obtained was a generalized decrease of the thickness of the extraocular muscles. In these cases, we found, together with a reduction in the thickness of the muscle, an irregular increase of the reflectivity. This was the first demonstration of the resolution of the ocular pathology. In our study, the reflectivity was low in the initial stages of the disease and became medium or high, with an irregular internal structure, during the course of the disease – a finding that reflected the progression of the muscle fibrosis. In fact, the metaplastic changes determine the formation of new intramuscular septa and these muscle fibres are replaced by fat tissue.

Consequent to the reduction of muscle thickness, we observed a reduction of the exophthalmos and an improvement of visual acuity. In the cases treated with IVIG, the disease of the optic nerve did not cause important and persistent damage of either visual acuity or the visual field.

The modifications of the ocular motility did not show great improvement after the IVIG therapy. In fact, the reduction of the extraocular muscle thickness and also of the orbital oedema paralleled an improvement of the irregularity of the echographic pattern caused by the fibrosis. However, the fibrosis caused the formation of pseudoparesis, which required correction by means of prism or surgery.

If supported by other studies, on larger populations, treatment with IVIG may be an important step forward in the cure of Basedowian ophthalmopathy, particularly as it does not cause the serious side effects that occur with steroid therapy. In fact, no relevant side effects were recorded in our study which included a follow-up of 2 years from the beginning of the treatment. However, because these therapeutical cycles are costly, we have not been able to treat a large number of patients (at present only patients with high ATA index have been given this treatment). Studies on larger populations may help to establish the most favourable time to begin therapy.

References

[1] M. Schrooyen. Signes ophtalmologiques de la maladie de Basedow. Bull. Soc. Belge Ophtalmol. 1988;226:9–19.

[2] G. Cennamo, G. Bonavolontà and A. Bizzarro. Echography optic nerve study in Graves' ophthalmopathy. Orbit. 1984;3(1):47–50.

[3] S. Morax, M.L. Herdan, M. Schaison *et al.* Neuropathies optiques compressives au cours de l'ophtalmopathie basedowienne problemes therapeutiques. Bull. Soc. Ophtalmol. France. 1987;3(87):341–348.

[4] R. Winand, J. Etienne-Decerf, G. Cornet and P.H. Mahieu. Aspects immunologiques de la maladie de Basedow. Bull. Soc. Belge Ophtalmol. 1988;226:9–19.

[5] A. Bizzarro, G. Cennamo and G. Bonavolontà. T-lymphocyte subsets in euthyroid Graves' ophthalmopathy. Orbit. 1984;3(4):223–227.

[6] F. Dorey and G. Strauch. Traitement par la ciclosporine de l'ophtalmopathie basedowienne. Bull. Soc. Belge Ophtalmol. 1988;226:65–70.

[7] D. Glinoer. Le traitement médical de l'exophtalmie endocrinienne. Bull. Soc. Belge Ophtalmol. 1988;226:59–64.

[8] G. Lamas, B. Girard *et al.* Traitement des séquelles de l'ophtalopathie basedowienne. Ann. Oto-Laryng. 1988;105:309–312.
[9] O. Bergers. Maladie de Basedow: diagnostic ochographique. Bull. Soc. Belge Ophtalmol. 1988;226:51–57.
[10] V. Mazzeo. L'ecografia dell'apparato oculare. Milano: Fogliazza Ed., 1987.
[11] R. Guthoff. Ultrasound in ophthalmological diagnosis. New York: Thieme Medical Publishers Inc., 1991.
[12] L. Sabetti, M.G. Serra, N. Furcese, S. Gentile and E. Balestrazzi. Correzione tra le alterazioni della motilità oculare e le modificazioni dei muscoli extraoculari nell'oftalmopatia basedowiana. Clin. Ocul. e Pat. Ocul. 1993;14(2):133–135.
[13] L. Sabetti, M.G. Serra, I. Baschieri and E. Balestrazzi. Uso delle immunoglobuline nell'oftalmopatia basedowiana: risultati clinici ed ecobiometrici. Clin. Ocul. e Pat. Ocul. 1993;14(2):130–132.
[14] A. Antonelli, A. Saracino *et al.* Trattamento combinato con immunoglobuline e.v. e radioterapia retrobulbare nella oftalmopatia basedowiana. Farmaci 1991;15(5).

Lelio Sabetti
Department of Surgery, Eye Clinic
University of L'Aquila
Viale della Croce Rossa
L'Aquila, Italy

[1]Department of Biological Science and Technology and Biometry
Chair of Nuclear Medicine
University of L'Aquila
L'Aquila, Italy

41. Echographic and electrophysiologic examinations in endocrine orbitopathy

Á. SZABÓ, M. JANÁKY and Z. VALKUSZ[1]
(Szeged, Hungary)

Abstract

Endocrine orbitopathy (EO) is the most frequent cause of compressive optic neuropathy (CON). The posterior thickening of the superior rectus, the medial rectus and the superior oblique muscles causes such optic nerve compression. The increased apical compression of the optic nerve results in Graves-related optic neuropathy.

The aim of this study was to correlate the echographic measurements of the medial rectus thickness with visual evoked potentials (VEP) in 17 patients with EO. Eleven patients suffered from long-standing EO, six patients had acute EO. Each patient had a visual acuity of 20/20 in both eyes. Medial rectus thickness was evaluated in the frontal section using contact A/B-mode echography performed with an Ultrascan Digital B instrument with a 10 MHz probe. The VEPs were evoked by pattern reversal stimulation and they were monopolarly recorded over the Oz site.

The VEPs were abnormal when the thickness of the medial rectus muscle was increased in cases of long-standing EO. The echographic and electrophysiological data were not correlated in cases of acute EO.

We suggest VEPs be recorded when a thickened medial rectus is detected by ultrasound in patients with EO, because VEPs can reveal the presence of dysthyroid optic neuropathy (DON).

Key words: Endocrine orbitopathy, compressive optic neuropathy, visual evoked potentials, echography

Introduction

Visual loss caused by compression of the optic nerve at the orbital apex by the enlarged extraocular muscles occurs in less than 5% of the cases of endocrine orbitopathy (EO) [1–3]. An important sign of dysthyroid optic neuropathy (DON) is the decrease of visual acuity; however, visual evoked potentials (VEP) are objective and more sensitive indicators of neuropathy [4–6].

Extraocular muscle enlargement can be determined by computed tomography [1,7]; echography is also a valuable technique for the evaluation of

G Cennamo and N. Rosa (eds.), Ultrasonography in Ophthalmology 15, pp. 355–359.

extraocular muscles [8–10]. Feldon *et al.* reported a linear relationship between worsening ophthalmopathy and extraocular muscle volumes [1]. Because DON develops insidiously, it seems of interest to search for subclinical lesions of the optic nerve. The aim of our examination was to find a correlation of echographic and electrophysiologic alterations.

Patients and methods

Seventeen patients with Graves' disease underwent orbital ultrasound scanning and electrophysiologic examination (5 males, 12 females aged 17 to 64 years, average 42.5 years). At the time of the examination 11 patients were euthyroid, five hyperthyroid and one hypothyroid. All the patients had the eye signs of class 4 of the classification of the American Thyroid Association [11].

Eleven patients (group I) had long-standing EO (duration of EO 2-6 years) and six patients (group II) had acute EO (duration of EO 5–11 months). All patients had normal visual acuity (20/20) in both eyes. Ultrasound examinations were carried out using Ultrascan Digital B System IV equipment with a 10-MHz probe. The diameter of the medial rectus muscle was measured by contact B-scan, in frontal section according to the method of Guthoff [9]. Our control group consisted of 17 normal individuals.

To record VEP, the different electrode was placed on the Oz point (according to the international EEG system), and the indifferent electrode was clipped to the right earlobe. To elicit VEP a black and white checkerboard pattern with 40′ and 20′ checksize was displayed on a TV screen. One hundred responses were averaged. Normal range of the latency: P100 = 110–125 msec. The difference between the latency recorded in patients and 'normal' latency was compared to the data of the medial rectus diameters.

Results

The data of 22 eyes of 11 patients with long-standing EO (group I) are shown in Table 1. The medial rectus thickness was normal in 11 eyes and enlarged in 11 eyes (mean: 3.9 ± 0.28 mm). The mean medial rectus thickness of control patients was 3.33 ± 0.28 mm. The mean medial rectus of group I was higher than in the control group, but the difference was not significant.

The latency of VEP was delayed in 16 eyes (Fig. 1), borderline in 2 eyes and normal in 4 eyes. The VEP were abnormal when the thickness of the medial rectus muscle was increased in group I. The results were not significant because of the small number of the patients, but clinically this seemed to be the tendency.

The data of the 12 eyes of six patients with acute EO (group II) are shown in Table 2. Each medial rectus was significantly ($p < 0.05$) thicker (mean: 4.11 ± 0.37 mm) compared with control values (3.33 ± 0.38). The latency was delayed in three cases, borderline in four cases and normal in five cases.

Table 1. **Medial rectus thickness and VEP values of patients with long-standing endocrine orbitopathy in group I**

Medial rectus thickness		**VEP**		
Normal	**Enlarged**	**Normal**	**Borderline**	**Abnormal**
11	11	4	2	16
Total: 22 eyes		**Total: 22 eyes**		

Table 2. **Medial rectus thickness and VEP values of patients with acute endocrine orbitopathy in group II**

Medial rectus thickness		**VEP**		
Normal	**Enlarged**	**Normal**	**Borderline**	**Abnormal**
0	12	5	4	3
Total: 12 eyes		**Total: 12 eyes**		

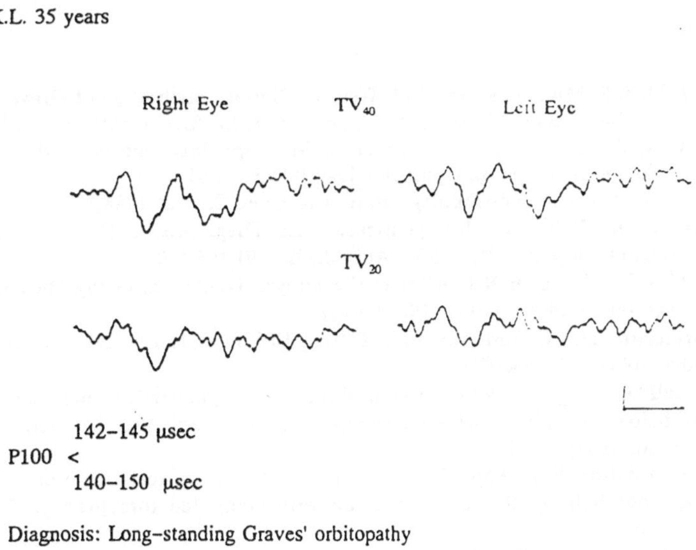

Fig. 1. **Visual evoked potentials of K.I. (38 years) with long-standing endocrine orbitopathy. The latencies are delayed using checksizes of 40′ and 20′ on both sides. The medial rectus thickness was 3.5 mm in the right eye and 5.8 mm in the left eye**

Discussion

Dysthyroid optic neuropathy may be a consequence of optic nerve compression by the enlarged extraocular muscles. Feldon *et al.* reported a linear relationship between worsening ophthalmopathy and extraocular volumes [1]. Given-Wilson *et al.* found a correlation between the medial rectus measurements obtained using orbital computerized tomography [8]. Setälä *et al.* reported a correlation between VEP values and the changes in the external eye muscles as visualized on CT scans in 15 patients with EO [7].

Our results obtained in cases of long-standing EO are similar to the findings of Setälä *et al.* We did not find a correlation between the thickening of medial rectus muscle and the lengthening of the latency in the acute EO group, probably because of the muscle fiber elasticity of the patients with acute EO. Feldon *et al.* postulated that apical optic nerve compression was more likely to occur with noncompliant, fibrotic muscle, than with more supple muscle of the same total volume [1].

Because VEP examination is an objective indicator of optic neuropathy that can detect subclinical lesions, we suggest VEP be recorded when medial rectus is thickened in patients with long-standing EO. In cases of acute EO VEP should be recorded if the clinical signs of EO worsen or do not improve despite appropriate treatment. Dysthyroid optic neuropathy can be detected by VEP in the early stages of EO, when visual acuity is 20/20 and the damage of the optic nerve is reversible.

References

[1] S.E. Feldon, S. Muramatsu and J.M. Weiner. Clinical classification of Graves' ophthalmopathy: identification of risk factors for optic neuropathy. Arch. Ophthalmol. 1984;102:1469.

[2] J.R. Guy, S. Fagien, J.P. Donovan *et al.* Methylprednisolone pulse therapy in severe dysthyroid optic neuropathy. Ophthalmology 1989;96:1048.

[3] J.J. Kansky. Clinical ophthalmology. Butterworth and Co. Ltd. 1984;2,7.

[4] B. Heinemann, P. Bischoff, J. Jörgensen *et al.* Zur Diagnostik der Opticus, Neuropathie bei endokriner Orbitopathie. Klin. Mbl. Augenheilk.1991;198:460.

[5] J.M. Neigel, J. Rootman, R.I. Belkin *et al.* Dysthyroid optic neuropathy. The crowded orbital apex syndrome. Ophthalmology 1988;95:1515.

[6] R. Wijngarde and G.H.M. Van Lith. Pattern EPS in endocrine orbitopathy. Documenta Ophthalmologica 1979;48(2):327.

[7] K. Setälä, C. Raitta, M. Välmäki *et al.* Visual evoked potentials in Basedow's ophthalmopathy before and after. Orbital decompression or retrobulbar irradiation. Exp. Clin. Endocrinol. 1991;97:344.

[8] R. Given-Wilson, R.M. Pope, M.J. Michell *et al.* The use of real-time orbital ultrasound in Graves' ophthalmopathy: a comparison with computed tomography. Br. J. Radiol. 1989;62:705.

[9] R. Guthoff. Ultraschall in der ophthalmologischen Diagnostik. Stuttgart: Ferdinand Enke, 1988;109.

[10] K.C. Ossoinig. Ein neues echographisches Merkmal zur verlässlichen Differentialdiagnostik der endokrinen Exophthalmus. Klin. Mbl. Augenhelik. 1982;180:189.

[11] S.C. Werner. Modification of the classification of the eye changes of Graves' disease. Am. J. Ophthalmol. 1977;83:725.

Ágnes Szabó
Department of Ophthalmology
Szent-Györgyi Albert Medical University
POB 407
6701 Szeged, Hungary

[1]Endocrine Unit
Szent-Györgyi Albert Medical University
POB 407
6701 Szeged, Hungary

42. Dynamic echography of extraocular muscles

T. AVITABILE, V. RUSSO and F. MARANO
(Catania, Italy)

Abstract

The role of dynamic echography in the study of the optic nerve is well established and thanks to this technique it is easy to differentiate solid and fluid lesions. The study of the extraocular muscles, on the contrary, has been mainly static thus far. The problem is that it is difficult to evaluate the absolute thickness of a muscle because despite numerous percentile tables, muscle thickness is affected by various factors (sex, age, weight, height, occupation, etc.). We have measured the thickness of the muscle in the primary position, in contraction and relaxation, and have evaluated the differences in normal subjects and in various kinds of disorders that affect muscles (Graves' disease, myasthenia, abducens paralysis, atrophy, strabismus, etc.).

Key words: Dynamic echography, extra-ocular muscles, muscle thickness, Graves' disease

Introduction

Among the various techniques used to image the orbital structures (magnetic resonance imaging, computerized tomography), echography provides the greatest amount of information about the movements of muscles and the optic nerve located in the orbital space. These data can be obtained using the standardized A-scan examination and the fast scanning B-scan instruments, which allow the operator to evaluate the movements of these structures in almost real time. There are two kinds of fast-scanning B-scan probes.

1) *B-scan probes with a single piezoelectric element transducer*: in this fast scanning instrument the crystals have a higher frame rate than the normal B-scan probes. There is also a faster elaboration of the signals. Furthermore, it is possible to freeze the images on the screen. This system increases the imaging of the real movements of the structures.

2) *Electronic linear array*: this transducer head consists of a large number of strips of piezoeletric material laid side by side, but acoustically isolated from

G Cennamo and N. Rosa (eds.), Ultrasonography in Ophthalmology 15, pp. 361–364.

one another. The linear array scanner utilizes electronic focusing. It is also possible to perform a dynamic echography using these probes.

With these two probes we obtain only qualitative information. Therefore, we are able to study the anatomical relationships between the different orbital structures, but we can only speculate, based on the echographer's experience, the dynamic process that can affect muscles and optic nerve. The bidimensional image reveals muscle incarceration following severe fractures of the orbital bones or sinus surgery [1,2].

Differently, 8 MHz standardized A-scan echography provides quantitative information, so that one may obtain a dynamic biometry of extraocular muscles and the optic nerve. Therefore, this type of echography provides data about the normal or pathological conditions and consequently about the functionality of the muscle. This biometry is called 'dynamic' or 'functional' in order to distinguish it from traditional biometry – it measures muscles and optic nerve size only in primary gaze – [3].

The new instruments, equipped with a standardized A-scan probe and amplification, can show almost 2000 images per second. Therefore it is also possible to study the dynamic processes of the orbital structures with this new A-scan instrument. Tamburelli et al. [4] showed that it is also possible to evaluate ophthalmic artery pulsations. Working with both B-scan and standardized A-scan instruments it is possible to differentiate the most common disorders that affect the motility of the extraocular muscles.

Dynamic Echography of the Extraocular Muscles

Generally, echography is the main technique used to measure muscle thickness and to evaluate the internal structure. This is done by observing the internal reflectivity. The technique also reveals exactly where the muscle is affected, either in the tendon or in the belly. All these different factors should be considered when making a diagnosis.

The principal factor is muscle thickness. Muscle thickening will suggest a thyroid ophthalmopathy, myositis, tumors (metastatic carcinoma, lymphoma, sarcoma, metastatic melanoma, amyloidosis) and an eventual contracture. Muscle thinning can be observed in very long globes with large posterior staphylomas [5,6], also with atrophy and paresis.

The normal values for the rectus muscles have been widely studied [7–11]. Most tables are referred to 90-95% of the normal population (expressed in 'percentile'). All authors caution that these normal values do not truly reflect all age and population groups. Ossoinig [12] suggested that the affected and the controlateral muscle be compared to determine whether a muscle is really enlarged. Values must be greater or lesser than 0.15 mm at the tendon and 0.3 mm at the muscle belly. Byrne and Green [13] found, in thyroid disease, that it is useful to add the value of all four rectus muscles and to compare this total to a normal overall value.

Tamburelli et al. [14] introduced a new approach for the evaluation of the extraocular muscles. This method is based on the dynamic aspect of each muscle examined. According to this theory, an abnormal muscle precociously changes its contraction and relaxation capacity. Therefore, the contraction thickening and the relaxation thinning are very different between normal individuals and patients. It appears that this method is not affected by the factors (age, weight, height, sex, race, occupation) that can disturb biometric measurements.

The dynamic evaluation of the medial rectus is performed as follows: first, using standardized A-scan echography, the muscle is measured in primary gaze. Then, the same muscle is measured, before abducting it by 30-40° and after adducting it by the same angle. The adduction causes a contraction of the medial rectus, whereas the abduction causes a relaxation of the same muscle. The values obtained from these measurements are converted to increasing and decreasing percentage in relation to the value obtained in primary gaze.

According to the method proposed by Tamburelli et al. [14], we dynamically studied the medial rectus of 15 healthy subjects (30 eyes) and 37 patients (74 eyes) affected by the following disorders: 20 patients: Graves' disease (without fibrosis); five patients: myasthenia; five patients: restrictive strabismus; four patients: abducens paralysis; and three patients: muscular atrophy.

Results

The highest per cent of thickening (23.7%) occurred the healthy subjects when the medial rectus was abducted (the muscle was contracted). The per cent of increase in thickening of the medial rectus during abduction was lower (13.3%) in patients affected by Graves' disease than in patients affected by other disorders (7.9%). The lower increase of the thickness in the patient groups is due to a loss of the contractile capacity of the muscular myofibrils. It is also due to an involvement of the interstitial muscular space that makes the muscle less elastic, and hence unable to shorten along the longitudinal axis.

The greatest per cent of thinning (21.5%) was obtained in the healthy subjects. Relaxation, according to Sherrington's law, depends on both the contraction capacity of the agonist, and the muscular and interstitial resistance of the examined muscle. On the contrary, we found a lower thickness reduction in patients affected by Graves' disease (15.1%) and those affected by the other disorders (10.9%). The lower decrease of the thickness in the diseased eyes could be due to lower contraction capacity of the agonist (not important) and to lower elasticity of the interstitial structure of the examined eyes.

Conclusions

The echographical study of eye disorders (extraocular muscles, optic nerve) is difficult. However, new typical echographic signs have been found to characterize these complicated disorders. Various studies have been conducted using static thickness measurements and comparing these data with 'normal measurements' obtained using statistical methods. 'Dynamic echography' of extraocular muscles can help us to classify better these conditions. Our values are in agreement with those reported by Tamburelli et al. [14]. Lastly, this method will perhaps help distinguish subsets of Graves' disease because the relaxation capacity is lost during the last stages of this disease. Further studies will help echographers to understand better the validity of this new method.

References

[1] J.T. Flynn, K.B. Mitcell and D.G. Fuller Ocular motility complications following intranasal surgery. Arch. Ophthalmol. 1979;97:453.

[2] D.R. Buus, D.T. Tse and B.K. Farris. Ophthalmic complications of sinus surgery. Ophthalmology 1990:97:614.

[3] K.C. Ossoinig. The technique of measuring the extraocular muscles. In H. Gernet (ed.), Diagnostica ultrasonica in Ophthalmologica. Meunster: RA Remy, 1979;166.

[4] C. Tamburelli, A. Capobianco, F. Focosi, B. Falsini, M. Dicembrino and A. Canale. Valutazione mediante A-scan standardizzato del complesso arteria oftalmica-guaine del nervo ottico. Clin. Ocul. e Pat. Ocul. 1993;14:116.

[5] J.L. Demer and G.K. von Noorden. High myopia an unusual cause of restrictive motility disturbance. Surv. Ophthalmol. 1989;33:281.

[6] M.S. Ruttum, M.A. Lloyd and M.F. Lewandowski. Echography in the diagnosis of restrictive motility caused by severe myopia. Am. J. Ophthalmol. 1990;109:350.

[7] L.C. McNutt, S.L. Kaefring and K.C. Ossoinig. Echographic measurement of extraocular muscles. In D.N. White and R.E. Brown (eds), Ultrasound in Medicine. Vol. 3. New York: Plenum, 1977;972.

[8] S. Tane and A. Komatsu. Echographic measurement of extraocular muscles in normal persons and in patients with thyroid orbitopathy. Acta XXIV Int. Congr. of Ophthalmol., San Francisco, 1982;120.

[9] T. Avitabile, M.G. Uva and F. Fiordalisi. I nostri valori ecobiometrici normali per la misurazione dei muscoli retti. Clin. Ocul. e Pat. Ocul. 1987;8/1:47.

[10] A. Reibaldi, G. Assennato, T. Avitabile and M.G. Uva. The echobiometric measurements of the extraocular muscles in normal subjects. In J.M. Thijssen (ed.), Ultrasonography in Ophthalmology. Dordrecht: Kluwer Academic Publisher, 1989.

[11] S.F. Byrne, E.K. Gendron and J.S. Glaser. Diameter of normal extraocular recti muscles with echography. Am. J. Ophthalmol. 1991;112:706.

[12] K.C. Ossoinig. The role of standardized ophthalmic echography in the management of Graves' ophthalmopathy. Dev. Ophthalmol. 1989;20:28.

[13] S.F. Byrne and R.L. Green. Ultrasound of the eye and orbit. St. Louis: C.V. Mosby Year Book, 1992;361.

[14] C. Tamburelli, F. Focosi, E. Buratto and M. Dicembrino. Biometria funzionale dei muscoli extraoculari. Clin. Ocul. e Pat. Ocul. 1990;5:377.

T. Avitabile
Catania University
Institute of Ophthalmology
Catania, Italy

43. A new approach to the study of Graves' ophthalmopathy: standardized A-scan echography and octreotide scintigraphy as possible parameters for disease activity

A. BIZZARRO, L. MANSI,[1] P.F. RAMBALDI,[1] S. DI MARTINO,[2] A. DE BELLIS,[2] N. ROSA[3] and G. CENNAMO[3]

(Naples, Italy)

Abstract

Eight patients, two male and six female, aged between 24 and 48 years, with Graves' disease and severe ophthalmopathy were included in the study. A standardized A-scan echography was performed to evaluate the reflectivity of the extraocular muscles (EOMs); a planar scintigraphy (PS) and/or a single photon emission computed tomography (SPECT) were also performed at various times after endovenous injection of 111 MBq In-111 OCT, a somatostatin analogue.

Reflectivity of EOMs was demonstrated by A-scan echography in four patients with active Graves' ophthalmology (GO) (group 1) and in four patients with non active GO (group 2). Scintigraphic results were in accordance with echographic findings. The reflectivity was higher in the former four patients than in the latter four. In patients of group 1, there was a significant labelled OCT accumulation in orbital tissue, while an orbital accumulation was not observed in group 2.

High reflectivity of EOMs as demonstrated by standardized A-scan echography and accumulation of In-111 OCT in orbital tissue as shown by scintigraphy are parameters of disease activity in GO. Standardized A-scan echography and In-111 OCT scan are useful, easy to perform and non invasive methods. They reveal the presence of flogosis and/or fibrosis in orbital tissue, and define the severity of the disorder in patients with ophthalmology.

Key words: Octreotide, Graves' disease, ophthalmopathy, echography, autoimmune disease

Introduction

The role of the immune system in the pathogenesis of Graves' disease has been well established, whereas the pathogenesis of this disorder has yet to be

G Cennamo and N. Rosa (eds.), Ultrasonography in Ophthalmology 15, pp. 365–370.

completely clarified [1]. Recently, Indium-111 Octreotide (In-111 OCT) [2], a somatostatin analogue able to bind specific somatostatin receptors, has been proposed for the clinical study of patients with autoimmune thyroid diseases [3,4]. The aim of the present study was to investigate the relationship between the involvement of the immune system and the uptake of In-111 OCT in patients with Graves' disease affected by thyroid-associated ophthalmopathy (TAO) [5]. Standardized A-scan echography was performed in all patients to evaluate the four extra-ocular muscles (EOMs).

Patients

Eight patients, two males and six females, age range 27–61 years, were included in the study. All had bilateral ophthalmopathy. Seven were affected by Graves' disease. One was affected by bilateral ophthalmopathy not related to autoimmune thyroid disease; some months later a non small cell lung carcinoma was diagnosed in this patient.

At the time of the study two patients (#1 and 2) were hyperthyroid, three patients (#3, 4 and 8) were euthyroid after a three-month interruption of methymazole therapy; patient #5, subtotally thyroidectomized three years before, was hypothyroid because of the suspension L-thyroxine therapy. Patient #6, who had undergone total thyroidectomy for multinodular goiter hyperfunctioning with autoimmune components, at the time of the examination was euthyroid because of L-thyroxine therapy. Patient #7 was not affected by evident thyroid disease, so he was euthyroid. As mentioned above, a lung carcinoma was later diagnosed in this patient; in this case bilateral ophthalmopathy was probably related to a paraneoplastic syndrome.

Material and methods

All these patients underwent a complete thyroid hormone evaluation. To study the index activity of bilateral ophthalmopathy, we assessed the Clinical Activity Score, and performed A-scan standardized echography and In-111 OCT scintigraphy. The Clinical Activity Score is based on seven signs (0–7) of active ophthalmopathy: spontaneous retrobulbar pain, pain on eye movement, eyelid erythema, conjunctival injection, chemosis, swelling of the caruncle, eyelid edema or fullness [6].

With A-scan standardized echography, we studied the thickness of extraocular muscles (EOMs) and their degree of reflectivity. High reflectivity of the EOMs indicates the presence of an active ophthalmopathy (non fibrotic aspect). More irregular or low reflectivity is correlated to fibrotic aspect [7].

The radionuclide study was performed using a large field-of view digital rotating gamma camera (Siemens Orbiter 75). It was positioned so as to include in the field the head and the neck of the patients in anterior view. All patients were given an intravenous injection of 111 MBq of In-111 Pentatreotide (Octreoscan, Mallinckrodt-Pettern Netherland) [8] after which a 20-minute dynamic flow study was performed. Two 30-minute scans were also obtained at 4 and 24 hours. Five-minute planar images were obtained at 25, 60 and 120 minutes. Five hours after the injection, a single photon emission computed tomography (SPECT) was obtained with 32 projections, 64*64 matrix, lasting 60 seconds each. Together they covered a 180° arc extending clockwise from 90° to +90°. Tomographic images were processed on a Siemens Maxidelta system nuclear medicine computer. After the acquisition, head volumes were reconstructed with a butterword filter, on the three orthogonal planes and in 3-display projection to obtain a better resolution of the distribution of activity over the structures.

Data analysis

A qualitative analysis was performed on all scintigraphic data. Regions of interest (ROIs) were set on thyroid, orbits, brain; the blood pool ROI was taken on the longitudinal venous sinus; the background ROI was traced close to the thyroid ROI avoiding the salivary glands. A semiquantitative ratio was calculated by comparing the average counts on thyroid, orbits and brain ROIs with background and blood activity (measured at the level of the longitudinal venous sinus).

Results

Six of the eight patients showed thyroid tracer uptake at early and delayed images. Standardized A-scan echography demonstrated differing degrees of enlargement of EOMs in all patients. Reflectivity differed among patients (Table 1).

Patient #1, hyperthyroid at the time of the study, showed non active ophthalmopathy; the Clinical Activity Score equalled 1, and A-scan standardized echography showed enlargement of EOMs with a low reflectivity. In this patient there was no In-111 OCT uptake. In patients #2 and 3 the Clinical Activity Score was low (= 1), and EOM reflectivity was low; there was a faint orbital uptake of In-111 OCT. In patient #4, the Clinical Activity Score was intermediate (= 3), EOM reflectivity was high and there was moderate uptake of the tracer at the level of the orbits. In patient #8 affected by Graves' disease who at the time of the study was euthyroid, and in patient #5 who was hypothyroid, there was severe ophthalmopathy; the Clinical Activity Score was 5, there was high reflectivity of EOMs and an intense In-111 OCT orbital uptake that was more evident at the SPECT study. In the patient who had undergone a total thyroidectomy (#6) and the patient (#7) affected by non thyroid associated ophthalmopathy (TAO), both the Clinical Activity Score and reflectivity were low. The In-111 OCT scans were negative at the level of the orbits and the thyroid.

Table 1. Characteristics of patients

Patients (n.)	Clinical activity score	A-scan standardized echography reflectivity aspect	In-111 OCT SCAN Thyroid	Orbits
1	1	Low	+	–
2	1	Low	+	±
3	1	Low	+	–
4	3	High	+	++
5	5	High	+	+++
6	2	Low		
7	0	Low		
8	4	High	+	+++

Table 2. Characteristics of patients

Patients (n.)	Thyroid disease	Clinical status	Previous therapy
1	GD	Hyperthyroidism	
2	GD	Hyperthyroidism	
3	GD	Euthyroidism	Me
4	GD	Euthyroidism	Me
5	GD	Hypothyroidism	S
6	GD	Euthyroidism	S, L-T4
7	LC	Euthyroidism	
8	GD	Euthyroidism	Me

From these data it is possible to identify two groups of patients. The first group (patients #4, 5 and 8) showed a clinically active ophthalmopathy, with a high reflectivity of the EOMs at A-scan standardized echography and tracer uptake at the level of the orbits. The second group, patients #1, 2, 3, 6 and 7, had a low Clinical Activity Score, low reflectivity at A-scan standardized echography and insignificant orbital tracer uptake.

Thyroid uptake was higher in patients with the active form of Graves' disease (first group) than in those with non active disease (second group). In the first group, there was an intense uptake regardless of the functional state of the gland. Low uptake was observed in three of the four patients of the second group. Orbital uptake was more difficult to analyze than thyroid uptake because of the low uptake in comparison to background and because of the presence of an aspecific activity due to the bone, blood and mucosa. An intense orbital accumulation was found in three patients with Graves' disease, who had clinically active ophthalmopathy. SPECT clearly showed the orbital uptake location. Mild accumulation was observed in three cases. A slight activity, not univocally evaluable, was observed in two other subjects. No orbital uptake was found in a patient affected by Graves' disease who had active exophthalmos, and in the patient with lung cancer, despite the presence of bilateral ophthalmopathy. Standardized A-scan echography showed high reflectivity in all patients with clinically active Graves' disease and provided information about the different involvement of the EOMs.

The temporal analysis of orbital uptake, expressed as ratio with respect to brain, showed the highest value at 4 hours, with decreasing activity at the 24-hour control. Lastly, we evaluated cerebral uptake in comparison to blood activity and found a lack of a significant blood brain barrier permeability for OCT over 24 hours.

Conclusion

Standardized A-scan echography is a useful, inexpensive and reproducible technique for the study of ocular, orbital and periorbital diseases. It allows the diagnosis of TAO, even in the early stage, and the follow-up of these patients. Moreover, it permits an early diagnosis of compressive optic neuropathy that may occur in Graves' ophthalmopathy (GO) [7]. A-scan findings help to differentiate between various diseases and so allow timely therapy.

In this study, A-scan standardized echography and the Clinical Activity Score were useful in demonstrating that In-111 OCT is a good method with which to evaluate ophthalmopathy activity [9]. We demonstrated the uptake of In-111 OCT at the level of thyroid and orbits in patients with active TAO. In-111 OCT accumulation at the level of orbits and high reflectivity of EOMs demonstrated by standardized A-scan echography are parameters of disease activity in patients with GO. These data are well correlated with the Clinical Activity Score in patients with active disease. Therefore, In-111 OCT scan could be proposed as a screening test for the selection of patients who could benefit from somatostatin treatment [10,11].

In-111 OCT orbital uptake in GO seems to be strictly related to the activity of the ophthalmopathy [12,13]. The entity of the thyroid uptake, and the tracer kinetics at the level of the orbits and the thyroid, suggest the hypothesis that the orbital uptake is due to the presence of a somatostatin receptor-positive mononuclear cell infiltration, while the thyroid uptake is due to the presence of somatostatin receptor at the level of the gland [14].

The discrepancy in the entity of the thyroid and the orbital uptake in GO may also be related to different stages of the pathology. Moreover, the different kinetics observed at the level of thyroid and the orbits suggest the possibility of other uptake mechanisms, not necessarily 'cell-mediated', like in the patient affected by lung cancer.

References

[1] P. Perros and P. Kendall-Taylor. The pathogenesis of the thyroid associated ophthalmopathy. J. Endocrinol. 1989;122:619–624.

[2] E.P. Krenning, D.J. Kwekkeboom, W.H. Bakker, W.A.P. Breeman, P.P.M. Kooij, H.Y. Oei, M. van Hagen, P.T.E. Postema, M. de Jong, J.C. Reubi, T.J. Visser, A.E.M. Reijs, L.J. Hofland, J.W. Koper and J.C. Lambert. Somatostatin receptor scintigraphy with [111 In-DTPA-d-Phe) and [123-I-Tyr] octreotide: the Rotterdam experience with more than 1000 patients. Eur. J. Nucl. Med. 1993;20:716–731.

[3] K. von Wender and G. Faglia. Potential indications for octreotide in endocrinology, Metabolism 1992;2(41):91–98.

[4] H.N. Wagner. Annual Meeting Highlight: Molecules with Message. J. Nuclear Med., 1992;33(8):10–12.

[5] E. Henze. Scientific highlight of the EAMN Congress 1992. J. Nucl. Med. 1993;34(2):17–20.

[6] L. Wartofsky. American Thyroid Association. Thyroid 1992;2(3):235–236.

[7] K.C. Ossoinig. The role of standardized echography in Graves' disease. Acta Ophthalmol. 1992;204:81.

[8] E.P. Krenning, W.H. Bakker, P.P.M. Kooij, W.A.P. Breeman, H.Y. Oei, M. de Jong, J.C. Reubi, T.J. Visser, C. Bruns, D.J. Kwekkeboom, A.E.M. Reijs, P.M. van Hagen, J.W. Koper and S.W.J. Lamberts. Somatostatin receptor scintigraphy with Indium-111-DTPA-D-Phe-1-Octreotide in man: metabolism, dosimetry and comparison with Iodine-123-Tyr-3-Octreotide. J. Nucl. Med. 1992;33:652–658.

[9] R.S. Bahn, R.S. Garrith and C.A. Gordman. Diagnosis and management of Graves' ophthalmopathy. J. Clin. Endocrinol. Metab. 1990;71:559–563.

[10] B. Tricojevi, M. Nesovi, J. Ciri, C. Vasjlievi, M. Stojanovi, M. Zarcovi and D. Slijepevi. The treatment of Graves' ophthalmopathy with synthetic somatostatin analogue (octreotide). J. Endocr. Invest. 1991;14(14):155.

[11] T.C. Chang, S.C.S. Kao, K.M. Huang. Octreotide and Graves' ophthalmopathy and mykoedema. Br. Med. J. 1992;304:158.

[12] P.T.E. Postema, G. Henneman, P.P.M. Kooy, H.Y. Oei, R. Wijngaarde, W.A. Vandenbosch, R.M.L. Poublon, W.M. Wiersinga, S.W.J. Lamberts and E.P. Krenning. Orbital 111-In-DTPA octreotide (10) accumulation in Graves' orbitopathy is not based on blood pool activity radioactivity. Thyroidal 10 accumulation and AO are correlated with disease activity in untreated Graves' disease. J. Nucl. Med. 1993;34(5):41.

[13] M. Tsao, M. Ferrarini, C. Evans, M. Ambro and T.L. Whiteside. Purification of glycosaminoglycan-stimulatory of lymphokine from supernatants of in vitro activated human mononuclear cells. Clin. Immunol. Immunopathol. 1989;50:122–31.

A. Bizzaro
Dipartimento di Internistica Clinica e Sperimentale "F. Magrassi"
Seconda Università di Napoli
Naples, Italy

[1]Istituto Scienze Radiologiche – Medicina Nuclear
[2]Istituto di Endocrinologia
Seconda Università di Napoli
Naples, Italy

[3]Istituto di Oftalmologia
Università di Napoli Federico II
Via S. Pansini 5
80131 Naples, Italy

44. Thyroid-associated ophthalmopathy: a new sign

P.E. GALLENGA, L. MASTROPASQUA, A. MANCINI,
M. CIANCAGLINI, E. ZUPPARDI and L. LOBEFALO
(Chieti, Italy)

Abstract

The authors describe a new sign in thyroid ophthalmopathy, i.e., sovraorbital and retroocular pain together with increased intraocular pressure in upgaze. This is a very early sign which tends to disappear in the late phases. The sign is correlated with the dynamics of the extraocular muscle enlargement.

Key words: Thyroid-associated ophthalmopathy, pain in upgaze, IOP increase

Introduction

Thyroid-associated ophthalmopathy, together with a multinodular hyperfunctioning goiter, is one of the manifestations of Graves-Basedow disease. Ophthalmopathy can be clinically detected in 40–50% of cases of thyroid dysfunction [1]. The main pathological alterations in thyroid ophthalmopathy occur in the orbital fat tissue (type I) and in the extraocular muscles (EOMs) (type II). In the early phases of the disorder there is an enlargement of the EOMs with edema and lymphocytic infiltration [2]. Later, after the immunomediated activation of the fibroblasts, there is fibrosis and atrophy of the EOMs [3]. Enlarged EOMs are echographically evident in more than 90% of dysthyroid patients, and this finding often precedes the onset of the symptoms [1].

The American Thyroid Association (ATA) classification of thyroid-associated ophthalmopathy consists of six classes based on signs and symptoms (Table 1) [4,5]. Glioner [6] suggested adding a seventh item to the classification, i.e., high intraocular pressure, which can result from altered outflow of the aqueous due to the orbital involvement. Increased intraocular pressure, which was not correlated to EOM thickness, was described in upgaze in patients with Graves' ophthalmopathy (GO) [7] and later shown to be 6 mmHg [8].

We have identified a new sign in GO: sovraorbital and retroocular pain in upgaze. This sign is very precocious and tends to disappear as the disease progresses. The aim of this study was to use echographic imaging [9–11] to detect orbital structural alterations and so attempt to define the characteristics and the pathogenesis of this new sign.

G Cennamo and N. Rosa (eds.), Ultrasonography in Ophthalmology 15, pp. 371–376.

Material and methods

Fifty-eight patients with Graves-Basedow disease (41 males: 70.7%, and 17 females: 29.3%) were enrolled in the study for a total of 116 eyes. The mean age was 42.72 years (SD ±13.37). Graves-Basedow disease was diagnosed on the basis of a clinical examination, hormonal dosage, thyroid scintigraphy and echography. All patients underwent ophthalmic morphofunctional evaluation, and exophthalmometry according to Hertel; diplopia was also recorded. Patients were classified according to the ATA classification modified by Werner (Table 1). Patients with lagophthalmos keratitis (ATA class 5) and/or signs of compression-induced optic neuropathy (ATA class 6) were excluded from the study.

Table 1. American Thyroid Association Classification of Graves-Basedow Disease*

Class	
0	No sign or symptoms
1	Signs only
2	Signs and symptoms without exophthalmos (grading)
3	Exophthalmos 3 mm (grading)
4	Muscle involvement with diplopia (grading)
5	Corneal involvement (grading)
6	Loss of visual acuity (optic neuropathy) (grading)

*Modified from: American Thyroid Association (Mod. by S.C. Werner SC 1977 and H.J.L.van Dyk 1981)

The patients remaining in the study underwent the following tests: 1) measurement of the thickness of the EOMs with standardized A-scan (mean value); 2) measurement of the superior oblique muscle thickness; 3) complete orbital echographic examination with both A- and B-scan [12], in particular we checked for the presence of dilation of the orbital venous system (superior ophthalmic vein and medial vertical vein), lacrimal gland alteration and direct or indirect signs of optic nerve compression; 4) tonometry, according to Goldmann, in primary position gaze and in upgaze – the patients were divided into two subgroups (Δ IOP <6 mmHg and Δ IOP $\geqslant 6$ mmHg); and 5) presence or absence of pain in upgaze. The data were evaluated with the χ^2 test.

Results

The subdivision of the patients according to the ATA classification is reported in Table 2. The incidence of pain in upgaze position was less than 22.41% (26

Table 2. Distribution of the studied eyes according to the American Thyroid Association classification

Grade	Signs	Symptoms	Exophthalmos	Diplopia	Eyes	%
0	-	-	-	-	24	20.69
1	+	-	-	-	22	18.97
2	+	+	-	-	8	6.90
3	+	+	+	-	52	44.83
4	+	+	+	+	10	8.61

Table 3. Pain in upgaze

Grade	Total eyes	Eyes with P.I.S.	%
0	24	7	29.17
1	22	6	27.27
2	8	5	62.50
3	52	7	13.46
4	10	1	10.00
Total	116	26	22.41

Table 4. Intraocular pressure increase in upgaze (Δ IOP $\geqslant 6$ mmHg)

Grade	Total eyes	Eyes with Δ IOP $\geqslant 6$ mmHg	%
0	24	5	20.83
1	22	3	13.64
2	8	5	62.50
3	52	22	42.31
4	10	6	60.00
Total	116	41	35.34

Table 5. Pain in upgaze vs Δ IOP $\geqslant 6$ mmHg ($p < 0.001$)

Pain	Δ IOP $\geqslant 6$ mmHg	Δ IOP < 6 mmHg
Presence	21	5
Absence	20	70

Table 6. Results pain in upgaze vs superior oblique muscle (thickness) ($p = 0.029$)

Pain	Thickness > 2.8 mm	Thickness $\leqslant 2.8$ mm
Presence	21	5
Absence	49	41

eyes) with a peak (62.5%) in patients in ATA class 2 (Table 3). As shown in Table 4, IOP was $\geqslant 6$ mmHg in upper gaze position in 41 out of 116 eyes (35.34%). We found a statistically significant correlation between increased IOP and pain in upgaze ($p < 0.001$) (Table 5), and between increased thickness of superior oblique muscle and pain in upgaze ($p = 0.029$) (Table 6). In agreement with our earlier study [7], there was no correlation between pain and mean EOM thickness. Enlargement of orbital venous system and/or lacrimal gland alteration was not correlated with pain in upgaze. However, the latter finding could be due to the limits of our methodology (resolution $\geqslant 2$ mm in the III Benedict space) [12].

Discussion

The presence of pain in upgaze was correlated to the thickness of the superior oblique muscle and with the increase of IOP in upgaze. This symptom is not correlated with the thickness of the other EOMs, with alteration of the lacrimal gland or with the enlargement of the orbital venous system.

The anatomical and topographic characteristics of the superior oblique muscle suggest the muscle could be involved in the pathogenesis of the pain and of the increased IOP in upgaze. In fact, in upgaze the enlarged belly of the superior oblique muscle (Fig. 1) is stretched and pushed forward into the trochlear ring thereby stretching the tendon [13]. The compression of the muscle and the stretching of the tendon give rise to the pain. In this situation the eye,

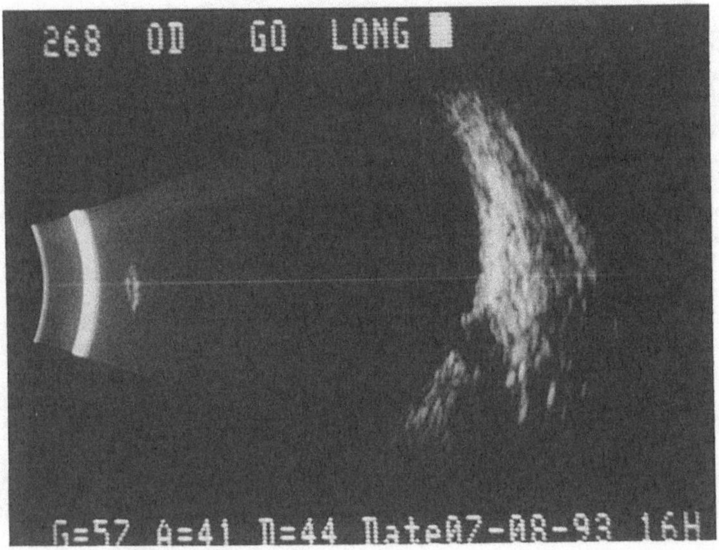

Fig. 1. B-scan: superior oblique muscle; longitudinal section

already compressed by the thyroid ophthalmopathy, is compressed by the posterior (because of the enlarged rectus muscle) and anterior (because of the enlarged belly of the superior oblique muscle and its tendon) complex. The latter situation could cause the increase in IOP in upgaze by a direct mechanism of compression or by compression of the orbital venous system.

This new sign is relevant because it has a high prevalence (62.5%) in the early phases of the disease, before the exophthalmos develops. In fact, the pain is characteristic of the edematous and inflammatory stage of the disease, which often coincides with the period when the increase in muscle thickening is fastest. The subsequent partial regression of the edema, and the onset of fibrotic processes, together with the saturation of the pain receptor, facilitates sliding of the superior oblique muscle into the trochlea, and hence explains the disappearance of the pain in upgaze. This hypothesis is based on the tridimensional and dynamic reconstruction of the echographic data. Studies with magnetic resonance imaging will probably throw more light on the dynamics of the involved orbital structures. A study in this sense is now underway in our Department.

References

[1] V. Sridama and L.J. De Groot. Treatment of Graves' disease and the course of ophthalmopathy. Am. J. Med. 1989;87:70–73.

[2] A.P. Weetman, S. Choen, K.C. Gatter, P. Fells and B. Shine. Immunohistochemical analysis of the retrobulbar tissue in Graves' ophthalmopathy. Clin. Exp. Immunol. 1989;75:222–227.

[3] A.P. Weetman. Thyroid associated eye disease: Pathophysiology. The Lancet 1991;388:25–28.

[4] S.C. Werner. Modification of the classification of eye disease changes in Graves' disease: recommendation of the ad hoc committee of the American Thyroid association (editorial). J. Clin. Endocrin. Metabol. 1977;44:203–211.

[5] H.J.L. Van Dyk. Orbital Graves' disease: a modification of the NOSPECS classification. Ophthalmology 1981;88:479–488.

[6] D. Glioner, J. Etienne-Decerf, M. Schrooyen, G. Sand, P. Hoyoux, P. Maheieu and R. Winand. Beneficial effects of intensive plasma exchange followed by immunosuppressive therapy in severe Graves' ophthalmopathy. Acta Endocrinol. 1986;111:30–38.

[7] P.E. Gallenga, G.F. Parmiani, L. Lobefalo, S. Sensi, L. De Remigis, G. Di Marzio and A. Troiano. Oftalmopatia di Graves ed oftalmotono. Clin. Ocul. e Patol. Ocul. 1989;10(5):353–357.

[8] P. Fells. Thyroid associated eye disease: clinical management. The Lancet 1991;338:29–32.

[9] K.C. Ossoinig. Die Ultraschalldiagnostik der Orbita. Klin. Mbl. Augenheilk. 1966;149:817–821.

[10] D.D. Coleman. Reliability of ocular and orbital diagnosis with B-scan ultrasound: II Orbital diagnosis. Am. J. Ophthalmol. 1972;174:843-847.

[11] A. Reibaldi, G. Assennato, T. Avitabile and M.G. Uva. The echobiometric measurements of the extraocular muscle in normal subjects. In J.M. Thijssen (ed.), Ultrasonography in ophthalmology. Dordrecht: Kluwer Academic Publishers, 1988.

[12] P.E. Gallenga and V. Mazzeo. La posizione ecografica in confronto alle altre metodiche diagnostiche. Indicazioni e limiti. In Ultrasuoni in medicina: Atti II Congresso Naz. S.I.S.U.M. (Rome). 1976;65–74.

[13] E. Dal Ponte. Il problema trocleare. In E. Dal Ponte (ed.), Cefalea primaria e occhio. Turin: SMO Publisher. 1992;107–14.

Prof. Pier Enrico Gallenga
Istituto di Oftalmologia
Università 'G D'Annunzio'
via Tiro a Segno, 2
66100 Chieti, Italy

45. Ultrasound diagnostics of lacrimal sac diseases

M. VÉGH, J. NÉMETH[1] and I. BERECZ
(Szeged and [1] Budapest, Hungary)

Abstract

We report our seven-year experience with Ultrascan Digital B® System IV ophthalmic ultrasound equipment in the diagnostics of lacrimal sac diseases. The following disorders were diagnosed by means of ultrasound: anatomical disorders (no. 2), inflammations (no. 85), mucoceles (no. 3), tumors (no. 3) and foreign bodies (no. 2). Ultrasound examination proved useful in indicating the surgical procedure in most cases of lacrimal sac disease, and in the examination of unsuccessful cases after operation without need to use any other diagnostic imaging method. Only in complicated cases was computed tomographic dacryocystography also used, or in cases of tumor, computed tomography with intravenous contrast material. The recently introduced color-coded Doppler ultrasound method was also applied for the differential diagnosis of tumors and for planning tumor therapy. The advantages of ultrasound diagnostics of the lacrimal sac over conventional or computed tomographic dacryocystography are that it is simple, quick and inexpensive; the patient is not exposed to radiation; it can be used without any contrast medium; and it is useful when the common canaliculus is occluded. Ultrasound examinations are suggested as first choice in the diagnostics of lacrimal sac diseases.

Key words: Lacrimal sac, ultrasound diagnostics, color-coded Doppler ultrasound, computed tomography

Introduction

For the everyday diagnostics of lacrimal sac diseases, dacryocystography is routinely applied worldwide [1,2]. However, this method is not always simple to use, especially in children. With the advance of technology, more approaches have become available for the diagnostic imaging of lacrimal drainage system diseases [3–10], including ultrasound diagnostics [11–18]. We use ultrasound in the routine diagnostics of lacrimal sac diseases, and in this study we describe the experience gained over a seven-year period.

G Cennamo and N. Rosa (eds.), Ultrasonography in Ophthalmology 15, pp. 377–382.

Material and methods

The indications of the use of ultrasound diagnostics were: 1) Pathological changes on the skin surface corresponding to the site of the lacrimal sac; these included swelling, pressure sensitivity and changes in the color of the skin. 2) Tearing with or without inflammatory content in adults. In infants, the examination was performed only in complicated cases. 3) To examine unsuccessful cases after operation.

The ages of the patients varied widely. The examinations were made with an Ultrascan Digital B™ System IV (Cooper Vision), at 10 MHz. The examinations were performed on patients lying on their back with their eyes closed. In most cases we used our own examination method [19–21], in which a water-filled sterilized rubber tube is placed between the transducer and the skin surface. The upper part of the rubber tube and the medial lid region of the skin were coated with 2% methylcellulose solution to attain a better contact. The ultrasound probe was fixed on the upper part of the rubber tube, correctly directioned towards the structure to be examined. In cases in which we examined the deeper layers, direct contact [11,14] and transocular contact examination methods [12,22] were used.

The A and B scan echograms were recorded on video-tape and pictures were copied by a Mitsubishi Video Copy Processor, Model P6OB. In complicated cases a Siemens Somatom DRG computed tomograph scanner was used with Omnipaque (Iohexol) contrast material for computed tomographic dacryocystography [10], and in tumor cases computed tomographic diagnostics with Omnipaque (Iohexol) intravenous contrast material was also applied [23]. For tumor diagnostics a color-coded Doppler ultrasound examination was performed with an Acuson 128 [17,18].

Results

During the past seven years, the following lacrimal sac disorders were diagnosed by ultrasound: two cases of anatomical disorders (diverticulum and congenital absence of the lacrimal sac; Fig. 1); 85 cases of inflammation (acute in 9 cases, chronic in 74 cases), three cases of mucocele, three cases of tumor (histology: adenocarcinoma, anaplastic carcinoma and nodular non-Hodgkin lymphoma), and two cases of foreign bodies.

In two cases of unsuccessful dacryocystorhinostomy the site of obstruction was identified by ultrasound: in one case a membrane-like echogram at the site of the bone 'window', and in the other case an abnormal situation of the middle turbinate bone caused a leakage obstruction (Fig. 2).

In the tissue surrounding the lacrimal sac, the following diseases were detected by ultrasound: inflammation with abscess in two cases, granuloma in one case (histology: pyogenic granuloma), dermoid cyst in two cases, and tumor in three cases (histology: basal cell carcinoma in two cases, hemangioma in one case).

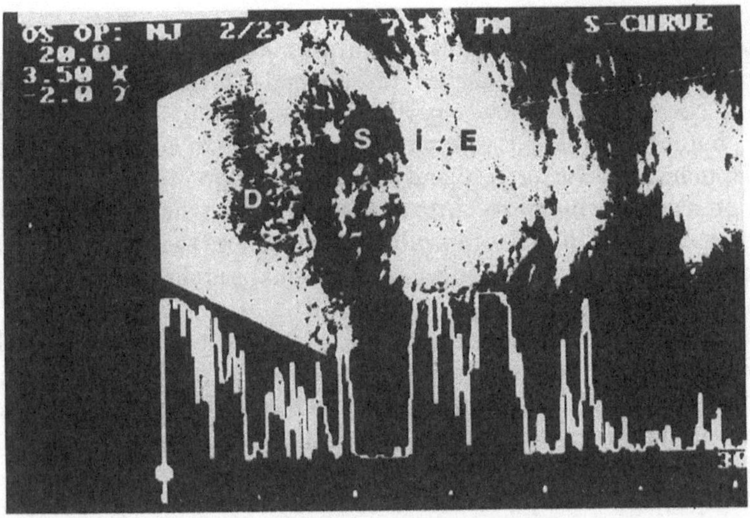

Fig. 1. A- and B-scan echograms of lacrimal sac diverticulum with signs of chronic inflammation. The diverticulum (D), cavity (S) and posterior wall (i) of the lacrimal sac, the discharge within, and phlogistic process in the ethmoidal cells (E) are well visible

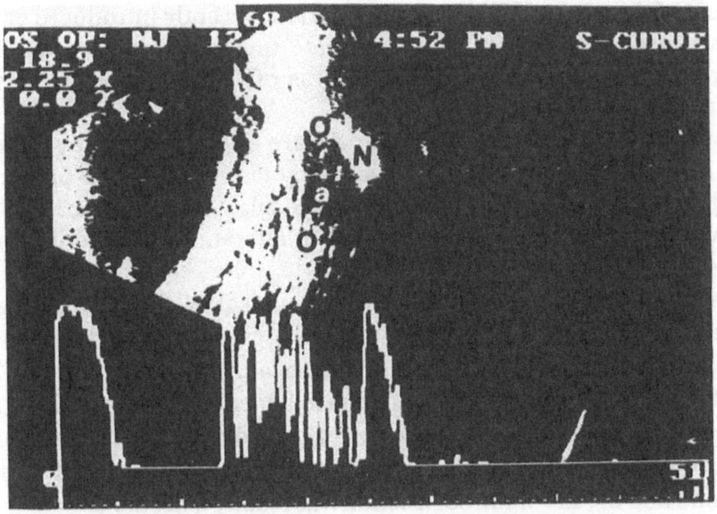

Fig. 2. A- and B-scan echograms of unsuccessful dacryocystorhinostomy, using the rubber tube method. The artificial cavity (a), the edges of the bone window (o), and the tip of the middle turbinate bone (N) in the nasal cavity can be clearly seen

Discussion

As reported previously [15,24], ultrasound examination of the lacrimal drainage system was not able to visualize the normal-size lacrimal canaliculi, the common canaliculus, the lower part of the nasolacrimal duct or the lacrimal ostium, but it can be used as routine for the diagnosis of lacrimal sac diseases. It provides indications for surgery, and can be used to monitor the patient after the operation, usually without recourse to other expensive diagnostic methods. It is important that the most technically advanced ophthalmologic ultrasound equipment be used in the diagnostics of lacrimal sac diseases [25,26], and for differential diagnoses.

We used the rubber tube method [19–21] for most examinations. This is a more comfortable procedure, especially for children, and it avoids infection by the ultrasound probe after surgery. The rubber tube method is as easy to perform as the direct contact method, and the echograms are of the same quality as those obtained with the water bath method.

In complicated cases, a Siemens Somatom DRG computed tomograph scanner was used with Omnipaque (Iohexol) contrast material for computed tomographic dacryocystography. With this method and using different sections, we were able to identify the exact site of the obstruction [5–7,10,23].

Ultrasound can be used to differentiate inflammation from a tumor [22]. In tumor cases, computerized tomography was also used to visualize better bone destruction, and with intravenous contrast material for a better visualization of the extent of the tumor [10,23]. We also used the recently introduced color-coded Doppler ultrasound [17,18] to differentiate tumors. This procedure provides information about the hemodynamic status of the tumor, which is useful for planning tumor therapy.

Anterior and middle ethmoidal air cells are also detectable by ultrasound in cases in which the air content is replaced by discharge, blood or tumor tissue [25–27]. Direct contact [11,14] and transocular contact [12,22] ultrasound procedures provide a better visualization of alterations of anterior and middle ethmoidal cells in deeper layers (Fig. 1).

Ultrasound diagnostics is also useful in the clinical follow-up after surgery of the lacrimal sac. After dacryocystorhinostomy echography revealed the bone window (Fig. 2), whereas the artificial cavity is not visualized if it contains air [25,26]. In cases of postoperative passage failure due to a membrane-like obstruction at the site of the bone window, the artificial cavity (formed by nasal mucosal and lacrimal sac flaps) was filled with fluid, in which case the cavity was well visualized by ultrasound and the site of the obstruction was readily detectable.

The advantages of ultrasound diagnostics of the lacrimal sac over conventional or computed tomographic dacryocystography are that it is simple, quick and inexpensive; the patient is not exposed to radiation; it can be used without any contrast medium; and it is useful when the common canaliculus is occluded. We suggest ultrasound examinations as first choice in the diagnostics of lacrimal sac diseases.

Reference

[1] J.J. Hurwitz and W.H. Victor. The role of sophisticated radiological testing in the assessment and management of epiphora. Ophthalmology 1985;92:407–413.

[2] F.J. Steinkogler, F. Karnel and G. Canigiani. Die digitale Dacryozystographie. Klin. Mbl. Augenheilk. 1987;191:55–57.

[3] M.H. Becker. The lacrimal system. In C.F. Gonzalez, M.H. Becker and J.C. Flanagan (eds), Diagnostic imaging in ophthalmology. New York: Springer-Verlag, 1985;81–91.

[4] W. Wiegand. Kernspintomographie von Auge, Orbita und Sehnerv. Bücherei des Augenarztes, Vol. 122. Enke, 1990;38–40.

[5] S.J. Zinreich, N.R. Miller, L.N. Freeman, L.W. Glorioso and A.E. Rosenbaum. Computed tompographic dacryocystography using topical contrast media for lacrimal system visualization. Orbit (Amsterdam) 1990;9:79–87.

[6] A. Ashenhurst, N. Jaffer, J.J. Hurwtiz and S.M. Corin. Combined computed tomography and dacryocystography for complex lacrimal problems. Can. J. Ophthalmol. 1991;26:27–31.

[7] H.J. Glatt, A.C. Chan and J. Barett. Evaluation of dacryocystorhinostomy failure with computed tomography and computed tomography dacryocystography. Am. J. Ophthalmol. 1991;112:431–436.

[8] W. Fein, L. Daykhovsky, T. Papaioannou, C. Beeder and W.S. Grundfest. Endoscopy of the lacrimal outflow system. Arch. Ophthalmol. 1992;110:1748–1750.

[9] R.A. Goldberg, G.W. Heinz and L. Chiu. Gadolinium magnetic resonance imaging dacryocystography. Am. J. Ophthalmol. 1993;115:738–741.

[10]M. Végh and E. Tanács. Computed tompographic dacryocystography. In M. Miglior, O.P.V. Bijsterveld and D. Spinelli (eds). The lacrimal system. Proceeding of the VII International Symposium on the Lacrimal System, Bruxelles, 1992. Milano: Ghedini, 1993;149–153.

[11] A. Oksala. Diagnosis by ultrasound in acute dacryocystitis. Acta Ophthalmol. (Kbh) 1959;37:176–179.

[12] K. Ossoinig. Die Ultraschalldiagnostik der Orbita. Mbl. Augenheilk. 1966;149:817–839.

[13] W.E. Scott, J.A. Fabre and K.C. Ossoinig. Congenital mucocele of the lacrimal sac. Arch. Ophthalmol. 1979;97:1656–1658.

[14] R. Rochels and R. Hackelbusch. B-Bild-Echographie bei Erkrankungen der ableitenden Tränenwege. Klin. Mbl. Augenheilk. 1982;182:181–183.

[15] M. Végh, J. Németh and P. Bordás. Dacryocystography or echography. Orbit (Amsterdam) 1988;7:191–195.

[16] J.J. Dutton. Standardized echography in the lacrimal drainage dysfunction. Arch. Ophthalmol. 1989;107:1010–1012.

[17] R. Guthoff. Ultrasound in ophthalmic diagnosis. A practical guide. Stuttgart: Thieme, 1991.

[18] J. Németh, Z. Morvay, Z. Horóczi and E. Nagy. A színkódolt Doppler ultrahangvizsgálat szemészeti alkalmazása. Szemészet 1992;129:34-37.

[19] M. Végh and J. Németh. A new device in ultrasound diagnostics of the lacrimal sac. Orbit (Amsterdam) 1988;7:197–200.

[20] M. Végh and J. Németh. j segédeszköz a saccus lacrimalis és ductus nasolacrimalis ultrahanggal való vizsgálatára. Szemészet 1988;125:116–120.

[21] M. Végh and J. Németh. Ultraschalldiagnostik des Tränensackes. Fortschr. Ophthalmol. 1990;87:638–640.

[22] R. Rochels, W. Lieb and A. Nover. Echographische Diagnostik bei Erkrankungen der ableitenden Tränenwege. Klin. Mbl. Augenheilk. 1984;185:243–249.

[23] M. Végh and E. Tanács. Use of computed tomographic dacryocystography in the elevation of lacrimal drainage system obstruction. Orbit (Amsterdam) 1993;12:105–109.

[24] M. Végh, J. Németh and P. Bordás. A könnyelvezet rendszer ultrahangvizsgálata. Szemészet 1988;125:90–95.

[25] M. Végh and J. Németh. Use of ultrasound diagnostics in lacrimal sac disease. Intern. Ophthalmol. 1991;15:397–399.

[26] M. Végh and J. Németh. Importance of ultrasound diagnostics in lacrimal sac disease. In P. Till (ed.), Ophthalmic echography. Proceedings of the 13th SIDUO Congress, Vienna, 1990. Dordrecht: Kluwer Publishers, 1991;193–197.
[27] G.V. Geyer. Nasennebenhöhlen. In R. Rochels (ed.), Ultraschalldiagnostik in der Augenheilkunde. Landsberg: Ecomed, 1986;131–145.

Mihály Végh
Department of Ophthalmology
Albert Szent-Györgyi Medical University
P.O. Box 407
H-6701 Szeged, Hungary

[1]Department of Ophthalmology
Medical University
Budapest, Hungary

46. Intraorbital wooden foreign body: wood can be isodense with air by computed tomography

V. GERMINETTI and M. IOSSA
(Biella (VC), Italy)

Abstract

A wooden foreign body inside the orbit may be difficult to diagnose. In fact, wood is not radiopaque and direct identification with computed tomography is rarely possible. In CT scans, a wooden foreign body can appear with the same density as air or fat and it can be indistinguishable from orbital tissues. We report a case in which computed tomography revealed a linear area of about 3 cm of extremely low attenuation in the left orbit of a middle aged man who had a facial trauma. Initially, the appearance and attenuation of the area suggested air, leading to the diagnosis of orbital emphysema. Further studies revealed a wooden foreign body, which was subsequently surgically removed from the orbit. We stress that echography plays a prime role in the management of orbital trauma.

Key words: Wood, foreign body, orbit, computed tomography, echography

Introduction

A wooden foreign body in the orbit may present considerable diagnostic difficulty because it is radiolucent. However, with the advent of ultrasonography, CAT scanning and magnetic resonance imaging the likelihood of identification is increased.

The management and diagnosis of a wooden foreign body inside the orbit is difficult, especially in cases of minor trauma. Only in a few cases is it clear from the history and the clinical examination that a foreign body is present within the eye or the orbit. Often, periorbital wounds occur in patients consequent to a low-velocity puncture with a sharp wooden object. These wounds may appear minor and superficial, unaccompanied by major symptomatology, and may be considered trivial by examining physicians. Therefore, penetration of the orbit by a small object can pass unnoticed.

Moreover, penetrating wounds of the upper eyelids have a greater tendency for intracranial extension because of the thin orbital roof, temporal squama and cribriform plate that allow access to the intracranial cavity of objects not strong enough to penetrate other regions of the skull.

G Cennamo and N. Rosa (eds.), Ultrasonography in Ophthalmology 15, pp. 383–389.

Because of its nature, wood is a particularly dangerous wounding agent. Being of porous organic material it is a natural reservoir for microbial agents. Moreover, it is not detectable by X-rays [1,2]. Consequently, an immediate diagnostic evaluation should be performed when a penetrating orbital wound is suspected. Numerous diagnostic techniques are now available, but echography and computed tomography [3] are fundamental in localizing the foreign body and in defining the orbital conditions and the most appropriate surgical approach.

We report a case of a patient with a retained wooden foreign body diagnosed by echography. The advantages and limits of echography and computed tomography are discussed.

Case report

A 56-year-old white man attended the first aid department after sustaining an injury to his left eye. While running, he fell and was struck by a reed. The first aid surgeon had superficially explored the wound of the left inferior eyelid and closed it, prescribed antibiotic ointment and advised the patient to seek specialist advice if the eye did not improve.

During the next two days the patient's left eye became increasingly painful and swollen, and so he attended the department of ophthalmology.

On examination his best corrected visual acuity of the left eye was 20/200. There was marked chemosis of the lower bulbar conjunctiva and the eye was proptotic. The motility of the left eye was severely limited in all fields of gaze. Ophthalmologic examination revealed a diagonal corneal abrasion. Both pupils were equal in size, round, and reactive to light. Fundus examination of the left eye was performed with binocular indirect ophthalmoscopy and revealed only a modest Berlin's oedema. The intraocular pressure was 14 mmHg. Hertel exophthalmometry with a base of 110 mm, measured 18 mm in the right eye and 27 mm in the left eye. The best corrected visual acuity of the right eye was 20/20; the anterior segment was normal; fundoscopic examination was also normal. Intraocular pressure was 18 mmHg.

The patient was admitted to the ophthalmology department and systemic and topical antibiotic therapy was started after a conjunctival swab was taken of the discharge of the wound. The swab of the discharge grew *Escherichia coli*, *Enterobacter cloacae* and *Klebsiella oxitoca*. The patient was given tetanus immunization.

Orbital X-rays did not reveal any evidence of a radiopaque foreign body or fracture. Orbital CAT scans were performed: axial and coronal 3 mm scans were obtained through the orbit with a General Electric CityPace CT scanner. These revealed, in the lower temporal orbit, a linear area of extremely low attenuation that resembled the path of a penetrating wound. The cranial contents appeared to be normal, with no evidence of foreign bodies. The area of attenuation, similar to that due to air, was considered to be caused by orbital emphysema (Figs. 1 and 2).

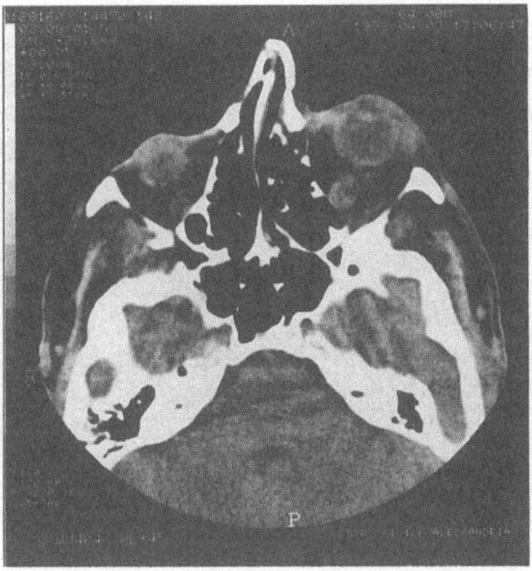

Fig. 1. Computed tomography, horizontal section, showing a linear area of extremely low attenuation in the lower temporal left orbit

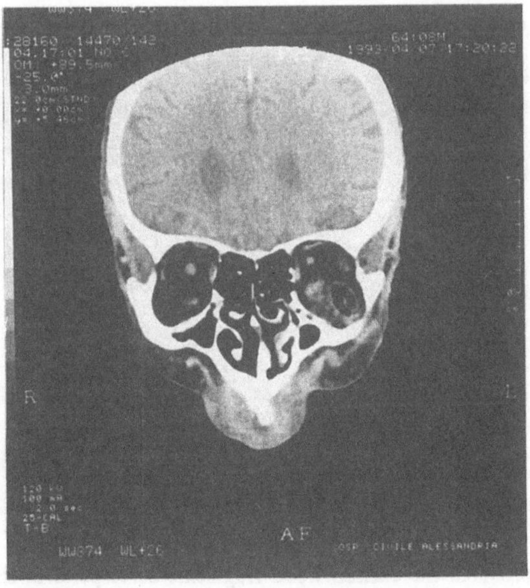

Fig. 2. Computed tomography, coronal section, demonstrating the area of extremely low attenuation in the left orbit

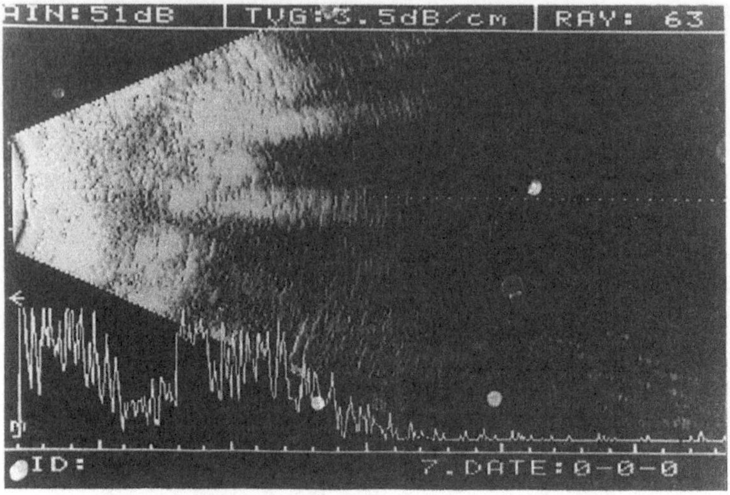

Fig. 3. Echography of the left eye (PB 5): the orbital foreign body is clearly evident

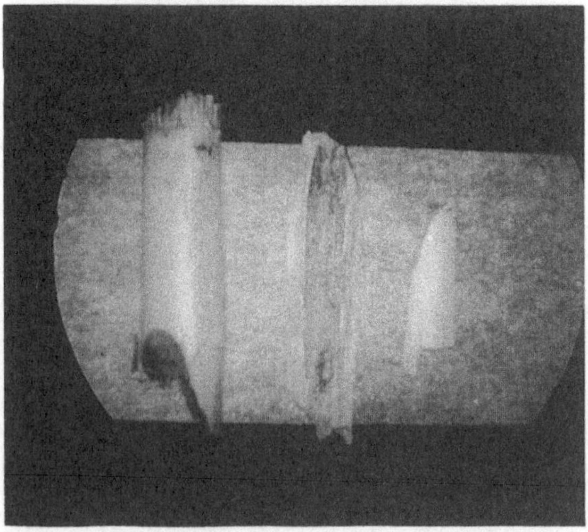

Fig. 4. Surgical specimen: the excised wood fragments correspond in shape and size to their appearance on echography and computed tomography

Because of the doubtful diagnosis, B-scan echography was performed with a Sonemed 3000. Echography identified a cylindrical foreign body with a diameter of 4 mm; it had a very high reflectivity.

The surgeon decided that, despite the possibility of damage to the structures of the orbit, the foreign body should be removed. The patient underwent exploratory surgery under local anesthesia. The wound was reopened and the foreign body (reed) was grasped with forceps and withdrawn. The foreign body broke during surgery. The total length of the fragments were 3 cm. A catheter drain was applied. Postoperatively, the fistula gradually stopped draining and closed. Over the next 15 days acuity returned to 20/20. Ocular motility gradually improved and after 4 months were normal.

Discussion

We describe a case of direct orbital trauma and minor lid laceration initially considered trivial. Orbital penetration was not suspected. Further investigations led to the diagnosis of an intraorbital foreign body. The case history suggests that in ocular injury caused by organic material such as wood, the possibility of a retained foreign body must be considered, particularly when proptosis, inflammatory signs and limitation of ocular movements persist. All periorbital punctures warrant a careful radiologic and echographic evaluation. The indication of a normal orbit by orbital radiography does not exclude a foreign body. Numerous instruments are now available for the diagnostic imaging of the orbit. The case reported demonstrates the importance of echography in cases of suspected radiolucent foreign body of the orbit.

Computed tomography is the single radiological tool of choice in evaluating head trauma, and is considered the primary diagnostic examination in cases of penetrating wounds of the orbit with suspected foreign bodies [4–6] because it allows early detection of retained ocular or intracranial foreign bodies, bone fractures, brain abscesses. However, CT has some significant limitations. In fact, many foreign bodies, especially those consisting of organic material, have densities very close to those of soft tissues. Wood can have a surprisingly low density. In fact, in our case the wooden foreign body was initially misinterpreted as air. This diagnostic error has been described by various authors [7–9]. Computed tomographic attenuation ranges from 556 to 54 Hunsfield Units (unit of density relative to an assigned air density value of 0). Thus, wood can easily be mistaken for air, particularly in the presence of fractures or sinus communications. Low attenuation seems to be due to trapped air.

It is difficult to find a foreign body using A-scan ultrasonography; indeed, it takes a long time to scan the whole orbit, because the difference between the high spikes of fat and of foreign bodies is small, and because of the poor penetration of the orbit apex. It is easier to find a foreign body using A-scan when one already knows the exact location of the foreign body.

On the contrary, B-mode ultrasound is easier because the whole orbit scanning is less time-consuming. In our case the intraorbital wooden foreign body was successfully diagnosed only by B-scan echography. Moreover, echography is less expensive than other diagnostic imaging instruments and should be applied first.

Recently, magnetic resonance imaging has been introduced in the diagnosis of orbital wooden foreign bodies [10]. Magnetic resonance imaging depends on the density of protons in the tissues and their relaxation time. These properties of wood and tissues are different. On the other hand, the radiodensity of wood is similar to that of soft tissues and therefore computed tomographic imaging is not always useful in the diagnosis of wooden foreign bodies. Magnetic resonance imaging should be used to confirm a diagnosis of a radiolucent foreign body already diagnosed by ultrasound [11].

All periorbital puncture wounds should be treated for possible intracranial penetration because the consequences of a retained intracranial foreign body may be very dangerous. In fact, the anatomy of the orbit plays an important role in the pathogenesis of orbital injuries with intracranial penetration. The orbit is shaped like a horizontal pyramid on a posteromedial axis, and tends to deflect foreign bodies toward the orbital apex. Moreover, the superior plate is easily penetrated. The globe has self-protective features, and is rarely ruptured, but it also tends to direct objects toward the orbital apex.

Once a foreign body is diagnosed, it is necessary to take a sample of the discharge, and specimens of the wound and foreign body for culture, and to start immediately systemic antibiotic therapy. It is mandatory to establish adequate tetanus immunization because wood is often contaminated with *Clostridium tetani*. An embedded organic foreign body must be removed because it may lead to abscess formation.

References

[1] J.E. Hansen, S.K. Gudeman, R.C. Holgate and R.A. Saunders. Penetrating intracranial wood wounds: clinical limitations of computed tomography. J. Neurosurg. 1988;68:752–756.

[2] P. Foy and M. Sharr. Cerebral abscesses in children after pencil-tip injuries. Lancet 1980;2:662–663.

[3] D.G. Charteris. Posterior penetrating injury of the orbit with retained foreign body. Br. J. Ophthalmol. 1988;72:432–433.

[4] R.A. Weisman, P.J. Savino, L. Schut and N.J. Shatz. Computed tomography in penetrating wounds of the orbit with retained foreign bodies. Arch. Otoryngol. 1923;109:265-268.

[5] S. Lindahl. Computed tomography of intraorbital foreign bodies. Acta Radiologica 1987;28:235–240.

[6] S.J. Zinreich, N.R. Miller, J.B. Aguayo, C. Quinn, R. Hadfield and A.E. Rosenbaum. Computed tomographic three-dimensional localization and compositional evaluation of intraocular and orbital foreign bodies. Arch. Ophthalmol. 1986;104:1477–1482.

[7] F.R. Cameron and P.J. Lechey. III. Intraorbital wood foreign body mimicking air at C. Radiology 1992;185:507–508.

[8] D. Bodne, S.F. Quinn and C.F. Cochran. Imaging foreign glass and wooden bodies of the extremities with CT and MR. J. Comput. Assist. Tomogr. 1988;12:608–611.

[9] C.S. Specht, J.H. Varga, M.M. Jalali and J.P. Edelstein. Orbitocranial wooden foreign body diagnosed by magnetic resonance imaging. Dry wood can be isodense with air and orbital fat by computed tomography. Surv. Ophthalmol. 1992;36:341–344.
[10] B.F. Green, S.P. Kraft, K.D. Carter, J.R. Buncic, J.A. Nerad, D. Amstrong. Intraorbital wood: detection by magnetic resonance imaging. Ophthalmology 1990;97:608–611.
[11] K.C. Ossoinig. Detection of wood foreign bodies. (Letter) Ophthalmology 1991;98:274.

V. Germinetti
Department of Ophthalmology
Ospedale degli Infermi
Biella (VC), Italy

Mario Iossa
via Alessio Baldovinetti 15
00142 Rome, Italy

47. Echographic features of the benign osteolytic lesions of the orbit in pediatric patients

J. FUKIYAMA, N. NAO-I, F. MARUIWA, Y. FUTAMI, I. OZUNO and A. SAWADA

(Miyazaki, Japan)

Bone defect on imaging studies often implies malignancy. However osteolysis can also be associated with benign lesions. We treated three children with benign osteolytic lesions. They were treated first by local physicians but later referred to us because orbital bone defects were found on computerized tomography. The initial symptom in these patients was upper lid swelling with pain. Soft tissue-density mass with underlying bone defects was found in the superotemporal aspect of the orbit on imaging studies. The lesions became smaller in size after the admission. Biopsy was performed in all cases and a yellowish brown friable mass was found in each. Histopathological diagnosis was probable eosinophilic granuloma. Resolution of the soft tissue-density mass with reconstruction of the bone defects occurred after the biopsy.

J. Fukiyama
Department of Ophthalmology
Miyazaki Medical College
5200 Kihara Kiyotake
Miyazaki 889-16, Japan

G Cennamo and N. Rosa (eds.), Ultrasonography in Ophthalmology 15, p. 391.

48. Dilated orbital veins. A clinical series with emphasis on ultrasound findings

H.C. FLEDELIUS, H. DAHL and J. THYSTRUP
(Hillerd, Denmark)

Abstract

We report on 8 patients with 'dilated orbital veins' seen over a 10-year period. Six were females aged 51–81 with carotico-cavernous fistula, three traumatic and three spontaneous. In five out of the six, retrobulbar dilated orbital veins could be typically demonstrated by ultrasound. The clinical features – among them a doctor's delay – are given. The remaining two patients were males. One had an orbital varix behind the eye, the other a complex of enlarged orbital veins, with arterialized blood flow, along the medial orbital wall, presenting anteriorly as a soft tumour. The issue of dilated orbital veins is a rewarding field for ultrasound diagnosis.

Key words: Orbital veins, carotico-cavernous fistula, echography

Introduction

The present review of 8 patients from a 10-year period was prompted by two recent cases of carotico-cavernous fistula (the last two cases of Table 1), where ultrasound eventually gave the diagnosis. Prior to that, however, there had been a considerable delay on the part of the doctor. Both patients presented with 'red eye' and diplopia due to abducens weakness.

Clinical reports

The first of the two recent patients, case no. 5 of Table 1, a nurse aged 62, complained of a rhythmic noise in her right ear. There was no head trauma in the history. Tinnitus being suspected, and with a systolic bruit auscultated on the neck, she was referred from the regional ENT department to the University Clinic for Vascular Surgery. Doppler examination indicated a fair flow in both carotid arteries. Aortico-cervicography and repeated CT-scans revealed no vascular abnormalities. Eventually she developed redness of the eye, small paracentral scotomas (due to minute retinal bleedings), and diplopia due to abducens weakness with esotropia.

G Cennamo and N. Rosa (eds.), Ultrasonography in Ophthalmology 15, pp. 393–398.

Table 1. Clinical features of the six cases reported – 1984–93

	EHC f, 78 1984	AP f, 81 1984	RC f, 71 1985	KH f, 51 1988	GG f, 62 1993	JV f, 51 1993
Head trauma	–	–	+	+	–	+
Protrusion	+	+	+	++	+	+
Injection	++	late+	+	++	late+	+
Unilateral visual loss	–	++	–	–	–	–
Abducens palsy	–	+	+	+	+	++
'Elevator palsy'	+	+	–	–	–	+
IOP rise	+	+	+	(+)	+	(+)
Bruit:						
Subjectively	–	–	+	+	+	+
Auscultation	–	–	+	+	+	+
Ultrasound diagnosis	–	(+)	+	+	+	+
Doctors' delay (months)	7	5	1-2	1-2	18	2

When we first saw her, auscultation and ultrasound evaluation (Fig. 1) immediately gave the diagnosis. Subsequently, a carotid angiography confirmed the diagnosis. Revision of the most recent CT-scan revealed a dilated upper orbital vein, which was not described at the time of the examination.

Figure 1 demonstrates the collapse of the dilated upper orbital vein after compression via the lower eye lid. On that occasion the patient informed us that during the first months of her disease, fingerpressing towards the infero-nasal anterior orbital tissue – similar to the transducer pressure applied during the test – caused the bruit to disappear. Later during the disorder, this was not possible.

The second patient (case no. 6, Table 1), a female aged 51, had received a blow with a fist near the left orbital region. After having been examined at the emergency ward she was sent home without follow-up. There was a black eye and she became aware of a continuous rhythmic sound. When redness of the eye and diplopia developed, she was referred to our clinic. At referral, markedly dilated retrobulbar veins were demonstrated by ultrasound (Fig. 2), which a few weeks later were also seen on the contralateral side. Carotid angiography confirmed the diagnosis.

Table 1 summarizes the clinical features of the 6 female cases of carotico-cavernous fistula. Evidently, auscultation of the orbital regions and ultrasound examination are the diagnostic procedures of choice. Three cases were spontaneous, and three were traumatic. The clinical spectrum is varied [1–3]. One patient had been subjected to long-term corticosteroid treatment on the assumption of orbital pseudotumour. The ultrasound examination was not

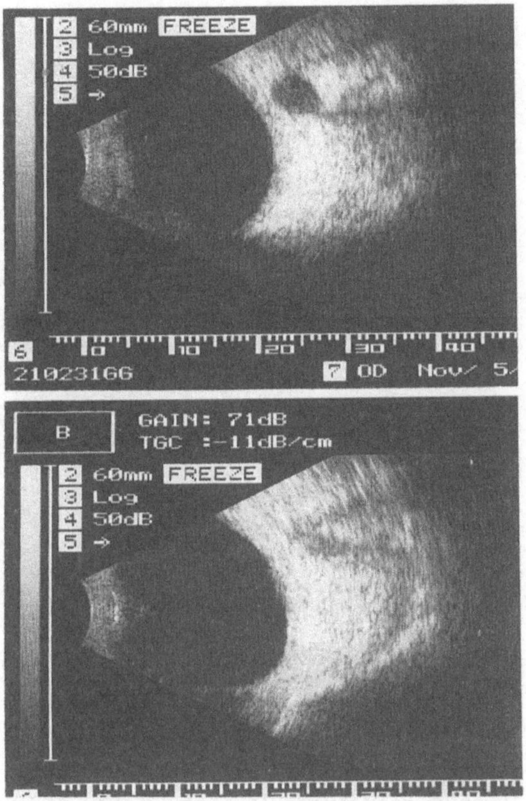

Fig. 1. Compression test in case no. 1. The venous lumen upwards in the orbit (top) collapses on transducer pressure from below, via lower lid, and directed posteriorly (bottom)

unambiguous, or, in 1984 we were not yet familiar with the typical ultrasonic features [4–7].

In the two male patients (case nos. 7 and 8) there was no bruit, and ultrasound findings were different. A 24-year-old male presented with a typical unilateral (left) orbital varix. When resting supine on the left side a marked proptosis of the eye appeared. He could produce it also by way of a Valsalva manoeuver during which the normal A-scan retrobulbar echogram changed to a cystic lesion causing a 10 mm forward shift in eye position; ophthalmoscopically there was arterial blink pulse, associated with transient visual loss.

The last patient, a 47-year-old man presented with a soft swelling in the upper nasal anterior orbit. Correspondingly, B-scan ultrasound demonstrated broad branching trunks with medium inner reflectivity. On A-scan arterial 'Schwirren' could barely be demonstrated. Clinical and ultrasonic appearance was not

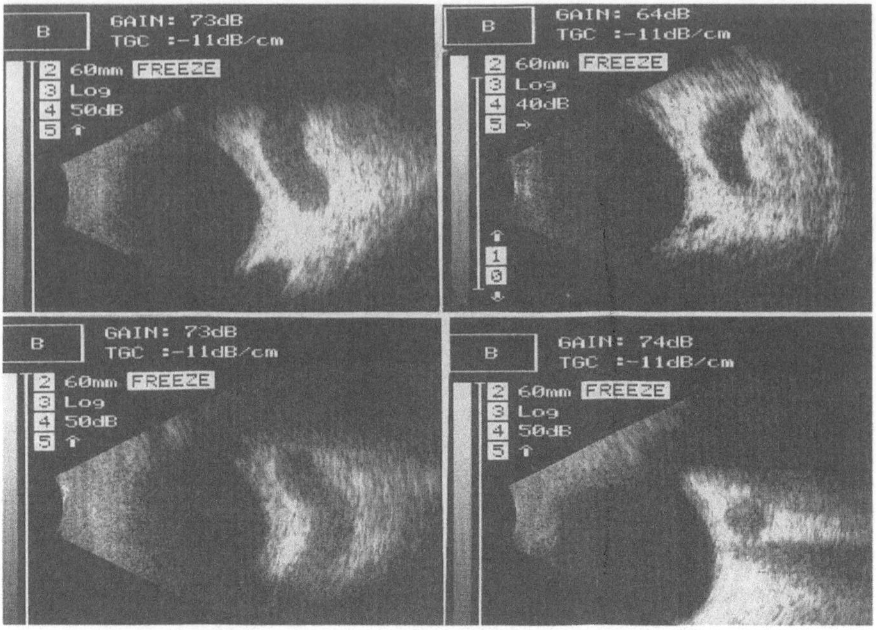

Fig. 2. Dilated sinuous orbital venous structures behind the bulb, in various sections, some transversely cut, some longitudinal. Case no. 2

influenced by a Valsalva manoeuver. Echographically, trunks were also seen behind the eye, together with an area with calcification (Fig. 3). Except for the latter finding, CT-scan showed no obvious lesions, but magnetic resonance-angiography amply imaged the venous plexes from the bridge of the nose, anteriorly, and backwards to the apex of the orbit and further back. The contrast pattern on magnetic resonance-scan suggested arterialized flow.

Concluding remarks

Ultrasound evaluation of the orbit should be performed early when assessing 'red eyes' if not otherwise explained. Anatomically the sinuous echographic trunks with smooth walls have no other natural correlate than venous structures. They are either varicose of nature, or mechanically distended in case of carotico-cavernous fistulas with reverse blood flow and increased pressure. Classical auscultation is still an essential procedure in diagnosing such cases.

Though primarily stressing the importance of the atraumatic ultrasound examination during clinical work-up, the present clinical report also emphasizes the usefulness of other imaging procedures, in particular for the planning of specific therapy when a conservative approach will not suffice [6].

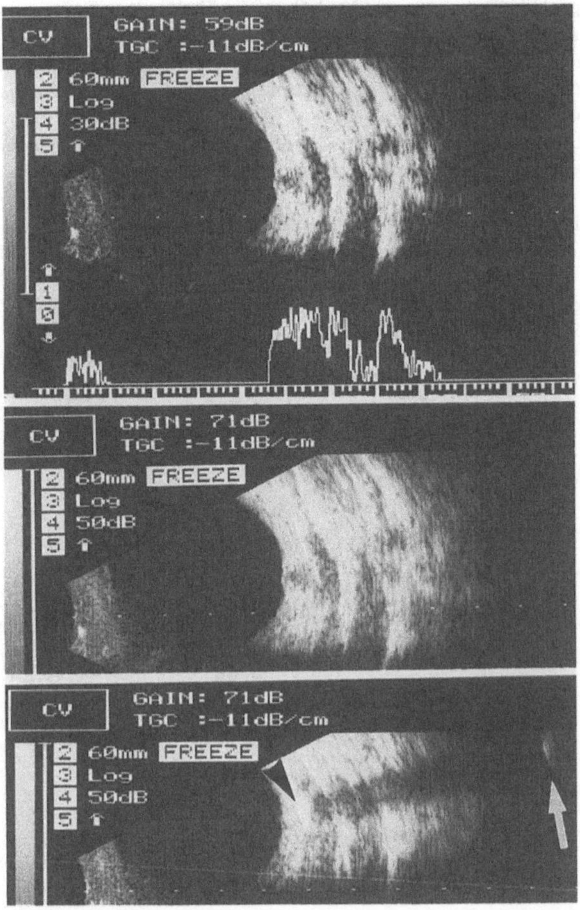

Fig. 3. Retrobulbar echograms (B-scan) in the last patient (case no. 8). The lumina of the vertically depicted structures show higher reflectivity than in Figs 1 and 2. A false optic nerve shadow is produced by a calcification just outside the eyewall (at bottom, black arrowhead; note also 'foreign body' duplicate echo far right, white arrow). Gains 59 db (top) and 71 db (middle and bottom)

References

[1] P.H. Madsen. Carotid cavernous fistulae. A study of 18 cases. Acta Ophthalmol. 1970;48:731.

[2] G. Brismar and J. Brismar. Spontaneous carotid-cavernous fistulas: Clinical symptomatology. Acta Ophthalmol. 1976;54:542.

[3] M.M. Slusher, B.R. Lennington, R.G. Weaver and C.H. Davis. Ophthalmic findings in dural arteriovenous shunts. Ophthalmology 1979;86:720.

[4] K.C. Ossoinig. Echographic differentiation of vascular tumours in the orbit. Docum. Ophthalmol. Proc. Ser. 1981;29:283.

[5] C.D. Phelps, H.S. Thompson and K.C. Ossoinig. The diagnosis of atypical carotid-cavernous fistula. Amer. J. Ophthalmol. 1982;43:423.
[6] D.L. Barrow, R.H. Spector, I.F. Braun, J.A. Landman, S.C. Tindall and G.T. Tindall. Classification and treatment of spontaneous carotid-cavernous sinus fistulas. J. Neurosurg. 1985;62:248.
[7] J.S. Jørgensen and R. Guthoff. 24 cases of carotid cavernous fistulas: frequency, symptoms, diagnosis and treatment. Acta Ophthalmol. 1985;63 Suppl. 173:67.

Hans C. Fledelius
University Eye Department E 2061
Rigshospitalet
2100 Copenhagen
Denmark

Axial eye length biometry and IOL calculations

49. Personalized intraocular lens power calculation. Importance of the optical profile

G.P. DESTRO, P.G. TOSCHI[1] and V. MAZZEO

(Ferrara and [1] Feltre (BL), Italy)

Abstract

Determination of intraocular lens power calculation for each surgeon and type of lens implant is the method of choice to obtain an accurate postoperative refraction prediction. Holladay and co-workers devised a personalized 'surgeon factor' that adjusts for any consistent bias in surgeon performance, whatever the source, based on a reversed application of their formula. In Sanders *et al.*'s method of calculating personal A-constants, the refraction factor is essential. Aflalo proposed different values for the refraction factor for various combinations of lens position and optic design. We compacted the actual and predicted refractions in 381 pseudophakic eyes, after surgery for posterior chamber implant performed by four different surgeons: 195 lenses were plano-convex, 186 biconvex. Each surgeon used plano-convex and biconvex implants. Postoperative refraction was calculated with four formulas: Holladay, SRK II, SRK II with personalization of A-constant obtained with the refraction factor proposed by Sanders *et al.* and by Aflalo (SRK II S, SRK II A). The A-constant, was related to lens design. The calculation error was the difference between the actual and predicted refractions for each eye. Plano-convex implants presented lower mean absolute errors than biconvex lenses using either individualized formulas (Holladay, SRK II S and SRK II A) or conventional SRK II (for plano-convex IOL, 0.64, 0.66, 0.66 and 0.75 diopters respectively versus 0.77, 0.87, 0.79 and 1.12 diopters for biconvex design). There was a significant difference between results obtained with various optical designs only for the SRK II ($p = 0.0009$) and SRK II S ($p = 0.002$) formulas. The personalized calculation with the Holladay surgeon factor and SRK II A reduced the error related to different lens design. This suggest that the Holladay surgeon factor and the more accurate determination of implant principal planes for the A-constant calculated with SRK II A led to a better postoperative refraction prediction.

Key words: Surgeon factor, A-constant, refraction factor, optic profile

G Cennamo and N. Rosa (eds.), Ultrasonography in Ophthalmology 15, pp. 401–407.

Introduction

Technological progress has led to new techniques for cataract surgery and for aphakia correction. Various types of intraocular lenses (IOL) are now available i.e. plano-convex, meniscus, laser-ridge plano-convex and biconvex. Intraocular lens power calculation formulas have been updated and prediction is now fairly accurate. Accuracy can be improved further with the personalization, for each surgeon and lens style, of some parameters of each formula [1,2]. The purpose of this study was to demonstrate the importance of personalizing the surgeon factor of the IOL power calculation and to investigate whether the implant optic profile affects postoperative refraction. We evaluated the SRK II and Holladay's formulas [2].

Materials and methods

From a database of 1470 cataract surgery cases, we selected 381 pseudophakic eyes for this study. Surgical procedures were performed at the University Eye Department of Ferrara (Italy) (U) and at the Ophthalmic Service of Feltre Hospital (Belluno, Italy) (H). All received a posterior chamber implant: 195 had plano-convex laser-ridge and 186 had biconvex (1:1) lenses (Table 1). Each of the four selected surgeons used lenses with the two different optical profiles and implanted at least 20 lenses of each type (Table 1).

The enrolled pseudophakic eyes fulfilled the following criteria: 1) postoperation best corrected visual acuity was at least 20/40 12 months after surgery; 2) no macular pathology, retinal detachment, corneal oedema and/or implant displacement. The mean age of the patients at surgery was 71 years (SD:11.1; ages between 46 and 87). The averaged keratometry (K) was measured with a Javal ophthalmometer (refractive index of 1.3375), the value obtained was transformed to the averaged corneal radius r with the formula: $r = 337.5/K$.

Table 1. Intraocular lenses used in this study. Type of optic design, medical center in which cataract surgery was performed and surgeon

Optic Design	Number (Center)	Manufacturer	Model	Number (Surgeon)
Plano-Convex	195 (U = 91; H = 104)	Cilco Cooper Vision	Sk21RU	91 (A = 47; B = 23; C = 21)
		Iolab	G756B	104 (D = 104)
Biconvex	186 (U = 102; H = 84)	Domilens	JB72	102 (A = 44; B = 26; C = 32)
		Pharmacia	155A	49 (D = 49)
		Amo	PC26TB	35 (D = 35)

U = Department of Ophthalmology, University of Ferrara; H = Ophthalmic Service, Feltre Hospital: A, B, C, D: surgeons

The contact technique was used for axial length (AL) measurements, with two different instruments according to the place of operation: 1) Ophthascan S (Biophysic Medical S.A., Clermont Ferrand, France) with A-scan contact biometry at 8 MHz at the Hospital Service (H); and 2) Ophthalmoscan Model 200 (Sonometrics System Inc. New York N.Y., U.S.A.) with an A-scan water-tip 17.5-MHz probe, at the University (U). In each patient the AL value was obtained from at least three measurements, chosen by the operator. Extra-capsular extraction with implants in the bag was the surgical technique used in both centers.

The spherical equivalent was calculated with two second-generation formulas: a regression formula SRK II [1] and a theoretical formula [2]. For each surgeon and for each IOL model, based on the data we have of almost twenty patients, we personalized the A-constant [3] using Sanders' original refraction factor (RF) or by calculating Holladay's surgeon factor. Personalization of these values is recommended for the regression formula, but is mandatory for Holladay's formula. Three SRK formulas were examined: simple SRK, where the A-constant is given by the manufacturer; SRK II S, where the A-constant is calculated using Sanders' refraction factor; SRK II A where the personalization was calculated using Aflalo's refraction factor.

The value of the real error of prediction (RErr) of each formula personalized or not for each eye (RErr = AR-PR, where: AR = spherical equivalent of postoperative correction that assures the best correct visual acuity; PR = predicted refraction) takes into consideration the signs (+) or (–), while the absolute error (AErr) takes into consideration the absolute value of this difference (AErr = I AR-PR I). The real errors were divided into positive and negative. The positive value indicated the tendency of the formula to overvalue the refractive effect of the implanted IOL. We determined the means of the absolute and real errors (MAR and MRE), and their standard deviations (ASD and RSD).

We divided the study population into two groups according to the type of IOL: plano-convex laser-ridge or biconvex, and evaluated the MAE (and ASD) for each group and for each formula.

The constant A of SRK II was personalized for each surgeon and type of lens with the Sanders formula [3]. For this individualized calculation of the constant A, we used the Sanders refraction factor [3], that takes account of the implant power (I) (RF = 1 if the power of the IOL is <= 16 D and RF = 1.5 if I >16) and the Rf proposed by Aflalo [6] that account of the optical profile and the implant site (Rf = 1.33 if plano-convex lens in the posterior chamber; Rf = 1.5 if biconvex in the posterior chamber; and Rf = 1.25 if meniscus or in the anterior chamber). Finally, we obtained, as mentioned above, three regression formulas: two personalized (SRK II S and SRK II A) arising from the use of the Sanders value of RF or that proposed by Aflalo, respectively, and one SRK II without personalized constant A.

To evaluate the predicted accuracy we compared the means and SD of the absolute errors using the one-sided variance test, and the Benferroni and

Student, and Newman and Keuls tests. For data collection and processing we used a IBM PC with the software Lotus 123 and SPSS.

Results

The mean axial length of the group was 23.12 mm (SD 1.06 mm), while the mean corneal power was 43.4 D (SD 1.435 D). We adopted Hoffer's method [5], to compare the results obtained with the three formulas. This method gives, for each formula, the percentage of the cases with absolute previsional errors ⩽ 1 or 2 D (Table 2) and the range between extreme positive and negative errors (RER, real error range). Moreover, we show the MRE and MAE, with RSD and ASD (Table 3).

As shown in Table 3, the mean of the absolute error was significantly greater with the non-personalized method (SRK II) than with the two personalized formulas (SRK II S and Holladay). The percentage of absolute error < 1 D, shown in Table 2 provides a more immediate comparison of the values obtained.

The mean of the absolute errors for plano-convex laser-ridge implants went

Table 2. Absolute error distribution for three formulas and two different optical profiles of IOL

	Optic design			
	Plano-convex		Biconvex	
Formula	AErr ⩽ 1D	AErr ⩽ 2D	AErr ⩽ 1D	AErr ⩽ 2D
SRK II	69.7%	96.4%	48.3%	88.2%
SRK II S	79%	98%	68.8%	90.4%
Holladay	79%	96.9%	75.2%	93%

AErr = absolute error

Table 3. Comparison between three formulas in all 381 eyes

Formula	MAE* (ASD*)	MRE* (RSD*)
SRK II	0.93 (0.72)	– 0.59 (1.02)
SRK II S	0.76 (0.68)	0.09 (1.01)
Holladay	0.70 (0.64)	– 0.05 (0.95)
	($p = 0.001$)	($p = 0.000$)

SRK II S = SRK II formula with A-constant personalized for each surgeon and type of IOL using Sanders refraction factor; MAE = mean absolute error; ASD = standard deviation of absolute error; MRE = mean real error; RSD = standard deviation of real error; * in diopters

Table 4. Correlation between optic design and predictive formulas

	Optic design			Optic design	
	Plano-convex	Biconvex	Statistics	Plano-convex	Biconvex
Formula	MAE (ASD)	MAE (ASD)	p	MRE (SD)	MRE (RSD)
SRK II	0.75 (0.61)	1.12 (0.78)	0.000	–0.42 (0.87)	–0.77 (1.12)
SRK II	0.66 (0.55)	0.87 (0.78)	0.002	0.06 (0.85)	0.18 (1.15)
Holladay	0.64 (0.57)	0.77 (0.7)	0.06	–0.07 (0.86)	–0.04 (1.04)
	(p = 0.115)	(p = 0.000)			

MAE = mean absolute error, ASD = standard deviation of absolute error, MRE = mean real error and RSD = standard deviation of real error, in diopters, for three formulas and two optical profiles. SRK II S = SRK II formula with A-constant personalized for each surgeon and type of IOL, using Sanders refraction factor

Table 5. Comparison between results obtained with personalized A-constant of SRK II formula with refraction factor Rf (5) by Retzlaff et al. [3]

	Optic design			Optic design			
	Plano-convex	Biconvex	Analysis	Plano-convex		Biconvex	
Formula	MAE* (SD)*	MAE* (SD*)	p	AErr ≤ 1D	AErr ≤ 2D	AErr ≤ 1D	AErr ≤ 2D
SRK II	S0.66 (0.55)	0.87 (0.78)	0.002	79%	98%	68.8%	90.4%
SRK II A	0.66 (0.55)	0.79 (0.74)	0.051	79.5%	98.5%	73.2%	93.1%

(SRK II S) and those using the same formula, but different Rf according to the optical profile of IOL by Aflalo; MAE = mean absolute error; SD = standard deviation; p = result of statistical analysis; AErr = absolute error. *in diopters

from 0.64 D (Holladay) to 0.75 D (SRK II); the difference was not significant (Table 3). The mean of absolute errors for the biconvex lenses, was higher with all three formulas: from 0.77 D (Holladay) 1.12 D (SRK II); the difference was significant ($p = 0.0009$). The personalization of the formula reduced the possibility of error with the plano-convex implants and, particularly, with the biconvex implants; therefore with the Holladay formula (unlike formulas SRK and SRK II S), the difference between the optical profiles was not significant. The ratio of absolute errors 1 D (Table 2) confirmed this observation.

Personalization of the A-constant for each surgeon and IOL model, obtained by substituting the original Sanders refraction factor [3] with that proposed by Aflalo [4] (SRK II A), improved the previsional accuracy of the SRK II personalized formula, especially in the case of biconvex lenses (Table 5). The comparison with laser-ridge plano-convex IOL was not statistically significant ($p = 0.051$); the mean of the absolute errors was reduced (from 0.87 to 0.79 D) and the ratio of these errors ≤ 1 D was increased from 68.8% to 73.2%.

Discussion

This study demonstrates that personalization of formulas for each surgeon and each type of lens results in a high predictive accuracy of the postoperative refraction and of the implant power. High predictive accuracy was obtained with the regression type calculation of IOL (SRK II S, personalized using the Sanders refraction factor, and SRK II using the Aflalo Rf) and with Holladay's theoretical approach (see Tables 3 and 5).

The optical profile of the implant is crucial in the individual regression formula, while it does not influence the Holladay formula. In any event, the prediction errors were higher with the biconvex profile than with the laser-ridge plano-convex lenses (Tables 4 and 5). This finding contrasts with Shammas' report of more accurate calculations with biconvex IOL [6,7].

Through the data obtained from the values of the postoperative refraction and from the IOL implanted, each surgeon who uses a single type of implant can know the relation that these have with the preoperative variables (axial length and mean corneal power).

Aflalo suggests relating the refraction factor to the IOL position and optical profile to account for the different positions of the principal planes of the implants. According to the different profiles of the lenses used, the principal image planes are: near the anterior face with the plano-convex, more to the back if biconvex, and in front for the meniscus lenses with convex anterior surface.

Using different refractions based on the profile of IOL, we studied personalized A-constants for each surgeon and each kind of lens. This calculation reduces the prediction error of the biconvex implants of non statistically significant values in contrast with the laser-ridge plano-convex IOL used (Table 5).

The Holladay formula ensured the best accuracy, for the whole group and for the optical profiles of the implanted IOL. Personalization of the surgeon factor reduces the effect of various sources of errors (position and type of implant, biometry, corneal power, suture, surgeon ability, reliability of the calculation, postoperative use of steroids). Because the surgeon factor compensates for the difference in the optical profile of IOL, individualization of the formula of the lens used would appear to be unnecessary. However, calculation of the surgeon factor is still very difficult.

References

[1] D. Sanders, J. Retzlaff and M. Kraff. Comparison of SRK II formula and other second generation formulas. J. Cataract Refract Surg. 1988;14:136–141.

[2] J.T. Holladay, T.C. Prager, T.J. Chandler, K.H. Musgrove, J.W. Lewis and R.S. Ruitz. A three-part system for refining intraocular lens power calculation. J. Cataract Refract. Surg. 1988;14:17–24.

[3] J. Retzlaff, D. Sanders and M. Kraff. A manual of implant power calculation including SRK II formula. Oregon: Medford, 1988.

[4] G. Aflalo. Evaluation du coefficient de refraction par la formule théorique de calcul de puissance d'implant. J. Fr. Ophthalmol. 1991;14:455–461.
[5] K.J. Hoffer. Accuracy of ultrasound intraocular lens calculation. Arch. Ophthalmol. 1981;99: 1819–1823.
[6] H.J. Shammas. Accuracy of lens power calculation with the biconvex and meniscus intraocular lenses. Am. J. Ophthalmol. 1988;106:613–615.
[7] H.J. Shammas. Accuracy of lens power calculation with the biconvex and meniscus intraocular lenses (Reply to correspondence). Am. J. Ophthalmol. 1989;107:309.

Prof. Vincenzina Mazzeo
via Polonia 79
44100 Ferrara, Italy

[1]Comunità Montana Feltrina
Presidio Ospedaliero
Divisione di Oculistica
Unità Locale Socio-Sanitaria, n. 4
32032 Feltre, Italy

50. Biopen, Ophthascan S and Biovision: comparison between the various biometric measurements

T. AVITABILE, M.G. UVA, L. FRANCO and R. GHIRLANDA
(Catania, Italy)

Abstract

We compared the measurements of the antero-posterior and latero-lateral eye diameter obtained with a hand-held biometric ruler (Biopen) and with contact biometry using the Ophthascan S instrument (Biophysic Medical) in 30 patients (60 eyes) affected by various ocular conditions, i.e., cataract, surgical aphakia), myopia and hypermetropia. Biopen proved to be as accurate as the traditional equipment, and unlike other equipment, it can be used by non-echographers, and in cases in which the patient cannot be moved.

Key words: Biometry, Biopen, Biovision, Ophthascan S, antero-posterior and latero-lateral diameters

Introduction

In recent years, ocular biometry has reached excellent levels of precision and accuracy. These procedures have been largely automated and simplified. Early biometric evaluations were somewhat complicated. The biometry performed by Kretz, for example, lacked the possibility of freezing the image; there was no immediate conversion of microseconds into millimeters; it was necessary to carry out the measurements on Polaroid and to resort to the immersion technique using A-scan. Nowadays more practical and faster biometers have been developed, leading to the advent of computerized equipments able to perform contact biometries without immersion technique A-scan and equipped not only with auto-freezing and automatic calculation but also probes with a light that provides a better fixation of the patient (1–3).

Among this new generation of biometers is the hand-held battery-run Biopen. This is roughly the size of a pen and it enables us to measure the antero-posterior and latero-lateral diameter of phakic and aphakic eyes simply and quickly. This apparatus is particularly useful in cases where it is necessary to perform a biometry at the patient's bedside. It emits ultrasounds at a frequency

G Cennamo and N. Rosa (eds.), Ultrasonography in Ophthalmology 15, pp. 409–414.

of 12 MHz and a speed of 1555 m/sec in phakic eyes and 1537 m/sec in aphakic eyes.

Biopen contains an internal microprocessor that records and stores the numerous measurements obtained after applanation and hence after the return of the ultrasonic waves, reflected by the lens and retina. The final measure, which is an average of all the others, is obtained within a few seconds (4–7).

We have evaluated the accuracy of the biometries performed with this new equipment by comparing them with those obtained with the Ophthascan S equipped with the standard 8 MHz A-scan probe, and with the Biovision instrument equipped with a 13 MHz contact probe.

Materials and Methods

Before beginning the study, we carried out 20 examinations, including ones performed with tissue model, in order to acquire a degree of dexterity with this new instrument. The results of these 20 examinations were not included in this evaluation.

We examined 60 eyes of patients ranging from 35 to 76 years of age, suffering from such eye conditions as emmetropia, cataract, surgical aphakia, myopia and hypermetropia. In particular, six eyes were emmetropic (without eye disease), 27 were suffering from cataract, six from surgical aphakia, 12 from myopia and nine from hypermetropia. None of them were affected by corneal disorders of any kind.

We measured the antero-posterior and latero-lateral diameter of each of these eyes, first with the Ophthascan S and the Biovision instruments, then with the Biopen instruments, and recorded the values obtained.

The technique used with the Ophthascan S was the classic immersion technique with A-scan and image freezing at the maximum reflectivity. The contact technique was used for the latero-lateral diameter. With the Biovision instrument, on the other hand, measurements of the antero-posterior and latero-lateral diameter were taken using the contact technique. Five measurements of the antero-posterior diameter and five measurements of the latero-lateral diameter were made with both instruments, and their respective average was calculated. The same procedure was performed with the Biopen.

After a local anaesthetic, the Biopen must be placed perpendicularly on the patient's cornea. Contact between it and the instrument is signalled by a beep which represents the start of the ultrasound emissions. Then the different measurements begin, but only those that remain perpendicular are picked up by the sound signal and shown in millimetres on the display. After working out their average, the instrument stops automatically and the value obtained appears on the display. However, it must be stressed that, in measurements of the antero-posterior diameter, one must take into account only those values beneath which four lines appear. These lines indicate that both the anterior and posterior surface of the lens and the retino-choroidal complex measurements may be considered reliable.

To measure the latero-lateral diameter, the Ophthascan S standard A-scan probe, the Biovision probe and the Biopen must be placed in contact with the eyeball on the equatorial meridian at about 13 mm from the limbus, after measurement with a compass. However, the Biopen's start button must be pressed twice consecutively, and measurements can be taken only after the display shows the letters 'APHC' (aphakic).

For a comparison of the data, we began by considering the average and the standard deviation of all the values obtained respectively with the biometry of the antero-posterior and the latero-lateral diameter performed with the different instruments (Table 1). Subsequently we calculated the range in which these values fluctuated and then took into account the different groups singly (emmetropia, cataracts, aphakia, myopia and hypermetropia) repeating the above method for each of them (Tables 2–6). We then compared the results obtained with these three instruments.

Table 1. All the eyes

	Ophthascan S	Biovision	Biopen
(A.P.)			
Average	23.94	23.92	23.84
SD	1.99	1.98	2.01
(L.L.)			
Average	23.58	23.53	23.48
SD	1.70	1.68	1.73

Table 2. Emmetropic eyes

	Ophthascan S	Biovision	Biopen
(A.P.)			
Average	23.30	23.22	22.85
SD	0.36	0.30	0.51
(L.L.)			
Average	23.30	23.25	23.07
SD	0.17	0.24	0.39

Table 3. Eyes with cataract

	Ophthascan S	Biovision	Biopen
(A.P.)			
Average	23.64	23.67	23.58
SD	1.18	1.22	1.20
(L.L.)			
Average	23.52	23.5	23.28
SD	1.05	1.01	1.02

Table 4. Aphakic eyes

	Ophthascan S	Biovision	Biopen
(A.P.)			
Average	23.55	23.48	23.24
SD.	0.92	1.05	1.20
(L.L.)			
Average	23.05	22.98	22.75
SD	1.34	1.25	1.72

Table 5. Myopic eyes

	Ophthascan S	Biovision	Biopen
(A.P.)			
Average	27.50	27.45	27.41
SD	1.46	1.37	1.52
(L.L.)			
Average	26.35	26.42	26.48
SD	1.35	1.30	1.21

Table 6. Hypermetropic eyes

	Ophthascan S	Biovision	Biopen
(A.P.)			
Average	22.37	22.35	22.38
SD	0.41	0.38	0.45
(L.L.)			
Average	22.07	22.05	22.17
SD	0.44	0.41	0.34

Results

The differences between the average values considered both globally and in the single groups with all three instruments were not statistically significant. The *t* and *p* values of the antero-posterior and latero-lateral diameter respectively were:

		Biopen vs OPHTH.	Biopen vs Biovision
– All the eyes:	A.P.	*t* =\0.274 *p* =\0.785	*t* =\0.220 *p* =\0.287
	L.L.	*t* =\0.319 *p* =\0.750	*t* =\0.161 *p* =\0.873
– Emmetropic eyes:	A.P.	*t* =\1.766 *p* =\0.108	*t* =\1.532 *p* =\0.157
	L.L.	*t* =\1.324 *p* =\0.215	*t* =\0.963 *p* =\0.358
– Eyes with cataract:	A.P.	*t* =\0.192 *p* =\0.849	*t* =\0.273 *p* =\0.786
	L.L.	*t* =\0.852 *p* =\0.398	*t* =\0.796 *p* =\0.429
– Aphakic eyes:	A.P.	*t* =\0.502 *p* =\0.626	*t* =\0.369 *p* =\0.720
	L.L.	*t* =\0.337 *p* =\0.743	*t* =\0.265 *p* =\0.796
– Myopic eyes:	A.P.	*t* =\0.148 *p* =\0.884	*t* =\0.068 *p* =\0.947
	L.L.	*t* =\-0.248 *p* =\0.806	*t* =\-0.117 *p* =\0.908
– Hypermetropic eyes:	A.P.	*t* =\-0.049 *p* =\0.961	*t* =\-0.153 *p* =\0.880
	L.L.	*t* =\-0.540 *p* =\0.597	*t* =\-0.676 *p* =\- 0.509

Discussion and Conclusions

The past decade has seen enormous progress in the surgical methods used in cataract surgery with IOL implants. In this context, ultrasonography has played a decisive role with regard to the measurement of the axial length for the purpose of calculating the power of the IOL to be implanted. In fact, the measurement must be accurate because even the slightest difference can determine a refractive error which may qualitatively alter the success of the surgery. In this context, we did not find any significant differences between the values obtained with the Ophthascan S and with the Biovision, which are widely approved instruments, and those obtained with the Biopen instrument. Indeed, the latter has the advantage not only of the accuracy, demonstrated in the comparison above, but also of being a hand-held, fairly manageable instrument that does not require extensive training, methylcellulose or complex techniques for its use. As the instrument is placed in direct contact with the cornea, the minimum pressure possible is obviously necessary to avoid affecting the measurement of the axial length of the eyeball.

References

[1] R.D. Binkhorst. The accuracy of ultrasonic measurements of the axial length of the eye. Ophthalmic Surg. 1981; 12:363.

[2] H.J. Shammas. A comparison of immersion and contact techniques for axial length measurement. Am. Intraocul. Implant. Soc. J. 1984; 10:444.

[3] J.M. Thijssen. Instrumentation and techniques for biometry. Doc. Ophth. Proc. Ser. Ophthalmic Echography. Edited by K.C. Ossoining, Martinus Nijhoff Dr Junk Publishers 1987; 48:1–5.

[4] S.E. Feldon and D.A. Wallace. A new generation of diagnostic ultrasonic instrumentation: the Biopen biometric ruler and Pachpen pachymeter. Kugler, Berkeley: Ghedini Ed. 1988; 1:602–608.

[5] R.M. Kristensen, D.A. Lee, R.E. Kristensen and L. Wynbrandt. A clinical evaluation of the Biopen. Am. J. Ophthalmol. 1989; 107:596–600.

[6] W. Hauff. Biometry. An exact method for the measurement of the axial length of the eye. Wien Klin. Wochenschr. 1983; 95:271.

[7] K.C. Ossoining. Standardized echography. Basic principle, clinical applications, and results. Int. Ophthalmol. Clin. 1979; 19:127.

T. Avitabile
Institute of Ophthalmology
Catania University
Catania, Italy

51. Unexpected ametropia after intraocular lens implantation: The role of different factors of ultrasound biometry and surgery

A. SERES, J. NÉMETH and I. SÜVEGES
(Budapest, Hungary)

Abstract

We analysed the data of 389 patients aged 68 years ($\pm$12 SD) to investigate the role of technical and biological factors on the final refractive results of patients with extracapsular cataract extraction and intraocular lens (IOL) implantation. We use the term of 'unexpected ametropia' for the difference between the final refractive result and the value theoretically expected according to the biometry, keratometry and IOL data (SRK-II formula). Using analysis of variance or, in one case, the two-tailed T-test, the following factors were analysed: implanted lens type, surgeon, biometry operator, waveform of the vitreoretinal spike on the biometry scans and cataract density.

On average, there was an unexpected shift of +0.32 D in the final patient refraction. Although the skills of the 18 surgeons differed greatly, we found a significant difference between recalculated (personalised) A-constants of only 3 colleagues. Cataract density and biometry operator did not significantly affect the result. Surprisingly, there was a statistically significant difference between the two IOL types implanted in 92% of our cases for the recalculated A-constants. These two lens types are produced by the same company and claimed to have the same A-constants by the manufacturer. Although the unexpected refractive error was found to be acceptable and similar to the data in the literature, our results underline the need of constant systematic control of all the factors influencing the IOL power calculations and the IOLs used.

Key words: Intraocular lens power calculation, SRK-II, personalized A-constant

Introduction

A review of the literature and our own experience suggests that implanting an intraocular lens (IOL) during cataract surgery with a power predicted by ultrasound biometry generally gives satisfactory results. However, there are inevitably some sources of errors, which, if one knows their origin, can be avoided.

G Cennamo and N. Rosa (eds.), Ultrasonography in Ophthalmology 15, pp. 415–420.

Different surgical techniques (different surgeons) can result in different refractive results when implanting IOL of the same power. To overcome this it was suggested that the A-constant for the different surgeons be recalculated [1,2]. Not only technical factors but also biological factors such as accuracy and precision of the device used for biometry, the keratometer, the way they are used, and the condition of the eye of the patient can cause significant differences as well as systematic deviations from the presumed result [3]. The aim of this study was to investigate the influence of some of these factors on the final refractive outcome of our patients who had undergone cataract surgery with IOL implantation.

Patients and methods

We reviewed the files of all patients who had undergone cataract surgery in our Department from January 1 to the end of September 1993 ($n=582$). The average age of the patients was 67.5 ± 12.2 years (mean $\pm$ SD). For this study we applied strict inclusion and exclusion criteria: only patients who had undergone extracapsular cataract extraction with posterior chamber lens implantation (ECCE+PCL) were included, phakoemulsifications, secondary or suture fixated intraocular lens implantations, combined procedures (ECCE+PCL+perforating keratoplasty, triple procedure) were excluded. We also excluded patients if the biometry or follow-up data in the files were incomplete or if the follow-up was less than 5 weeks. Thirdly, we excluded all eyes with best corrected visual acuity (BCVA) less than 0.3 since we believe that if the spherical component of the final refraction of the patient is measured by reading charts, in cases in which BCVA is below this limit the refraction data can be unreliable for our purposes. A total of 389 eyes were included in this study.

The preoperative ultrasound biometry was performed by 11 colleagues, mostly residents. We used the Ultrascan Digital System 2000 device with a 10 MHz, focused, soft-tip hand-held probe and the contact method. The system gain was kept at 48 dB. The keratometry readings were done by using a Javal-Schiöt type ophthalmometer. For the IOL power calculations the SRK-II formula with the software built in the ultrasound device was used. Because we have no digital archive of the biometry scans, we used the printouts of our ultrasound device for the analysis of the waveform of the vitreoretinal spike.

We classified the eyes into groups according to the density of the cataract before surgery using a Volk 90 D lens. The groups were as follows: 1) fundus structures can be clearly seen; 2) parts of the fundus are visible; 3) only red reflex; 4) no red reflex; and 5) special types of cataract (congenital, traumatic).

As mentioned earlier, all the 389 eyes were operated using the standard extracapsular method, by 17 different surgeons. The skill of the surgeons differed greatly because they included specialists with several hundreds cataract operations per year, and residents with less than 10 operations a year. We have implanted 20 different types of IOL from different manufacturers; two of these were implanted in 91.5% of the cases, so only the results obtained with these two models were used for this study.

The postoperative refraction was recorded as the correction giving the best results in reading charts from 5 meters. For patients with astigmatism the spherical equivalent was used. The average postoperative follow-up for refraction was 9.3 weeks, all exceeding 5 weeks.

Our patients are not necessarily planned to be corrected to emmetropia, so the term 'unexpected' ametropia was introduced, i.e., the difference between postoperative refraction and the refraction the patient should have had with the IOL that had been implanted (expected refraction, calculated using the SRK-II formula). Therefore, we eliminated the errors that can arise from mistyping data or misselection of the lens during operation by attaching an information sheet to the patients' files immediately after the implantation. However, this procedure does not eliminate doubts arising from the manufacturer's mislabeling [4].

To investigate the role of the above-mentioned factors in causing unexpected deviations in refraction we performed analyses of variance (ANOVA), or in one case, the two tailed t-test for the unexpected refraction error. We also recalculated the A-constant for all the eyes and by applying ANOVA for the recalculated A, we obtained an individual A-constant for the specific factor (surgeon, biometry operator, quality of vitreoretinal spike, lens type, cataract density). The unexpected refraction error in diopters and the recalculated A-constants cover the same phenomenon and are strongly related to each other. Refraction error is usually given in diopters; however, in this paper we mainly use the individual A-constants, because if the different factors differ significantly from the theoretical values, this kind of data can easily be used to select the correct lens diopters prior to surgery.

Results

From January 1 to the end of September, 1994, 389 patients underwent ECCE+PCL surgery, having BCVA acuity better than 0.3. The average unexpected refraction error was $+0.32 \pm 1.05$ (mean $\pm$ SD). This difference from 0 was significant ($p < 0{,}001$). Of the 389 patients, 286 (74%) had an unexpected refraction error below 1 D, 363 (93%) below 2 D, 380 (98%) below 3 D. Only 9 of these patients (2%) had an unexpected refraction error above 3. Figure 1 shows the distribution of the unexpected refraction errors. Our results correlate well with data in the literature [5,6].

Two models of IOL produced by the same company were implanted in most of the cases (91.5%). The factory A-constant is the same (118.9) for both. After recalculating the A-constant for the two types of IOL we found that the recalculated A-constants differed significantly from each other and also from the factory value (Table 1).

As a measure of proper alignment of the transducer and consequently of the perpendicularity of the ultrasound beam to the retinal surface, we analyzed the

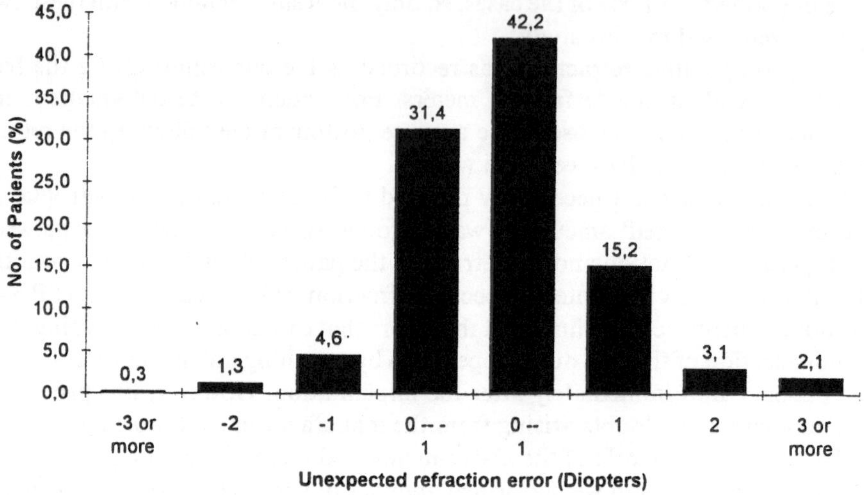

Fig. 1. The distribution of the unexpected refraction error (diopters)

Table 1. Results for different IOL models (A, B)

	All lenses	IOL - A	IOL - B
No. of eyes	389	145	211
Unexpected error (D)	0.32	0.50	0.18
Recalculated A	119.37	119.65	119.17
Intergroup differences			
All lenses	–	$p < 0.001$	$p < 0.001$
IOL – A	–	–	$p < 0.001$

posterior wall waveform on the reprints of the A-scans. Theoretically the number of breakpoints correlate to the perpendicularity of the ultrasound beam. Dividing the eyes into groups according to the number of breakpoints, no significant difference was found in the unexpected error or in the recalculated A-constant. There was no significant difference as to cataract densities between the groups mentioned earlier.

We also recalculated the A-constant for the different surgeons. In Fig. 2 the surgeons are listed from left to right according to the number of cases they operated in the study period. Although the recalculated A-constant varied between surgeons, a significant difference was found only between surgeons A, I and N.

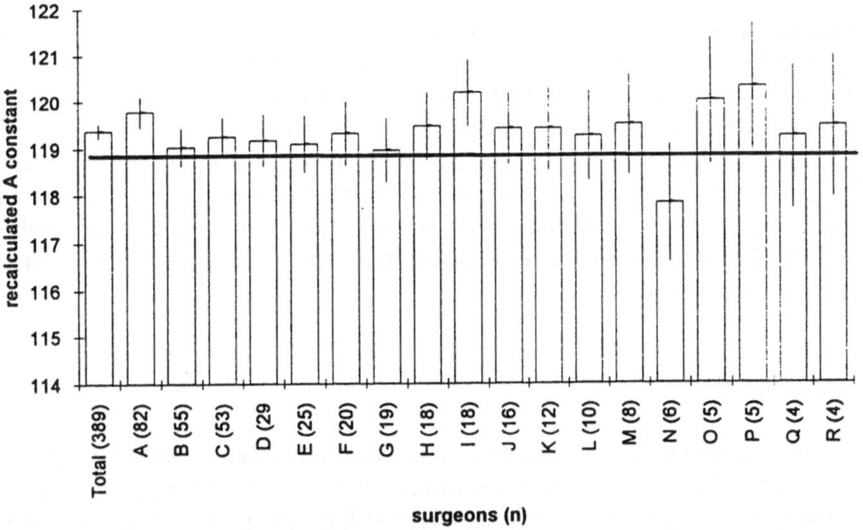

Fig. 2. Recalculated A-constants for different surgeons. The surgeons are listed from left to right according to the number of operations performed in this series. The vertical lines on the bars are the 95% confidence intervals of ANOVA. The horizontal line represents the factory A-constant (118.9)

Discussion

An overall + 0.32 D unexpected refractive error was found in this series of cases. For the A-constant it is equivalent to 0.47, so the difference in the IOL power to be implanted is close to +0.5 diopters. The distribution of the unexpected refraction error of the patients is very similar to other reports. In this paper we shall not review the possible causes of the systematic error. However, using a practically modified A factor we can shift the difference between our expected and final refraction results towards 0 D.

Since a soft tip contact method was used for the biometry, the indentation of the cornea is a possible source of error. The significant differences found in between axial length measurements made with the contact and immersion methods [7,8] are probably due to the indentation of the cornea using the contact method. An incorrect technique, and the excessive indentation may be specific of the biometry operator. Anyway, there were no significant differences between the examiners.

Turning to the results on other factors that can, in theory, influence the success of IOL power calculation, similar to other authors [9], we compared the different types of lens implanted. The significant difference between two IOL models, claimed by the manufacturer to have the same A-constant, casts doubts on these factory data. We suggest that not too many types of IOL be used and that regular statistic controls be made so that any differences can be detected.

The fact that we did not detect significant differences between groups of A-scans that differed in the number of vitreoretinal spikes means that the 'built-in expert' of our biometry device and the judgement of the examiner (in our practice the examiner selects from five stored scans, all accepted by the machine) are sufficiently efficient to avoid gross errors.

The recalculation of the A-constant for surgeons is a longstanding practice. Similar recalculation for the biometry examiners is important to control their work. Any significant differences between examiners are indicative of methodical mistakes and represent a reminder that these colleagues need constant control and training.

Conclusion

From the statistical analysis of the refractive results of 389 eyes that had undergone cataract surgery it seems that the whole system of keratometry – ultrasound biometry, lens selection and surgery, works well in our clinic. A systematic shift of 0.32 D was found in the refraction results which seems to be acceptable, although it can easily be taken into consideration in the future. The factors most responsible for variability were the surgeon and the IOL type. Variability arising from the surgical technique has long been known, but we did not expect to find significant differences between the IOL types. Similar regular controls are needed to keep the variability of our postoperative refraction within an acceptable range.

References

[1] J. Retzlaff, D. Sanders and M. Kraff. A manual of implant power calculation, SRK TM formula. Chicago: 1982.

[2] H.J. Shammas. Atlas of ophthalmic ultrasonography and biometry. St. Louis, Toronto: The C.V. Mosby Company, 1984;292–293.

[3] J. Németh. Sources of Errors in Intraocular Lens Power Calculation. In: Ravalico (ed.) Iatrogenic Damage in Ophthalmology. Trieste: 1992;185–189.

[4] T. Olsen and H. Olsen. IOL power mislabeling. Acta Ophthalmologica 1993;71:99–102.

[5] M.S. Dang and P.P. Sunder Raj. SRK II formula in the calculation of intraocular lens power. British Journal of Ophthalmology 1989;73:823–826.

[6] E. Frisch, G. Chaine, A. Gaudric and G. Coscas. Validité de prédiction après implant standard et implant calculé selon la formule SRK. Jr. Fr. Ophthalmol. 1989;12:13–16.

[7] H.J. Shammas. A comparison of immersion and contact techniques for axial length measurements. Am. Intraocul. Lens Implant. Soc. J. 1984;10:444–447.

[8] T. Olsen and P.T. Nielsen. Immersion versus contact technique in the measurement of axial length by ultrasound. Acta Ophthalmologica 1989;67:101–102.

[9] H.J. Rouhainen. Intraocular lens power calculation. A retrospective analysis of its practical value. Acta Ophthalmologica 1989;67:79–82.

András Seres
SOTE 1st Department of Ophthalmology
1083 Budapest, Töm u. 25–29
Hungary

52. On the importance of the ratio between axial eye length and corneal curvature radius for intraocular lens prediction after cataract surgery. Further investigations, with the emphasis on low-ratio eyes

H.C. FLEDELIUS and M. FICH
(Hillerød, Denmark)

Abstract

Previous studies have indicated the importance of the ratio between axial length (AL) and corneal curvature radius (Crad) for the size of the intraocular lens calculation error in cataract series. Skew Al:Crad ratios being found, in particular, in very long and very short eyes, this anomalous finding may be (at least partly) responsible for the reduced prediction accuracy often reported in eyes that are either short or long.

A low ratio <2.8) has been reported in 5–6% of all eyes. We compared 10 such eyes with 15 mid-ratio and 10 high-ratio eyes and found that even updated theoretical formulas appear to have difficulty in correctly assessing intraocular lens power prior to cataract surgery.

Key words: Cataract surgery, axial eye length, corneal curvature, intraocular lens prediction

Introduction

In an attempt to identify eyes likely to give prediction error after cataract surgery with intraocular lens (IOL) insertion, we previously focused on the importance of the ratio between axial length (AL) and corneal curvature radius (Crad). In the context of SIDUO, the paper given in Tokyo in 1992 described a sample of patients with a discrepancy between empirical and theoretical IOL prediction formulas. Completely different AL:Crad ratio values were obtained in this group when compared with a series of cataract patients in whom there was fair agreement between empirical and theoretical IOL prediction formulas.

Eyes with a fair prediction agreement between methods were characterized by a correlation between the two parameters (resulting in an around-median ratio range of 2.80–3.05) and prediction error was generally small. In contrast, the prediction discrepancy group showed AL:Crad values outside the range given

G Cennamo and N. Rosa (eds.), Ultrasonography in Ophthalmology 15, pp. 421–425.

above, predominantly on the high side (mainly in long eyes), and prediction error was more evident. In particular, this held for the theoretical formula then used in our clinic (Binkhorst).

Here we focus on low-ratio eyes, i.e. eyes with relatively short axes and flat corneae. Having replaced the Binkhorst formula as chosen routine, the Catrefract IOL prediction program [1] is compared to SRK II.

Material and methods

Ten consecutive eyes with a low AL:Crad ratio (2.61–2.79) were identified from the Catrefract database. A mid-ratio group (n = 15, actual ratio range 2.83–3.05) and a high ratio group (n = 10; 3.11–3.68) were also selected for comparison purposes. Median ages were 71–74 years in the three groups; 23 were females, 12 males.

Keratometry and axial ultrasound measurements were performed by NIDEK KM-800 and Echoscan US-3000, respectively. All patients had posterior chamber lenses, of only a few brands. Follow-up time concerning final refraction was 4–14 months. Prediction error evaluated with the methods under study was given as predicted minus actual refractive value, in D.

Results

Table 1 shows the mean values and standard deviation, median values, and ranges, for the three ratio groups. The AL and Crad values, taken separately, overlap considerably from group to group. This is particularly true of Crad values. However, the selection of a low-ratio group implies a feature of small eyes with less steep corneae. Contrarily, the high-ratio group trend is towards long axes and corneal curvatures that 'have not followed the axial length'.

In contrast to the mid- and high-ratio groups, there were obvious prediction errors in the low-ratio group, and there was a significant systematic trend associated to the prediction method. Typically, Catrefract predicted to the high side, towards plus, while SRK II slightly underestimated. This can be clearly seen in Figure 1.

Discussion

The possible role of the AL:Crad ratio in routine IOL prediction has been analysed by various approaches. Initially, in a follow-up series we found that prediction error (then by Binkhorst and SRK) correlated stronger to the AL:Crad ratio than to its two constituents, axial length and corneal curvature radius taken separately [2].

Next, a poor fit between Binkhorst and SRK II made up the selection basis

Table 1. Oculometry, keratometry, and prediction error results in the three subgroups, as defined by a low, a mid, and a high ratio between AL and Crad, respectively. Mean value (SD) at top, median value (range) below

	Low ratio AL: C-rad n = 10	Mid-ratio n = 15	High ratio n = 10
Axial length (mm)	21.43 (0.82) 21.36 (20.25–22.74)	23.26 (0.79) 23.33 (21.76–24.6)	25.28 (2.11) 24.65 (23.3–29.9)
C-rad (mm)	7.93 (0.23) 7.99 (7.52–8.20)	7.88 (0.21) 7.89 (7.51–8.35)	7.70 (0.29) 7.69 (7.17–8.15)
Ratio AL:C–rad	2.70 (0.06) 2.70 (2.61–2.79)	2.96 (0.06) 2.96 (2.83–3.05)	3.27 (0.17) 3.23 (3.11–3.68)
Refraction (D) after IOL	0.95 (1.95) 0.63 (–1.5 – 4.25)	–0.23 (0.90) –0.25 (–2 – 2.25)	–1.46 (1.10) –1.32 (–3.25 – 0.5)
Prediction error (D) by Catrefract	1.39 (0.86) 1.36 (–0.15 – 2.67)	0.18 (0.52) 0.26(–0.61 – 1.49)	0.02 (0.63) 0.03 (–1.49 – 0.81)
Prediction error (D) by SRK2	–0.65 (0.80) –0.48 (–2.01 – 0.34)	–0.23 (0.60) –0.29 (–1.19 – 1.25)	0.25 (1.03) 0.59 (–1.62 – 1.62)

for the study reported at SIDUO XIV [3,4]. Marginal AL:Crad values were important for (lack of) agreement between prediction methods (the more marginal, the poorer fit), and also for prediction error. The higher the ratio, the more marked the underestimation by Binkhorst; SRK II came closer to the zero-line, however, with plus values in the high tail of the AL:Crad distribution.

No low-ratio eyes were included in the 1992 material, but if the prediction error regression lines are extended to the left, on a graph with AL:Crad ratio on the x-axis and error (in D) on the y-axis [4], the trend is in keeping with Figure 1 of this paper. Though close to zero, for low-ratio eyes the theoretical formula (Catrefract) would be on the plus side, and SRK II towards minus.

The updated Catrefract program entails an empirical assessment of IOL position-to-be, as calculated from eye size and anterior segment dome shape (including as parameters the corneal curvature and the pre-operative anterior chamber depth). Because the oculometric distributions are numerically dominated by near-to-norm eyes, it is not surprising that aberrant oculometry in the very few (mainly short) eyes cannot be safeguarded in the prediction formulas, in general. In particular, one might expect an IOL-position with a more shallow anterior chamber depth than given by the manufacturer of the IOL actually

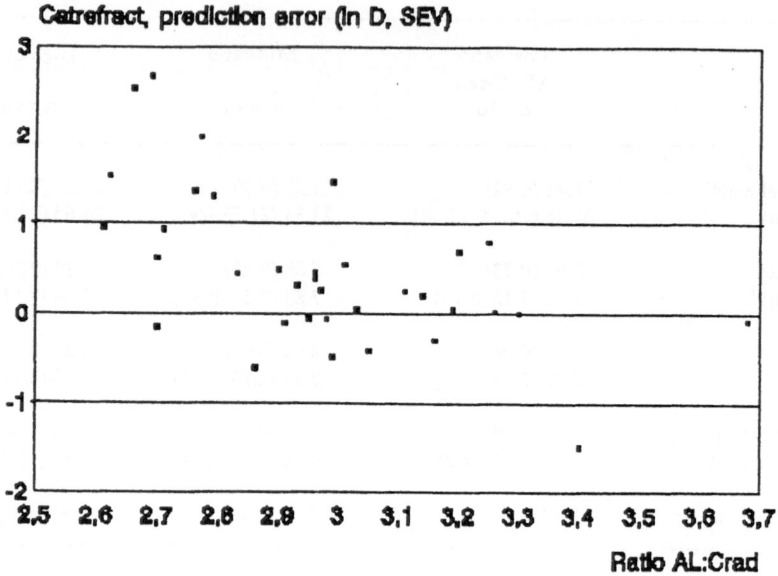

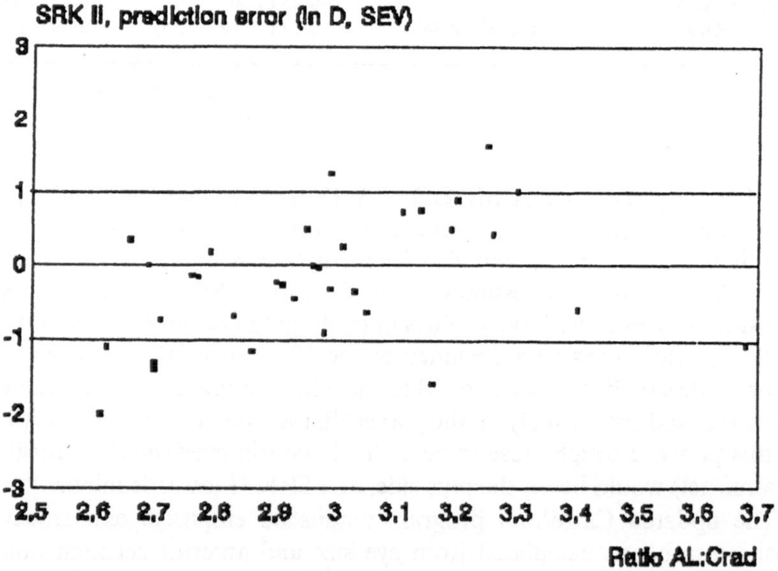

Fig. 1. Prediction error (in D, spherical equivalent value) as a function of AL:Crad ratio value, on x-axis, with Catrefract (top) and SRK II (bottom). The horizontal lines delimit prediction error within ±1 D from zero

chosen for surgery, to result in a 'more plus' prediction error than otherwise predicted.

Recently we had the opportunity of re-measuring the operated eyes of three patients from the low-ratio group, who presented with prediction errors of 2.7, 2.5, and 2.0 D, respectively. Encountering the difficulties in measuring eyes with the strongly sound-reflecting intraocular lens in place, grossly we found that axial length measurements had been correct while anterior chamber depths were 0.25 and 0.36 mm shorter than predicted by Catrefract during pre-operative assessment in two, out of 3. There was no measurement error in the corneal curvature radius.

Correction factors in low-ratio eyes?

Will the present results lead to the introduction of fudge factors when selecting IOL power in eyes oculometrically considered at risk of a significant prediction error? We cannot yet tell. Moreover, only a few per cent of patients will show ratios on the very low side. On the other hand, a very low ratio might serve as a warning to the surgeon. By subsequent follow-up the surgeon could then establish whether practical measures should be taken or not.

References

[1] T.H. Olsen, K. Thim and L. Corydon. Accuracy of the newer generation intraocular lens power calculation formulas in long and short eyes. J. Cataract Refract. Surg. 1991;17:187.

[2] H.C. Fledelius, P.H. Alsbirk and E. Goldschmidt. Intraocular lens calculation. An evaluation of Binkhorst and SRK estimates. Acta Ophthalmol. 1987;75:579.

[3] H.C. Fledelius and M. Fich. The ratio axial eye length: corneal curvature radius and IOL calculation. SIDUO XIV, Tokyo, October, 1992. In Docum. Ophthalmol. Proc. Ser. 58. Boston: Kluwer Academic Publishers, 1995;69–74.

[4] M. Fich and H.C. Fledelius. Intraocular lens prediction and oculometric harmony. With special reference to skew ratios between axial length and corneal curvature radius. Acta Ophthalmol. 1993;71:408.

H. Fledelius
Eye Department
Hillerød Sygehus
Hillerød, Denmark

53. Corneal power choice for lens calculation in keratoplasty with cataract extraction and lens implantation

L. PIERRO, E. CONFORTO, E. ZAGANELLI, L. GUARISCO and R. BRANCATO

(Milan, Italy)

Abstract

In keratoplasty with cataract extraction and intraocular lens (IOL) implantation, preoperative keratometry is the major source of error in lens power selection. Different keratometry readings are used. To find the most accurate reading, IOL power values for emmetropia (IOL1), calculated in 100 normal eyes, were compared with those obtained using the following keratometry values: of the fellow eye (IOL2), Katz Foster value 42.6 D (IOL3), Hoffer value 43.8 D (IOL4). IOL2 was the closest to IOL1 (p = n.s.), IOL3 the furthest ($p = 0.001$). Fellow eye keratometry is advised if available (if not use Hoffer value).

Key words: Keratoplasty, keratometry value, IOL calculation, biometry

Introduction

The selection of an appropriate intraocular lens (IOL) depends on accurate measurements of the corneal power, of the anterior chamber and of the axial length (axl) [1]. When a triple procedure is planned (combined keratoplasty, cataract extraction and IOL implant) it is difficult to predict the refractive outcome because the exact postoperative keratometry of the cornea curvature is unknown [2]. It is impossible to obtain accurate preoperative keratometry from the preoperative eye. Some surgeons use the preoperative keratometry of the eye to be operated, and some use the fellow eye in their calculations [2]. Others use average keratometric values derived from their own series, on the assumption that there is no correlation between pre- and postoperative K values [2–4]. The aim of this study was to find the most accurate keratometric value to obtain the most precise intraocular lens power. The aim of this study was to find the keratometric value that resulted in the most precise intraocular lens power.

G Cennamo and N. Rosa (eds.), Ultrasonography in Ophthalmology 15, pp. 427–430.

Materials and methods

We selected 100 patients (100 eyes) for cataract surgery. Exclusion criteria were: corneal abnormalities; intraocular pressure >20 mmHg; previous eye surgery, and axl > to 26 mm. All patients underwent keratometry and axl measurements were taken. Keratometry was performed with the Javal keratometer produced by Haag-Streit. After adjusting the eye-piece to correct possible ametropia of the examiner, measurements were taken. Axial length measurements were calculated with an ultrasound biometer (Sonomed a 2000) equipped with a linear amplifier and a solid 10 MHz focused probe with an axial resolution of ±0.1 mm. The refractive power of the lens was estimated using the SRK programme for IOL calculation. We estimated the emmetropic power of the fictive IOL, using different K values but maintaining the same axl value. We used: 1) the K value of the operated eye; 2) the K value of the fellow eye; 3) a K of 42.6 D (main keratometry value obtained by Katz and Foster); and 4) a K of 43.8 D (average mean value obtained by Hoffer).

Statistical analysis was performed using the one sample t-Test, testing whether the mean differences were significantly different from zero. The Bonferroni correction was taken into account. The differences were obtained by subtracting each IOL value from IOL1.

Results

The mean axl value of the operated eye was 23.026 (SD: ±0.975). The mean value of IOL1 was 19.850 (±2.741); IOL2: 19.691 (±2.279), IOL3 20.604 (±2.472), IOL4: 19.430 (±2.527). The mean value of the keratometry readings of the operated eye was 43.73 D (±0.870), and of the fellow eye, 43.72 D (±0.870). Comparing IOL2-4 with IOL1, it was found that IOL2 was the closest to IOL1 (p = n.s); IOL3 was the most dissimilar ($p = 0.001$) and IOL4 was in the middle ($p = 0.039$). IOL2 and IOL4 tend to be lower than IOL1, and IOL3 higher than IOL1. IOL3 had the highest absolute value among the differences considered.

Discussion

Today many corneal surgeons recognize the advantages of lens implantation during keratoplasty [2–5]. In addition to the numerous problems involved in the calculation of implant power for standard cataract surgery, the surgeon is faced with the problem of not knowing the postoperative keratometry readings. This may result in errors in the calculation of IOL power and the spherical equivalent refraction and in undesirably high amounts of corneal astigmatism. To improve the predictability of the refractive outcome some surgeons have used the recipient eye for lens implant calculations, while others have used the mate keratometry readings. Taylor estimated a standard +18 diopter lens implant power [6]. Katz-Foster and Gabel [2,6–8] used keratometry readings from the mate eye, the recipient eye, or used the average keratometry readings obtained from a recent concurrent series of corneal transplantations. Binder performed lens implant power calculations based on estimated postkeratoplasty corneal curvatures which were obtained from recent concurrent series using the same donor/recipient diameter combination [7]. Troutman calculated a 0.67 D increase in K for every 0.1 mm increase of donor button size over recipient bed size [9]. According to Casey, a 0.5 mm discrepancy between donor and recipient may reduce hypermetropia by a diopter or two [10]. Olson, on the other hand, reported a statistically insignificant difference between the refraction after same-size grafts and after over-size grafts [11]. Kozansky and Cavanagh found no relationship between preoperative and postoperative corneal powers, and suggested that the true relation is between the donor keratometry and the postoperative recipient keratometry [12]. According to Amr Salah-Eddin Abdel-Hakim, the relationship between postoperative and donor corneal power exists only when certain trephine sizes are used and when the recipient cornea is not excessively scarred [13]. These different theories give some idea of the importance of reducing post-operative astigmatism, and of the current state of confusion as to the choice of which preoperative keratometry value to use. The average postoperative corneal power reading for each surgeon (based on previous series of cases) and a personalized A-constant update are, in our opinion, the best techniques to improve the predictability of refractive results. Our study may be helpful in cases in which these techniques are not available and the surgeon does not have his own average of preoperative corneal values. This theoretical study strongly indicates that the fellow eye keratometry (when available) results in the best choice of corneal power. If unavailable we advise using Hoffer's 43.8 D keratometry value.

References

[1] J. Retzlaff, D. Sanders and M. Krass. A manual of implant power calculation. Oregon: Medford, 1981.

[2] P.S. Binder. The triple procedure. Refractive results, 1985, Update. Ophthalmology 1986; 93(12):1482–1488.

[3] P.S. Binder. Intraocular lens implantation after penetrating keratoplasty. Refractive and Corneal Surgery 1989;5:224–229.

[4] P.S. Binder. Refractive errors encountered with the triple procedure. Cornea, refractive surgery and contact lens: transaction of the New Orleans academy of ophthalmology. New York: Raven Press, 1987:111–120.

[5] G.J. Crawford, R.D. Stulting, G.O. Waring, W.S. Van Meter and L.A. Wilson. The triple procedure. Analysis of outcome, refraction, and intraocular lens power calculation. Ophthalmology 1986;93(6):817–824.

[6] D.M. Taylor. Keratoplasty and intraocular lenses. Ophthalmic Surg. 1976;7(1):31–42.

[7] H.R. Katz and R.K. Foster. Intraocular lens calculation in combined penetrating keratoplasty, cataract extraction and intraocular lens implantation. Ophthalmology 1985;92(9): 1203–1207.
[8] M. Gabel, R. Meyer and D. Musch. Intraocular lens power. In F.S. Brightbill (ed.), Corneal surgery theory, technique, and tissue. St. Louis: C.V. Mosby, 1986;153–157.
[9] R.C. Troutman. Microsurgery of the anterior segment of the eye: the cornea, optics and surgery. St. Louis: C.V. Mosby, 1977;2:107.
[10] T.A. Casey. Corneal grafting and intraocular lenses. In E. Rosen, W.M. Haining and E.J. Arnott. Intraocular lenses implantation, St. Louis: C.V. Mosby, 1984:609.
[11] R.J. Olson, T.P. Mattingly, S.R. Waltman and H.E. Kaufman. Refractive variation and donor tissue size in aphakic keratoplasty. A prospective randomized study. Arch. Ophthalmol. 1979;97:1480-1481.
[12] A. Kozansky and H.D. Cavanagh. The triple procedure: cataract extraction, intraocular lens insertion and corneal transplant. In W.A.C. Ntark and A.E. Maumenee (eds), Anterior segment surgery. Baltimore: Williams and Wilkins, 1987:260–266.
[13] A.H. Amr Sah-Eddin and K. Ahmmad. Intraocular lens power calculations in the triple procedure. Br. J. Ophthalmol. 1989;73:709–713.

Prof. R. Brancato
Department of Ophthalmology and Visual Sciences
University of Milan
Istituto Scientifico Ospedale S. Raffaele
Via Olgettina 60
Milan, Italy

54. Age-related changes of axial length and configuration of progressive myopic eyes

V. HIDASI and L. KOLOZSVÁRI[1]
(Debrecen and [1]Szeged, Hungary)

Abstract

The enlargement of progressive myopic eyes can last many years. Between 1988–1992 we studied more than 600 myopic patients (years of age: 4–76) with ultrasound. We measured axial lengths and determined the configurations of the eyeballs. The aim was to investigate whether the axial length and/or the configuration showed an age-related change. In this population the axial length increased continuously with age and in older individuals there was a higher incidence of staphylomatous eyes.

Key words: Progressive myopia, age, axial length, configuration

Introduction

Myopia is divided into three groups according to the refractive error: low, moderate and high degree. However, as shown in Table 1, there is no consensus as to the number of diopters that represent the cut-off point between these groups [1,2].

According to the presence or the lack of degenerative changes, myopia is classified benign or physiologic, and malignant or pathologic. The benign form never reaches high refractive powers, there are no degenerations, the stabilization ensues relatively soon and the visual acuity remains good. Consequently, some authors call it 'physiologic myopia' supposing it to be a normal variant up to 6 diopters. In contrast, in malignant or pathologic myopia the refractive error may reach high, sometimes extreme values, and finally severe degenerative changes develop (fundus degenerations, staphyloma formation, etc.). This form is also known as 'degenerative myopia'. The enlargement of the globe is continuous and sometimes lasts for many years, and the visual acuity is generally very impaired. Because in these cases the pathologic changes progress, it is sometimes called 'progressive myopia'. We use the latter term in the obviously progressing cases regardless of the refractive power or of other changes at the time of examination because we consider the main criterion of progression to be the rapid lengthening of the axis of the eyeball.

G Cennamo and N. Rosa (eds.), Ultrasonography in Ophthalmology 15, pp. 431–436.

Table 1. Classifications of myopia according to the refractive error

	MYOPIA		
	Low	Moderate	High
Thompson [2]	<3 D	3–6 D	>6 D
Kettesy [1]	<7 D	7–12 D	>12 D
Nagy [7]	<4 D	4–8 D	>8 D

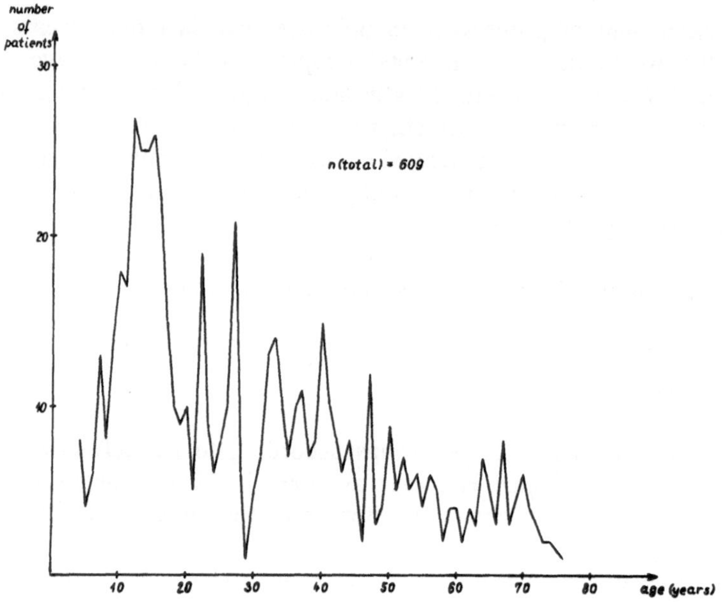

Fig. 1. Number of patients according to age

The normal eye stops growing at about 6–8 years [1,4]. On the contrary, the myopic eye does not stop growing at this time. Generally, the later the manifestation of myopia, the sooner its stabilization.

Materials and methods

Between 1988–1992 more than 600 myopic patients were examined with ultrasound in our clinic; particular attention was paid to axial length and the shape of the eyes. We used the Cooper Vision Digital B IV machine. The axial

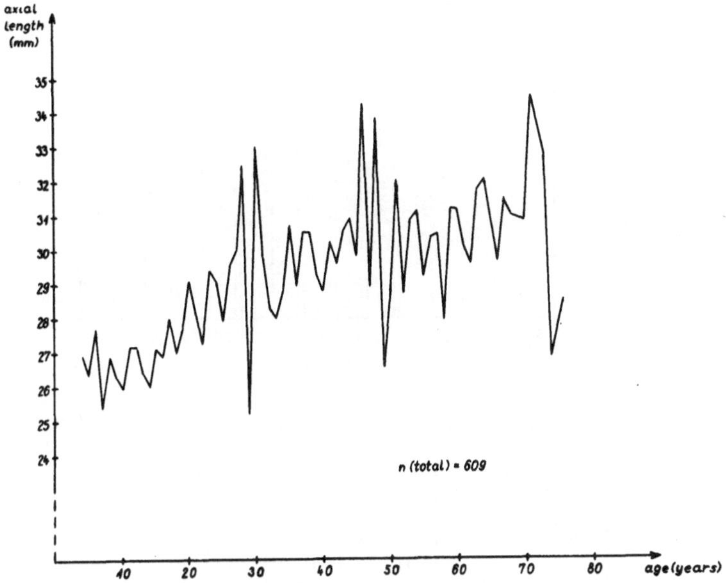

Fig. 2. Axial length averages according to patient age in annual breakdown

length measurements were performed with the immersion A-method. At least three values were recorded in each eye; if these values deviated widely, other measurements were made. We used the contact B-method to establish the shape of the eyeballs. The patients' age ranged between 4 and 76 years (Fig. 1).

Results

The axial length changes of this population in relation with age is shown annually (Fig. 2) and in 5- and 10-year breakdowns (Figs. 3a,b). There was a continuous increase in axial length.

Utkin [5] distinguished three types of myopic eyes: spherical, oval, and irregular. Svirin et al. [6] described five groups: regular pear-shaped, irregular pear-shaped, angular, diffuse spherical, and with small but peripheral staphylomas. In 1990 in our clinic we distinguished two main types and within them seven subtypes, which was modification of Utkin's classification (Table 2). In accordance with Fledelius [7], the regular spherical form accounted for most of our patient material (Fig. 4). In the elderly the rate of this shape diminished while that of oval, staphylomatous eyeballs increased. The latter form was hardly ever observed in patients below the age of 13 years (Figs. 5a,b).

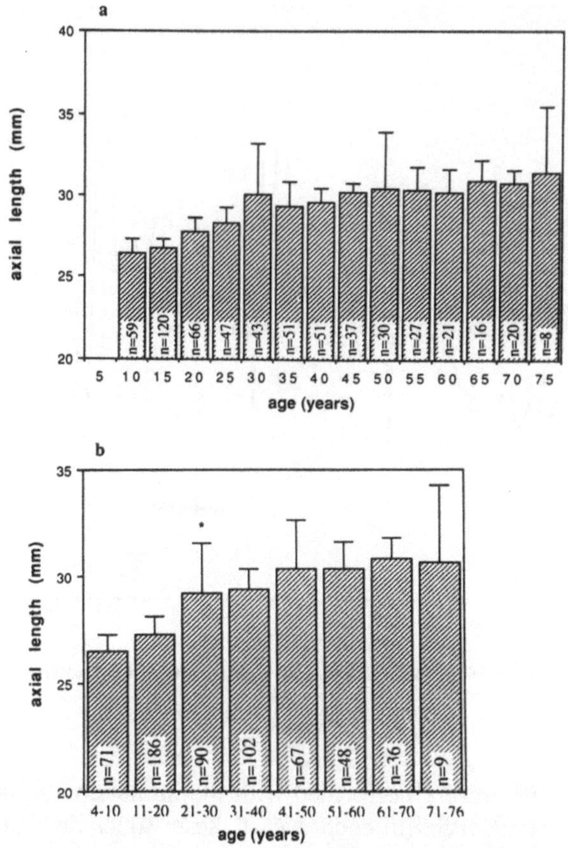

Fig. 3. Axial length averages according to patient age: a) in 5-year breakdown; b) in 10-year breakdown

Discussion

Based on our findings we conclude that: 1) the malignant (i.e., degenerative) myopia may progress throughout the patients lifetime thus is may be worth performing scleral reinforcement in any age; 2) the long-lasting the enlargement of the bulb, (a) the more probable that 'there is not enough room' for it in the orbit and thus it assumes an antero-posteriorly lengthened oval form, and (b) the more frequent the staphyloma formation thereby providing a variety of forms of the posterior pole.

Finally, the echographic axial length measurement is probably the least harmful and the most accurate and less expensive method with which to establish if the eyeball is lengthening or if it has already stabilized, because visual acuity is frequently deteriorated by macular degeneration and the objective refraction measurements may be influenced by phacosclerosis in older age.

			number of eyes	%	
I. (spherical)	1.		275	45.5	(1.)
	2.	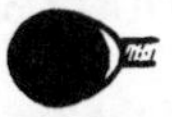	109	18.0	(2.)
	3.	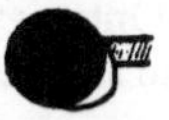	66	11.0	(3.)
	4.	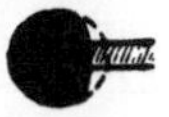	12	2.0	(7.)
II. (oval)	1.	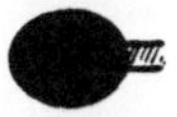	45	7.4	(6.)
	2.	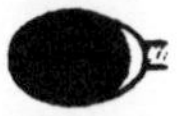	51	8.4	(4.)
	3.	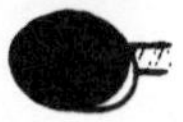	47	7.7	(5.)
		total:	605	100.0	

Fig. 4. Breakdown by the shapes of the examined myopic eyes

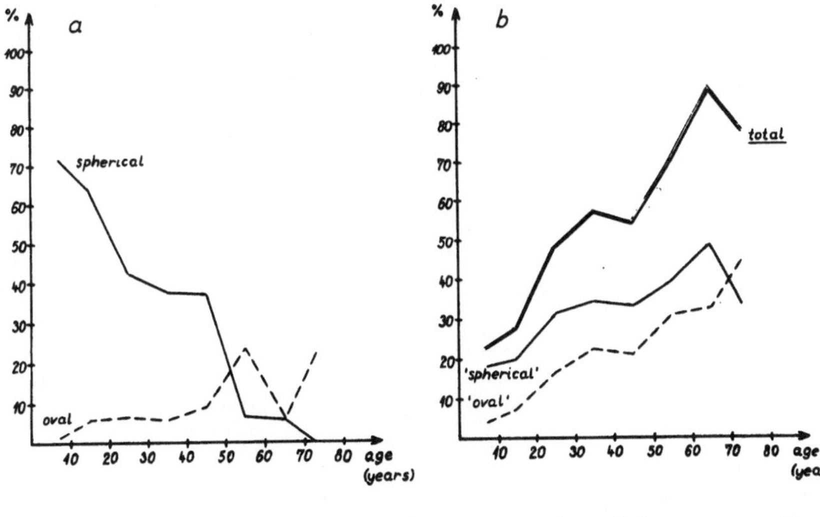

Fig. 5. The time course of configurational changes of a. regular, b. staphylomatous myopic eyes in 10-year breakdown

References

[1] B. Boros, A. Kettesy and K.F. Rövidlátás. Kközellátóság, myopia. In Szemészet. (ed.), Medicina, Budapest, 1967;76–80.
[2] B. Ward and F.B. Thompson. Pathology of myopia. In F.B. Thompson (ed.), Myopia Surgery. New York: Macmillan Publishing Co. Inc., 1990;8–9.
[3] V. Hidasi, L. Kolozsvári and Z. Nagy. Posterior pole configurations in progressive myopia. In P. Till (ed.), Proceedings of the 13th SIDUO Congress. Dordrecht: Kluwer Academic Publishers, 1990;385-392.
[4] F.K. Tabbara. Anatomy and embryology of the eye. In Appleton & Lange (ed.), General Ophthalmology. East Norwalk: Prentice-Hall International Inc., 1989;18.
[5] V.P. Utkin. Nekatorie dannie biometrii glaz so sferitseskoj i asferitseskoj miopiei. Oftalm. Z. 1979;160:34–38.
[6] A.V. Svirin, T.V. Serebriakova, U.E. Batmanov and A.P. Nesterov. Dvuhmernaia echografia v issledovanii glazs miopiei. Vestnik Oftalm. 1982;5:40–42.
[7] H.C. Fledelius. Ultrasound (A-mode) in a case of nasal posterior scleral extasy. Acta Ophthalmol. 1970;48:502–507.

Vanda Hidasi
Department of Ophthalmology
University School of Medicine,
P O Box 30
H-4012 Debrecen, Hungary

55. Measurement and prediction of the postoperative anterior chamber depth for intraocular lenses of different shape and material

W. HAIGIS, J. KAMMANN,[1] G. DORNBACH[1] and R. SCHÜTTRUMPF[1]

(Würzburg and [1]Dortmund, Germany)

Abstract

We compared four models used to predict the postoperative anterior chamber depth (ACD) after intraocular lens (IOL) implantation. Of these, only our model and Olsen's were able to predict correctly the ultrasonically measurable postoperative ACDs. The SRK/T and Holladay algorithms fail, since they give optical rather than acoustical ACDs. Optical ACDs, which cannot be measured acoustically, are required as input parameters in the popular IOL formulas of these authors. Acoustical ACDs, on the other hand, are needed for thick lens formulas.

The correlation between predicted and true postoperative ACDs is better in the Haigis and in the Olsen models, than in the SRK/T and Holladay models. Contrary to others, our prediction model is completely based on (ultrasonically) measurable data.

Key words: IOL formula, anterior chamber depth, ACD lens shape, optical ACD, acoustical ACD

Introduction

Intraocular lens (IOL) formulas may be divided into theoretical formulas based on an optical model and empirical formulas, which are derived with the help of statistical methods. Another classification distinguishes between different *formula generations*. In a recent paper Hoffer [1] described the present generation [1–3] as the third one, defined by an anterior chamber depth (ACD), which is dependent on axial length and corneal curvature. Earlier formula generations were characterized by different degrees of functional 'variability' of the ACD (or A-constant).

When popular theoretical IOL formulas are analyzed [e.g., 4], it can be shown that they all may be reduced to:

G Cennamo and N. Rosa (eds.), Ultrasonography in Ophthalmology 15, pp. 437–447.

$$(1)\qquad D_L = \frac{n}{L-d} - \frac{n}{n/z-d}$$

$$\text{with } z = D_C + \frac{Ref}{1 - Ref\, d_{BC}} \quad \text{and } D_C = \frac{n_C - 1}{R}$$

D_L: refractive power of IOL
D_C: corneal refractive power
Ref: refraction
n: index of refraction of aqueous and vitreous (1.336)
R: corneal radius
d_{BC}: vertex distance between spectacles and cornea
d: 'anterior chamber depth'
L: axial length
n_C: (fictitious) corneal refractive index

This formula (1) is valid for infinitely thin plano-convex lenses or 'lenses' consisting of just one spherical refracting surface. Other lens shapes, e.g., biconvex lenses, were *literally excluded* from this formula. To cope with the IOL of the real world, those theoretical formulas differ in the *meaning*, that the individual formula parameters have, and thus also in: the numerical value used for the (fictitious) refractive index n_C of the cornea; the numerical value L that has to be input for the axial length; and the value d of the 'anterior chamber depth' ACD.

Since all (theoretical) formulas expect a number to be input for the ACD, the true postoperative ACD and the quality of different algorithms, by which the ACD may be predicted, are of interest.

Material and methods

Pre- and postoperative ultrasound biometry (at least one month after surgery) using a BMS 811 Echocomp in immersion technique was performed on 542 eyes. Corneal curvatures were measured with a Javal type keratometer. All eyes had received a posterior chamber lens in the bag after capsulorhexis. Surgery had been done by one surgeon (JK) from August 1989 to August 1992; from May 1991 a no-stitch-technique had been used.

The lenses implanted were all of biconvex style from Adatomed GmbH (Munich, Germany), consisting of 34 PMMA lenses type 75 st (10° angulated, 5.5–6 mm optic, diameter 10–11 mm), 64 PMMA lens type 88 ti (angulation 0°; 6 mm optic; overall diameter 11 mm) and 444 silicone lenses type 90D. Due to slight differences in design, these silicon lenses are subdivided into three groups 90D-a (n = 230), 90D-b (n = 84) and 90D-c (n = 130).

Results and discussion

Mean pre-and postoperative ACDs

The results of the pre- and postoperative measurements of the ACDs are listed in Table 1 and shown in Figure 1. The means are shown for all five lens types. Generally, postoperative ACD is roughly 1 mm longer than preoperatively. While the mean preoperative ACD is more or less the same for all patients, slight differences due to individual IOL designs may be observed in the postoperative data.

Prediction of postoperative ACDs

The measured postoperative data has to be compared to calculated values as given by different prediction formulas. Four prediction models were used to calculate the expected postoperative ACD: the algorithms of the Holladay [2] and SRK/T [3] formulas, a model published by Olsen [5] and a statistical model of our own [6, 7]. These models were as follows:

Holladay ACD prediction

The algorithms for the ACD prediction of the Holladay formula are

$$AC_{HOLL} = 0.56 - 3.595 + 0.9704\ ACD_{const} + r - SQRT\ (r^2 - D^2/4)$$

where

$r = R$ for $R \geqslant 7$	$D = 0.533\ AL$	for $AL \leqslant 25.326$
$r = 7$ for $R < 7$	$D = 13.5$	for $AL > 25.326$

($AL = AL_{pre}$: preop. axial length; R: mean corneal radius).

Table 1. Mean pre- and postoperative acoustically measured ACD [mm] (s.d.: standard deviation) for different IOL types. PMMA: combined results for lenses 75st and 88ti; SILI: results for all 90D silicon lenses; all: results for all lenses

Mean AC/IOL	75st	88ti	90D-a	90D-b	90D-c	PMMA	SILI	All
Total n	34	64	230	84	130	98	444	542
Mean AC_{pre}	3.29	3.37	3.30	3.22	3.28	3.34	3.28	3.29
±s.d.	0.51	0.45	0.41	0.39	0.43	0.47	0.41	0.42
Mean AC_{post}	4.32	4.38	4.22	4.19	4.22	4.36	4.22	4.24
±s.d.	0.33	0.35	0.36	0.31	0.31	0.34	0.34	0.34

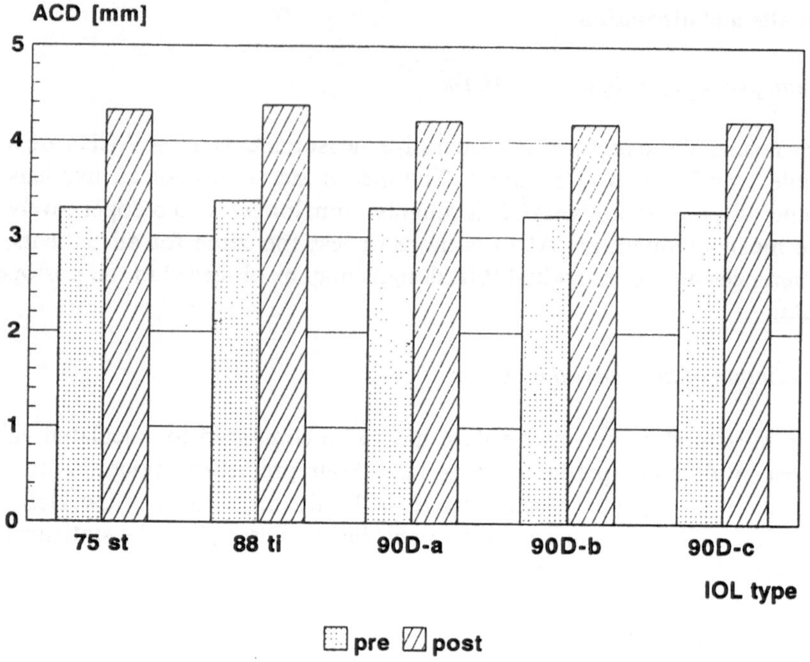

Fig. 1. Mean pre- and postoperative acoustically measured ACD for the five lens types of this study

SRK/T ACD prediction

With the same notation as above, the ACD calculation in the SRK/T formula is given by

$$AC_{SRK} = -3.336 + ACD_{const} + r - SQRT\,(r^2 - D^2/4)$$

where

$r = R$
$D = -5.41 + 0.58412\ AL + 33.075/R$ for $AL \leqslant 24.2$
$D = -7.42 + 1.002\ AL - 0.0138\ AL^2 + 33.075/R$ for $AL > 24.2$

The geometry underlying the ACD prediction in both the Holladay and SRK/T formula is plotted in Figure 2. Both formulas utilize the height t_1 of the corneal dome as previously used by Fyodorov and Kolonko in the late 1960s [8].

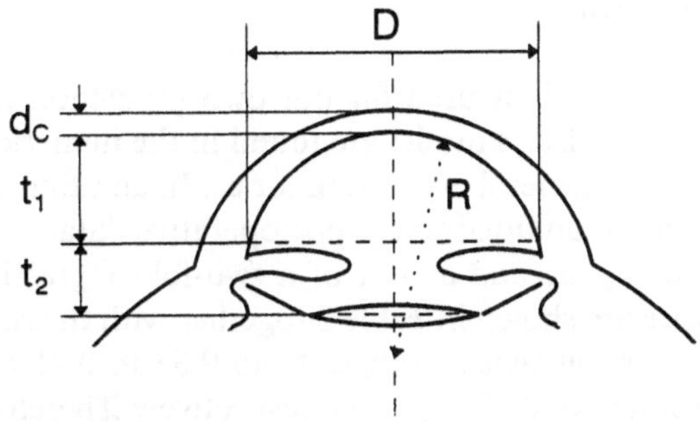

$$t_1 = R - \sqrt{R^2 - \frac{D^2}{4}}$$

Fig. 2. Geometry for ACD calculations in the Holladay and the SRK/T formulas

Olsen ACD prediction

Our own statistical model as well as that of Olsen is based on a multiple linear regression analysis correlating the postoperative ACDs with preoperative values for ACD and axial length. This approach has been used previously [6,9,10]. Its general form is

$$AC_{post} = a_0 + a_1\, AC_{pre} + a_2\, AL_{pre} \tag{2}$$

where

AC_{post}: postop. ACD by ultrasound
AC_{pre}: preop. ACD by ultrasound
AL_{pre}: preop. axial length by ultrasound

and a_0, a_1, a_2: fit parameters out of the statistical analysis.

The specific parameters for a_0, a_1 and a_2 as published by Olsen [5] lead to

$$AC_{OLS} = \overline{AC_{post}} - 3.56 + 0.25\, AC_{pre} + 0.12\, AL_{pre}$$

where

$\overline{AC_{post}}$ denotes the mean of AC_{post}.

Haigis ACD prediction

The same statistical basis is used for our own prediction model. As is shown below, differences to Olsen's model are found in the numerical values for a_0, a_1, and a_2 and also in the general expression for a_0. In addition, this parameter may be calculated rather than fitted to the postoperative data.

The coefficients a_0, a_1 and a_2 out of a two-fold regression analysis for the different lens types are shown in Table 2 together with the respective correlation coefficients. It turns out that a_1 ranges from 0.33 to 0.41 and a_2 from 0.05 to 0.11 with mean values of 0.37 and 0.08, respectively. Therefore, we took $a_1 = 0.4$ and $a_2 = 0.1$ to characterize our model. (Not yet published studies with other IOL types yield quite similar results for a_1 and a_2). From Table 3 it can be seen that the correlation coefficients for this specific choice for a_1 and a_2 are virtually identical to that of Table 2.

Table 2. Regression coefficients a_0, a_1 and a_2 and correlation coefficient R for the dependance $Ac_{post} = a_0 + a_1$ ACpre + a_2 AL_{pre} for the different IOL of this study

Coeff./IOL	75st	88ti	90D-a	90D-b	90D-c	PMMA	SILI	All
a_0	0.92	0.82	0.30	1.96	1.93	0.87	1.09	1.12
a_1	0.41	0.37	0.37	0.37	0.33	0.38	0.36	0.37
a_2	0.09	0.10	0.11	0.05	0.05	0.10	0.08	0.08
R [%]	74.4	64.1	62.6	53.4	56.7	67.6	58.9	60.0

Table 3. Regression coefficient a_0 and correlation coefficient R for the dependance $AC_{HAI} = a_0 +$ 0.4 Ac_{pre} + 0.1 AL_{pre} for the different IOL of this study

Coeff./IOL	75st	88ti	90D-a	90D-b	90D-c	PMMA	SILI	All
a_0	0.71	0.68	0.55	0.58	0.55	0.67	0.55	0.58
R [%]	74.4	64.0	62.5	52.6	56.2	67.6	58.9	60.0

With a_1 and a_2 thus given, there is only a_0 left to individually characterize the ACD for a given IOL. This parameter can easily be determined by calculating the respective means from equation (2):

$$a_0 = \overline{AC_{post}} \quad - 0.4 \quad \overline{AC_{pre}} \quad 0.1 \quad \overline{Al_{pre}}$$

Thus our own prediction model for the ACD calculation is given by

$$AC_{HAI} = \overline{AC_{post}} - 0.4 \quad \overline{AC_{pre}} - 0.1 \quad \overline{AL_{pre}} + 0.4 \; AC_{pre} + 0.1 \; AL_{pre}$$

Predicted vs measured individual postoperative ACDs

For all 90D silicone IOL (n = 444), the predicted postoperative ACDs of all four models are plotted against the true measured values in Figure 3. It can be seen that the Holladay and SRK/T algorithms yield values by far too high. Only our own model and the one of Olsen give reasonable agreement between calculated and measured data.

The quality of a prediction algorithm may be judged from the absolute values that it produces and also from the functional dependance between calculated and measured data. Therefore, the correlation coefficients for this dependance were calculated for all lens types and all prediction models and plotted in Figure 4. It follows that, with the exception of lens 75 st, where all models yield comparable and relatively high correlations, the Holladay and SRK/T predictions give smaller correlation coefficients than the other two models thus indicating the better performance of the regression algorithms.

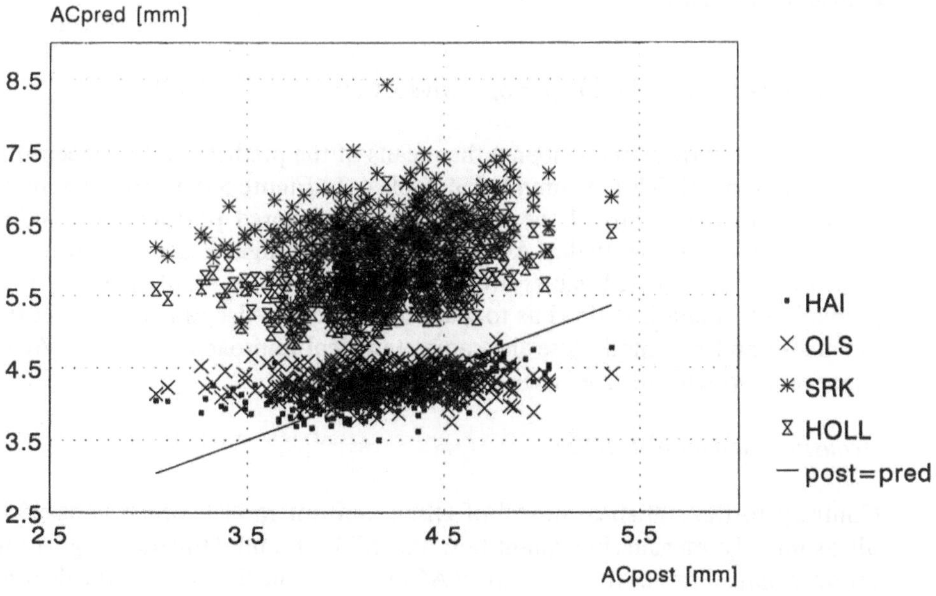

Fig. 3. Predicted vs measured individual postoperative ACD for silicone IOL type 90D (n = 444) for all four ACD prediction models

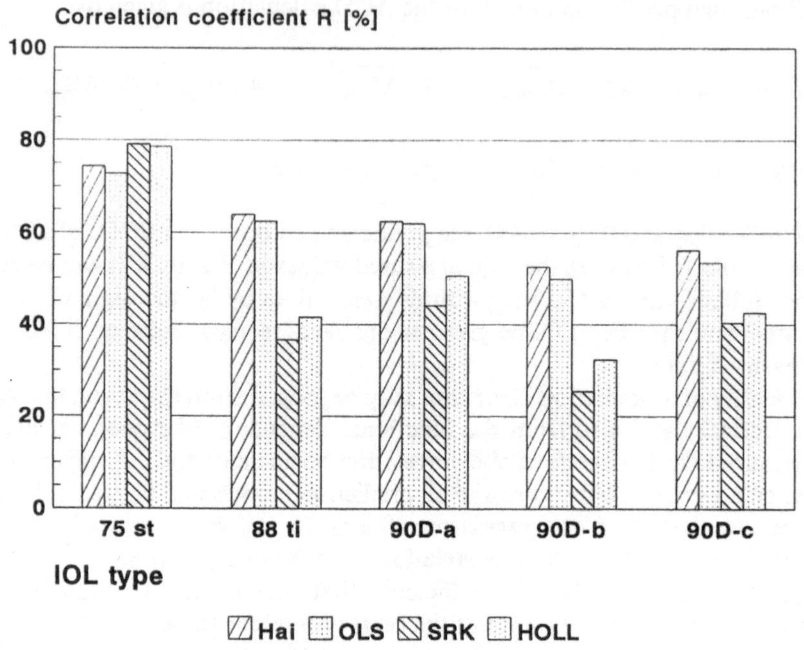

Fig. 4. Correlation coefficient for the dependance between predicted and true ACD for all IOL and all ACD prediction models

Predicted vs measured mean postoperative ACDs

For all IOL (PMMA and silicone) the means of the predicted ACDs according to the different models are compiled in Table 4. In Figure 5 these predictions are compared to the means of the ultrasonically measured postoperative ACDs. Again, SRK/T and Holladay ACDs are much too high. For our own model, measured and predicted values are identical. This is not surprising, since our prediction formula is defined as to yield this identity. Also, due to the fact that his model and our model use the same statistical approach, the Olsen ACDs come very close to the true measured values.

Acoustical and optical ACDs

Contrary to the statistical model of Olsen and our model, which is based on ultrasonically measurable quantities, the SRK/T and Holladay algorithms produce *optical* rather than *acoustical* ACDs. By 'acoustical ACDs' the distance from the anterior corneal vertex to the anterior vertex of the IOL is understood (Fig. 6). This distance ACD_{ac} is directly measurable by ultrasound. In fact, ACD_{ac} is what ultrasonographers refer to when they are talking about the 'anterior chamber depth'. It includes the vertex distance d_{CL} as well as the

Table 4. Mean predicted postoperative ACDs according to the different models for all lenses of this study (s.d.: standard deviation; R: correlation coefficient)

Mean AC/IOL	75st	88ti	90D-a	90D-b	90D-c	PMMA	SILI	All
Mean AC_{HAI}	4.32	4.38	4.22	4.19	4.22	4.36	4.22	4.24
±s.d.	0.25	0.24	0.23	0.21	0.24	0.24	0.23	0.24
R [%]	74.4	64.0	62.5	52.6	56.2	67.7	58.9	62.0
Mean AC_{OLS}	4.35	4.49	4.32	4.22	4.31	4.44	4.30	4.32
±s.d.	0.19	0.20	0.19	0.18	0.20	0.21	0.19	0.20
R [%]	72.8	62.5	62.0	49.9	53.5	64.6	57.0	59.9
Mean AC_{SRK}	5.31	4.86	6.49	6.37	5.69	5.02	6.23	6.01
±s.d.	0.27	0.38	0.36	0.26	0.41	0.41	0.50	0.67
R [%]	79.1	36.7	44.1	25.5	40.4	36.1	28.6	9.8
Mean AC_{HOLL}	5.08	4.81	5.84	5.72	5.47	4.90	5.71	5.56
±s.d.	0.23	0.32	0.33	0.24	0.38	0.32	0.36	0.47
R [%]	78.6	41.6	50.5	32.4	42.6	43.3	40.7	19.9

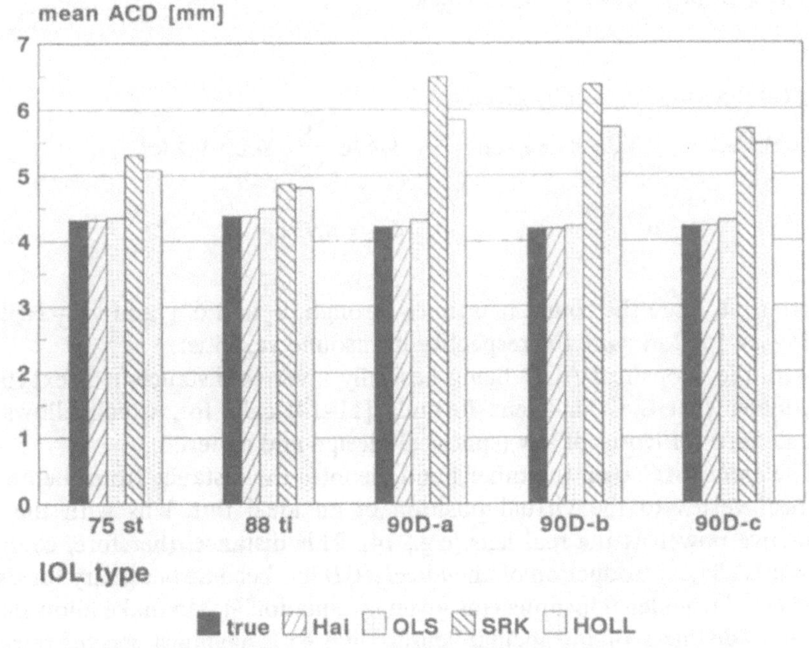

Fig. 5. True and predicted mean ACD for all IOL and all ACD prediction models

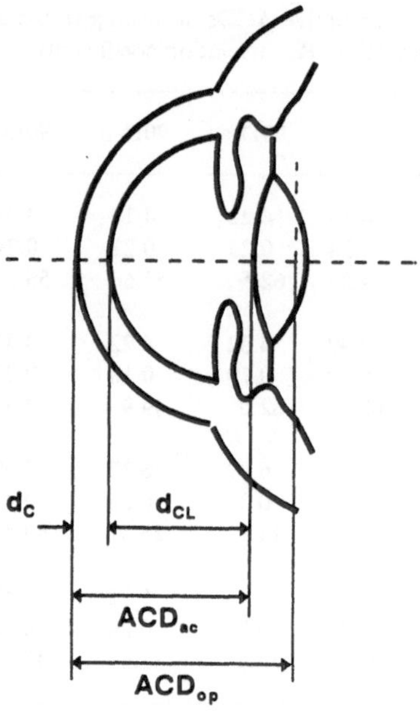

Fig. 6. Definition of *acoustical* and *optical* ACD: the *acoustical ACD* includes also the corneal thickness d_C and is directly measurable by ultrasound. The unmeasurable *optical ACD* serves as a fudge factor in popular theoretical IOL formulas

corneal thickness d_C and is given by

$$ACD_{ac} = 0.5\,(t_C + t_{CL})\,v_{CL} = 0.5\,t_C\,\frac{v_C}{v_C}\,v_{CL} + 0.5\,t_{CL}\,v_{CL}$$

$$= d_C\,\frac{v_{CL}}{v_C} + d_{CL} = d_{CL} + 0.93\,d_C$$

where t_C, t_{CL} are the round trip times through d_C and d_{CL} and $v_C = 1639$ m/s and $v_{CL} = 1532$ m/s are the respective ultrasound velocities.

With the acoustical ACD being basically a vertex distance, it is exactly the parameter that the thick lens formula [11–14] calls for, which allows IOL calculations for lenses of any (spherical) design and material.

The *optical ACD*, on the other hand, denotes the distance from the anterior corneal vertex to the virtual position of an ideal thin lens with the same refractive power as the real lens [e.g., 14]. This distance, therefore, cannot be measured. The introduction of an *optical ACD* has become necessary for today's theoretical (thin lens) formulas (as given by equation (1)) to make allowance for the non-idealness of intraocular lenses (like e.g., having a *second* refracting surface as in a biconvex lens): the *optical ACD* has to serve as a fudge or fit factor, since, as pointed out earlier, these formulas are still based on ideal, infinitely thin plano-convex lenses.

References

[1] K.J. Hoffer. The Hoffer Q formula: a comparison of theoretic and regression formulas. J. Cataract. Refract. Surg. 1993;19:700–712.

[2] J.T. Holladay, K.H. Musgrove, T.C. Prager, J.W. Lewis, T.Y. Chandler and R.S. Ruiz. A three-part system for refining intraocular lens power calculations. J. Cataract Refract Surg. 1988;14:17–24.

[3] J. Retzlaff, D.R. Sanders and M.C. Kraff. Development of the SRK/T intraocular lens implant power calculation formula. J. Cataract Refract. Surg. 1990;16(3):333–340.

[4] W. Haigis. Kritische Hornhautradien gefährden bei Verwendung der SRK/T-Formel die korrekte IOL-Berechnung. Ophthalmologe 1993;90:703–707.

[5] T. Olsen. Über die Schätzung der postoperativen Vorderkammertiefe mit den modernen Formeln zur Kunstlinsenberechnung. In M. Wenzel, M. Reim, H. Freyler and Ch. Hartmann (eds.), Kongr. d. Deutsch. Ges. f. Intraokularlinsen Implant. Aachen 1991. Berlin, Heidelberg, New York: Springer, 1991:156–165.

[6] W. Haigis, W. Waller, Z. Duzanec and W. Voeske. Postoperative biometry and keratometry after posterior chamber lens implantation. Eur. J. Implant. Refract. Surg. 1990;2:191–202.

[7] W. Haigis, J. Kammann, G. Dornbach and R. Schüttrumpf. Vorhersage der postoperativen Vorderkammertiefe bei Implantation von PMMA - und Silikonlinsen im Kapselsack. In Kongr. d. Deutsch. Ges. f. Intraokularlinsen Implant., Zürich 1993. Berlin, Heidelberg, New York: Springer, 1993;505–510.

[8] S.N. Fyodorov and A.I. Kolonko. Estimation of optical power of the intraocular lens. Vestnik Oftalmologic (Moscow) 1967;4:27.

[9] R.D. Lepper and H.G. Trier. Refraction after intraocular lens implantation: Results with a computerized system for ultrasonic biometry and for implant lens power calculation. The Hague: Junk, Doc. Ophthal. Proc. Ser. 1984;38:243–248.

[10] T. Olsen. Prediction of intraocular lens position after cataract extraction. J. Cataract Refract. Surg. 1986;12(7):376–379.

[11] C.D. Binkhorst and L.H. Loones. Intraocular lens power. Trans. Am. Acad. Ophthalmol. Otolaryngol. 1976;81:70–79.

[12] G. D. Barett. Intraocular lens calculation formulas for new intraocular lens implants. J. Cataract Refract. Surg. 1987;13:389-396.

[13] W. Haigis. Strahldurchrechnung in Gauβ'scher Optik zur Beschreibung des Sustems Brille-Kontaktlinse-Hornhaut-Augenlinse (IOL), 4. Kongr. d. Deutsch. Ges. f. Intraokularlinsen Implantation, Essen 1990. In K. Schott, K.W. Jacobi and H. Freyler (eds). Berlin: Springer, 1991;233-246.

[14] W. Haigis, Z. Duzanec and P. Fischer. Refraktionsbilanz bei Implantation von Bikonvex-Hinterkammerlinsen. 5. Kongr. d. Deutsch. Gesellsch. f. Intraokularlinsen Implant., Aachen 1991. In M. Wenzel, M. Reim, H. Freyler and Ch. Hartmann (eds). Berlin, Heidelberg, New York: Springer, 1991;198–210.

W. Haigis
Kopfklinikum Würzburg
Universitätsklinik und Poliklinik für Augenkranke
Josef-Schneider-Straβe
970820 Würzburg, Germany

[1]Eye Clinic
St. Johannes Hospital
Dortmund, Germany

56. Echobiometric and morphometric study of the orbit and eyeball of the neonate. Possible pathogenesis of essential infantile esotropia

C. TAMBURRELLI, A. CAPOBIANCO, T. TARTAGLIONE and B. BAGOLINI

(Rome, Italy)

Abstract

The etiology of essential infantile esotropia is not yet known. Various strabismogenic factors may influence the immature sensory system so inducing the development of strabismus. Oculo-musculo-skeletal mechanical anomalies may cause strabismus in newborns with craniofacial dysostosis and in adults with severe myopia. Several structural characteristics of the orbit of a group of patients with essential infantile esotropia and a control group have been studied by means of echography, magnetic resonance imaging and computerized tomography scan. We measured temporal orbital spaces between bone and sclera with echography, and calculated the angle between the lateral orbital walls on computerized tomographic and magnetic resonance imaging scans.

There was a decreased space at the level of the most anterior portion of the temporal side of the orbit in patients. The angle formed by the posterior intersection of the lateral orbital walls was significantly smaller in the group of patients affected by essential infantile esotropia than in the control group. The differences detected could be among the factors responsible for essential infantile esotropia.

Key words: Echography, esotropia

Introduction

A theory regarding the mechanical etiopathogenesis of strabismus in patients with severe myopia has recently been proposed [1,2]. This condition, known as "heavy eye syndrome", is characterised by the gradual development of deviations which may be so marked as to be occasionally defined "monstrous strabismus". Diplopia is absent.

Echographic and tomographic evaluations have revealed a marked reduction of the orbital space consequent to excessive enlargement of the eyeball. This

G Cennamo and N. Rosa (eds.), Ultrasonography in Ophthalmology 15, pp. 449–456.

results in a gradual and progressive compression on the lateral rectus muscle and causes paresis with consequent contraction of the medial rectus and esotropia. An association between horizontal and cyclovertical strabismus resulting from oculo-musculo-skeletal mechanical anomalies occurs in cranio-facial dysostosis (oxycephaly, Crouzon's disease, plagiocephaly) [3].

Essential infantile esotropia develops during the first six months of life. The term 'essential' is used because the etiology of the condition is not known. It seems that various strabismogenic agents affect the still immature and sometimes functionally imperfect sensory system, thus inducing the development of strabismus.

Given the pathogenetic hypothesis regarding the development of strabismus consequent to alterations in the relationships between the eyeball and the orbital bone structures as occurs in cranio-facial dysostosis and in severe myopia of the adult, we have evaluated, using imaging techniques, some structural characteristics of the orbit of the neonate suffering from essential infantile esotropia. The aim of this study was to ascertain whether anatomical conditions that may favour the development of oculo-motor anomalies are present in this condition. In particular and in view of the possible damage of the lateral rectus muscle resulting from compression of this structure against the bony wall of the orbit during postnatal development, we have evaluated the lateral orbital spaces. All patients were assessed using orbital echography as well as nuclear magnetic resonance and computerised axial tomography.

Materials and methods

We determined the dimensions of the space between the lateral wall of the orbit and the eyeball. Special attention was paid to the lateral rectus muscle which lies between the sclera and the orbital bone.

The lateral spaces were evaluated using B-scan echography (Mini B; Biophysic Medical). To study the relationships between the eyeball, the lateral rectus muscle and the lateral wall of the orbit, we performed two scans, perpendicular to each other, along the lateral wall of the orbit (Fig. 1): i) T-transverse scan, which permits the evaluation of the lateral orbit when scans are performed perpendicularly to the long axis of the lateral rectus muscle; and ii) L-longitudinal scan, which permits the evaluation of the orbit when scans are taken parallel to the long axis of the lateral rectus muscle. The lateral orbital spaces were evaluated at three sites: anterior, center and posterior, which are denoted L1, L2 and L3, respectively (Fig. 2). Biometry of the axial eye length was performed together with evaluation of the sites indicated above.

Twenty-two normal neonates with a mean age of 0.6 months (range: few hours to five months) and 12 infants suffering from essential infantile esotropia with a mean age of 7 months (range: four to 13 months) were evaluated using the technique described above. Besides the orbital spaces, we also evaluated the direction of the lateral orbital wall as related to the visual axis of the eyeballs. Special attention was paid to variations in the obliquity of the wall with respect

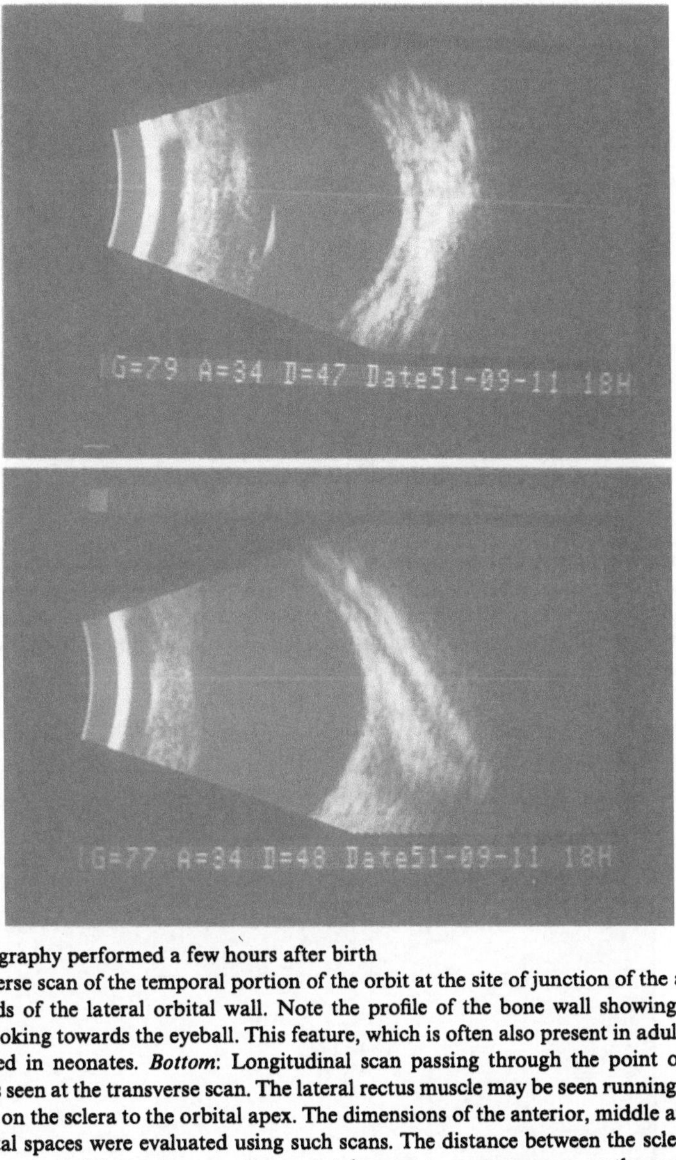

Fig. 1. Echography performed a few hours after birth
Top: Transverse scan of the temporal portion of the orbit at the site of junction of the anterior and middle thirds of the lateral orbital wall. Note the profile of the bone wall showing an internal convexity looking towards the eyeball. This feature, which is often also present in adult subjects, is more marked in neonates. ***Bottom***: Longitudinal scan passing through the point of maximum convexity as seen at the transverse scan. The lateral rectus muscle may be seen running from its site of insertion on the sclera to the orbital apex. The dimensions of the anterior, middle and posterior lateral orbital spaces were evaluated using such scans. The distance between the sclera and bone surface was measured for each space. Care was taken not to exert pressure on the eyeball so as to avoid artifacts

to the visual axis. In particular, we calculated the angle formed between the lines of posterior prolongation of the lateral orbital walls at the point of intersection. We have arbitrarily defined this, angle "α" (Fig. 3).

The angle between the lateral orbital walls was calculated using images obtained at computed tomography and magnetic resonance. Axial scans were

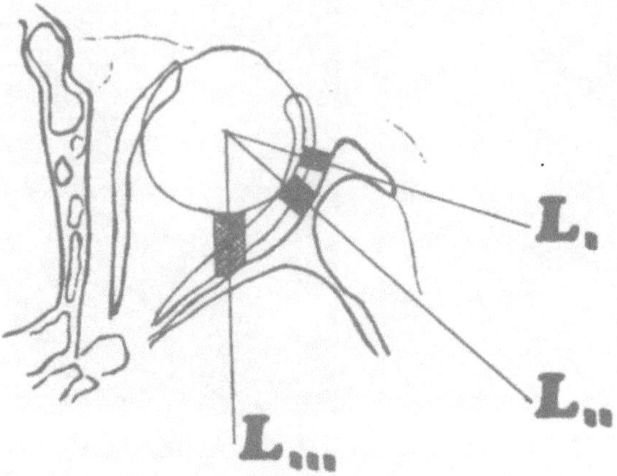

Fig. 2. Schematic representation of points L1, L2 and L3. Biometric evaluation of the lateral orbital spaces was performed at these sites. L1: Most anterior site lying just posterior to the lateral orbital margin. L2: Point at which the lateral rectus muscle no longer passes tangentially to the surface of the sclera.L3: Maximum width between the temporal portion of the posterior pole and the bone surface

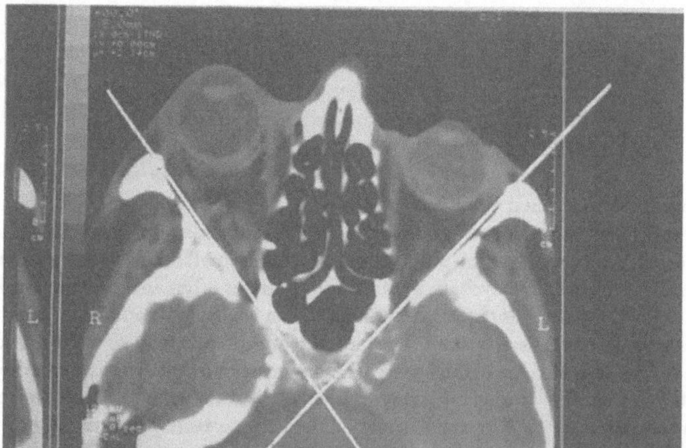

Fig. 3. Orbital computerized tomography. Axial scan showing the neuro-ocular plane passing simultaneously through the corneal apex, the apex of the orbit, the optic chiasma and through the occipital cortex. The superimposed white lines are parallel to the surfaces of the lateral orbital walls. We have defined the angle formed at the line of intersection of the posterior prolongations of the latter "α". The size of angle α is indicative of the obliquity of the lateral orbital walls. Similar observations were made at magnetic resonance axial scanning

performed and the spatial plane of reference was that running from the apex of the cornea through that of the orbit, through the optic chiasma and reaching the occipital cortex as defined by Cabanis and Salvolini [4].

We also evaluated 42 neonates aged from one to 18 weeks (mean 3.8 weeks) and submitted, as part of the work-up of various neonatal cerebral disorders, to magnetic resonance imaging of the cranium. No alterations of the orbit and/or eyeball were detected in these patients.

Seven children with a mean age of 18.3 months (range: 13 to 28 months) and suffering from essential infantile esotropia and 40 adults with a mean age of 56 years (range: 19 to 73 years) suffering from various extraorbital disorders were also evaluated at computed tomography. The data are reported in Table 1.

Table 1.

Echographic evaluation of the lateral orbital spaces
- 22 normal neonates (age range: few hours to 1 month)
- 12 infants suffering from essential infantile esotropia

MRI and CT scan evaluation of the angle "α"
- 42 normal neonates
- 7 children suffering from essential infantile esotropia (age range: 13 to 28 months)
- 40 adult patients with no pathology of the orbit and/or eyeball (age range: 19 to 73 years)

Results

The echographic measurements of the lateral orbital spaces and of axial lengths in normal subjects and in patients suffering from essential infantile esotropia are shown in Tables 2 and 3, respectively. We have analysed the data regarding L1, L2 and L3. With regard to the dimensions of the orbital space a significant difference was observed only for position L1 which is reduced in patients suffering from essential infantile esotropia ($p = 0.005$).

Table 4 shows the values of angle α (i.e., the angle at the intersection of the posterior prolongations of the lateral orbital walls) in the three groups of patients (normal neonates, neonates with essential infantile esotropia and normal adults). There was no significant difference between normal neonates and normal adults. On the other hand. angle α was significantly decreased in neonates suffering from congenital infantile esotropia ($p = 0.001$) (Fig. 4).

Table 2. Echographic measurements of the lateral orbital spaces (mm) in normal neonates and in neonates suffering from essential esotropia

	Normal			Infants with essential infantile esotropia		
	L1	L2	L3	L1	L2	L3
Mean	2.87	3.7	66.08	2.01	2.99	6.28
St. Deviation	1.20	1.1	1.26	0.8	1.25	1.31
Minimum	1.20	1.98	3.85	1.23	1.76	3.97
Maximum	4.5	5.5	8.8	2.81	4.21	7.67

L1, L2 and L3 are, respectively, the anterior, central and posterior sites along the lateral orbital space.

Table 3. Axial lengths in normal patients and in those suffering from essential infantile esotropia and who were submitted to determination of the lateral orbital spaces

	Normal Axial length	Essential infantile esotropia Axial length
Mean	17.39	17.98
Standard Dev.	0.76	0.89
Minimum	16.11	16.86
Maximum	18.90	19.78

Table 4. Angle α was measured in 89 cases at the line of intersection of the posterior prolongations of the planes through the lateral orbital walls

	Normal neonates angle α	Normal adults angle α	Infants with essential infantile esotropia angle α
Mean	84.11	82.37	71.4
S.D.	4.65	6.89	7.81
Minimum	65.5	67.6	61.5
Maximum	100.5	102.3	82.5

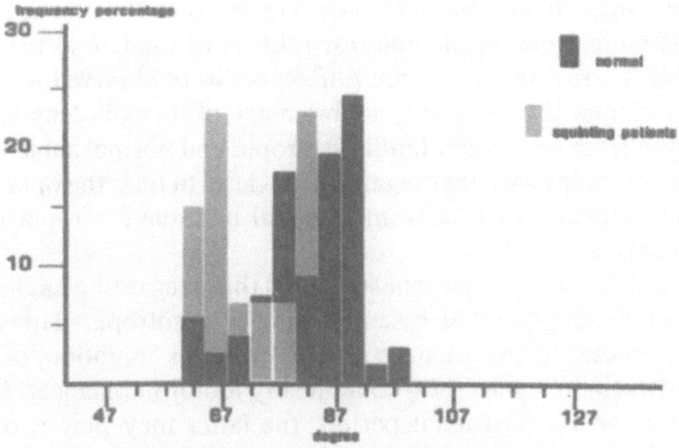

Fig. 4. **Histogram showing the relative incidences of angle α (expressed as percentage) both in patients suffering from essential infantile esotropia (dark) as well as in control subjects (white). On the abscissa, angle α is expressed in degrees. Note that the group of patients with essential infantile esotropia presents lower values of angle α**

Discussion

Essential congenital esotropia is an esodeviation that develops before six months of age. The term "essential" is used because the etiology of the pathology is unknown and to distinguish this condition from other forms of esodeviation. In fact, the differential diagnosis includes "nystagmus block syndrome" (which is a refractive accommodative esotropia characterised by bilateral paralysis of the sixth cranial nerve) and also type I of Duane's retraction syndrome.

Von Noorden [5,6] has hypothesised that stabismogenic factors could exert an influence on the as yet normal sensory system during the first three months of life when the sensory and motor systems are still functionally immature. This influence results in a defective motor fusion and consequently the fusional vergences do not develop.

Among the factors suggested, we consider the evaluation, both echographically and by other imaging techniques, of one aspect of the anatomical conditions of the orbit and eyeball during the first six month of life to be particularly important. In view of the obliquity of the lateral wall of the orbit, the lateral rectus muscle, which lies approximately 45° to the visual axis of the eyeball, is particularly subject to alterations and compressions exerted by the latter [1,2]. This might occur even when there are slight disproportions during the first months of life. It is important to bear in mind that, post-natally, even transitory alterations of muscle dynamics may influence the immature sensory and motor fusions thus transforming a transitory defect into a permanent deficit.

The data obtained in the present study suggest that there is a significant decrease in the dimensions of the anterior portion of the lateral orbital space (L1). On the other hand, no significant differences were observed in the size of the eyeball, as evaluated at echographic biometry of its axial length, between patients suffering from essential infantile esotropia and normal subjects.

This finding correlates with that regarding angle α. In fact, the opening of the lateral walls in patients suffering from essential infantile esotropia is smaller than that of normal subjects.

The echographic data of the present study and those regarding angle α cannot account for the development of essential infantile esotropia. However they demonstrate the presence, in patients suffering from this condition, of anatomical alterations which, in some cases, could justify motor imbalances. Occurring during the critical early post-natal period, the latter may play a role in the development of essential infantile esotropia. We thus conclude that some anatomical anomalies of the orbit should be included among the possible factors contributing to the development of essential infantile esotropia.

References

[1] B. Bagolini, C. Tamburrelli, A. Dickmann, L.C. and C. Colosimo. Convergent strabismus fixus in high myopic patients. Doc. Ophthalmol. 1990;74:309–320.

[2] B. Bagolini, A. Dickmann, C. Tamburelli and C. Colosimo. Origin of the lateral rectus paresis in strasbismus of high myopic patients. In E. Campos (ed.), Strabismus and ocular motility disorders. London/New York: The Macmillan Press Ltd., 1990; 215–218.

[3] B. Greaves, J. Walker and K. Wybar. Disorders of ocular motility in craniofacial dysostosis. J. Roy. Soc. Med. 1979;72:21.

[4] E.A. Cabanis, U. Salvolini, A. Rodallec, F. Manichelli, U. Pasquini and P. Bonnin. Computed tomography of the optic nerve. Part II. Size and shape modifications in papilledema. J. Comput. Assist. Tomograph. 1978;2:150–155.

[5] G.K. von Noorden. Infantile esotropia a continuing riddle (Richard C. Scobee Memorial Lecture). Am. Orthopht. J. 1984;34:52.

[6] G.K. von Noorden. Current concepts of infantile esotropia (Bowman Lecture). Eye 1988;2:343.

Ciro Tamburelli
Via Filippo Nicolai 91
00168 Rome, Italy

57. Intraoperative axial length biometry in esotropia surgery

P. PERISSUTTI, A. VINCIGUERRA and S. PENSIERO
(Trieste, Italy)

Abstract

Intraoperative axial length biometry was carried out in 30 patients treated for esotropia with posterior fixation suture and/or recession of the medial rectus muscles. The exact intraoperative determination of the location of the equator is recommended in order to prevent: 1) Excessive medial rectus recessions with consecutive postoperative muscle underactions (usually a recession of 10.5–11 mm from limbus is considered safe, but this location could be too posterior to the equator); 2) A significant limitation of rotation in eyes treated with posterior fixation sutures. In fact, the placement of these sutures based on an arbitrary number of millimeters from the limbus (or from the insertion of the medial rectus muscle, usually 13 mm) again creates an excessive slack in the muscle and remarkably decreases its contractile force; and 3) high rates of undercorrections in esodeviations exceeding 60 prism diopters when traditional bimedial rectus recessions are performed as initial treatment.

Axial length biometry determination represents a substantial improvement over the arbitrary choice of some set distance from the limbus as the site of the equator irrespective of axial length. Intraoperative biometry could prevent errors in axial length determination caused by restlessness of the awake child, or by intraocular pressure changes following the administration of anaesthetic and preliminary surgical procedures (i.e., placement of the lid speculum). In the treatment of congenital or convergence excess esotropia, intraoperative biometry leads to more accurate surgery because the planned suture locations can be adjusted intraoperatively.

Key words: Esotropia, strabismus surgery, axial length biometry

Introduction

Most surgical formulas for rectus muscle recessions are based on grading the operation in millimeters of surgery per prism diopters of deviation or by recessing the muscle to a given distance from the limbus or the muscle insertion [1,2]. To our knowledge, the importance of the size of the globe in determining

G Cennamo and N. Rosa (eds.), Ultrasonography in Ophthalmology 15, pp. 457–463.

the amount of surgery has received little attention.

Because of the considerable variation in the rectus muscle insertion-limbus distance, and in the limbus-equator distance [1,3,4,5], the amount of recession of rectus muscle necessary to place it at/or posterior to the equator will vary with axial length and the individual patient's rectus muscle insertion-limbus distance.

The purpose of this work was to assess the surgical results in esotropic patients with respect to the preoperative deviation, taking into account the globe's equator.

Materials and methods

The ocular axial length was determined in 30 esotropic patients treated with post-fixation suture and/or recession of medial rectus muscles. Of these, 12 had excess convergence esotropia. The preoperative deviation ranged: from 18 to 70 PD for distance, and from 25 to 70 PD for near vision. The age at surgery ranged from 18 to 180 months.

Axial length was determined with the Biophysic Medical Paxial Unit in the operating room, just before surgery. The axial length was the mean of three measurements made in each eye. To calculate the position of the equator, we used the formula proposed by Kushner et al. [1], which is shown in Figure 1.

In all cases of recession the scleral suture was located between the equator and 2 mm posteriorly, to prevent the excessive reduction of the muscular function reported in cases of more posterior sutures [6]. The post-fixation suture was placed in the muscle 2–4 mm posterior to the equator, so that all of the slack in the medial rectus occurred posterior to the post-fixation suture [7,8].

Results and discussion

Axial length was correlated with age and refractive error. As expected, bulb size tended to increase with age and decreased sharply as hypermetropia increased (Figs. 2 and 3).

Figure 4 shows cases in which only a monolateral or bilateral medial rectus muscle recession was performed. The graph represents the recession effectiveness (prismatic diopter per millimeter of surgery) in relation to preoperative deviation in distance vision. Effectiveness clearly increased with respect to the preoperative deviation.

Twelve cases of convergence excess esotropia were treated with Fadenoperation and/or medial rectus muscle recessions. There was a positive correlation between size of preoperative and amount of postoperative deviation, in near vision (Fig. 5). Figure 6 shows that there was a greater response to surgery for distance vision using only recession rather than posterior fixation suture, with the same linear regression slope. The posterior fixation suture reduced the

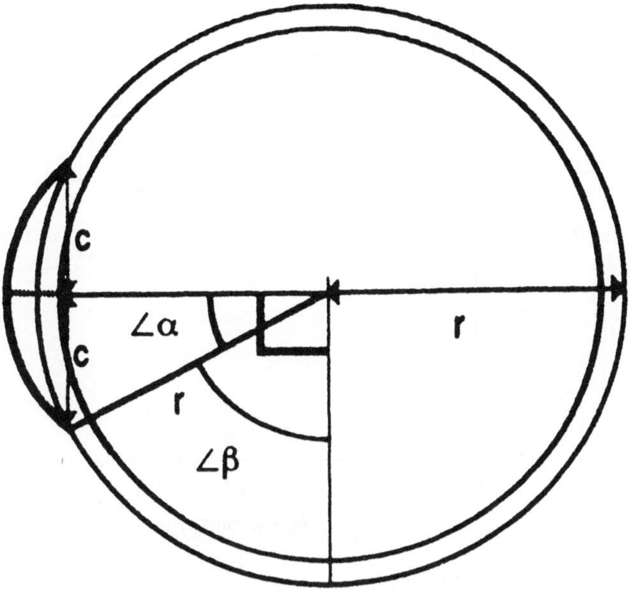

$\angle\beta$ = angle from limbus to equator

r = radius of globe in mm

c = 1/2 corneal diameter

$\angle\alpha + \angle\beta = 90°$

$\frac{c}{r} = \sin \angle\alpha$

$\angle\alpha = \arc\sin \frac{c}{r}$

$\angle\beta = 90° - \arc\sin \frac{c}{r}$

E = mm from limbus to equator

$E = 2 \pi r \left(\frac{\beta}{360°}\right)$

E

Fig. 1. Formula for the calculation of the position of the equator (Kushner et al. 1990)

effectiveness of the recessed muscle by 5 PD.

Based on these findings, we believe that posterior fixation suture does not lead to a slackness of the muscle, but, as shown in Figure 5, to a decrease in its contractile force.

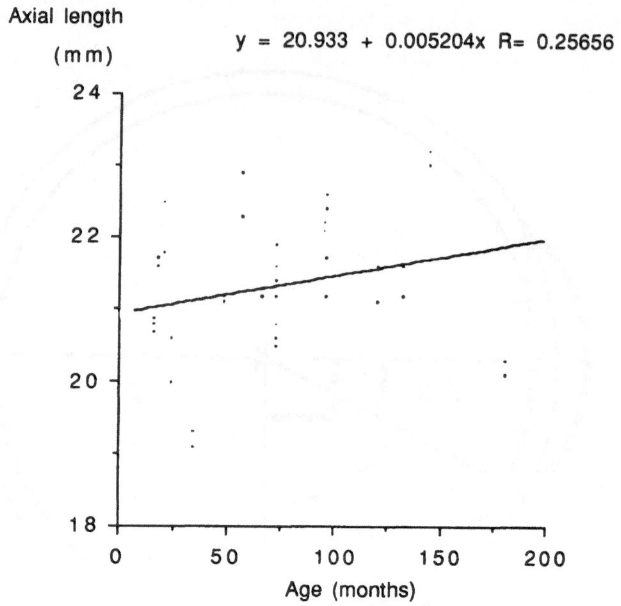

Fig. 2. Axial length in relation to age

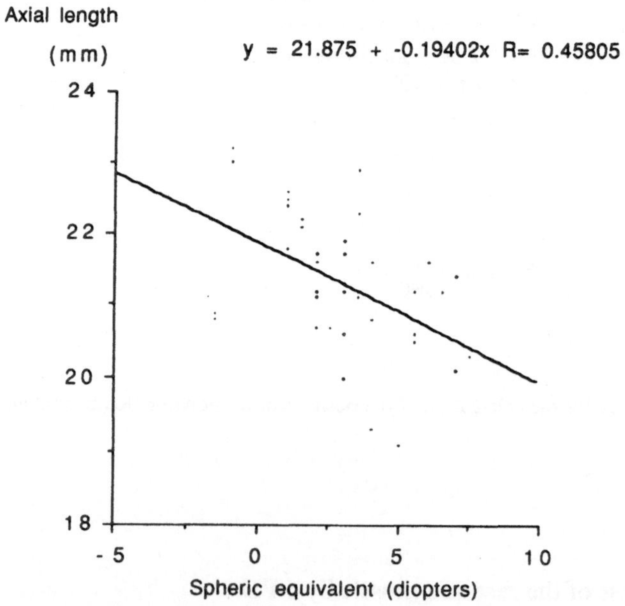

Fig. 3. Axial length in relation to hypermetropia

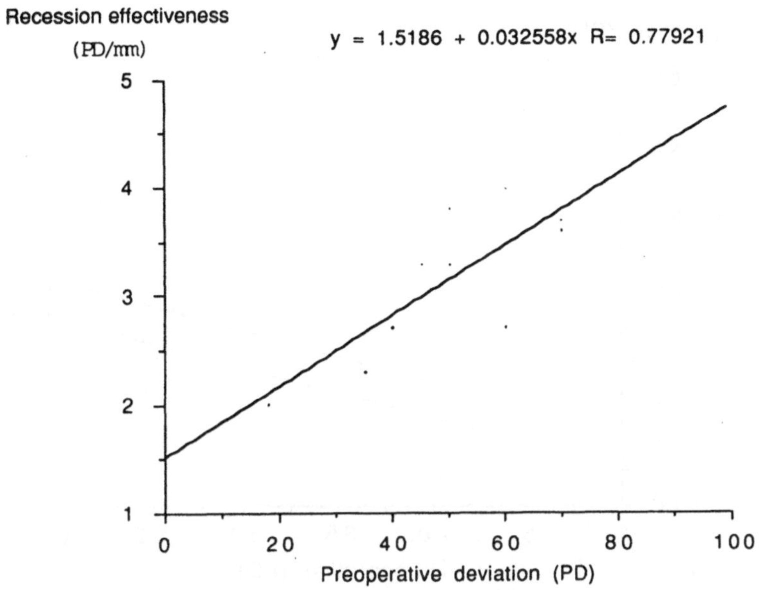

Fig. 4. Monolateral or bilateral medial rectus muscle recession. Recession effectiveness in relation to preoperative deviation

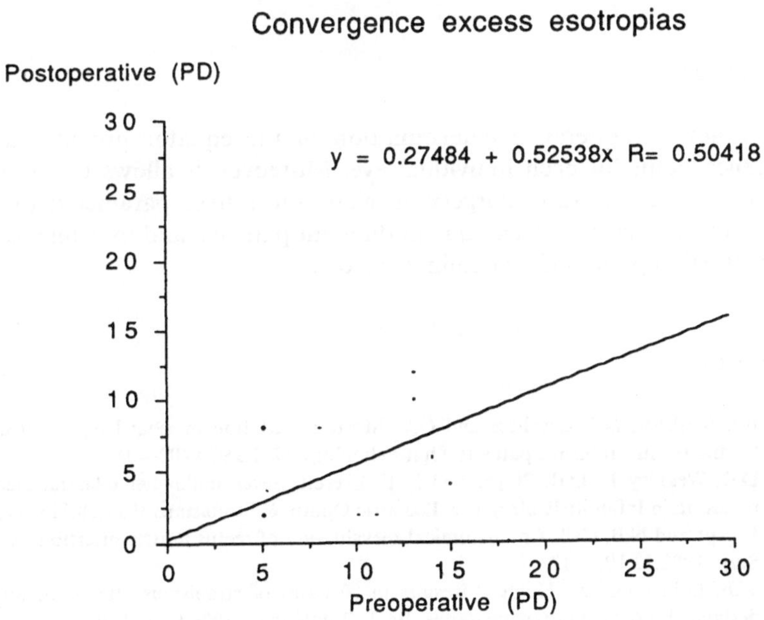

Fig. 5. Fadenoperation and/or medial rectus muscle recession. Post- and preoperative deviation in near vision

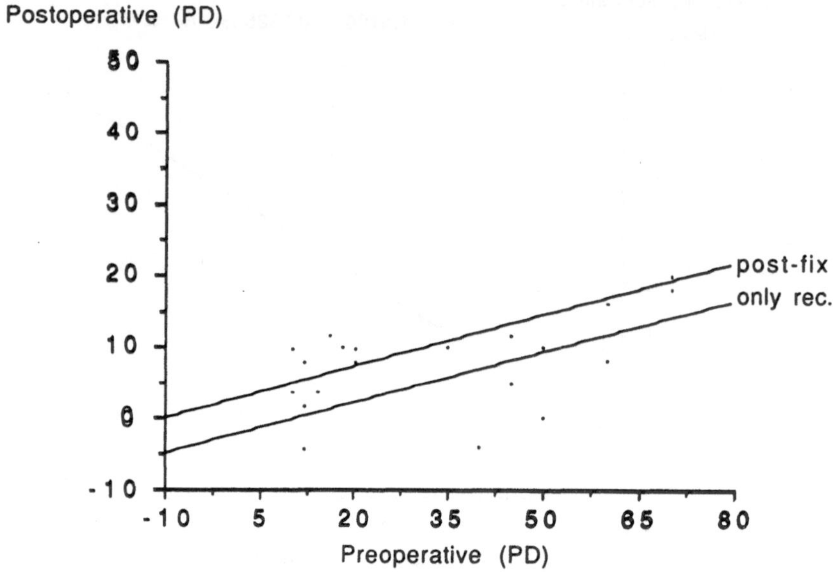

Fig. 6. Medial rectus muscle recession. Post- and preoperative deviation

Conclusions

The exact intraoperative determination of the equator provides a specific reference point for each individual eye. Moreover, it allows us to assess the effectiveness of esotropia surgery in relation to a fixed parameter; to compare the results of the same technique in different patients; and to define exactly the new insertion point and so eliminate errors.

References

[1] B.J. Kushner, N.J. Lucchese and G.V. Morton. Variation in axial length and anatomical landmarks in strabismic patients. Ophthalmology 1991;98(3):400–406.

[2] D.R. Weakley Jr, D.R. Stager and M.E. Everett. Seven millimeter bilateral medial rectus recession in Infantile Esotropia. J. Pediatric Ophth. & Strabismus 1991;28:113–115.

[3] L. Apt and N.B. Call. An anatomical reevaluation of rectus muscle insertions. Ophthalmic Surg. 1982;13:108–112.

[4] W.E. Gillies and A. Hughes. Results in 50 cases of strabismus after graduated surgery designed by A-scan ultrasonography. Br. J. Ophthalmol. 1984;68:790–795.

[5] W.E. Gillies and A. McIndoe. Measurement of strabismus eyes with A scan ultrasonography. Aus. J. Ophthalmol. 1981;9:231–232.

[6] B.J. Kushner and M. Vrabec. Theoretical effects of surgery on length tension relationship in extraocular muscles. J. Pediatric Ophth. & Strabismus 1987;24:126–131.
[7] B.J. Kushner. Evaluation of the posterior fixation plus recession operation with saccadic velocities. J. Pediatric Ophth. & Strabismus 1983;20:202–209.
[8] R.J. Leitch, P.J. Burke and I.M. Strachan. Convergence excess esotropia treated surgically with fadenoperation and medial rectus muscle recessions. Br. J. Ophthalmol. 1990;74:278–279.

Paolo Perissutti
Department of Ophthalmology
Children's Hospital of Trieste
Trieste, Italy

Instrumentation and techniques

58. Spectral maps from intraocular tumors by a new imaging technique using a modified echographic B-mode instrument

R. FREZZOTTI,[1] E. MOTOLESE,[1] A. BARTOLOMEI,[1] L. MASOTTI,[2] S. ROCCHI[3] and A. FORT[2]

([1,3]Siena and [2]Florence, Italy)

Abstract

A new imaging technique that combines spectral maps with the conventional B-mode display was applied to eyes affected by intraocular tumors in order to characterize tissutal structure. Here we describe a modular system for the evaluation of the application of the proposed technique in clinical practice. With a modified echographic B-mode equipment, the radio frequency ultrasound signal and the relative scanning transducer position are sampled, digitized and stored by a two-channel acquisition system for a whole scanning period (freezing function).

The data, digitized with an 8-bit resolution and 50 MHz sampling frequency, are processed by a personal computer, which, like a wholly digital echographic B-mode equipment, builds the B-mode image and combines it with the spectral map of the zone outlined by the physician.

Key-words: Radio frequency echo-signal, spectral map, intraocular tumors

Introduction

Conventional ultrasonography, based on both the A-mode and the B-mode technique was introduced in ophthalmology to differentiate intraocular tumors and related lesions and to evaluate tumor thickness for monitoring the growth pattern. Today, with the wide use of conservative treatments, it assumes a primary role in the management of intraocular tumors because the treatment effectiveness is strongly dependent on the tumor type, dimension and position inside the eye.

Conventional ultrasonography, whose principal characteristics for intraocular tumors are well known, is not able to provide sufficient data regarding histological characterization and tissutal structure for the filtering and averaging processes on the backscattered echo-signals, and therefore there is a loss

G Cennamo and N. Rosa (eds.), Ultrasonography in Ophthalmology 15, pp. 467–474.

of information. These processes are, however, necessary to visualize and analyze the signals as we can see in A and B-mode presentation [1].

To overcome this problem we can analyze the features conveyed by the radio frequency (RF) backscattered echosignal. Some of these features, depending on the mean size, shape, elastic properties and concentration of the scattering particles, can be extracted by estimating the power spectrum density (PSD). In fact, the pathological zones can be considered as a random distribution of particles, in a homogeneous fluid, characterized by mean size below the ultrasound wavelength and the particle medium features influence the PSD behaviour of the RF backscattered echoes. However, the information on the tissue microstructure is hidden in random components due to the stochastic nature of the tissue and the PSD of the zone being investigated must be statistically estimated [2,3].

The power spectral density (PSD) is commonly estimated via fast Fourier transform (FFT) followed by an averaging process on the investigated homogeneous zone. Different parameters extracted from the PSD have been proposed to characterize tissue zones, but they are no longer relevant when the zone of interest is not homogeneous, that is when calcified and necrotic zones are present. As described in previous articles, our group proposed the formation of topological maps based on the centroid of the echoes backscattered from limited tissue zones which can be considered homogeneous [4–8].

This technique aims to emphasize local inhomogeneities, in terms of particle mean size, typical of some intraocular tumors like retinoblastoma or neoformations with histological changes induced by conservative therapies.

The conventional approach to PSD estimation (via FFT) is not suitable because the short data windowing greatly reduces the averaging effectiveness and the related estimates of spectral parameters are affected by residual randomness. Therefore, the PSD is estimated through an auto-regressive (AR) modelling technique that is substantially insensitive to the above-mentioned windowing effects. Low order AR models are used because they smooth the spectrum peaks and pits due to the position of the random scatterers, while preserving the spectrum shift trend. The derived topological maps are proposed as a support to conventional A- and B-mode imaging because they emphasize the spectral features of the RF backscattered signals (which are completely lost in conventional ultrasonography) that demonstrate the differences in acoustic impedance.

Theoretical framework

The backscattered signal, x(t), is a stochastic process that, in the frequency domain X(f), can be written as follows:

$$(1) \quad x(f) = \sum_i T^2(f)\, A^2(f_i\, Z_i)\, B_i(f)\, e^{-jw2Zi\backslash c}$$

In Eq. 1, f is the frequency; z_i and B_i (f) are the axial position and the frequency response of the i-th scatterer which depends on its shape and size; T(f) is the transducer response and A(f, z_i) is the attenuation due to the biological medium. T(f) and A(f, z_i) are squared because ultrasonic pulse-echo systems are considered. When only the absorption phenomenon is considered, A(f, z_i) can be expressed by the following formula:

$$(2) \qquad A(f, z) = e^{-fz}$$

a being the absorption coefficient.

Assuming the validity of the Rayleigh-Born approximation, B_i (f) can be obtained as follows. The velocity potential 0 scatt of the acoustic field at point r scattered by an object placed at point r_i, is:

$$(3) \qquad \Phi_{scatt}(r, r_i) = \Phi_{inc}(r_i)\, f_i\, (K, K')\, \exp \frac{jK[r-r_i]}{[r-r_i]}$$

where Φ_{inc} is the velocity potential of the incident field; K is the propagation vector of the impinging field and K′ is the propagation vector of the scattered field. The backscattered field can be found by setting K′=–K:

$$(4) \qquad B(f) = F(K, K')_{[k'=-k]}$$

If the scatterers are assumed to be spherical fluid particles, B(f) can be approximated as the following function of frequency:

$$(5) \qquad B(f) = F(K, K') = \mu \frac{\sin(2ka)}{8k} - a\frac{\cos(2ka)}{4}$$

where μ is a parameter related to the particle acoustic impedance and a is the particle radius.

The information concerning the particle size contained in the backscattered ultrasonic signal is embedded in random components due to the random character of the tissue microstructure that is represented by the randomness of the scatterer positions.

The function B(f), in Eq. 1 is the only term dependent on the scatterer size and the average size of the scatterers and it can be obtained by evaluating the power spectrum density of the process, thus eliminating the noisy effect of the random phase shifts. It is well known that the power spectrum density is given by the following equation, when the process is ergodic and stationary:

$$(6) \qquad PSD = E\,[x\,(2f)\, x'\,(2f)]$$

where E [ ] is the expectation operator.

As a clarifying example, a tissue made up of identical scatterers with uniform spatial distribution can be selected. In this case by substituting Eq. 1 in Eq. 6, the PSD results as follows:

$$(7) \qquad PSD_{per}(K) = \frac{1}{L} \sum_{r=1}^{L} x^{r}_{per}(K)\, x^{*r}_{per}(K)$$

Experimental laboratory results

For ophthalmological ultrasonic diagnosis, one must differentiate among tissues made up of particles whose mean dimension ranges from about 20 µm to 100 µm. This differentiation is usually performed by ultrasonic transducer characterized by a 10 MHz central frequency, which implies a wave length of 150 µm, well above the mean particle diameter. This choice is determined by the trade-off between good resolution and low attenuation of the ultrasonic waves in tissue.

To validate the proposed imaging technique a laboratory set-up was prepared. The principle characteristics of this set-up are listed below:

Transducer

6 dB band width of 7 MHz
Central frequency equal to 3.9 MHz
12 dB focal spot of 0.8 mm at a distance of 35 mm

Pulser-receiver

Panametrics model 5052
35 MHz bandwidth

Acquisition system

Oscilloscope Tecktronics model TDS 540

Personal computer

The spectral imaging technique was applied both to the backscattered signals from a simulated tissue model and to the ultrasonic signals backscattered from a test-object and collected by using the laboratory set-up described above. In the latter case, a linear scanning was performed on a test-object made of a gel suspension of calibrated late spheres of 20–50–80–100 µm.

This model was verified on two *in vitro* specimens obtained from enucleated eyes affected by retinoblastoma (RTB) and choroidal malignant melanoma (CMM). These tumors do not present any problem for clinical diagnosis but they are substantially different as regards the histological characteristics. Therefore, they represent a good model with which to evaluate the reliability of the RF analysis. RTB is characterized by a very irregular internal structure while CMM presents a more regular internal structure.

Formation of spectral maps

The backscattered signals are split into segments, whose length is 1:4 times the transducer pulse length; with the ultrasonic equipment we have used, this corresponds to 250–1000 μm pathological segments (Fig. 1).

Each segment is processed by the AR technique and the spectrum centroid is evaluated. A topological map is built by associating a colour or grey level to each value obtained; the colour or grey scale ranges from the theoretical centroid value calculated for 80 μm spheres to that calculated for 20 μm spheres.

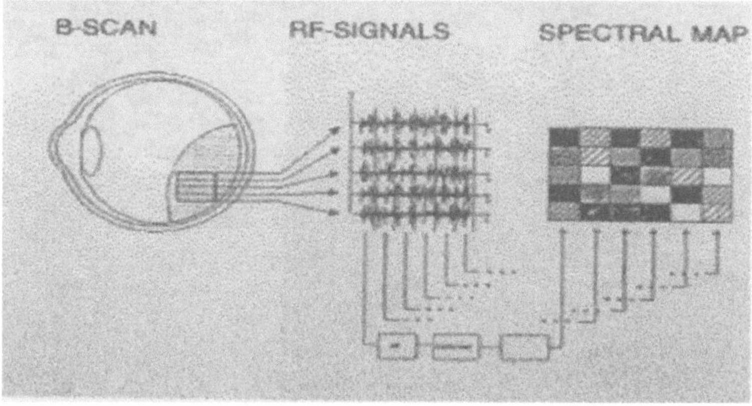

Fig. 1.

In earlier work, we presented the results related to the simulated model and the test object: particles characterized by small differences in diameters (from 20 to 100 μm) are differentiated on the spectral maps. Our experience is also based on pathological specimens related to RTB and CMM. The different histological characteristics of the two disorders, which cannot be determined by B-mode presentation, are detectable on the spectral maps [9].

Hardware modular solution to evaluate the proposed technique performances

An evaluation of the performance in ophthalmological diagnosis of the proposed technique requires completely digital echographic equipment. A modular solution has been assembled; this consists of a modified echographic apparatus, an acquisition system and a conventional personal computer. This hardware structure is somewhat cumbersome, but it allows the physician to evaluate the actual capability and effectiveness of the proposed technique in the clinical field, even though the system is not easy to handle and the imaging results are not on-line.

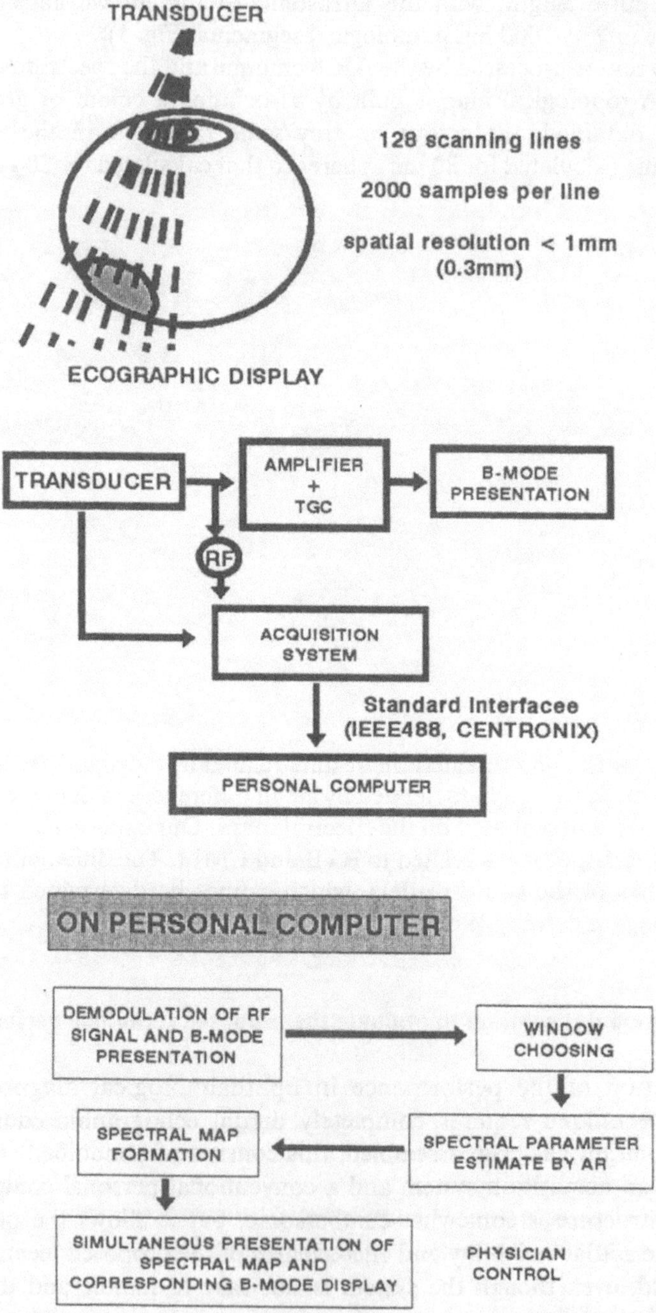
TRANSDUCER
128 scanning lines
2000 samples per line
spatial resolution < 1mm
(0.3mm)
ECOGRAPHIC DISPLAY
TRANSDUCER
AMPLIFIER
+
TGC
B-MODE
PRESENTATION
RF
ACQUISITION
SYSTEM
Standard Interfacee
(IEEE488, CENTRONIX)
PERSONAL COMPUTER
ON PERSONAL COMPUTER
DEMODULATION OF RF
SIGNAL AND B-MODE
PRESENTATION
WINDOW
CHOOSING
SPECTRAL MAP
FORMATION
SPECTRAL PARAMETER
ESTIMATE BY AR
SIMULTANEOUS PRESENTATION OF
SPECTRAL MAP AND
CORRESPONDING B-MODE DISPLAY
PHYSICIAN
CONTROL

Fig. 2

A block scheme of the assembled structure is shown in Figure 2 together with the technical requirements. An acquisition system digitizes and stores the amplified RF echosignals from a whole scanning section and the transducer position of each scanning line. The storing memory is updated at each scanning section; under the physician's control the memory data are frozen and the information is transferred to a PC. The proposed imaging technique is implemented on the PC according to the flow diagram.

Conclusions

A diagnostic support is proposed that combines spectral maps based on the extraction of a spectral parameter from the RF backscattered ultrasonic signal and conventional B-mode scan, both of which are simultaneously displayed because the topological references are retained.

Local tissue is characterized from the estimation of the frequency centroid related to the mean size of scatterers that constitute the tissue. The spectral maps give complementary information with respect to conventional B-mode imaging, thus a complete diagnostic support is provided when they are simultaneously displayed. The B-mode presentation exploits the information related to the echo amplitude, while the spectral maps outline the frequency behaviour of the backscattered signals which is hidden in the B-mode presentation. The spectral maps do not lead to an automatic diagnosis but they offer the advantage of preserving their relevance even when the investigated region is not homogeneous.

We propose a hardware configuration for the evaluation of the effectiveness of the imaging technique in the clinical field and for the estimation of the technical requirements of a new echographic equipment able in real time to provide the physician with relevant information about the spectral characteristics of the echoes backscattered from pathological zones.

References

[1] V. Mazzeo. Ecografia dell'apparato oculare. Milano: Fogliazza Editore 1987.

[2] A.T. Cheung, P.W. Buchen, C. Macaskill and D.E. Robinson. Backscattered spectrum of a ramdomly peffurbed regular array of discrete scafferers. J. Acoust. Soc. Am. 1989;86(1):40.

[3] D.J. Coleman, R.M. Silverman, M.J. Rondeau, F.L. Lizzi, I.W. McLean and F.A. Jakebies Correlation of acoustic tissue typing of malignant melanoma and histopathologic features as a predictor of death. Am. J. Ophthalmol. 1990;110:380–388.

[4] S.M. Kay and S.L. Marple. Spectrum analysis. A modern perspective. EEE Proc. 1981;69(1): 1380.

[5] M.F. Insana, R.F. Wagner, D.G. Brown and T.J. Hall. Describing small-scale structure in random media using pulse echo ultrasound. J. Acoust. Soc. Am. 1990;87(1):179.

[6] F.L. Lizzi, M. Greenbaum, E.J. Feleppa and M. Elbaum. Theoretical framework for the spectrum analysis in ultrasound tissue characterization. J. Acoust. Soc. Am. 1983;73(4):1366.

[7] F.L. Lizzi, M. Ostromogilisky, E.J. Feleppa, M. Rorke and M.M. Yaremko. Relationship of the ultrasound spectral parameters to features of tissue microstructure. IEEE Trans. on UFFC 1986;33(1):319.

[8] S.L. Marple. Digital spectral analysis with applications. Englewood Cliffs, N.J.: Prentice Hall, 1987.

[9] A. Bartolomei, S. Nardoni, S. Rocchi, E. Motolese, R. Frezzotti and L. Masotti. L'analisi spettrale del segnale ecografico a radiofrequenza nelle neoplasie oculari: risultati preliminari. In L. Falco and S. Esente (eds), Tumori Intraoculari. Proceedings of the International Symposium on Intraocular Tumors (Florence), 1990.

[1]Prof. Eduardo Motolese
Department of Ophthalmological and Neurosurgical Sciences
University of Siena
Siena, Italy

[2]Department of Electronic Engineering
University of Florence
Florence, Italy

[3]Department of Electronic Engineering
University of Siena
Siena, Italy

59. Methods in the echographic study of ocular tumors: indices of clinical follow-up of the disease

G. ADDABBO, E. MOTOLESE and R. FREZZOTTI
(Siena, Italy)

Abstract

We report our experience in evaluating volume and other indicators that can be used to monitor tumor growth. These data are easily read using three-dimensional echography developed by us.

Key words: Echography, three-dimensional, contour lines, tumors

Introduction

The progress that has been made in recent years in ocular echography has opened new frontiers in the field of ophthalmological diagnosis. Easy access to digital image processing techniques, and the ever increasing use of computers represent the departure point for a correct approach to modern ocular echography [1–4].

Today, many diagnostic systems are integral parts of computers and many other systems offer the capability of exchanging diagnostic information with the external microprocessor (CPU) of a personal computer (PC) [5–8].

Since 1987 in the Ophthalmological and Neurosurgical Sciences Department of the University of Siena (Italy) the diagnostic potentialities of the three-dimensional reconstruction of B-scan echograms, and the volume and areas of tumor lesion sections have been investigated. This technique is an important aid to the diagnosis and monitoring of ocular tumors and it offers a quantity of biometric data thus far unavailable with conventional echography [9–12].

With the increase of our experience, the technique has been extended to applications of image-elaborations with digital image-processing; this has considerably improved the information obtained with ultrasonographic imaging and consequently the diagnostic reliability of the technique [14,15].

G Cennamo and N. Rosa (eds.), Ultrasonography in Ophthalmology 15, pp. 475–482.

Material and methods

Clinical reports

In recent years we have produced the three-dimensional reconstruction of many tumors. In this paper we present 10 cases of choroidal malignant melanoma where we have calculated not only the volume but also other clinical indicators that we retain are relevant in monitoring the evolution or regression of the neoplasia. These cases with the respective indicators are shown in Table 1.

Principle

The technique is based on obtaining serial bidimensional sections of tumoral lesions. The tumor is divided into slices of a specific thickness, varying from 0.1 to 0.5 and 1 mm and the volume is calculated: the sum of the lesion areas in each scan slice, multiplied by the slice interval, is equal to the tumor volume.

We are currently evaluating the possibility of using the Gauss algorithm on the object-oriented images to calculate the volume using multiple integration; the advantage would be to have a calculation error tending to zero.

Instrumentation

Echograph Teknar, Ophthasonic Image 2000 A/B-scan System with a 10 MHz B-scan focused probe. A tracking mechanism that serves to anchor the probe and to acquire seriated scansions. This is motorized and managed electronically by means of a PC. With the software we can program the pace of the linear slide of the probe on the examined eye and the distance between the sections. We have projected, produced and registered patented (N. SI93U000004.) the tracking mechanism (Fig. 1). A personal computer (80486) 16Mb RAM with a video interface. A '3-D Echo-Analysis' software, which serves to obtain the three-dimensional reconstruction of the image and to analyze the B-scan echograms of the video-signal processing obtained from the echograph. With this software we can handle a quantity of data that could not be obtained with traditional echographic instruments.

More accurate algorithms allow us to calculate the volume of lesions that have an anomalous morphology. A rather precise measurement of tumor thickness can be obtained with the 'contour lines method'. All the data can be recorded on a 'physical memory' in the form of files for easy and quick consultation.

Table 1.

Cases	1	2	3	4	5	6	7	8	9	10
Basal Area (mm 2)	51.68	35.5	19	66.5	1.5	60.56	14.94	18.62	27.62	7.38
Thickness (mm)	9	5	5.87	11.37	2.5	16.75	12	5.62	8.31	1.89
Thickness/Basal area (mm 1)	0.17	0.14	0.31	0.17	1.66	0.27	0.80	0.30	0.30	0.24
External Surface (mm 2)	313.1	175.81	172	477	55.22	522.2	237.3	217.8	214	128.43
Area of section (mm 2)										
Average	35.32	27.76	31.57	55.97	11.02	34.43	74	19.32	35.5	11.74
Variance	13.15	6.83	10.25	23.29	5.05	17.9	12.6	8.54	4.81	10.81
Volume (mm 3)	441.48	144.49	217	829.18	7.61	1536.2	237.33	217.81	302.46	92.70

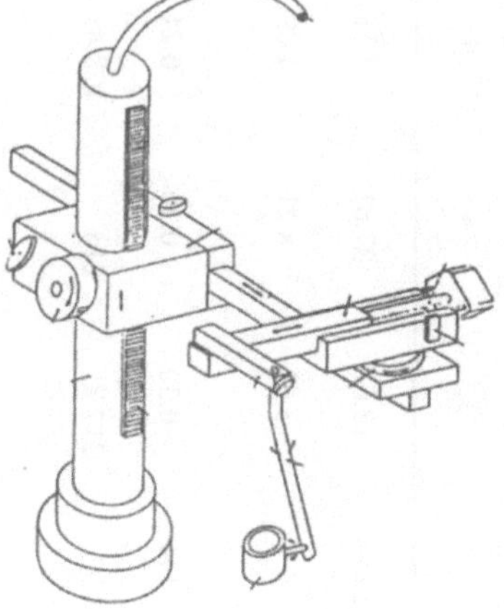

Fig. 1. Tracking mechanism

Technique

Three-dimensional B-scan images are elaborated in five steps:

Step 1. Acquisition: the images come from the video output or from the serial port RS232 and they are sent to the PC.

Step 2. Image Analysis: this filters and reduces the noise and increases the diagnostic quality of the image. We use *lowpass filters* to attenuate the abrupt changes of grey level in a selected zone and *highpass filters* to emphasize the changes and the contrasts and to emphasize the edges of the lesion (Fig. 2). We use bandpass filters to emphasize the intralesional grey levels and to attenuate those of the adjacent zones (Fig. 3). Wiener's algorithm is used to filter the noise. We sample the spatial frequency of the changes in grey level in a desired region of the image by means of the Fast Fourier Transformer (FFT). Using this software with digitized standardized A-scan one can estimate the signal attenuation by means of the K angle; it also allows us to study the internal structure and lesion reflectivity.

Step 3. Areas and volume calculation: we calculate the area of the sections, and their averages are represented in a graph that shows the morphological outline of the neoplasia (Fig. 4). The volume is calculated according to the following formula:

$$\Sigma \text{ area of the section x interval between the sections}$$

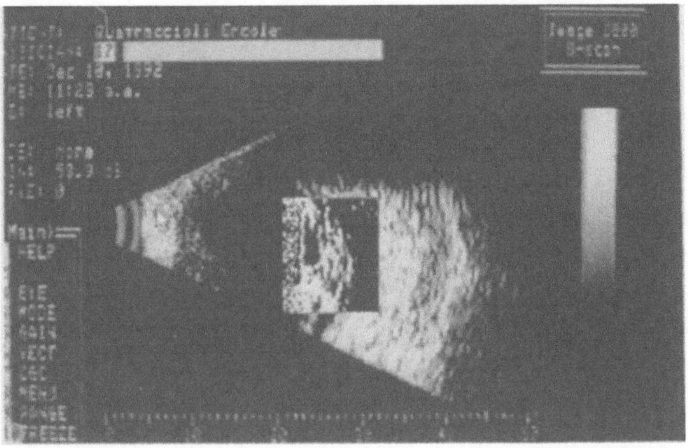

Fig. 2. **Highpass filtering**

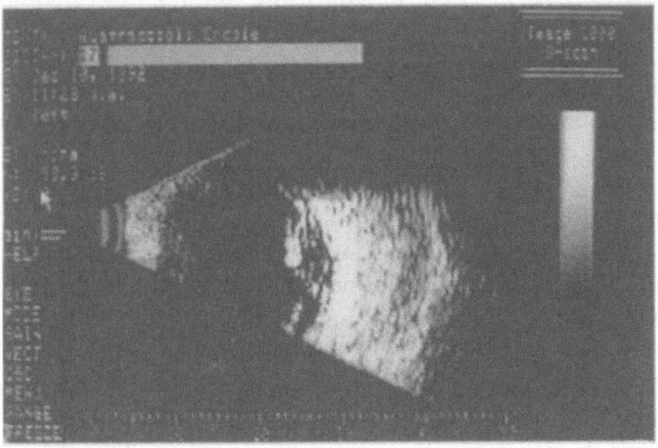

Fig. 3. **Bandpass filtering**

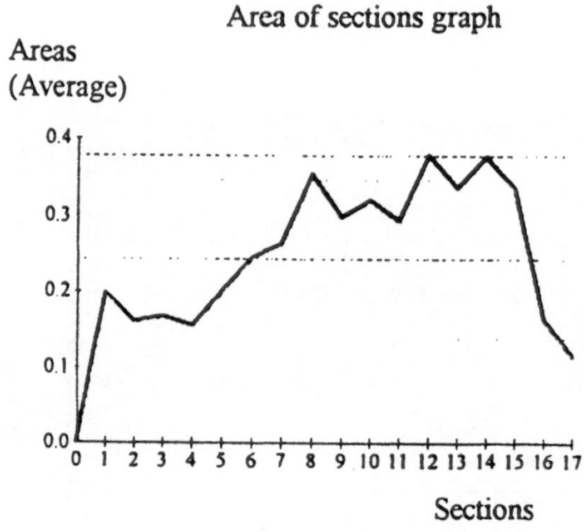

Fig. 4. Average areas

We also calculate the basal area of the tumor and the external surface. The tumor thickness on the retinal plain is evaluated by means of the 'contour lines method'. This consists in sampling the lesion in a series of planes that are parallel with respect to the basal area and that move from the base towards the apex of the lesion. Each plane is of a different colour and the sampling frequency increases with increasing proximity to the apex of the tumor according to an exponential law. In the map arising from contour lines method the various thicknesses are shown in different colours.

Steps 4 and 5. Statistical evaluation of the measurements obtained and the reconstruction of the three-dimensional graphics (Fig. 5).

Discussion

Among the numerous techniques available for ophthalmological investigation, echography plays an increasingly important role because it is a non invasive examination and because it can be used to monitor ocular and orbital tumors under conservative treatment. The studies conducted so far were devoted to the use of traditional ultrasonographic techniques to evaluate tumor thickness, and standardized A-scan to evaluate internal structures. Therefore, there are two approaches to tumor monitoring: on one hand, there is the evaluation of the qualitative ultrasonographic data that are produced from the analysis of the signal of the radio frequency; on the other hand, there is the quantitative approach that focuses on the biometric data of the lesion obtained through the elaboration of the video-signal, followed by the three-dimensional reconstruction of the tumor.

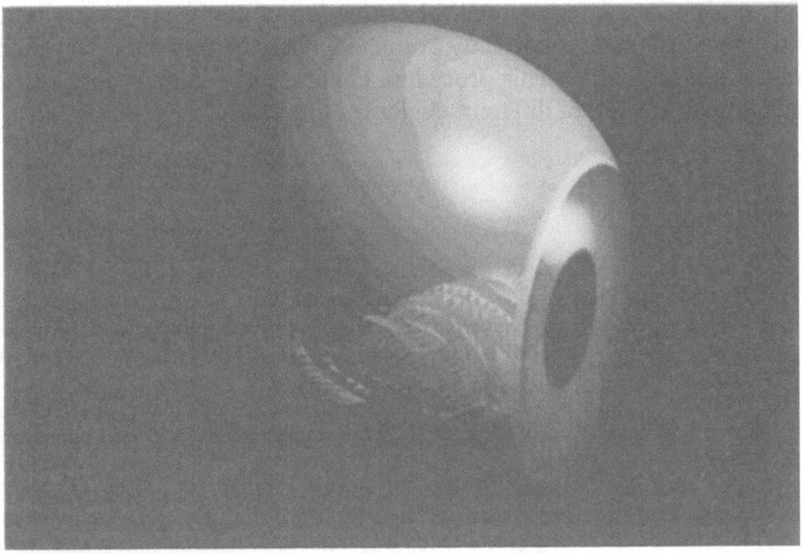

Fig. 5. Three-dimensional graphics

The cases reported by us present some peculiarities. After studying the correlation among the indicators, we conclude as follows:

1. There was not a significant linear correlation among the measurements of the tumor thickness performed by the standardized A-scan and volume ($r = 0.120$). If there is a correlation, it is not linear because, in such cases, slight changes of thickness would correlate with greater volume changes.
2. There is a highly significant linear correlation of the thickness using the contour lines method and volume ($r = 0.984$). However, it should be stressed that this finding cannot be extended beyond our sample, and that the object-oriented elaboration of the three-dimensional reconstruction is used to obtain both the volume and thickness measurements.
3. The external surface of the tumor and the volume are not correlated parameters.
4. There is a highly significant linear correlation between the basal area of the tumor and volume ($r = 0.919$). The averages of the area of the sections and of their variance are also useful parameters.
5. The value of the average of the area of the sections area could serve as reference values for subsequent sampling; the variance among the section areas may reflect the morphological pattern of the lesion and it could reveal changes in the shape of the tumor that occur without a significant increase of the volume.

This study seems to encourage the evaluation of all the suggested indicators because some of them, if correctly evaluated, could be important in the follow-up of the tumor [16–19]. This procedure could also be used to differentiate the kinetic growth models of different ocular tumors [20].

References

[1] R. Azriel and C.K. Avinash. Digital picture processing. Academic Press. 1982.
[2] V. Cappellini. Elaborazione numerica delle immagini. Turin: Boringhieri Ed., 1985.
[3] L. Cavalli Sforza. Analisi statistica per medici e biologi. Turin: Boringhieri Ed., 1983.
[4] D.J. Coleman, L.F. Lizzi and R.L. Jack. Ultrasonography of the eye and orbit. Philadelphia: Lea-Febiger, 1977.
[5] D.J. Coleman. Ultrasonic measurement of eye dimensions. International Ophthalmology Clinics. Ophthalmic Ultrasonography: comparative techniques. Boston: Little Brown and Co., 1979.
[6] T. Colton. Statistica in medicina. Padua: Piccin, 1983.
[7] C. Eichler, A. Herthel, P.K. Lommatzsch and P. Fuhrmann. Echographische Befunde vor und nach Beta-bestrahlung (106 Ru-106 Rh) von Aderhautmelanomen, Klin. Monatsbl. Augenheilk. 1987;190(1):17–20.
[8] L. Falco, G.L. Paladini, S. Utari, S. Esente and N. Passarelli. 3D (VXL-3D): Lo stato della ricerca (caratterizzazione tissutale, calcolo del volume). Clinic. Ocul. e Patol. Ocul. 1993;14(2):85–87.
[9] R. Frezzotti, E. Motolese, G. Addabbo, G. Dell'Eva, M. Burroni, E. Patacchini, B. D'Aniello and A. Gatti. Tentativi di ricostruzione tridimensionale dell'immagine ecografica. III S.I.E.O. Congress, Naples, 13 November 1988. Clin. Ocul. e Patol. Ocul. 1989;10(5).
[10] S. Harrington. Computer graphics. Mc Graw-Hill, 1983.
[11] M. Ito, T. Shiina, Y. Sugata and Y. Yamamoto. On two and three dimensional image processings applied to ophthalmic region. XXII S.I.D.U.O. Congress, 1988.
[12] V. Mazzeo. Testo atlante di ecografia oculare. Fogliazza Ed., 1988.
[13] V. Mazzeo. Recenti innovazioni nella strumentazione per diagnostica in ecoftalmologia. Clinic. Ocul. e Patol. Ocul. 1993;14(2):56–62.
[14] E. Motolese, G. Addobbo, B. D'Aniello, M. Burroni and G. Dell'Eva. Immagini tridimensionali in ecoftalmologia. Proc. LXIX S.O.I. Congress, Rome, 12-15 October, 1989.
[15] E. Motolese, B. D'Aniello, M. Burroni, G. Dell'Eva, G. Addabbo, and N. Paterra. Three-dimensional "images" in ophthalmology. XXXVI I.C.O., Singapore, 18-24 March, 1990.
[16] M. Nagao and T. Matsutama. Edge Preserve Smoothing. Computer Graphics and Image Processing. 1979;9.
[17] W.K. Pratt. Digital images processing, Wiley and Sons, 1978.
[18] J.A. Shields, C.L. Shields and L.A. Donoso. Management of posterior uveal melanoma. Surv. Ophthalmol. 1991;36(3):161–195.
[19] J. Teuber. Digital image processing. London: Prentice Hall, 1993.
[20] L. Zografos, C.L. Gailloud, C.H. Perret, L. Chamot, S. Raimondi and S. Carrel. Terapia conservativa dei melanomi uveali. In Proc. LXVII S.O.I. Congress, Rome, 26–29 November 1987.

Prof. Edoardo Motolese
Department of Ophthalmological and Neurosurgical Sciences
University of Siena
Siena, Italy

60. Acoustic characteristics of the eye lens

J.M. THIJSSEN,[1,4] C.L. DE KORTE,[1,5] A.F.W. VAN DER STEEN,[1,5]
J.J. DUINDAM,[2] C. OTTO[3] and G.J. PUPPELS[3]
([1]Nijmegen, [2]Amsterdam, [3]Enschede and [4]Rotterdam, The Netherlands)

Abstract

The purpose of this study is to characterize the eye lens (human and porcine) by acoustic measurements and to investigate whether relations exist with the local protein content. The acoustic measurements were performed with a 'scanning acoustic microscope' (SAM), operating at a frequency of 20 MHz. At this frequency the lateral resolution in the acoustic images was 150 mm. A double-transmission pulse-echo technique was employed to obtain acoustic parameter images of a central, 1-mm thick slice of the lenses. The two-dimensional images were derived by ultrasonic spectroscopy displaying the ultrasound velocity, the attenuation at 20 MHz and the slope of the attenuation coefficient between 17 and 213 MHz. The images were summarized by profiles along the optical and equatorial axes of these parameters.

Acoustic parameters were obtained from human lenses (n = 13) and porcine lenses (n = 10). The protein contents of human lenses were obtained from the literature. Additionally, Raman microspectroscopy was used to measure the local protein content of porcine lenses (n = 3). The relation between the protein content and the acoustic parameters was investigated by comparing the axial and lateral profiles.

There was a gradual decrease of the magnitude of the acoustic parameters from the centre to the periphery of the porcine eye lens, which is clearly equal to the decrease in protein content profiles. For the human lenses the acoustic characteristics and the protein content exhibit the same profile, fairly constant in the lens nucleus and decreasing towards the periphery of the lens cortex. Strong positive correlation coefficients for acoustic parameters and protein content for the porcine lens were found.

It is concluded that protein concentration-related phenomena can be investigated by measuring the acoustic parameters.

Key words: Eye lens, ultrasonic spectroscopy, ultrasound velocity, ultrasound attenuation, Raman microspectroscopy, protein content, correlation

G Cennamo and N. Rosa (eds.), Ultrasonography in Ophthalmology 15, pp. 483–496.

Introduction

To a certain extent, the eye lens forms an obstruction for the examination of the eye, because of its high reflectivity and absorption. In addition, the velocity of ultrasound propagation in the lens is considerably higher than in the surrounding media. Consequently, biometry equipment must be specifically calibrated for measurements of the axial eye length. We measured the local distribution of ultrasound parameters of the eye lens. In earlier studies [1,2] it appeared that the relatively strong curvature of the lens surfaces prevented an accurate measurement of the attenuation. Moreover, the velocity was only measured of the lens as a whole, i.e., no assessment of eventual inhomogeneities was made. The study by van der Steen *et al.* [3] was made with a custom-made SAM (scanning acoustic microscope) and a central, 1-mm thick slice of porcine lenses was measured. There was a large inhomogeneity of the porcine lenses both for the velocity and the attenuation parameters, which can be summarized as a systematic decrease of the parameters from the centre towards the periphery of the lens. It was

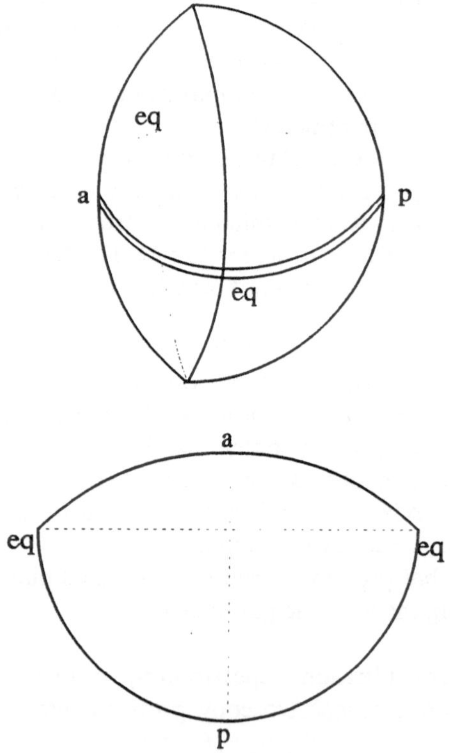

Fig. 1. Top: Scheme of lens with central slice indicated. Bottom: definition of axial profile (a–p) and equatorial profile (eq–eq)

hypothesized that the acoustic and optical parameters of the eye lens depend mainly on the local protein content. Here we report measurements of the local protein content in porcine lenses.

Measurement of the local protein content of porcine lenses was performed by means of Raman microspectroscopy [4,5] and the correlation with the local acoustic parameters was investigated. The local acoustic characteristics of human eye lenses were also measured. These results are compared with the data of the protein distribution in human lenses, also measured with Raman microspectrometry, as derived from an earlier paper [6].

Materials

Human eyes (n = 13) were obtained from donors whose age range was 19–85 years. For measurements of the acoustic parameters, the lenses were prepared by cutting the eye at the limbus and reaching the lens from the back. The lens was loosened by cutting the zonula fibres and the lens was removed. Next the lens was placed in a comb-like cutting device and a 1-mm thick slice was cut centrally [3]. Therefore, the lens slice contained the two geometrical axes (Fig. 1). The human lens slices were measured 24 to 36 hours post mortem.

Porcine eyes (n = 10) were obtained from the municipal slaughter house within 4 hours after the death of the animals and prepared in the same way as the human eyes. The porcine lenses used to measure the protein concentration (n = 3) were removed from eyes with the method described above, but then fixed in a physiological saline solution with the addition of 4% formalin solution, and buffered for 7 days. This preparation does not influence the protein content when measured with Raman microspectroscopy [7]. Thereafter, 1-mm thick slices were cut; these contained the two eyes axes as before.

Methods

Acoustic microscopy

The principle and the details of the scanning acoustic microscope (SAM) have been extensively described elsewhere [3,8–10]. The SAM is based on a double transmission measurement through a tissue specimen. The specimen is placed on a plane reflector in a water tank (filled with physiological saline solution at 20°C). The ultrasound transducer (20 MHz in this study) is directed perpendicular at the reflector and at its focal distance. The transducer is made to perform 2-D rasterscans (100 × 80 points, 0.1 mm steps). One scan is made without the lens slice, the second with the slice in place (Fig. 2). From the echoes (rf-acquisition by digital oscilloscope) reflected by the front of the slice and the plate echoes for the two conditions, it is possible to calculate the ultrasound velocity and the attenuation coefficient at each position. The attenuation

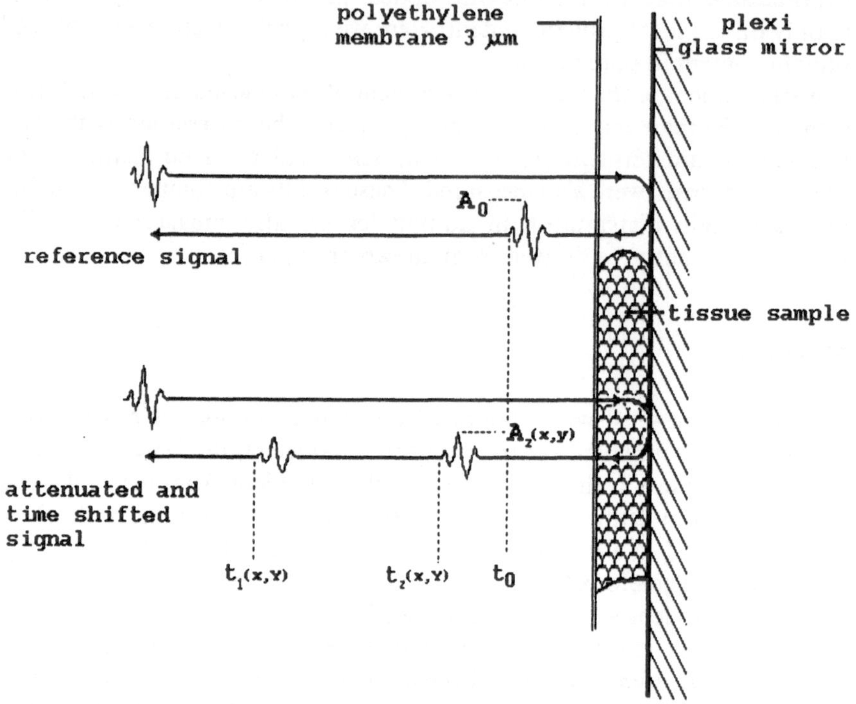

Fig. 2. Scheme of the SAM measurement technique (image rotated 90° counter-clockwise): at each position a reference measurement (yielding A_0, t_0) and a tissue measurement (A_2, t_1, t_2) are made

coefficient is approximated by a linear frequency dependence, and, therefore, the slope versus frequency and the value at 20 MHz can be calculated. In summary, three images (comparable to C-scans) are obtained for every lens slice. In order to enable the comparison with literature data and the correlation of acoustic data with protein concentration, the 2-D images were summarized in the axial and lateral (equatorial) profiles of the acoustic parameters.

Raman Microspectroscopy

Raman spectra were obtained with a confocal Raman microspectrometer (CRM, [4]), excited with a 630 nm laser source. The spectra were estimated at intervals 0.3 mm along the axial and equatorial axes of the lens slices. The absolute water content was calculated from the spectra and the local protein content was obtained by simple subtraction from 100%. This is allowed because the lipid content of mammalian eye lenses is less than 2%.

Relational Statistics

The profile of the acoustic parameters and the local protein contents along the optical and equatorial axes are displayed graphically, so a qualitative comparison can be made by the reader. A quantitative comparison was performed in two ways. The Pearson correlation coefficient between the acoustic parameter and protein content profiles of porcine lenses (n = 5) was calculated for the data points along the axial profile. The data of the local acoustic parameters and the local protein content of human lenses [6] are not normally distributed, so calculation of the Pearson correlation coefficient would be incorrect. In the second approach the velocity profile was calculated from the protein content profile. Due to the absence of collagen in the lens the protein concentration is fully determined by globular proteins, so the velocity can be calculated [11]:

$$c = 1500 + 3.2\,p\ [m/s] \quad (1)$$

For human lenses the protein profile measured by Siebinga *et al.* [6] was taken, after rescaling of the position axis (because of a difference in lens size).

Results

The 2-D images of acoustic parameters were 'cosmetically' enhanced by interpolation and smoothing. As an example, a picture of a slice of a human lens is shown in Figure 3A. The corresponding 2-D acoustic images in Figures 3B-D show the velocity of ultrasound (grey levels scaled from black to white over the range 1500 to 1650 m/s), the attenuation coefficient at 20 MHz (range: 0 to 30 dB/cm) and the attenuation coefficient slope (range: 0.0–2.0 dB/(cm MHz)).

The images are summarized in plots of the axial profiles (Fig. 4) and the equatorial halfprofiles (Fig. 5) of the same parameters [9]. In these figures the mean of the depicted parameter of all lenses (n = 13) and the lines of plus/minus one standard deviation are plotted (dashed lines). The irregularities at 2 mm and at 4 mm in Figures 4 and 5, respectively, are located at either the transition from the cortex to the nucleus, or from the cortex to the bathing fluid. The cortex could not be prevented from loosening from the nucleus in some cases. Similar results were obtained for the porcine lenses [3].

The local protein content in the porcine lens as measured in this study is shown in Figures 6A and B in axial and lateral profiles, respectively. These protein profiles appear to be very similar to the acoustic profiles as presented previously [3]. The protein content averaged over the axial profile was found to be approximately 60%.

The human acoustic parameters profiles in Figures 4 and 5 were compared to protein content data (Fig. 7) taken from the literature [6]. The data in the latter paper was obtained from an eight-year-old subject. The equatorial velocity half-

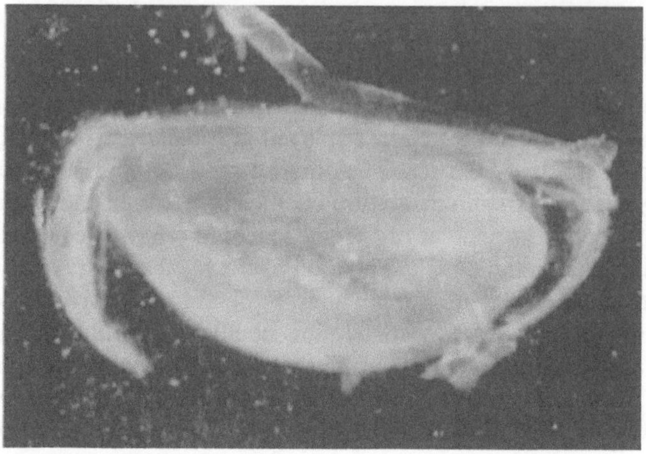

(A)

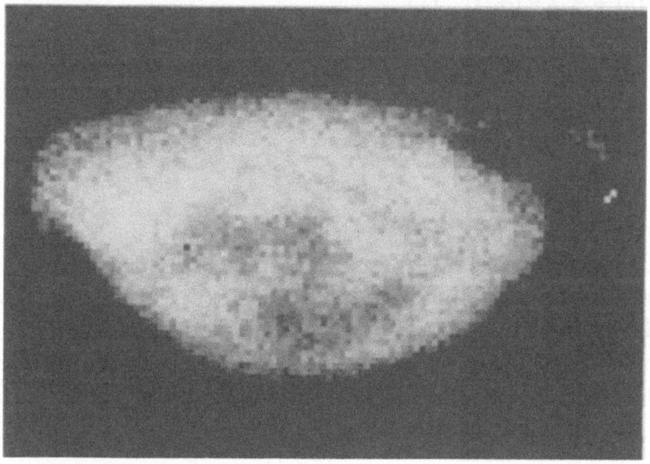

(B)

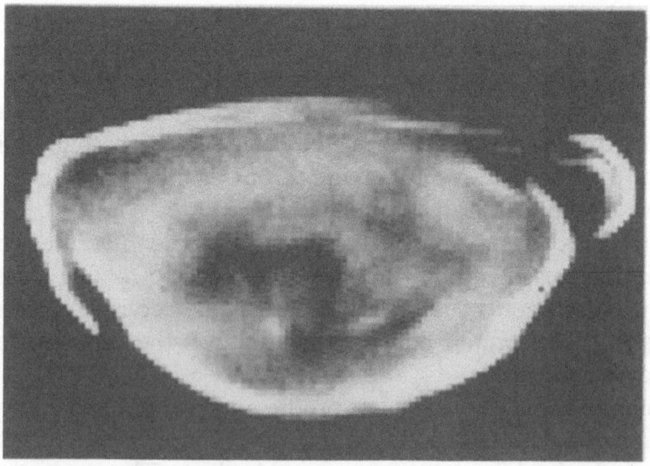

(C)

profile calculated from the protein content profile is shown in Figure 8 together with the velocity data from Figure 3.

The Pearson correlation coefficients, calculated for the porcine lens, are very high and significant both between the acoustic parameters ($r \geqslant 0.92$), and also between these parameters and the protein content ($r \geqslant 0.80$). The mean value of the axial profiles is particularly important because this is the direction of ultrasound propagation in clinical biometry and also because literature data (*in vitro* experiments) were generally obtained in axial measurements. The present data are summarized together with these literature data in Table 1. It can be concluded that the velocity measured in this study is lower than most literature data. The attenuation data from literature are not sufficient to permit a conclusion to be drawn.

Discussion

Three acoustic parameters were measured in human and porcine eye lenses. The results obtained show that the variation of the acoustic parameters in the human eye lens is less than in the porcine lens [3]. In the porcine lens the acoustic parameters decrease from the center to the equator, contrary to the human lens where the parameters have approximately the same value over a wide range (nucleus diameter).

(D)

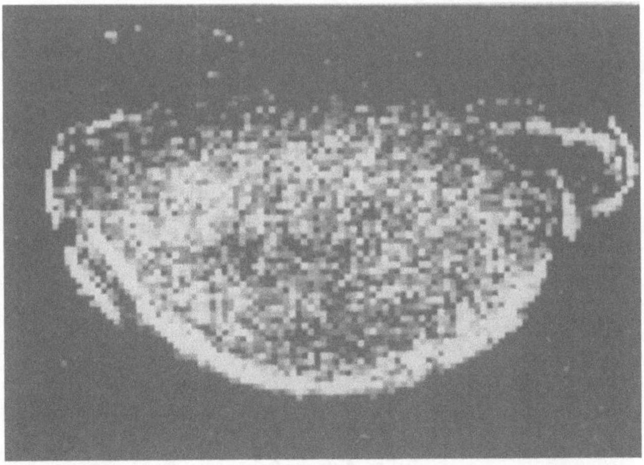

Fig. 3. A. Optical reflection image of 1-mm thick central slice of human lens; B. corresponding grey scale encoded image of local velocity of ultrasound (range 1500–1700 m/s); C. image of attenuation coefficient at 20 MHz; D. image of slope of attenuation coefficient [9] (see opposite page)

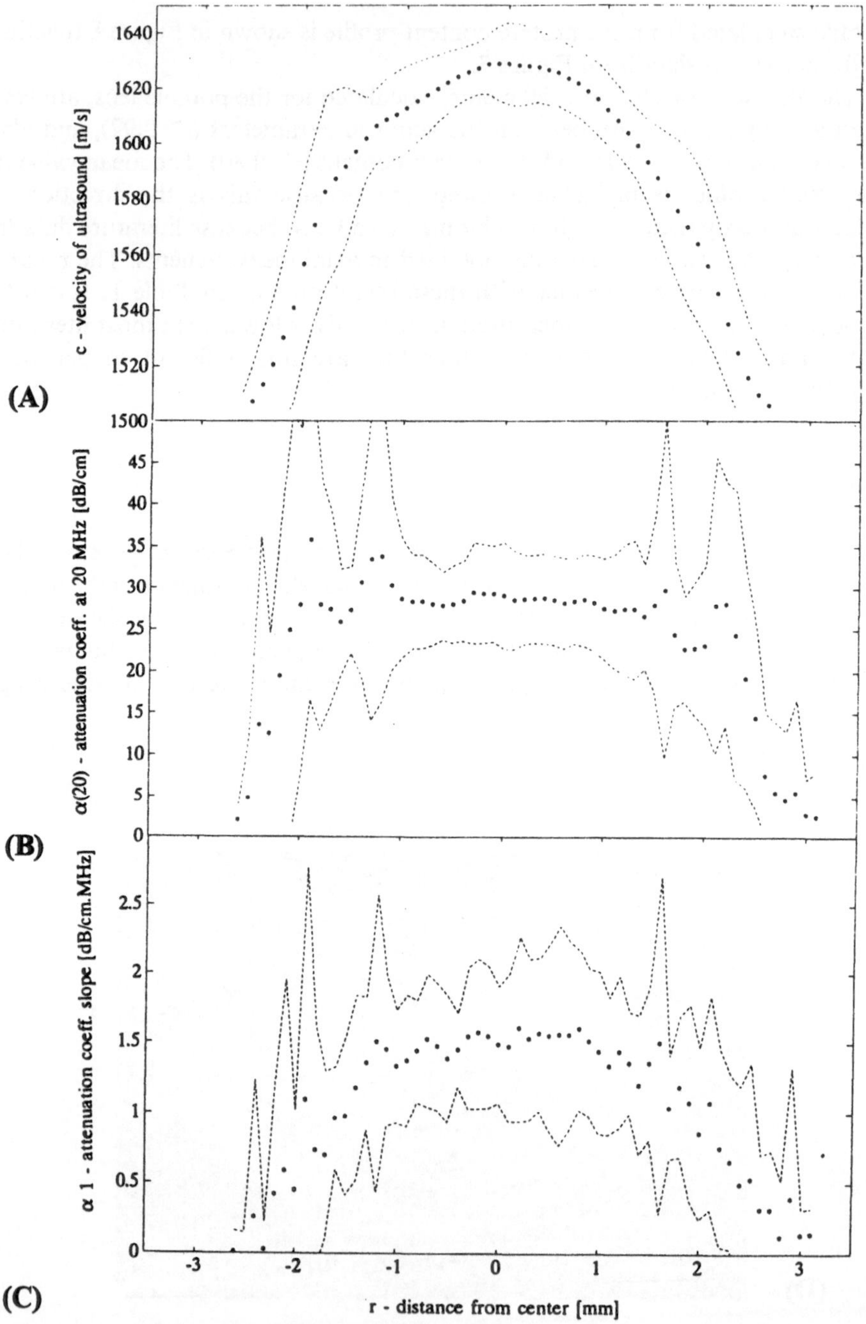

Fig. 4. Axial profiles of acoustic parameters in human lenses (n = 13), solid points: mean values, dotted lines: standard deviation: A. velocity of ultrasound; B. attenuation coefficient at 20 MHz; C. attenuation coefficient slope [9]

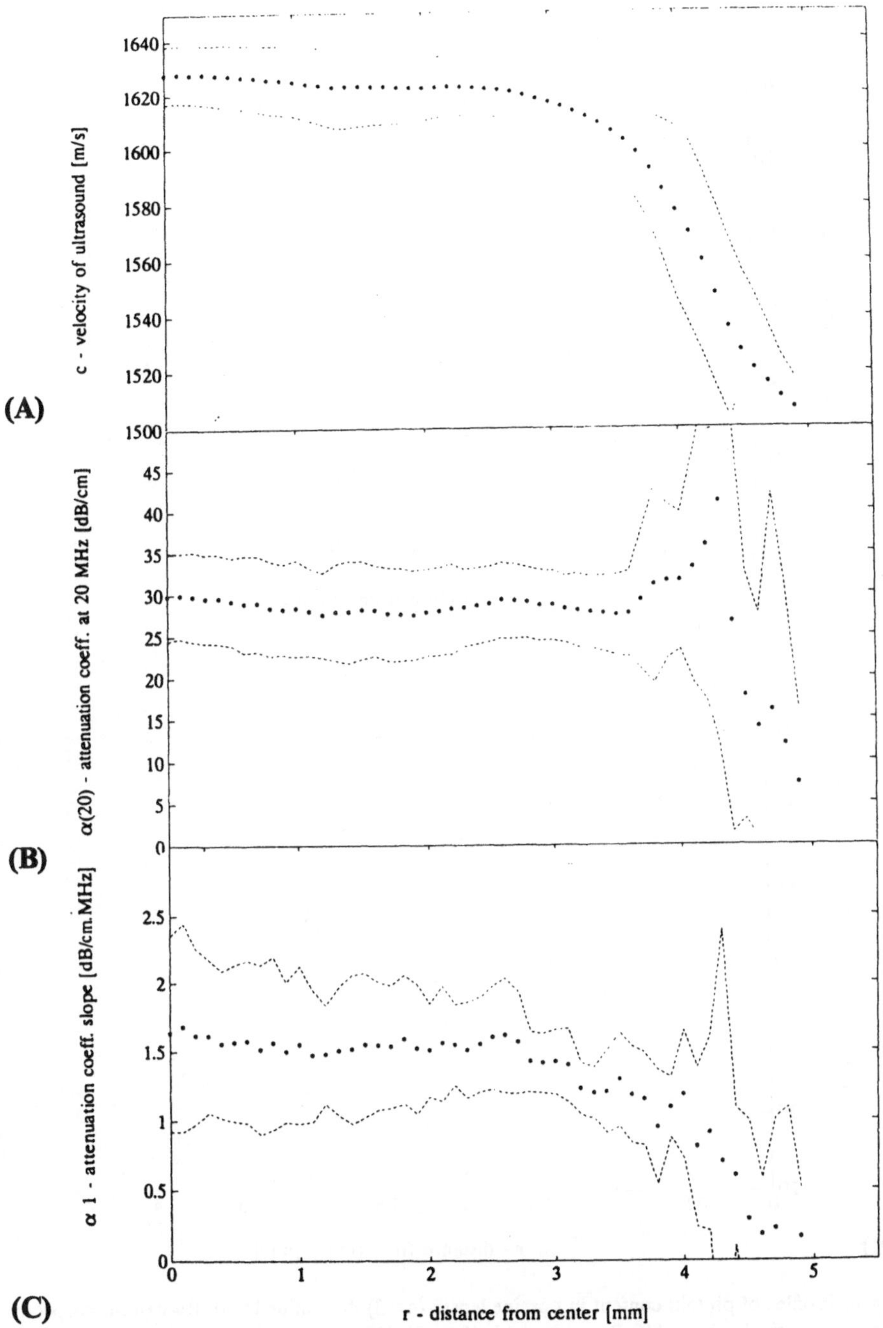

Fig. 5. (A, B, C): Half-profiles of acoustic parameters along equatorial axis in human lenses (n = 13); same parameters as in Fig. 4 [9]

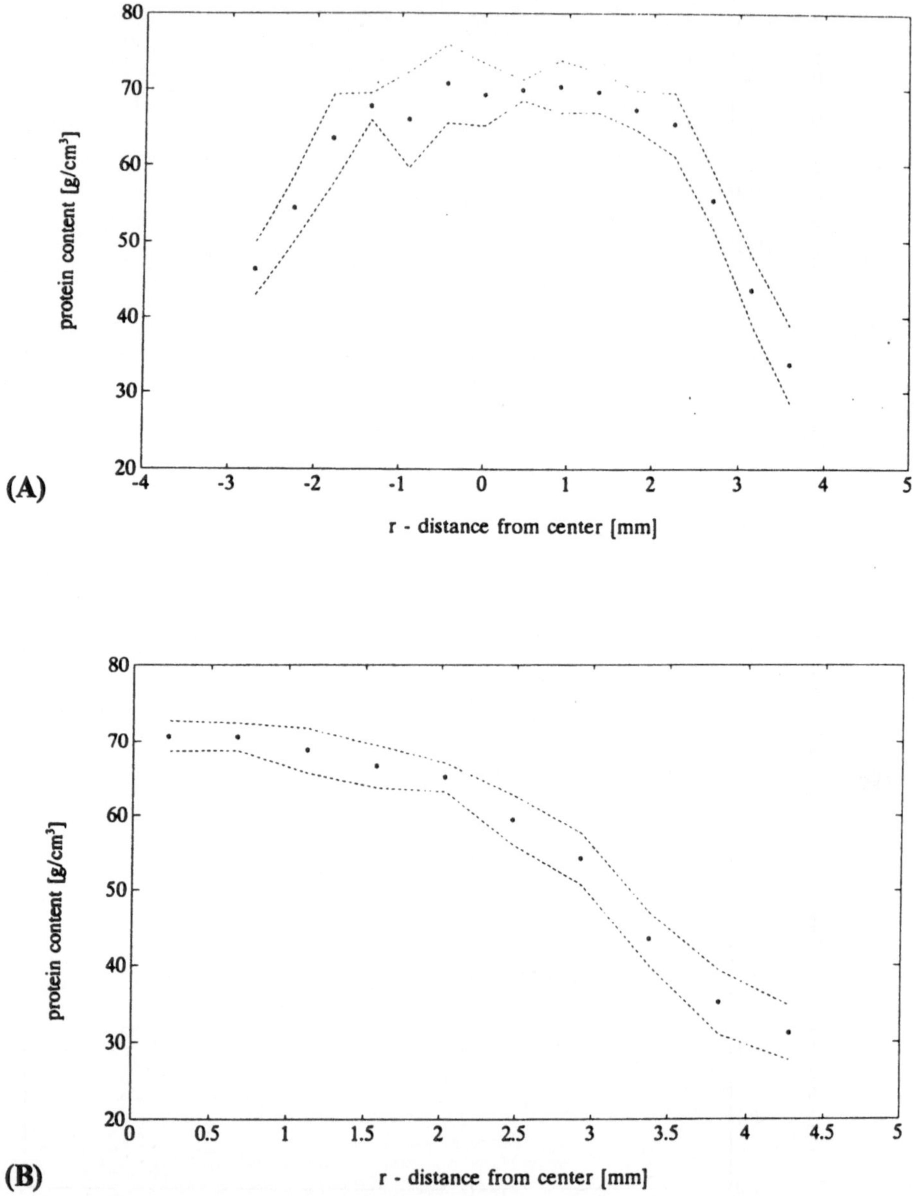

Fig. 6. Profiles of protein content in porcine lenses (n = 3) determined with Raman microspectroscopy: A. optical axis profile; B. equatorial half-profile [9]

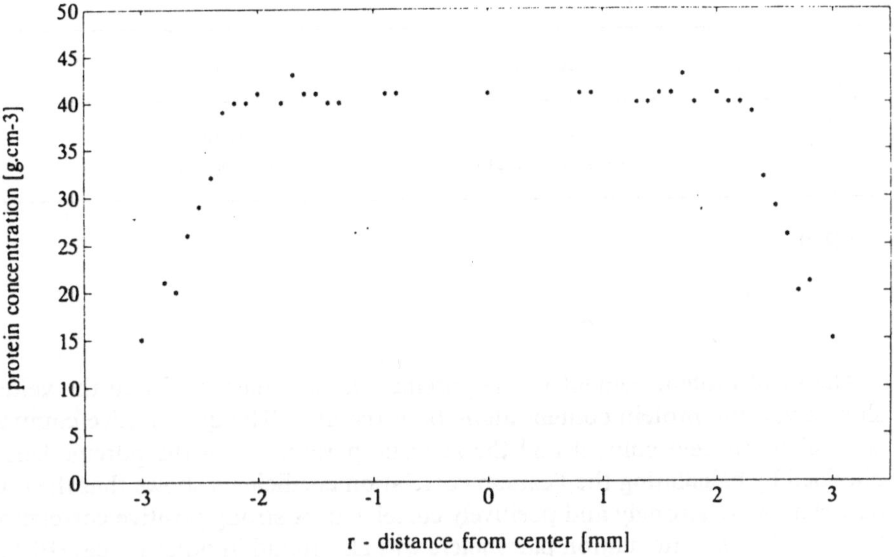

Fig. 7. **Protein concentration (equatorial half-profile) in 8-year-old human lens [11]**

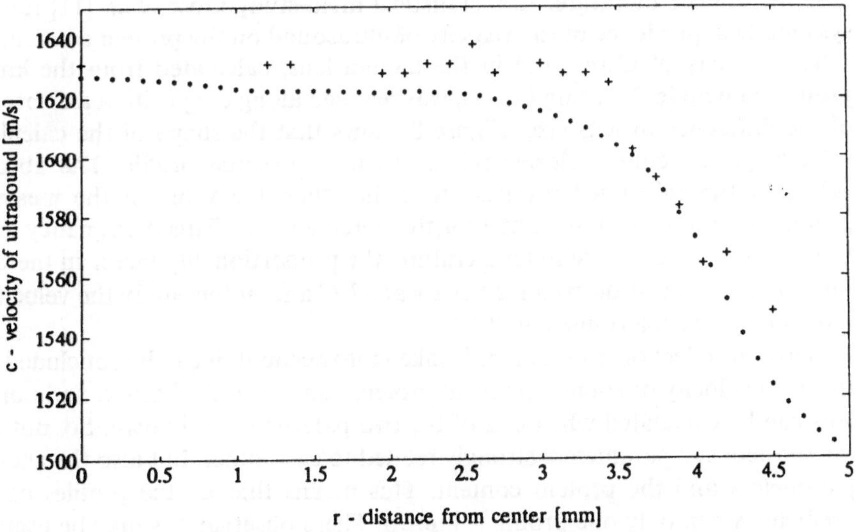

Fig. 8. **Equatorial half-profile of velocity of ultrasound, measured (*) and calculated (+) in the human lens [9]**

Table 1. Ultrasound velocity at 20C [m/s]

	Human	Porcine
This study	1590±6	1630±10
Literature	1631* (1620–38)	1644* (1627–57)

* Cf. [2, 3].

The local protein content in the porcine lens was measured and the values show a varying protein content along both the axes. The quantitative comparison of the protein content and the acoustic parameters of the porcine lenses obtained by calculating the Pearson correlation coefficients shows that the four parameters are strongly and positively correlated. A strong positive correlation between the two attenuation parameters was also found in other tissues [10,12–14]. The correlation between the ultrasound velocity and the attenuation parameters has not been reported previously. Recently, van der Steen *et al.* [15], found that there is no correlation between local velocity of ultrasound and the local attenuation parameters in liver. The strong correlation between the attenuation parameters and protein content, as found here in the lens, has been described in the literature. In a statistical meta-study Goss *et al.* [11] found a systematic dependence of the velocity of ultrasound on the protein content.

The velocity of ultrasound in the human lens, calculated from the known protein content [6] by using Eq. (1), was rescaled along the position axis because of the difference in lens size. Figure 8 shows that the shape of the calculated velocity profile cine is closely related to the measured profile. The absolute values of the calculated profiles are higher than the value of the measured profiles, both for the human and for the porcine lenses. This discrepancy might be caused by a difference in temperature: the proportionality factor in the Goss formula (Eq. 1) was derived for tissues at 27°C and in this study the velocity of ultrasound was determined at 20°C.

When the effect of temperature is taken into account, it can be concluded that the local velocity of sound and local protein content in the human and porcine lens can be calculated when one of the two parameters is known. So, not only are the acoustic parameters strongly related to each other, but also the acoustic parameters and the protein content. This means that all the profiles can be predicted when only one profile is known. These observations may be useful in studies of the aging of the eye lens.

Acknowledgement

This work has been supported by a grant from the Dutch Cancer Fund-Koningin Wilhelmina Fonds (NUKC 89-03). The human eye tissues were obtained from Eurotransplant and the cornea transplantation department of The Netherlands Ophthalmic Research Institute. The latter institutions are acknowledged for supplying donor material that was not suited for transplantation.

References

[1] J.M. Thijssen, H.J.M. Mol, M.J.T.M. Cloostermans and W.A. Verhoef. Acoustic parameters of ocular tissues. In J.S. Hillman and M.M. Le May (eds), Ophthalmic ultrasonography. The Hague, Boston, Lancaster: W. Junk Publisher, 1983:450–455.

[2] J.M. Thijssen, H.J.M. Mol and M.R. Timmer. Acoustic parameters of ocular tissues. Ultrasound Med. Biol. 1985;11:157–161.

[3] A.F.W. van der Steen, C.L. de Korte and J.M. Thijssen. Ultrasonic spectroscopy of the porcine eye lens. Ultrasound Med. Biol. 1994;20:177–186.

[4] G.L. Puppels, W. Colier, J.H.F. Olminkhof, C. Otto, F.F.M. de Mul and J. Greve. Description and performance of a highly sensitive confocal Raman microspectrometer. J. Raman Spectrosc. 1991;22:217–225.

[5] F.F.M. de Mul and J. Greve. Rampac: a program for the analysis of complicate Raman spectra. J. Raman Spectrosc. 1993;2:245–250.

[6] I. Siebinga, G.F.J.M. Vrensen, F.F.M. de Mul and J. Greve. Age-related changes in local water and protein content of human eye lenses measured by Raman microspectroscopy. Exp. Eye Res. 1991;53:233–239.

[7] A. Huizinga, A.C.C. Bot, F.F.M. de Mul, G.F.J.M. Vrensen and J. Greve. Local variation in absolute water content of human and rabbit eye lenses measured by Raman microspectroscopy. Exp. Eye Res. 1989;48:478–496.

[8] C.L. de Korte, A.F.W. van der Steen and J.M. Thijssen. Acoustic velocity and attenuation of eye tissues at 20 MHz. Ultrasound Med. Biol. 1994;20:471–480.

[9] C.L. de Korte, A.F.W. van der Steen, J.M. Thijssen, J.J. Duindam, C. Otto and G.J. Puppels G.J. Relation between local acoustic parameters and protein distribution in human and porcine eye lenses. Exp. Eye Res. 1994;53:617–627.

[10] A.F.W. van der Steen, J.M. Thijssen, J.A.W.M. van der Laak, G.P.J. Ebben and P.C.M. de Wilde. Quantitative correlation of acoustic and light microscopy, J. Microscopy. 1994;175: 21–33.

[11] S.A. Goss, L.A. Frizell and F. Dunn. Dependence of the ultrasonic properties of biological tissue on constituent proteins. J. Acoust. Soc. Am. 1980;67:423–457.

[12] B.J. Oosterveld, J.M. Thijssen, P.C. Hartman and G.J.E. Rosenbusch. Detection of diffuse live disease by quantitative echography: dependence on *a priori* choice of parameters. Ultrasound Med. Biol., 1993;19:21–25.

[13] R.L. Romijn, I.M. Thijssen, B.J. Oosterveld and A.M. Verbeek. Ultrasonic differentiation of intraocular melanomas: parameters and estimation methods. Ultrasonic Imag. 1991;13:27–55.

[14] J.M. Thijssen, B.J. Oosterveld, P.C. Hartman and G.J.E. Rosenbusch. Correlation between acoustic and texture parameters from RF-and B-mode liver echograms. Ultrasound Med. Biol. 1993;19:13–20.

[15] A.F.W. van der Steen, J.M. Thijssen, G.P.J. Ebben, J.A.W.M. van der Laak and P.C.M. de Wilde. Correlation of histology and acoustic parameters of liver tissue on a microscopic scale. Ultrasound Med. Biol. 1994;20:177–186.

Johan M. Thijssen
[1]Institute of Ophthalmology
Biophysics Laboratory
University Hospital
Nijmegen, The Netherlands
[2]Netherlands Ophthalmic Research Institute
Amsterdam, The Netherlands

[3]Department of Applied Physics
University of Twente
Enschede, The Netherlands

[4]Currently at the Clinical Physics Laboratory
Academic Children's Center – 435
University Hospital
P.O. Box 9101
6500 HB Nijmegen, The Netherlands

[5]Currently with the Erasmus University Rotterdam
and the Interuniversity Cardiology Institute
The Netherlands

61. Bacterial contamination of ultrasound probes

U. FRIES and C. OHRLOFF
(Frankfurt am Main, Germany)

Abstract

Bacterial contamination of probes is unavoidable in contact echography. Ultrasound probes are not made sterile by wiping with disinfection; this procedure only leads to a reduction in germs. Bacterial growth was found in 31% of swabs after 48 hours of culture. Some solid probes can be sterilized by soaking in peroxide solution (3%). However, some probes are damaged by strong disinfectants. Sterility can only be ensured by the use of a sterile cover.

Key words: Ultrasound probes, sterility, echography

Introduction

The correct disinfection of ultrasound probes is a problem in ophthalmic ultrasonography. Ultrasound is widely used in diagnostics and biometry prior to cataract surgery; the same probe may be used in many eyes, and some of these may carry an infection, e.g., endophthalmitis. A risk is also represented by patients affected by such multimorbid diseases as HIV^+ associated with progressive vitreoretinal disorders. Because these eyes are examined with the same probes used to examine other patients, strict rules of hygiene should be followed.

Ultrasound probes are highly sensitive precision mechanical instruments. Fluid should not come into contact with the region where the wire enters the probe. Also disinfection by heat or gas will damage the instrument. In most A-mode and some biometry probes the piezzoelectrical crystal lies uncovered fastened with adhesive to its setting. In pachymetry some probes are open (immersion technique) with a fluid meniscus held by the adhesion power of water. Some probes with fixation light have a solid plastic tip. There are various types of B-mode probes, e.g., with stiff or flexible plastic covers, or silicone covers.

Because of the sensitivity of ultrasound probes, disinfectants should be used with care; they could damage a probe, and the time required to be effective is not always compatible with office hours.

G Cennamo and N. Rosa (eds.), Ultrasonography in Ophthalmology 15, pp. 497–501.

Table 1. Disinfection of optometric devices to prevent the spread of AIDS

After cleaning, instruments may be disinfected by 10 to 30 minutes exposure to any of the following fresh solutions (sodium hypochlorite is preferred)
0.5% solution (1 to 10 dilution) of common household bleach (sodium hypochlorite)
3% hydrogen peroxide
70% ethanol
70% isopropyl alcohol

Table 2. Bacterial growth; germs 48 hours after wipe disinfection

Staphyloccocus albus	107
Staphyloccocus aureus	11
Staphyloccocus citreus	3
Corynebacterium	9
Hemophilus influencae	7
Proteus mirabilis	8
Spores	11

Tolon *et al.* [1] have studied the sterilization of ultrasound probes. Some countries, e.g., the USA [2] have produced guidelines for the disinfection of probes (Table 1) . The aim of this study was to evaluate the efficacy of the common wipe disinfection.

Method

After 500 examinations in our laboratory, a swab was taken before and after wipe disinfection. The same number of swabs was taken from each probe (A-mode, B-mode, and biometry). Swabs were taken both with chocolate and cooked blood agar plates, and incubated for 24 and 48 hours. The contact agent was sterile hydroxymethylcellulose in A- and B-mode and none in biometry. We tested bacterial growth; virus and fungus tests were not done. Routine wipe disinfection was done with hydromerfen solution 1:32000. Because gas or heat disinfection would damage our probes, the zero test was done with a sterile cover. We also tested the effect of soaking the probe in 3% peroxide solution for 10 minutes.

Results

Most swabs had no culture: 78% after 24 hours and 69% after 48 hours (Tables 2 and 3). Bacterial contamination was detected in one agar plate near to the swab.

Table 3. Bacterial growth; germs 48 hours after swab without disinfection

Staphylococcus albus	457
Staphylococcus aureus	42
Staphylococcus citreus	7
Corynebacterium	29
Hemophilus influencae	21
Proteus mirabilis	23
Pseudomonas aeruginosa	7
Diplococcus pneumoniae	15
Streptococcus pyogenes	11
Klebsiella pneumoniae	3
Escherichia coli	11
Spores	78
Fungi	5
No growth	791
	(n = 1500)

Table 4. Disinfectant recommendations provided by ultrasound distributors

Mild cleaning agent
Mild wipe disinfection, no soaking
Alcoholic swab
Disinfectants with a low per cent of alcohol
70% alcohol solution
3% peroxide solution
Special solutions (not always sufficient)

There was no growth in the tests done with a sterile cover, and after soaking in 3% peroxide solution for 10 minutes. There was little difference in quality, quantity or species of germs on the different probes, after wipe disinfection.

Discussion

The results show that the common wipe disinfection with mild agents does not guarantee sterility, only a reduction in the number of germs (Fig. 2). This is a problem because many patients are examined perioperatively. Studies should be conducted to investigate this aspect in greater detail. With the increase of AIDS, contact lenses, tonometers and contact glasses have been detected as routes of transmission. There are no guidelines for disinfection of ophthalmic probes that cover all the various types of probes. In case of product liability the respective manufacturer or distributer has to authorise the disinfectant as it potentially might destroy the probe by loosening or penetrating the adhesives. The various recommendations of distributors have been divided into groups and are listed in Table 4.

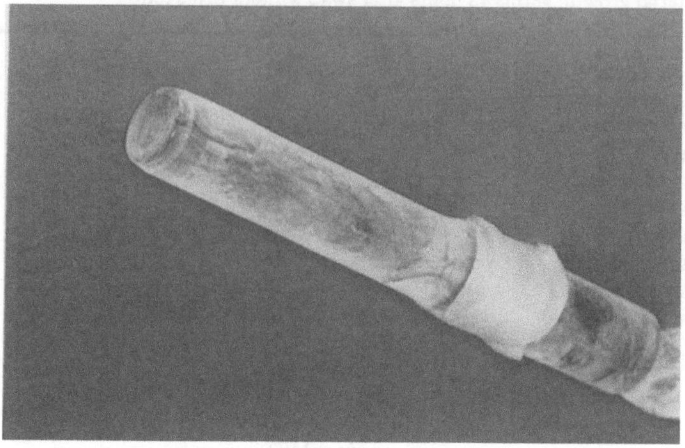

Fig. 1. B-mode probe with armed cover

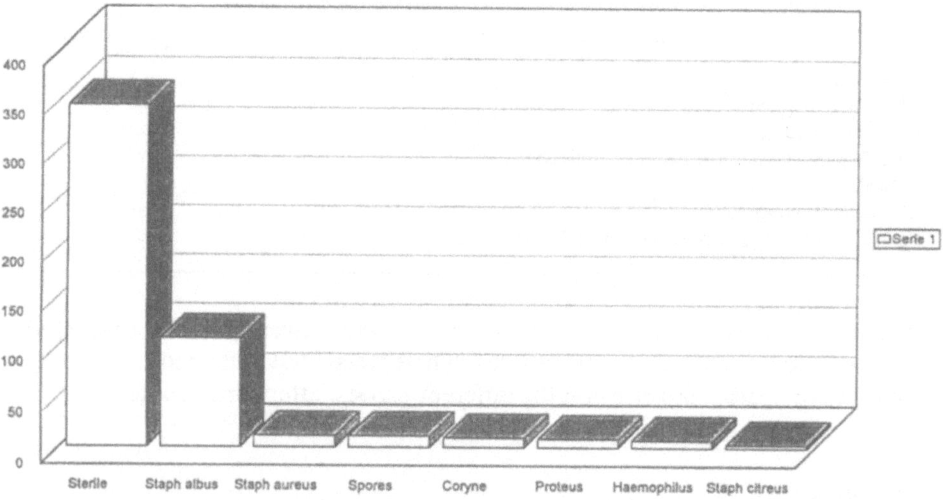

Fig. 2. Bacterial contamination in the wipe group

The use of sterile covers (Fig. 1) or probes [1,3,4] is very common in other fields. The use of a water-filled rubber as a pre-run for diagnosis of disorders of the lacrimal drainage system has been described [5]. This entails minimal little loss of gain, and when using the contact fluid, care should be taken not to contaminate the wires, and is best done by sealing the cover with a special lock.

Alcoholic disinfectants (70% isopropanol) will not kill all germs, and spores as from bacillus species might survive. Other types of disinfectants need more time, 3% peroxide takes 10 minutes to be effective.

O'Doherty *et al.* [6] described probe contamination and transmission of *Staphyloccocus aureus*, a problem germ in hospitals and also found in our study. The use of sterile covers has been recommended in general surgery and urology [3,4]. A sterile coupling agent has been suggested even for therapeutical ultrasound [7]; because the coupling agent is an ideal culture medium for bacteria, we used sterile methylcellulose.

References

[1] M. Tolon, H. Ohgke, R. Denning and M. Otte. Infektionsprophylaxe bei der Sonographie. Ultraschall in der Medizin 1984;5(2):77-79.

[2] American Academy of Optometry. 65(7):600.

[3] C. Nies, A. Zielke, C. Hasse, H. Sitter and H.J. Klotter. Sterilized single-use packing of ultrasound applicators for intraoperative use. Chirurg. 1992;63:526–527.

[4] J.B. Sloan. Two new applications for 3M Steri-Drape 'O'Conner rectal shield'. Urology 1991;37(3):269.

[5] M. Végh and J. Néhmet. Ultraschalldiagnostik des Tränensackes. Fortsch. Ophthalmol. 1990:87(6):638–640.

[6] A.J. O'Doherty, P.G. Murphey and R.A. Curran. Risk of *Staphyloccocus aureus* transmission during ultrasound investigation. J. Ultrasound. Med. 1989;8(11):619–620.

[7] R.N. Brueton and B. Cambell. The use of geliperm as a sterile coupling agent for therapeutic ultrasound. Physiotherapy 1987;73(12):653–654.

Dr. med. U. Fries
Universitäts-Augenklinik
Theodor-Stern-Kai 7, H8b
D-60590 Frankfurt am Main
Germany

62. Color Doppler and 3D. New techniques in eye and orbit investigation

A. VALLI and R. PROTTI
(Turin, Italy)

Abstract

Color Doppler imaging is a recent advance in ultrasonography. It allows simultaneous two-dimensional imaging of structure and blood flow evaluation. Doppler information is superimposed in colour over a conventional gray scale image. Using this technique we have examined the central retinal artery, the posterior ciliary arteries and the ophthalmic artery, and compared their average systolic speed with measurements taken in eyes affected by macular degeneration, diabetic retinopathy and glaucomatous pathology. We also describe a new procedure of three-dimensional image elaboration to demonstrate its potential in ophthalmic diagnosis.

Key words: Color Doppler, central retinal artery, three dimension, eye circulation

Introduction

The Doppler effect is an apparent change of frequency that an ultrasonic beam undergoes on reflection from a moving body [1]. Erythrocyte flow through blood vessels can produce such frequency changes in reflected ultrasound and those changes are proportional to the rate of flow. This is the origin of the Doppler signal. The interpretation of the Doppler signal takes into account the acoustic reading, the morphological analysis and the direction of the flow [2].

Materials and methods

We use a Duplex Scanner system which couples a pulsed Doppler system to the two-dimensional echograph and in this way enables a selective evaluation of the flow in blood vessels at different depths [3]. Therefore, at the orbit, the pulsed Doppler beam electronic cursor can be positioned so as to locate the ophthalmic artery and examine its behaviour as it bends around the optic nerve, the long and short posterior ciliary arteries and the central retinal artery as it passes inside the optic nerve and exits from the papilla [4–7].

G Cennamo and N. Rosa (eds.), Ultrasonography in Ophthalmology 15, pp. 503–507.

The patient lies supine for the examination. The probe has a frequency of 10 MHz and it is so positioned and oriented as to visualize the orbital area of interest. The vessel to be studied is selected by means of an electronic cursor. The flow rate, which in normal subjects is about 30 cm per second, and the flow, which is 28 mL per minute, is measured on the trace.

Where a vessel is traced in blue, that vessel has a flow in the opposite direction a condition found, for instance, in internal carotid artery occlusion. Therefore, also evidence of trace inversion is given graphically.

By placing the echodoppler cursor at the terminal part of the optic nerve, it is possible to analyze the actual flow in the arteries of the papillary and peripapillary circulation. The terminal branch of the central artery is visualized along its course to the optic nerve; the medial and lateral route of the long posterior ciliary artery can be followed.

Results

In the central retinal arteries of healthy subjects, we have measured a flow rate of 11.8 cm per second and a blood volume of 6 mL per minute; in the posterior ciliary arteries, the flow rate reaches 13 cm per second (Fig.1). In those areas we found marked changes of the Doppler morphology, of the flow and of the volume per minute in subjects affected by simple chronic glaucoma, where the mean systolic flow rate is 6.6 cm per second (2).

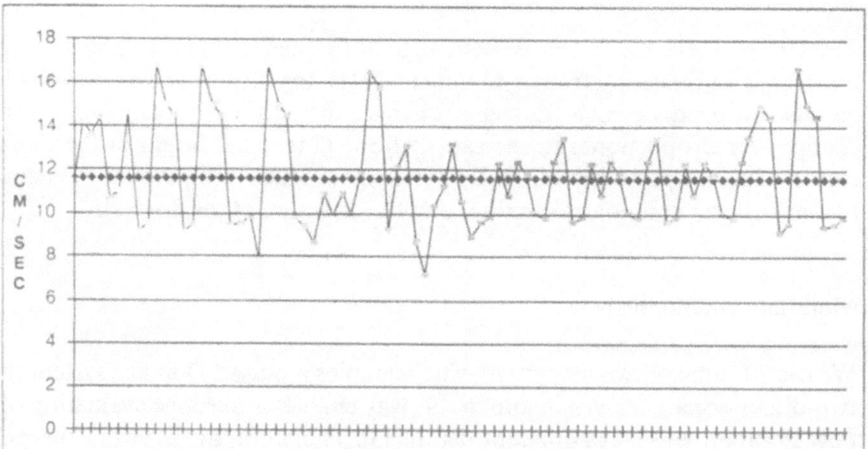

Fig. 1. Statistical calculations obtained from eyes of healthy subjects with a mean value of 11.8 cm per second

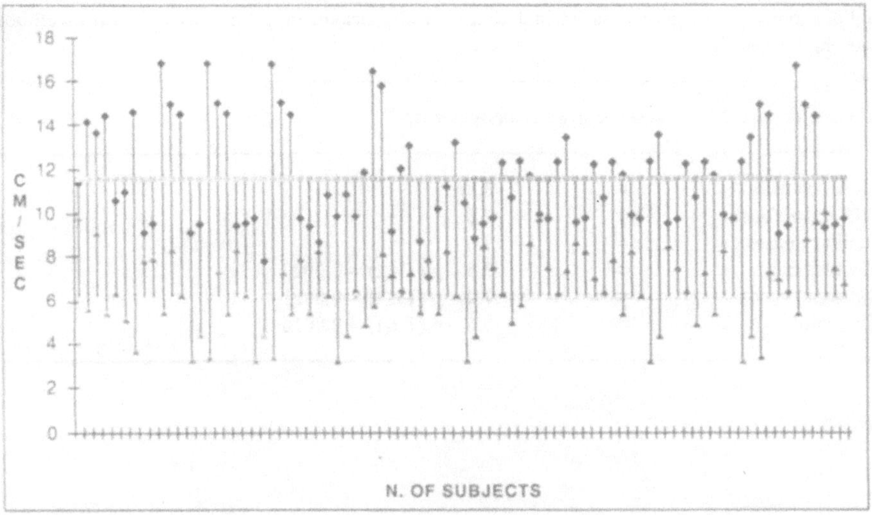

Fig. 2. Comparison between values found in healthy subjects and those found in eyes affected by glaucoma (a mean flow rate of 6.6 cm per second)

Often, in cases of glaucoma with advanced perimetral damage, there can be a marked slowing of the flow in proportion to the gravity of the perimetral damage (Fig. 2). This is associated with morphological alterations of the diastolic peak to the point where, in eyes with haemorrhagic glaucoma after retinal central vein thrombosis, there is a complete morphological alteration of the Doppler picture with a marked slowing in flow rate. Lowering of the flow rate is found in oedema of the papilla, papillary ischaemia, and in eyes affected by angioscleroticallybased dry macular degeneration. An interesting application of the color Doppler imaging consists in the exploration of vitreal content in case of haemovitreous. In such cases, it is possible to visualize the movements of the haematic corpusculature in the vitreous chamber, a prognostic application for eventual vitrectomy.

The possibility of having a two-dimensional model with high resolution enables, in the eyes of subjects with diabetic retinopathy and proliferative shoots, measurement of shoot thickness, its distance from the retina and, by coupling up the colour-doppler module, visualization and evaluation of the presence of neovascularization.

Color Doppler imaging permits measurements of retinal central artery flow and retinal central vein flow in cases of retinal central vein thrombosis, the mean values obtained being about 6.9 cm per second (Table 1). Also interesting is the possibility of evaluating in real time the effect of topical instillation of betablockers.

Subjects with retinal detachment have a slowed down flow rate with a mean of about 6.5 cm per second.

Table 1. Comparison between eyes of normal subjects and eyes affected by macular degeneration, diabetic retinopathy, glaucoma, retinal central artery occlusion, retinal central vein thrombosis and papillary oedema

Normal vs pathology – systolic peak velocity (cm/s)		
CRA occlusion	=	3.56
CRV thrombosis	=	7.8
Papillary edema	=	7.6
Macular deg.	=	7.5 – p (T⩽t) = 0.0027
Diabetic	=	7.2 – p (T⩽t) = 0.0021
Glaucoma	=	6.6 – p (T⩽t) = 0.0016

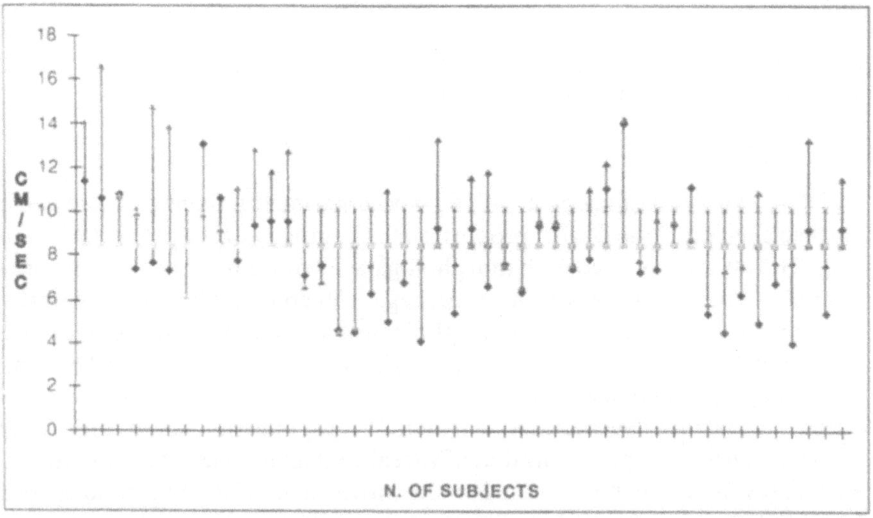

Fig. 3. The values obtained in subjects with macular degeneration and diabetic retinopathy who had received treatment with the peptide fraction of bovine factor VIII

Conclusions

Color Doppler is useful in clinical practice for the monitoring of the efficacy of ongoing therapy (see Fig. 5). Another interesting application is in the diagnosis of pre- and post-radiation treatment of endobulbar neoformations and in differentiating between neoformations and subretinally organized haemorrhage [8].

3D

An interesting innovation in instrumental diagnostics is the image processing systems for obtaining three-dimensional pictures. We are experimenting with a technique and the use of a processor, which 'extracts' high resolution two-dimensional figures from CAT, MNR and echograph images, to reconstruct two-dimensional sequential sections for the study of each single bulbar and peribulbar element from different angles. The images are processed to obtain three-dimensional views, from which the ensemble of the explored orbital structures can be assessed. At present, the study is being conducted on the bony parts, but we are in the process of applying these programmes to the study of soft tissue.

References

[1] C. Franceschi. L'investigation vasculaire pa ultrasonographie doppler. Paris: Ophthalmol. 1991;109:522–526.

[2] P. Arbeille, A. Benanou, S. Sales *et al.* Ectomographie et analyse spectral du signal doppler dans le bilan de la valutation du système carotidien. Journal des maladies vasculaires. 1984;9:171.

[3] M. Hemerici and H.J. Freund. Efficacy of C.W. Doppler and duplex-system examinations for the evaluations of extracranial carotid diseases. J. Clin. Ultrasound 1984;12:155.

[4] S. Duke-Elder. The ocular circulation: its normal pressure relationships and their physiological significance. Br. J. Ophthalmol. 1971;10:982.

[5] W.E. Lieb, S.M. Cohen, D. Merton, J.A. Shields, D.G. Mitchell and B.B. Goldberg. Color Doppler imaging of the eye and orbit. Arch. Ophthalmol. 1991;109:527–531.

[6] A. Valli, B. Brogliatti and A. Boles Carenini. Ecodoppler dell'arteria oftalmica. Clin. Oc. 1991;4:296–299.

[7] P.M. Flaharty, W.E. Lieb, R.C. Sergott, T.M. Bosley and P.J. Savino. Color doppler imaging. Arch. Ophthalmol. 1991;109:522–526.

[8] R.F. Guthoff, R.W. Berger, P. Winkler, K. Helmke and L.C. Chumbley. Doppler ultrasonography of the ophthalmic and central retinal vessels. Arch. Ophthalmol. 1991;109:532–536.

Andrea Valli
C.I.D.I.M.U. s.r.l.
Str. Alberoni, 18/26
10133 Turin, Italy

63. B-Scan color Doppler techniques in arterial/vein fistula

E. MORAGREGA-ADAME, C. VELASCO-BARONA,
G. GARCIA-BRIONES,[1] M. CRUZ-RIVERO[2] and
L. GARCIA-HIMMELSTEIN[2]
(México City, México)

Abstract

We present two cases of cavernous-carotid artery fistula monitored with B-scan color Doppler. One case corresponds to a traumatic fistula with high blood flow, and the other corresponds to a dural low blood flow fistula. We describe the ultrasonographic and flow characteristics of both cases.

Key words: Color Doppler-arterial/vein fistula, high flow, angiography, reversed blood flow

Introduction

In accordance with the findings of Guthoff [1], Tane [2], Wu [3], and Janev [4], we used color Doppler techniques to study vascular diseases of the orbit. Here we describe two cases of cavernous/carotid fistula. The first involves post-traumatic complications, while the second is a spontaneously formed dural fistula.The purpose of this study is to illustrate the usefulness of ultrasound, particularly color Doppler techniques, in the diagnosis and follow-up of such cases.

An arterial/vein (A/V) fistula is an abnormal communication between the cavernous sinus and the carotid artery system. The fistula can be classified according to its etiology as traumatic or spontaneous; according to its flow (low or high); and anatomically in post-traumatic or dural [5–7]. An important characteristic of some fistulas is a direct communication between the intracavernous portion of the internal carotid artery and the cavernous sinus (Type I of Parkinson, Type A of Barrow) [5].

Known as 'direct fistulas', these usually have a high blood flow and are caused by a traumatic rupture of the artery wall [7]. The dural type (Type 2 of Parkinson [5], Type B-C-D of Barrow [5]) are true congenital arterial/vein malformations that develop spontaneously or are associated with systemic hypertension, arteriosclerosis, and vascular collagenopathies, or with a traumatic delivery. The dural fistula is a communication between the cavernous

G Cennamo and N. Rosa (eds.), Ultrasonography in Ophthalmology 15, pp. 509–516.

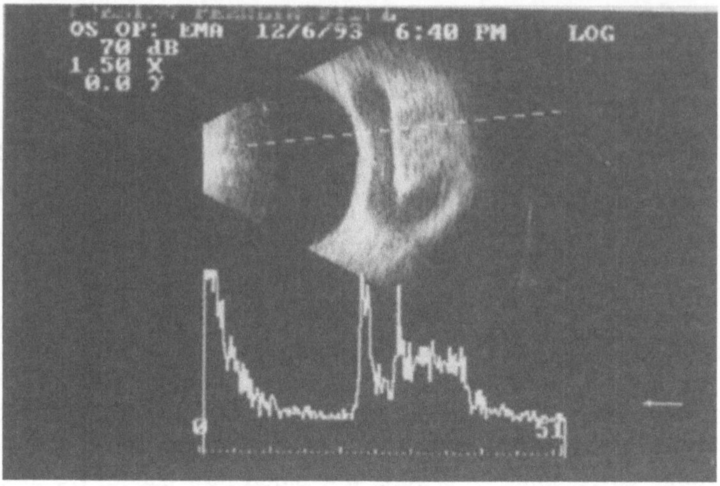

Fig. 1. Case 1. A-B echogram showing the enlargement of the superior ophthalmic vein, longitudinal plane

sinus and one or more meningeal branches of the internal carotid artery (Type B of Barrow) [5], of the external carotid artery (Type C Barrow), or both (Type D of Barrow). Generally these fistulas have a low artery flow and produce signs and symptoms spontaneously without any traumatic history.

Case No. 1

A 30-year-old male presented diplopia and an audible bruit on his left side two months after suffering a trauma on the left eye. When he was first seen by an ophthalmologist he had 20/20 vision in both eyes, hyperhemia and edema in the conjunctiva of the left eye and normally reactive pupils in both eyes. We found 22 prismatic diopters of exotropy and limitation of the abduction in the left eye. Visual fields were normal and a pulse in the left orbit was detected by simple palpation, and later confirmed with the use of a stethoscope. We performed ultrasound (Figs. 1 and 2), color Doppler B-scan (Figs. 3–5), carotid angiography, vertebral angiography and CT-scan (Fig. 6). The diagnosis made was a direct fistula, carotid/cavernous fistula (traumatic) with reversed blood flow in the superior ophthalmic vein. The intraocular pressure was 16 mmHg in the right eye and 26 in the left eye (Figs. 1–6).

Case No. 2

A 45-year-old female with no history of trauma, presented with pain, edema and hyperhemia of the left eye (Fig. 7). Visual acuity was 20/20 on the right eye and 20/60

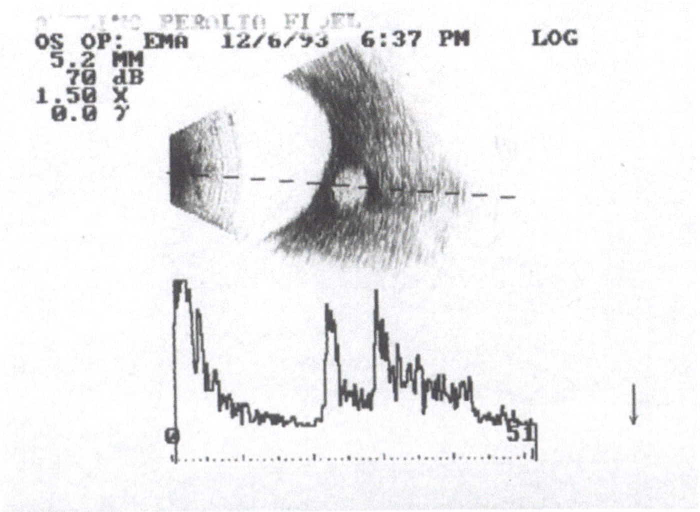

Fig. 2. Case 1. A-B echogram showing the enlargement of the superior ophthalmic vein, transversal plane

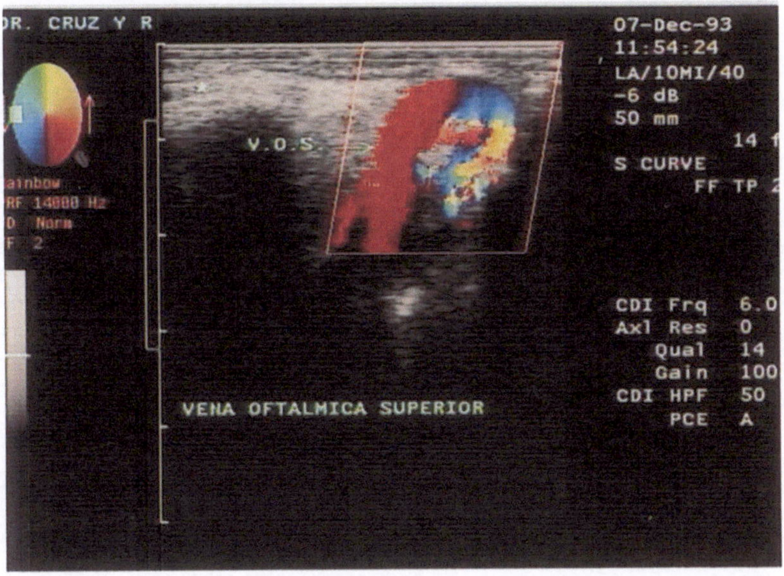

Fig. 3. Case 1. Color B-scan echogram showing the superior ophthalmic vein with red flow (to the transducer) and blue flow (away from the transducer)

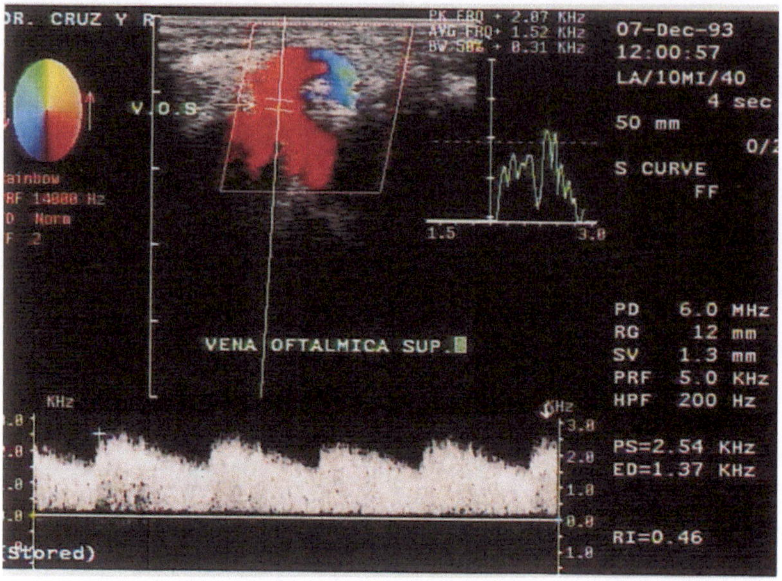

Fig. 4. Case 1. Same study as in Fig. 3, but with the Doppler vector, to show the spectrum of the flow. Superior ophthalmic vein

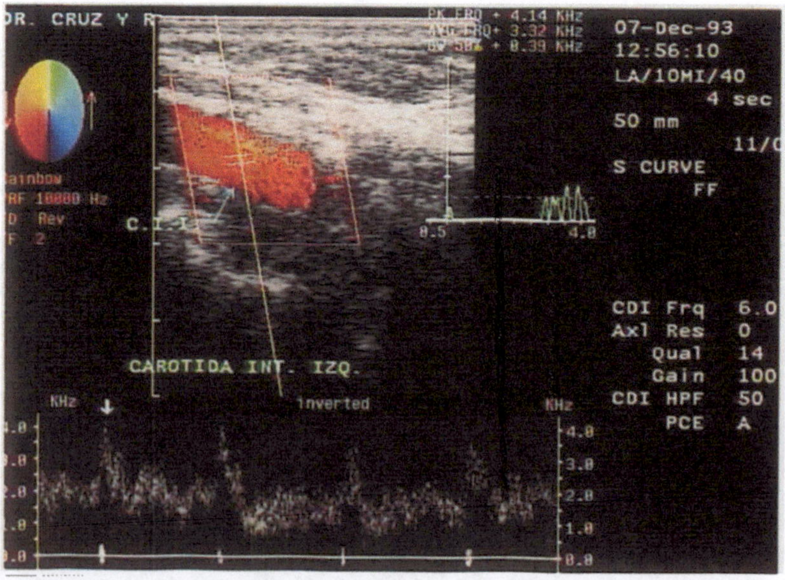

Fig. 5. Case 1. Color Doppler with spectrum of the flow in internal carotid artery

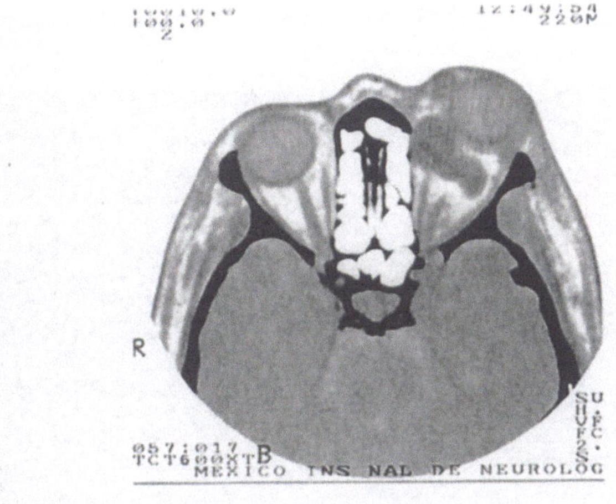

Fig. 6. Case 1. CT-scan showing the enlargement of the superior ophthalmic vein

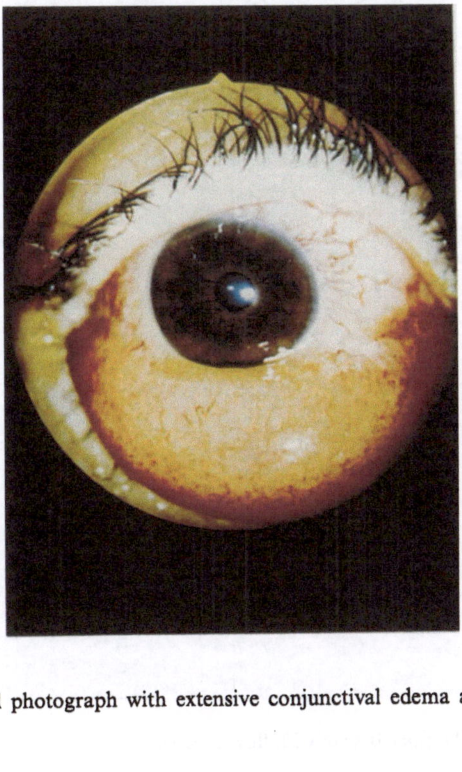

Fig. 7. Case 2. Clinical photograph with extensive conjunctival edema and enlarged episcleral vessels

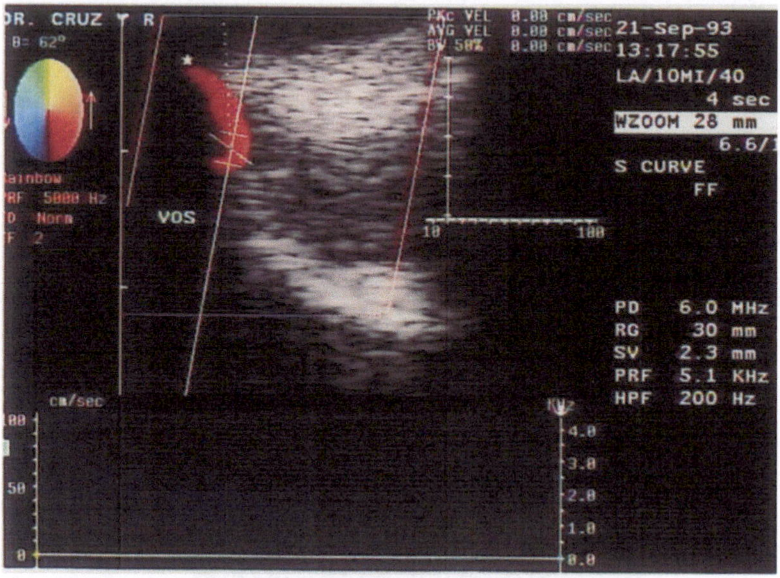

Fig. 10. Case 2. Color Doppler still showing blood flow in the superior ophthalmic vein

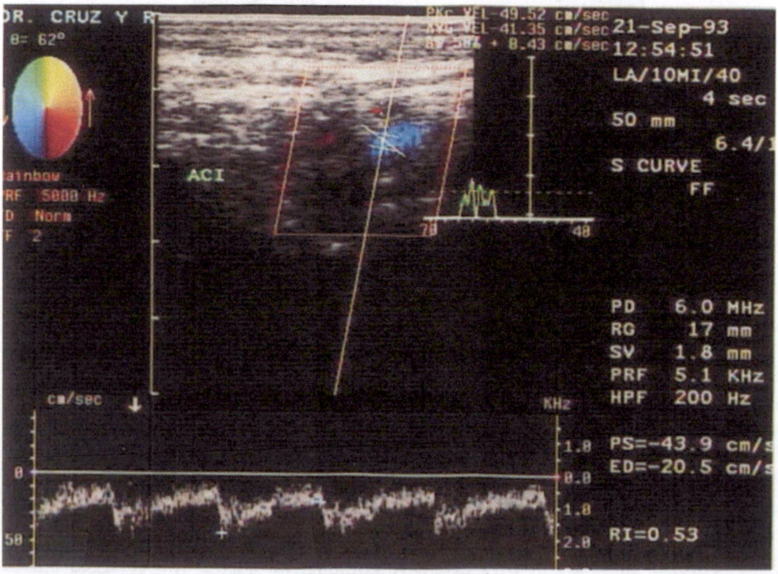

Fig. 11. Case 2. Color Dopper B-scan with flow spectrum

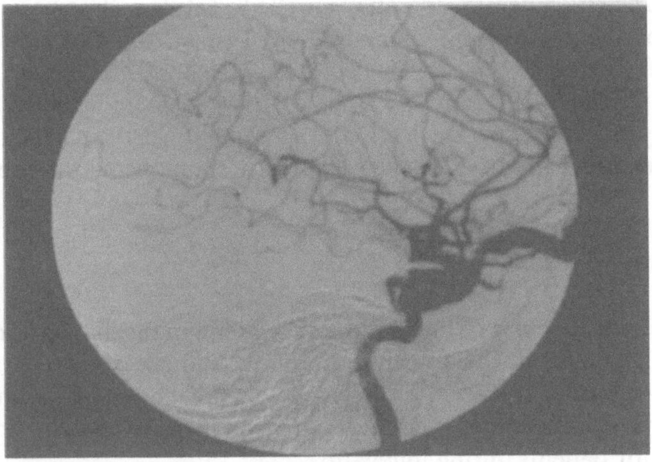

Fig. 8. Case 2. Carotid angiography showing the cavernous sinus

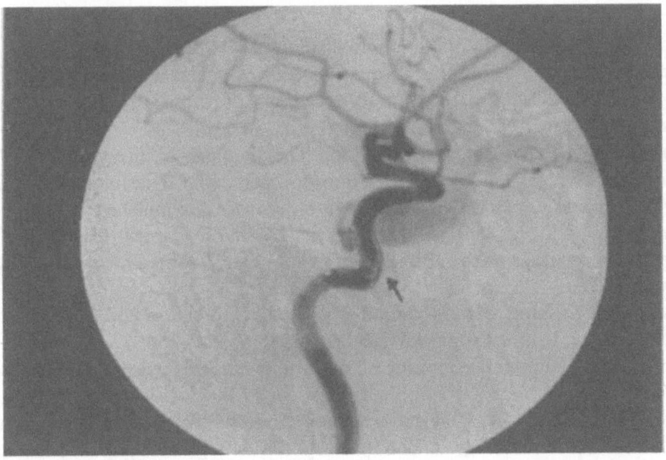

Fig. 9. Case 2. The angiogram shows the superior ophthalmic vein enlarged, and the catheter in the internal carotid artery during an attempt to place the balloon (arrow) in the sinus

on the left eye which improved to 20/40 with pinhole. In the upper eyelid of the left eye we found subdermic varix, conjunctival hyperhemia and chemosis. Intraocular pressure was 17 mmHg in the right eye and 29 mmHg in the left eye. Both eyes had a grade IV angle. Exophthalmometry was 13 in the right eye and 26 in the left eye. The ophthalmoscopic examination of the left eye revealed venous congestion with no optic disc alteration. Goldman perimetry visual fields were normal.

A diagnosis of spontaneous dural cavernous/carotid fistula was made by CT-scan and angiography (Figs. 8 and 9). There was thrombosis of the medial left cerebral artery. A new angiography revealed a fistula with some vessels that came from the meningohypophysiary branch. Two attempts at embolization were unsuccessful because of a severe decrease of the perfusion to the brain. A follow-up with ultrasound B-scan color Doppler showed that the fistula was still open, but the symptoms and signs are slowly disappearing (Figs. 10 and 11). This behavior is characteristic of the dural fistulas that present spontaneous thrombosis.

Discussion

B-scan color Doppler techniques are very useful in the diagnosis of A/V fistulas and in particular to demonstrate the flow, and measure such parameters as resistance index, spectrum, etc. which can not be studied with conventional ultrasonic examination. In addition, this non invasive examination can be used to monitor patients during follow-up.

References

[1] R. Guthoff. Ultrasound in ophthalmologic diagnosis. Stuttgart: Georg Thieme Verlag, 1991.
[2] S. Tane, M. Hirata and M. Hashimoto. Analysis of ocular circulatory kinetics in glaucoma using ultrasonic Doppler method. Proceedings of the 13th SIDUO Congress Vienna. Dordrecht: Kluwer Academic Publishers, 1990.
[3] Z. Wu, Y. Mo, Y. Pang, J. Lian and A. Zeng. The diagnosis of intracranial A/V malformation with orbital involvement by B-scan color-doppler and CT scan. Proceedings of the 13th SIDUO Congress, Vienna. Dordrecht: Kluwer Academic Publishers, 1990.
[4] K. Janev, K. Spahiv, N. Salihu and D. Perovic. Traumatic Carotid/Cavernous fistula affecting the orbit. Proceedings of the 13th SIDUO Congress, Vienna. Dordrecht: Kluwer Academic Publishers, 1990.
[5] D. Barrow, R. Spector, I. Brown and S. Tindall. Classification and treatment of spontaneous cavernous-carotid sinus fistula. J. Neurology 1985;62:248–256.
[6] T. Parkinson. Collateral evolution of cavernous-carotid artery-anatomy. Canad. J. Surv. 1964;7:251–266.
[7] E. Kwan, G. Hishima, R. Higashida, V. Halbach and S. Wolpert. International neuroradiology in neuro-ophthalmology. J. Clin. Neurophthalmology 1989;9:83–97.

Dr. Eduardo Moragrega-Adame
Dr. Cecilio Velasco-Barona
Asociación para Evitar la Ceguera en Mexico
'Hospital Dr. Luis Sanchez Bulnes'
Mexico City, Mexico

[1]Instituto Nacional de Neurologia
Mexico City, Mexico

[2]Gabinete de Ultrasonido Medico
México City, México

64. A case of reversed flow of ophthalmic artery confirmed by color Doppler imaging

K. EMI, H. ISHIKAWA[1] and Y. UJI[1]

(Yokkaichi, Mie, Japan)

Abstract

Color Doppler imaging (CDI) is a non invasive method with which to evaluate the velocity and flow volume of vessels. We found reversed flow in the ophthalmic artery of a 73-year-old female who had a cerebrovascular disorder. She was hospitalized 5 years earlier because of a cerebrovascular attack. Computerized tomography and magnetic resonance imaging indicated an old left parietal lobe infarction. We used the TOSHIBA SSA-260A apparatus and a 5-MHz electronic sector probe for CDI. Digital subtraction angiography showed no evidence of occlusion or narrowing of either carotid artery. Reversed flow in the ophthalmic artery represents a collateral blood flow from the external to the internal carotid artery.

Key words: Color Doppler imaging, ophthalmic artery, cerebrovascular disorder, magnetic resonance imaging, digital subtraction angiography

Introduction

Color Doppler imaging, which does not require the use of irradiation or radio-opaque agents, can illustrate the state of the vessels. Therefore, color Doppler imaging is often used to assess the hemodynamics of various vascular diseases. We found a reversed blood flow in the left ophthalmic artery of a 73-year-old female who had a cerebrovascular disorder.

Materials and method

We used the Toshiba SSA-260A apparatus and a 5-MHz electronic sector probe for color Doppler imaging (Figs. 1 and 2). The patient had been treated for heart failure and 5 years ago she had a cerebral infarction. During examination, she was in the supine position with the tested eye closed. The probe was carefully placed over the upper lid using a coupling gel. The blood flow toward the probe is depicted in red and that away from the probe in blue. Therefore, most arterial

G Cennamo and N. Rosa (eds.), Ultrasonography in Ophthalmology 15, pp. 517–522.

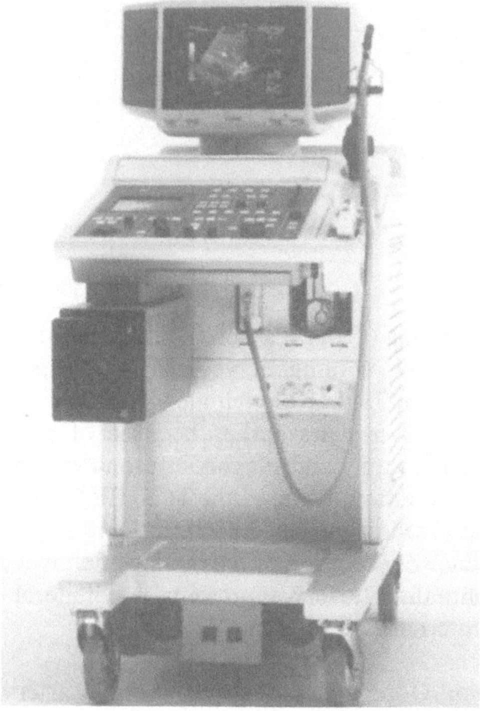

Fig. 1. Ultrasonic color Doppler diagnostic device, Toshiba SSA-260A

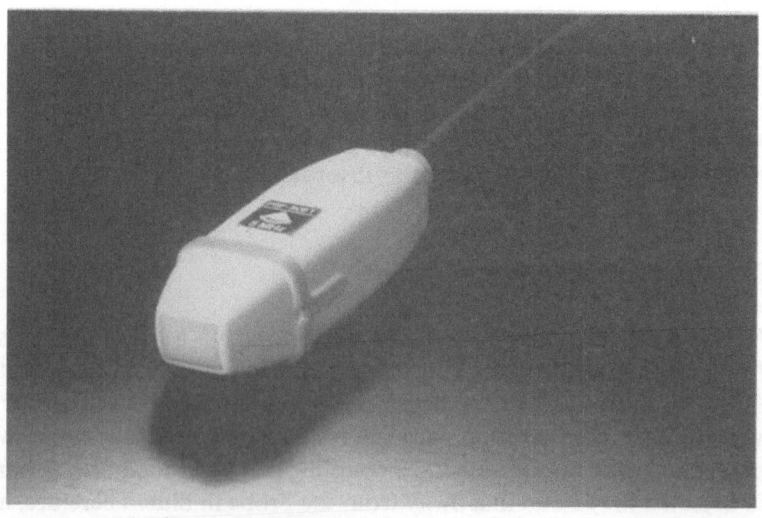

Fig. 2. 5 MHz electronic sector scanner for color Doppler imaging

flow is red and venous flow is blue. In the imaging mode, arteries can be distinguished from veins by their pulsatility. When examining the eye and orbit, we attempted to align the ultrasonic beam parallel to the optic nerve. The blood flow of the ophthalmic artery is identified as a pulsatile vessel adjacent and parallel to the optic nerve. Doppler frequency shifts within the ophthalmic artery were measured to determine the peak systolic velocity (V-max), end diastolic velocity (V-min) and mean-enveloped blood flow velocity (V-mean).

Results

The reversed blood flow of the left ophthalmic artery was detected by color Doppler imaging. V-max was 17 cm/s, V-min was 1 cm/s and V-mean was 8 cm/s (Fig. 3). Computed tomography showed a low density area in the parietal lobe (Fig. 4). T1-stressed magnetic resonance imaging showed a low signal area in the same lesion (Fig. 5), which indicated the old cerebral infarction. Intravenous digital subtraction angiography showed no closure or narrowing of either internal carotid artery (Fig. 6).

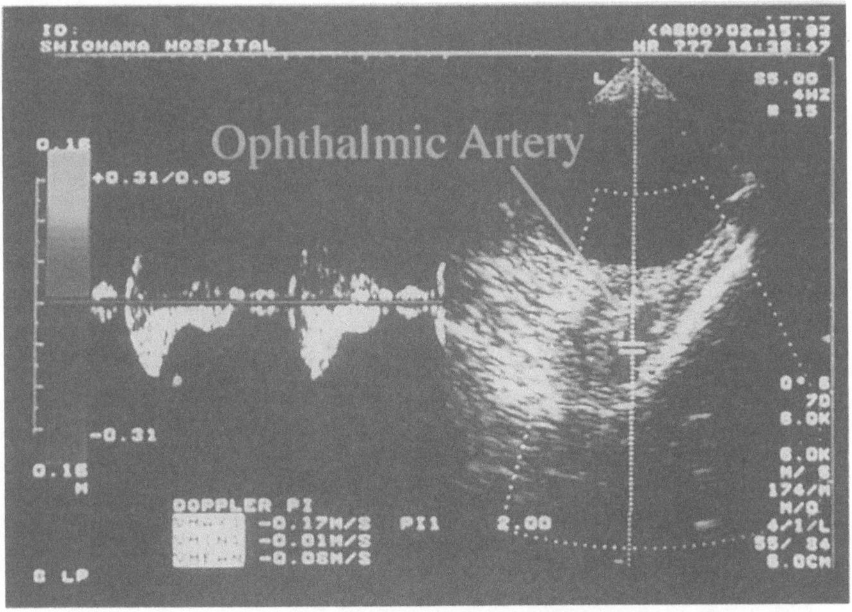

Fig. 3. Color Doppler image illustrating the reversal of flow in the ophthalmic artery

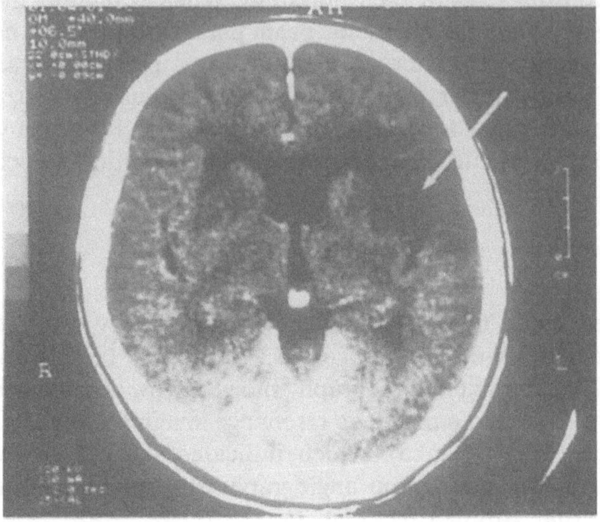

Fig. 4. Computed tomography illustrates the old cerebral infarction

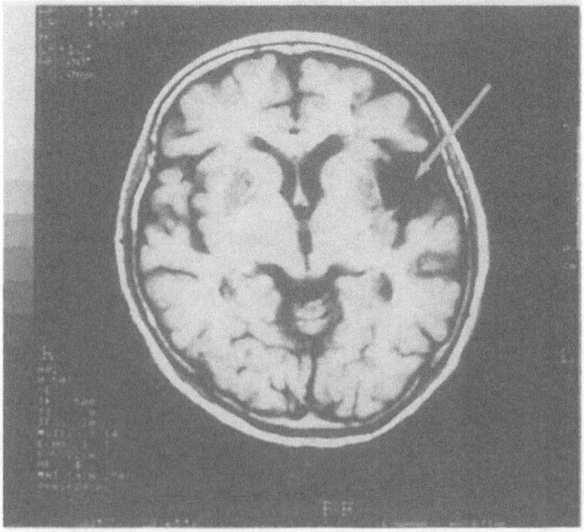

Fig. 5. Magnetic resonance imaging also detects the old cerebral infarction

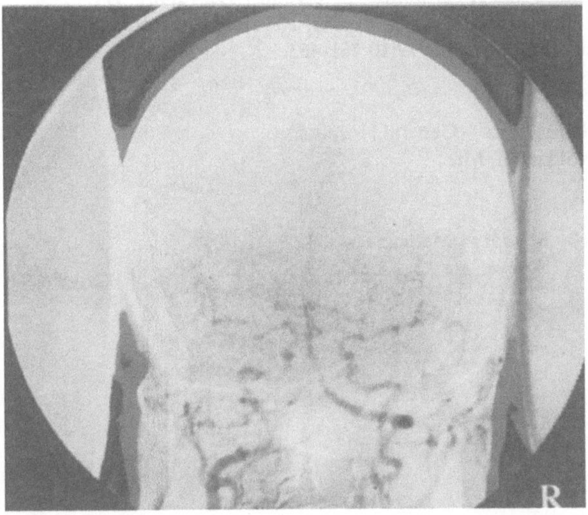

Fig. 6. Digital subtraction angiogram shows there is no occlusion of either internal carotid artery

Discussion

In 1990, Hashimoto [1] found a reverse blood flow in an ophthalmic artery in a patient whose internal carotid was completely occluded. In 1992, Ho [2] reported reversed ophthalmic artery flow in 12 eyes with ischemic ocular syndrome. Reversed flow in the ophthalmic artery is due to collateral blood flow from the external carotid to the internal carotid because of the low blood pressure in the latter.

Pitts [3] and Hodek-Demarin [4] reported that internal carotid stenosis or intracranial arterial stenosis causes the reversed flow. Our patient was not affected by stenosis of either internal carotid artery, but she had a history of cerebral infarction and heart failure. This suggests that the left internal carotid artery caused the reversal of flow in the left ophthalmic artery.

References

[1] T. Hashimoto, M. Hashimoto and S. Tane. Doppler flowmetry of carotid and intraorbital ophthalmic arteries. Jpn. J. Clin. Ophthalmol. 1990;44(11):1773–1777.

[2] A.C. Ho et al. Color doppler imaging of the ocular ischemic syndrome. Ophthalmology 1992;99:1453–1462.

[3] F.W. Pitts. Variations of collateral circulation in internal carotid artery occlusion. Comparison of clinical and X-ray findings. Neurology 192;12:467–471.
[4] V. Hodek-Demarin and H.R. Mueller. Reversed ophthalmic artery flow in internal carotid artery occlusion. Stroke 1979;10:461-463.

Kazuo Emi
Mie Prefectual Shiohama – General Hospital
1, Shiohama, Yokkaichi, Mie
Japan, 510

[1]Mie University – School of Medicine
Mie, Japan

65. Obstruction of the superior ophthalmic vein assessed by the colour Doppler imaging technique – value in differential diagnostics

Z. NAGY, J. NÉMETH, I. SÜVEGES and M. BODOSI

(Budapest, Hungary)

Abstract

We describe a case of a patient with a syndrome of paradoxical worsening of a dural-sinus cavernous arteriovenous malformation which was an iatrogenic consequence of previous embolization of the basal branches of a dural shunt with Yvalon. It is presumed that the thrombogenous Yvalon reached the basal branches of the medial meningeal artery of the superior ophthalmic vein, where it caused a complete thrombosis. The compromised ocular and orbital venous outflow caused a dramatic worsening of the ocular congestive symptoms: venous stasis retinopathy with dilated veins, flame and dot-shaped hemorrhages and secondary increase in intraocular pressure. The diagnosis of thrombosis of the entire superior ophthalmic vein was confirmed by color Doppler imaging. The pathomechanism is discussed. Although the ocular pathology is usually self-limiting after establishment of the collateral venous outflow channels, because of serious congestive ocular symptoms, argon laser photocoagulation and conservative antiglaucomatous local therapy were applied. In this patient, shortly after establishing the orbital collateral venous draining channels, the ocular symptoms improved. There was no other complication during the one-year follow-up.

Key words: Carotido-cavernous sinus fistula, dural shunt, superior ophthalmic vein, thrombosis, color Doppler

Introduction

Carotid-cavernous sinus fistulas and the dural shunt syndrome are quite rare in ophthalmological practice. Most cases are of spontaneous origin, or occur after a head trauma. The abnormal anastomosis between the internal carotid artery and cavernous sinus is the anatomical basis of the disorder. Due to the pressure gradient between the artery and the venous flow, arterial blood enters the venous system, this is the so-called 'venous arterialization'. The clinical features in such cases are the consequences of the altered intravascular hemodynamics.

G Cennamo and N. Rosa (eds.), Ultrasonography in Ophthalmology 15, pp. 523–528.

In 1987 Sergott [1] described an interesting clinical phenomenon, which he called the 'syndrome of paradoxically worsening of dural-cavernous sinus arteriovenous malformation'. The pathogenesis in this syndrome is basically different from the well known principle of 'venous arterialization' (direct or indirect communication between the internal or external carotid artery and the cavernous sinus). In these patients the entire superior ophthalmic venous outflow is compromised due to the complete venous thrombosis. The clinical symptoms occur suddenly and can be very frightening. Nevertheless, the conservative treatment should be used, because of the self-limiting processes.

The clinical features are: unexpectedly rapid worsening; mild, or overt exophthalmos; pain in the orbital region; 'red eye syndrome'; reduced ocular movement, in some cases ophthalmoplegia; diplopia; ptosis; visual deterioration; and vascular congestive signs in the fundus.

Here we present a case, where at the onset of the procedure the syndrome was due to the above-mentioned 'venous arterialization', but in the second stage of this malformation, caused iatrogenically, the pathogenesis basically altered. The objective and subjective complaints of the patient were so severe, that a second neurosurgical intervention was considered, before elucidating the exact pathogenesis.

Case report

A 55-year-old male patient, affected by insulin-dependent diabetes mellitus and hypertension for 5 years, in spring 1992 came to the outpatients department of our clinic with a progressing proptosis and symptoms of vascular congestion both in the anterior and posterior segment (Fig. 1). The symptoms had appeared some weeks before, and a computerized tomography, performed in another institute, showed mild protrusion of the globe and widening of the extraocular muscles (Fig. 2). A selective digital subtraction angiography was then performed and showed a vascular malformation of the right meningohypophyseal branch.

Upon completion of the diagnostic examinations, an invasive therapy was decided. A coaxial catheter was introduced to the right medial meningeal artery and its basal branches were embolized with Yvalon. After the operation a regular carotid compression massage was suggested to the patient.

Some days after leaving the hospital, the ocular symptoms started to worsen: the proptosis increased, a diplopia appeared, then a pain started around his right eye, and the anterior segment symptoms (gorgous episcleral veins and chemosis) frightened the patient. At his second admission to hospital the visual acuity on the right side was 0.15; the proptosis of the affected side was 6 mm greater than on the other side. The slit lamp examination showed dilated, arborized episcleral veins and severe chemosis; the cornea was normal. The proptosis prevented complete closure of the lid. The anterior chamber was shallow; during the gonioscopy the angle was opened, but the Schlemm-

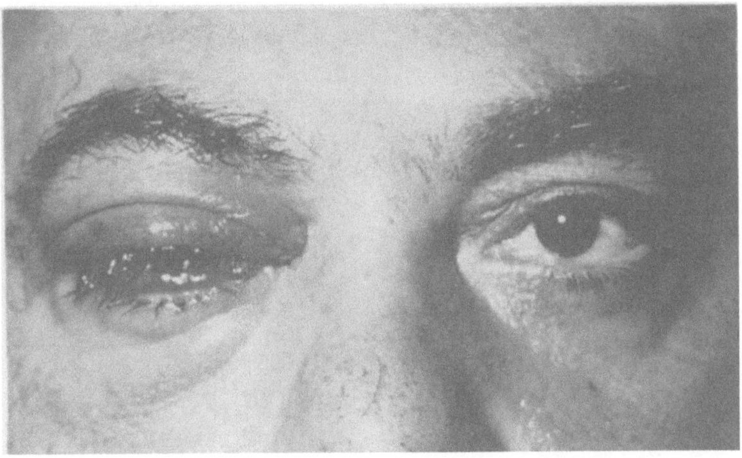

Fig. 1. Progressing proptosis and vascular congestion in the anterior segment

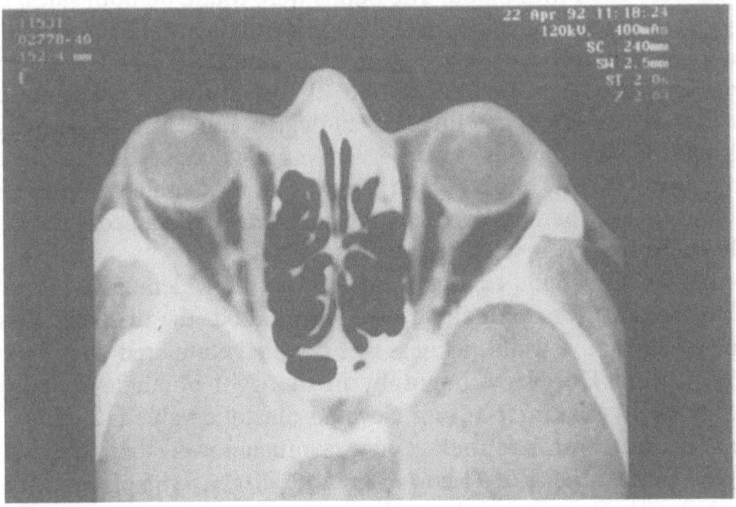

Fig. 2. Computerized tomographic scan showing slight protrusion of the eye and enlargement of the extraocular muscles

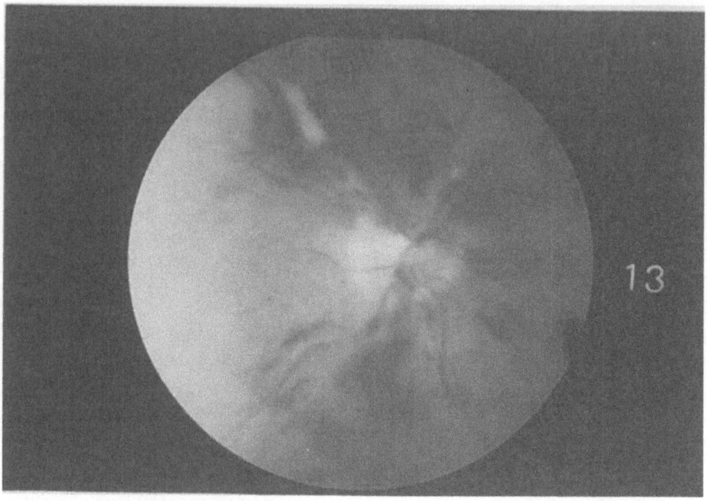

Fig. 3. Funduscopy showed hyperemic, slightly blurred optic nerve head, flame-shaped hemorrhage along the main venous vessels

channels were filled with blood. The pupils were round on both sides, but on the right side there was a relative afferent pupillary defect. The intraocular pressure with applanation tonometry was 28 mmHg, and on the other side 16 mmHg. The eye movements were reduced in all directions; Goldmann perimetry showed, with the small size target a 20-degree concentric constriction of the visual field. On the fundus we observed vascular congestion; the papilla was hyperemic and slightly blurred, but there was no measurable prominence. Along the venous vessels there was some flame and some dot-shaped hemorrhage, and a slight edema on the macular region (Fig. 3).

The ocular ultrasound examination showed the widening of the extraocular muscles; the superior ophthalmic vein was dilated, the diameter was 3.0 mm and the posterior eye wall thickness was doubled compared with the other side (Fig. 4). Colour Doppler echography in the right ophthalmic artery showed normal velocity (30 cm/s) but an elevated diastolic value (12 cm/s). The flow velocity in the central retinal vein was much lower than the normal and compared to the other side (1 cm/s versus 4 cm/s). In the place of the superior ophthalmic vein there was only a tubular structure, without any perfusion. The anatomical localization correlated very well with the result of the ophthalmic ultrasound examination. The tubular structure without perfusion proved to be an entirely thrombotized superior ophthalmic vein (Fig. 5).

The ocular symptoms progressed, so we requested a neurosurgical opinion. Before the decision, with the use of Tc 99 m HMPAO radiopharmakon a

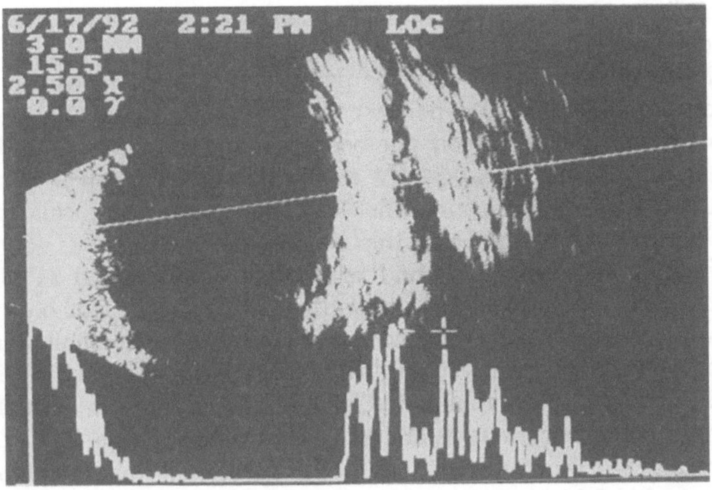

Fig. 4. The dilated superior ophthalmic vein

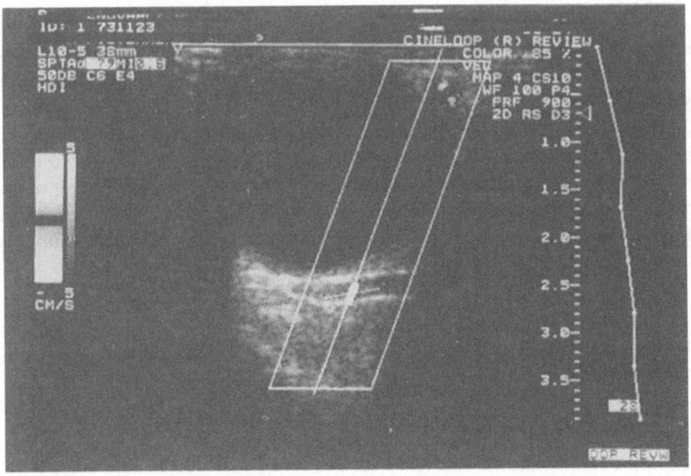

Fig. 5. The thrombotized superior ophthalmic vein, no perfusion can be detected

SPECT examination was performed to judge the collateral perfusion, which was normal. Because of the diabetes and the systemic hypertension, and because ophthalmic symptoms can persist after surgery, conservative treatment was decided.

In the ophthalmic literature some patients were reported with proliferative vitreoretinopathy [2,3] and neovascular secondary glaucoma [3,4], so we performed a panretinal argon photocoagulation with spots of 2–300 μm in diameter, 0.1 sec, with 0.25–0.34 mW energy. After a follow-up of 18 months the patient is in remission, his visual field is complete, the intraocular pressure is normal and no ophthalmological treatment is being given.

The pathogenesis of the second relapse can be explained as follows: the thrombotizing agent, Yvalon thrombotized iatrogenically not only the basal branches of the meningeal artery, but also the superior ophthalmic vein, so there was a complete block in the venous flow of the superior ophthalmic vein. In such cases the orbital drainage is impaired, and the venous flow can normalize only if the venous collaterals are re-established. According to Sergott, this takes from two weeks to two months, in our case the improvement started within 3 weeks.

The interest of this case is that, because of the severe progression, the different symptoms caused differential diagnostic problems. In this case only the colour Doppler imaging technique was of differential diagnostic value. The decision whether to use conservative or surgical treatment can only be decided in a diagnostically well-equipped institute.

References

[1] R.C. Sergott, R.I. Grossmann, P.J. Savino, T.M. Bosley and N.J. Schatz. The syndrome of paradoxical worsening of the dural-cavernous sinus arteriovenous malformations. Ophthalmology 1987;94:205–212.

[2] R.E. Kalina and W.A. Kelly. Proliferative retinopathy after treatment of carotid cavernous fistulas. Arch. Ophthalmol. 1978;96:2058–2060.

[3] M.J. Harris, S.L. Fine and N.R. Miller. Photocoagulation treatment of proliferative retinopathy secondary to carotid-cavernous fistula. Am. J. Ophthalmol. 1980;90:515–518.

[4] H.S. Sugar. Neovascular glaucoma after carotid-cavernous fistula. Ophthalmology 1979;86: 1521–1529.

Z.Z. Nagy
First Department of Ophthalmology
Semmelweis Medical School
Tömö u. 25–29
H-1081 Budapest, Hungary

66. Color Doppler imaging of orbital arteries in ischemic ocular syndrome

K. EMI, H. ISHIKAWA[1] and Y. UJI[1]

(Yokkaichi, Japan)

Abstract

Recently, ocular ischemic syndrome has been increasing together with hypertension, diabetes and cardiovascular and cerebrovascular disorders. Color Doppler imaging is a non invasive procedure with which to perform angiography and velocitometry of intra-orbital vessels. We used an SSA-260A (TOSHIBA Medical Co. Ltd.) and a 7-MHz electronic linear transducer for the examinations. Twelve normal subjects and thirteen patients were examined with the device. In normal subjects, the mean velocity of the ophthalmic artery was 24.9 cm/s and that of the central retinal artery was 7.9 cm/s. In patients, the mean velocity of the ophthalmic artery was 16.2 cm/s and that of the central retinal artery was 5.2 cm/s. Color Doppler imaging is useful for the estimation of ocular ischemic syndrome.

Key words: Color Doppler imaging, ischemic ocular syndrome, hemodynamics of the orbital arteries

Introduction

The condition of vessels can be evaluated with color Doppler imaging, without the use of irradiation or a radio-opaque agent. Therefore, color Doppler imaging is often used to assess the hemodynamics of cardiovascular, cerebrovascular and peripheral vascular diseases. We measured the blood flow velocity of the ophthalmic artery and the central retinal artery in patients with ischemic ocular syndrome using color Doppler imaging and compared the results with data obtained in normal subjects.

Materials and method

We used the Toshiba SSA-260A and a 7.5-MHz electronic linear probe for color Doppler imaging (Figs. 1 and 2). The study group consisted of 13 patients and 12 normal subjects, ranging in age from 53 to 77 years. The subjects were in the

G Cennamo and N. Rosa (eds.), Ultrasonography in Ophthalmology 15, pp. 529–534.

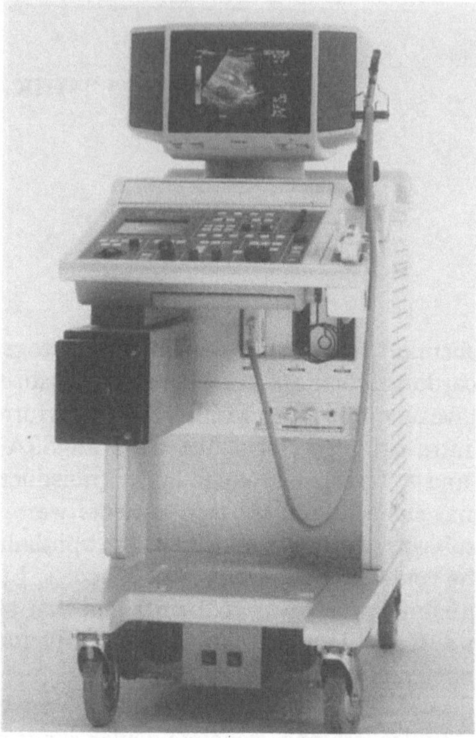

Fig. 1. Ultrasonic color Doppler diagnostic device, Toshiba SSA-260A

supine position with the tested eye closed. The probe was carefully placed over the upper lid using a coupling gel. The blood flow toward the probe is depicted in red and away from the probe in blue. Therefore, most arterial flow is red and venous flow is blue. In the imaging mode, arteries can be distinguished from veins by their pulsatility. When examining the eye and orbit, we attempted to align the ultrasonic beam parallel to the optic nerve. The blood flow of the central retinal artery is identified in the B-scan image of the optic nerve and the ophthalmic artery is identified as pulsatile vessel adjacent and parallel to the optic nerve. Doppler frequency shifts within the ophthalmic and central retinal arteries were measured to determine the peak systolic velocity (V-max), end diastolic velocity (V-min) and mean-enveloped blood flow velocity (V-mean). Gosling's pulsatility index was calculated to determine the vascular resistance of the orbital vessels.

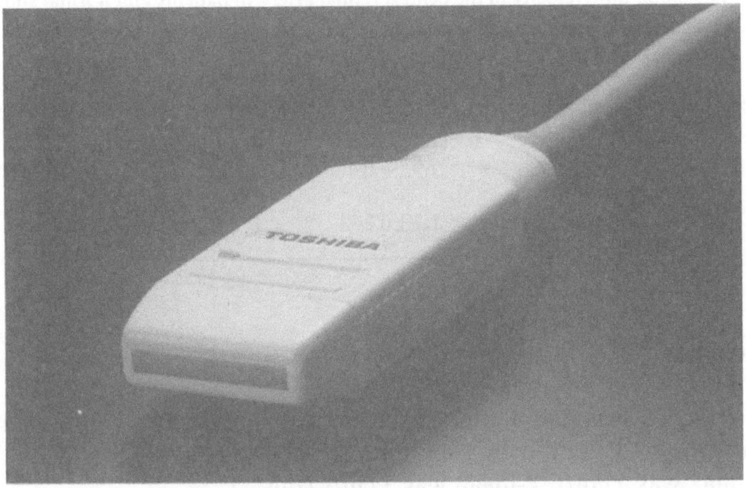

Fig. 2. 7.5 MHz electronic linear scanner for color Doppler imaging

Results

The blood flow velocity of 12 eyes of normal subjects and 17 eyes of patients could be measured in the ophthalmic artery. The blood flow velocity of 15 eyes of normal subjects and 16 eyes of patients could be determined in central retinal artery. The mean and peak blood flow velocities in normal subjects were faster than in patients in both the ophthalmic and the central retinal arteries ($p<0.01$). The pulsatility index in the ophthalmic artery in normal subjects was lower than in patients ($p<0.01$; Table 1). There was no significant difference between the groups regarding the central retinal artery (Table 2).

Table 1. The blood flow velocity in the ophthalmic artery in patients and normal subjects

	Normal	Patient
V-max	38.3 ± 1.0 cm/s	28.2 ± 3.7 cm/s
V-min	24.9 ± 6.9 cm/s	16.2 ± 4.4 cm/s
PI	1.1 ± 0.2	1.4 ± 0.2

Table 2. The blood flow velocity in the central retinal artery in patients and normal subjects

	Normal	Patient
V-max	12.5±3.7 cm/s	9.0±2.5 cm/s
V-min	7.9±2.0 cm/s	5.2±1.9 cm/s
PI	1.2±0.2	1.3±0.3

Case reports

Case 1. A 75-year-old female noticed a defect in the right visual field. Funduscopy and fluorescein angiography revealed hemi-CRAO of the right eye. V-max was 5 cm/s. V-mean was 3 cm/s (Fig. 3).

Case 2. A 61-year-old diabetic man was referred to us because of decreased vision. Ophthalmoscopic examination of both eyes showed proliferative changes in the retina. Panretinal photocoagulation was done. V-max was 8 cm/s. V-mean was 4 cm/s (Fig. 4).

Case 3. A 60-year-old normal male. V-max was 10 cm/s. V-mean was 7 cm/s (Fig. 5).

Discussion

Ho [1], Williamson [2] and Hashimoto [3] reported color Doppler imaging of ischemic ocular syndromes. Ocular circulation can be measured by means of fluorescein angiography, laser Doppler, the laser specle method, the ultrasonic pulse Doppler method and color Doppler imaging. The former three methods are used to evaluate the retinal circulation and the latter two methods can estimate the orbital circulation. An advantage of color Doppler imaging is that the blood flow in the ophthalmic and central retinal arteries is toward the probe, and so very little correction for the beam angle is needed. Color Doppler imaging cannot measure volumetric flow within the orbital vessels because of limitation in color Doppler spatial resolution of about 1 cm. But the peak systolic velocity may be a gauge of systolic blood flow and the pulsatility index may be a index of diastolic blood flow. Color Doppler imaging provides quantitative data about retrobulbar blood flow characteristics rapidly and non-invasively. Therefore, color Doppler imaging is useful to evaluate and monitor patients affected by such ischemic ocular syndromes as diabetes, hypertension, retinal artery occlusion and retinal vein occlusion.

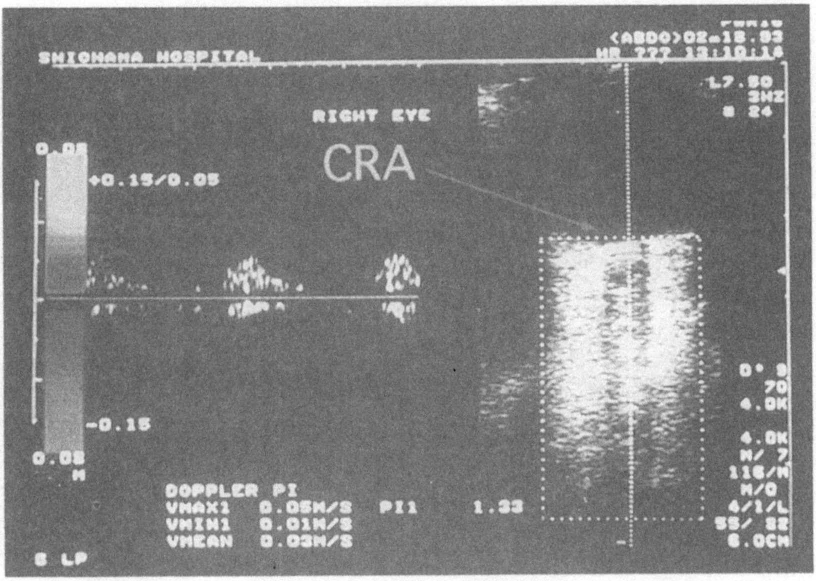

Fig. 3. Color Doppler imaging of case 1

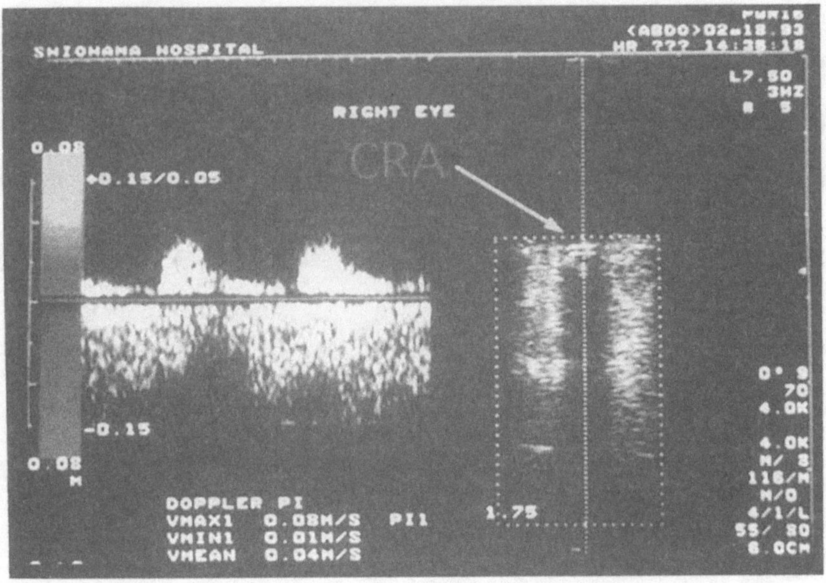

Fig. 4. Color Doppler imaging of case 2

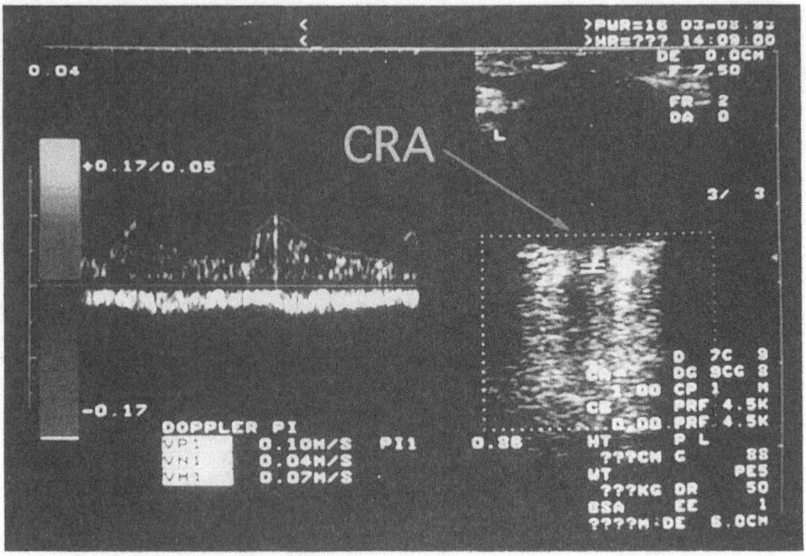

Fig. 5. Color Doppler imaging of case 3

References

[1] A.C. Ho *et al.* Color Doppler imaging of the ocular ischemic syndrome. Ophthalmology 1992;99:1453–1462.

[2] T.H. Williamson *et al.* Color Doppler velocitometry of the optic nerve head in arterial occlusion. Ophthalmology 1993;100:312–317.

[3] T. Hashimoto, M. Hashimoto and S. Tane. Doppler flowmetry of carotid and intraorbital ophthalmic arteries. Japan. J. of Clin. Ophthal. 1990;44(11):1773–1777.

Kazuo Emi
Mie Prefectual Shiohama – General Hospital
1 Shiohama, Yokkaichi, Mie,
Japan, 510

[1]Mie University – School of Medicine
Mie, Japan

67. Pilomatrixoma of the eyebrow

E. FRIELING and K. LÊ-RUPPERT
(Regensburg, Germany)

Abstract

A painless, circumscribed, reddish-blue lesion was found in the region of the right eyebrow of a 11-year-old girl. Standardized echography showed a round cystic lesion with an additional dome-shaped lesion at its base which was medium to highly reflective and showed a regular heterogeneous structure with medium sound attenuation and vascularity at the base. For diagnostic and cosmetic reasons the tumor was excised. Histopathologically the lesion proved to be a 'benign calcifying epithelioma Malherbe' (pilomatrixoma). The echographic and histological characteristics are described and correlated.

Key words: Standardized echography, histology, tumor of the eyebrow

Introduction

Pilomatrixoma are benign tumors originating from hair follicles. They were first described by Malherbe in 1880 as 'calcifying epithelioma' [1]. In the ophthalmic literature the first cases were reported by Ashton in 1951 [2]. The term 'pilomatrixoma' was initially proposed by Forbes and Helwig in 1961 [3] to emphasize the histogenesis of the tumor from hair matrix cells. The histological diagnosis is based on the presence of basophilic cells, shadow cells and foci of calcifications [4]. The most common sites of involvement are the upper extremities and the face, especially the upper eye lid, eye brow and canthal region [5]. The lesion tends to occur in children and young adults [6] with female predominance [5].

To our knowledge the echographic features of a pilomatrixoma have never been reported.

Case report

In August 1993 a 11-year-old girl was referred to us with a subcutaneous, painless lesion under her right eye brow. It had grown rapidly in a few days from a small reddish nodule to a large, bumpy lesion with blue-red discoloration of

G Cennamo and N. Rosa (eds.), Ultrasonography in Ophthalmology 15, pp. 535–540.

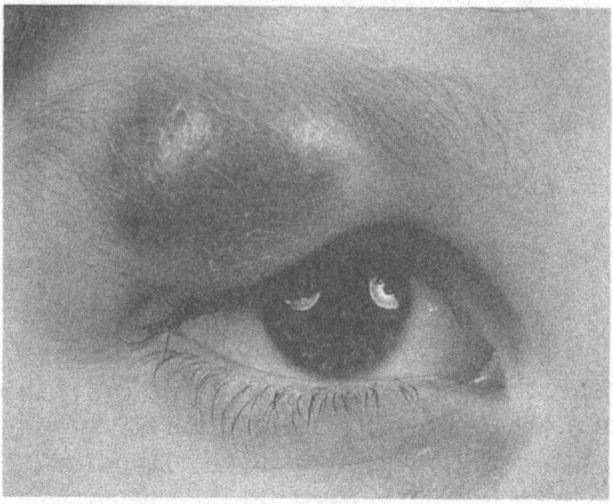

Fig. 1. Pilomatrixoma of the eyebrow (11-year-old girl)

the overlying skin (Fig. 1). At the time of examination there were no other dermatologic or ophthalmologic abnormalities.

Echographic examination was performed with standardized A-scan and with B-scan. Both eyes and orbits were normal. The evaluation of the region of the right eye brow showed a large round cystic lesion (Fig. 2b), sharply outlined with low reflectivity and regular internal structure (Fig. 2a). At the upper base of this cystic lesion there was a dome-shaped elevation, well-defined with medium high to high reflectivity, regular heterogeneous internal structure and medium sound attenuation (Fig. 2). The cystic part of the lesion was slightly compressible with a maximal diameter of about 14 mm. The diameter of the dome shaped elevation was 5.3 mm.

At the temporal side of the cyst another structure was detected: a straight line with low to medium reflective echoes below. This structure could be shifted by changing the head position, so that a layer of fluid blood was suspected.

Standardized A-scan revealed vascularity at the base of the solid lesion. To confirm and to document this vascularity Colour Doppler imaging was performed (Ultramark 6 HDI/Advanced Technology Laboratories). Colour coded B-scan showed the vessels at the temporal base of the solid lesion (Fig. 3a) which had been recognised before with A-scan. Other than that no vessels were detected.

After optimising the angle of incidence, Duplex Doppler scan allowed a semiquantitative assessment of the blood flow in the detected artery. Maximal systolic blood flow velocity was about 8 cm/sec (Fig. 3b). After further enlargement of the lesion the tumor was excised.

Histological evaluation revealed a multilobulated tumor involving the lower

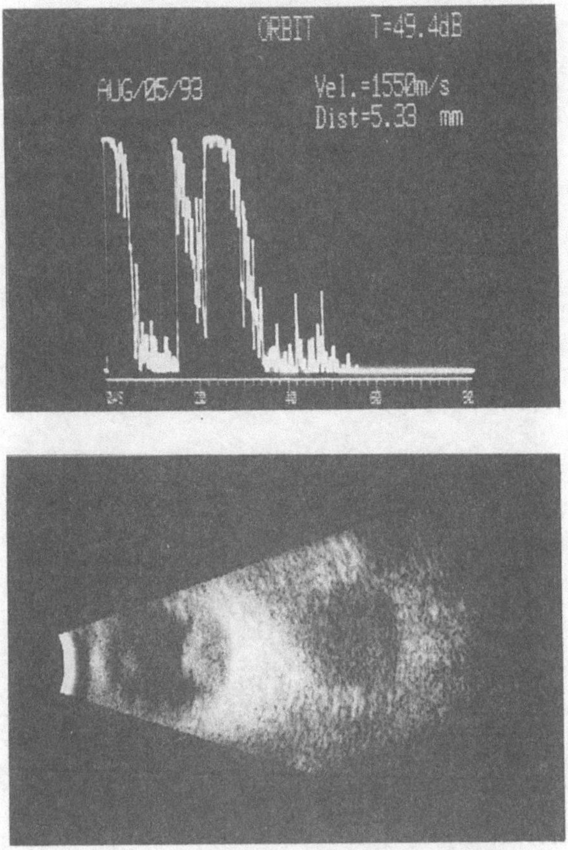

Fig. 2. **Standardized A-scan and corresponding B-scan of a pilomatrixoma**

dermis, surrounded by a pseudocapsule. Large parts inside the pseudocapsule were filled with blood cells, indicating an hemorrhage occupying large parts of the cystic lesion. At higher magnification, irregularly-shaped islands of epithelial cells were observed attached to the capsule. These islands were composed of basophilic cells at the periphery and so-called shadow cells toward the center of the island (Fig. 4). Nearby there were small foci of calcifications and a few small areas of bony lamellar indicating ossification. Because of this typical histologic appearance the diagnosis of a pilomatrixoma was made.

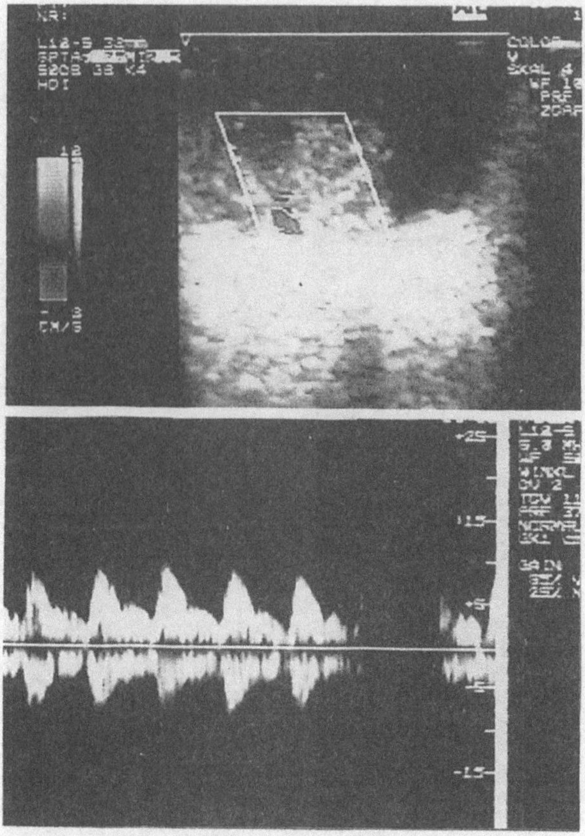

(a)

(b)

Fig. 3. a) Color Doppler Imaging: Localisation of a tumor artery at the temporal tumor base. b) Duplex Doppler: Documentation of blood flow velocity in the tumor vessel (8 cm/sec)

Discussion

Pilomatrixoma of the periorbital region are rare findings for ophthalmologists and to our knowledge their echographic characteristics have never been described.

Table 1 summarises the criteria of Standardized Echography for Pilomatrixoma as we found them in this case.

Trying to correlate echographic and histologic features, the cystic appearance of the lesion is explained by the well-defined borders of the pseudocapsule. The low reflective, regularly structured substance which filled most of the cyst was as we had suspected caused by an internal hemorrhage. This was probably the cause of the sudden enlargement of the lesion which, as reported by Swerlick et al. in 1982 [7] takes place in 15–20% of the cases.

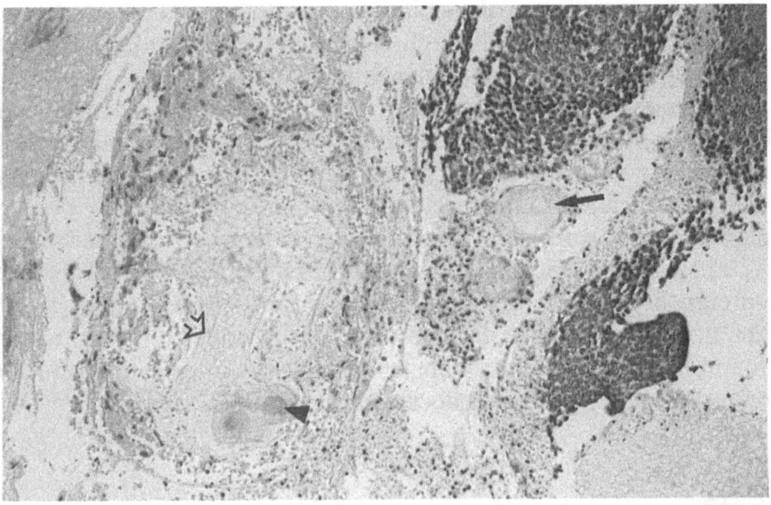

Fig. 4. Histological specimen of a pilomatrixoma (HE, 200 ×). Island of epithelial cells with basophilic cells in the periphery and the so-called shadow cells (open arrow) in the center of the islands. Small areas of calcifications (short arrow) and ossifications (arrow head) are further characteristics of this tumor

Table 1. Criteria of Standardized Echography in a case of pilomatrixoma

Quantitative Echography
- Reflectivity: medium high to high
- Internal structure: regular heterogeneous
- Sound attenuation: medium

Kinetic Echography
- Vascularity + (at the base)
- Mobility: immobile
- Consistency: firm to hard

Topographic Echography
- Shape: round to oval
- Borders: well outlined, encapsulated
- Location: subdermal (lids, eyebrows)

In the solid part of the tumor, the multilobulated structure with islands of epithelial cells, the areas of calcification and the foci of ossification are responsible for the relatively high reflectivity, the regular heterogeneous structure and the medium sound attenuation.

Calcium deposits beside the hemorrhages are further secondary changes, which are found in 75% of the histological specimens [8]. Calcifications and ossifications are signs of tumor aging. Our specimen showed small foci of ossifications, which are found in 15 to 20% of cases [3], probably developed by metaplasia from fibroblasts into osteoblasts, induced by calcium-rich shadow cells [9]. These foci of ossification are responsible for the few small areas of 100% high foreign body spikes in A-scan, as described by Ossoinig [10]. Colour Doppler Imaging helped us only to verify the vascularity which already had been found by A-scan. Colour Doppler Imaging did not detect any further area of vascularisation but helped to document the tumor vessels.

References

[1] A. Malherbe and J. Chenantais. Note sur l'épithéliome calcifié des glandes sébacées. Prog. Med. 1880;8:826–828.

[2] N. Ashthon. Benign calcified epithelioma of eyelid. Trans. Ophthalmol. Soc. U.K., 1951;71: 301–307.

[3] R. Forbis Jr. and E.B. Helwig. Pilomatrixoma (Calcifying epithelioma). Arch. Dermatol. 1961;83:608–618.

[4] P. Solanki, I. Ramzy, N. Durr et al. Pilomatrixoma. Arch. Pathol. 1987;111:294–297.

[5] M. Boniuk and L.E. Zimmerman. Pilomatrixoma (benign calcifying epithelioma) of eyelid and eyebrow. Arch. Ophthalmol. 1963;70:399–406.

[6] F. Moehlenbeck. Pilomatrixoma (calcifying epithelioma). Arch. Dermatol. 1973;108:532–534.

[7] R.A. Swerlick, P.H. Cooper and S.E. Mackel. Rapid enlargement of pilomatrixoma. J. Am. Acad. Dermatol. 1982;7:54–56.

[8] W.C. Peterson Jr. and A.M. Hult. Calcifying epithelioma of Malherbe. Arch. Dermatol. 1964;90:404–410.

[9] H. Wiedersberg. Das Epithelioma calcificans Malherbe. Dermatol. Monatsschr. 1971;157: 867–883.

[10] K.C. Ossoinig. Advances in diagnostic ultrasound. In P. Henkind (ed.), Acta: XXXIV International Congress of Ophthalmology. Philadelphia: J.B. Lippincott Company, 1983.

E. Frieling
Dept. of Ophthalmology
University of Regensburg
Franz-Josef-Strauß-Allee 11
93042 Regensburg, Germany

68. Colour Doppler imaging of endocrine ophthalmopathy

Z. HORÓCZI, Z. MORVAY and Á. SZABÓ
(Szeged, Hungary)

Abstract

Eleven patients suffering from endocrine ophthalmopathy for more than one year were examined with color Doppler imaging. Blood flow of the ophthalmic artery, the superior ophthalmic vein, and the central retinal artery and vein was determined. An Acuson 128 color Doppler imaging system equipped with a 7.5 MHz probe was used. Except in one case, values corresponding to the normal controls were obtained in the ophthalmic artery and in the central retinal artery. In the former case the velocity profile corresponds to generalized arteriosclerosis. In no case could Doppler shift be detected in the superior ophthalmic vein, whereas in normal controls the value was 13.1 cm/sec. We consider the lack of imaging of the superior ophthalmic vein flow to be characteristic of endocrine ophthalmopathy.

Key words: Central retinal artery, colour Doppler, Graves' ophthalmopathy, opthalmic artery

Introduction

The pathogenesis of the ophthalmopathy in Graves' disease has not yet been explained definitely. It is thought to be due to an autoimmune reaction against orbital tissue [1]. In addition, indirect signs indicate that vascular changes play an important role in this condition. In this study we examined the orbital circulation directly using colour Doppler imaging [2,3].

Eleven of our patients with endocrine ophthalmology were studied at the Department of Radiology of our university. The blood flow of the orbital vessels was examined by means of the colour Doppler technique that allows simultaneous two-dimensional imaging. This method requires little time, is non invasive, causes minimal discomfort and gives valuable information on the orbital circulation.

G Cennamo and N. Rosa (eds.), Ultrasonography in Ophthalmology 15, pp. 541–543.

Methods

All examinations were performed with an Acuson 128 colour Doppler unit, using a 7.5 MHz linear phased array transducer. Sterile electrode gel was applied as a coupling medium. Our 11 patients were chosen among the patients of our ultrasound laboratory. They all were suffering from bilateral endocrine ophthalmopathy of more than one year's duration, and the significant enlargement of the internal rectus muscles was detected by ultrasonography. Therefore, the ultrasonographic findings, and not the Hertel values determined our choice.

Our study population was as follows: 4 men and 7 women, mean age 41.3 years. One man had open angle glaucoma, compensated with eye drops. There was no more accompanying ophthalmologic disorder. Data of 10 healthy volunteers were used as controls.

The circulatory conditions of the central retinal artery and vein, the ophthalmic artery and the superior ophthalmic vein were evaluated in each case. The inferior ophthalmic vein was not examined because it is difficult to detect even in healthy controls.

Results

The blood flow values obtained in the ophthalmic artery and in the central retinal artery and vein in our patients affected by endocrine ophthalmopathy corresponded to the values obtained in the normal controls. In the superior ophthalmic vein, Doppler shift could not be detected in any case; the normal control value was 13.1 cm/sec. These values are shown in Table 1 together with the data of the control group. It is to be noted that in a 70-year-old patient the velocity profile indicated generalized arteriosclerosis.

During our examinations the eye was not pressed by the transducer. This is worth mentioning, because if the vein wall is compressed by the external pressure, results may be misleading.

Table 1. Results

	Ophthalmic artery	Superior ophthalmic vein	Central retinal artery	Central retinal vein
Blood flow velocity average ± SD (cm/sec)				
Endocrine ophthalmopathy	31.18.2/93.4	–	11.32.8/3.41.02	4.91.5
Healthy control	33.97.9/8.73.5	13.12.6	12.82.7/4.01.1	4.81.52

Discussion

In endocrine ophthalmopathy, superior ophthalmic vein flow cannot be detected by means of colour Doppler technique, or, alternatively, there might be only minimal flow. Our finding is in agreement with reports from colleagues of the Department of Ophthalmology in Mainz [4], who could not detect any shift in the superior ophthalmic vein in four cases out of 12; in the remaining eight cases, they obtained lowered velocities, average 7.1 cm/sec. Japanese colleagues obtained similar results [5].

These findings suggest that the superior ophthalmic vein is compressed by the enlargement of the volume of the orbital muscles and fat, which causes venous stagnation. Venous stagnation may produce edema thereby increasing the volume of the orbital content. This may worsen in time and obstruct the outflow. This seems to demonstrate that orbital circulation plays a role in endocrine ophthalmopathy. Naturally, the autoimmune reaction is considered to be the primary factor, but the clinical picture may be exacerbated by the decreased venous outflow.

References

[1] C.A. Gorman, R.R. Waller and J.A. Dyer. The eye and orbit in thyroid disease. New York: Raven Press, 1984.

[2] R.F. Guthoff, R.W. Berger, P. Winkler, K. Helmke and L.C. Chumbley. Doppler ultrasonography of the ophthalmic and central retinal vessels. Arch. Ophthalmol. 1991;109:532.

[3] W.E. Lieb, S.M. Cohen, D.A. Merton, J.A. Shields, D.G. Mitchell and B.B. Goldberg. Color doppler imaging of the eye and orbit. Technique and normal vascular anatomy. Arch. Ophthalmol. 1991;109:527.

[4] H. Benning, W. Lieb, W. Göbe, G. Kahaly and F. Grehn. Color doppler imaging in patients with Graves' disease. Congress of D.O.G., Mannheim, 1992.

[5] N. Yoshiko, H. Toshi, Y. Keiji and I. Yoichi. Color doppler imaging of orbital blood flow in dysthyroid ophthalmopathy. The 14th Biennal Congress of the International Society for Ophthalmic Ultrasound, Tokyo 1992, pp. 216–224.

Dr. Zoltán Horóczi
Albert Szent-Györgyi Medical University
Department of Ophthalmology
P.O. Box 407
H-6701 Szeged, Hungary

69. Color Doppler imaging in patients with unilateral glaucoma

M. NEUDORFER, A. KESSLER,[1] J. ALMOG, M. LAZAR, M. GRAIF[1] and O. GEYER

(Tel-Aviv, Israel)

Abstract

A reduced ocular perfusion is one possible explanation for the visual field loss in glaucoma. We have therefore compared the circulation dynamics of the glaucomatous eye and the contralateral normal eye of the same patient with unilateral glaucoma. Ten patients with unilateral open angle glaucoma (AOG) participated in the study. Inclusion parameters for OAG-patients were glaucomatous visual field defect, and a cup:disk ratio of more than 0.5. We used the Acuson (Mountain View, CA) apparatus together with a 7.5 MHz linear transducer to calculate the peak systolic, diastolic, and average blood flow velocities in the ophthalmic, central retinal, and short posterior ciliary arteries (PCAs). Blood flow velocities in the central retinal artery and PAs of the glaucomatous eyes, were significantly lower ($p < 0.001$). There was no significant difference between blood flow velocities in the ophthalmic arteries of the glaucomatous and normal contralateral eyes. This shows that the blood flow velocity of the arteries supplying the eye is reduced in OAG.

Key words: Central retinal artery, color Doppler, ophthalmic artery, short posterior ciliary arteries, unilateral glaucoma

Introduction

Vascular factors have been implicated in the pathogenesis of optic nerve damage and visual field loss in glaucoma [1]. To determine the role of these factors in glaucoma we compared the flow characteristics of glaucomatous vs. contralateral normal eyes in patients with unilateral pseudoexfoliation glaucoma.

G Cennamo and N. Rosa (eds.), Ultrasonography in Ophthalmology 15, pp. 545–548.

Material and methods

We studied 10 patients (5 men and 5 women) with unilateral pseudoexfoliation glaucoma, mean age 74 years (range, 66–84 years). Inclusion criteria were glaucomatous eyes: untreated intraocular pressure (IOP) of at least 22 mmHg, a cup:disc ratio of at least 0.6 and a visual field defect; normal eye: no ocular abnormality, normal discs and visual fields and IOP below 22 mmHg. A difference of at least 0.3 in cup:disc ratio between the normal and glaucomatous eye was also required. Topical β blockers and propine were stopped 2 weeks prior to entering the study. Topical pilocarpine, or echotiophate iodide, and carbonic anhydrous inhibitors were allowed to be used at the time of color Doppler imaging examination. Sonographic examination was performed using a color Doppler ultrasound machine (Acuson 128 XP10 Mountain View, CA) with a 7.5 MHz linear array transducer. Scanning was performed in the axial view thereby obtaining an overall view and identifying the precise location and direction of flow in the vessels. Vascular flow was evaluated by both color and spectral Doppler modes. The Doppler angle was kept below 60 degrees. Central retinal artery (CRA) measurements were performed at approximately 2 mm posterior to the globe. Posterior ciliary vessels were located temporally adjacent to the optic nerve. The resistance index (RI), a measure of peripheral vascular resistance, was calculated for the ophthalmic artery (OA), CRA, and the short posterior ciliary artery (SPCA).

Statistical comparisons of glaucomatous vs. paired normal eyes measurements were made using the standard paired two-tailed Student's t test. Statistical significance was set at p values less than or equal to 0.01.

Results

The mean RIs and IOPs in the OA, SPCA and CRA of the glaucomatous eye and paired normal eyes are given in Fig. 1. The RIs in the CRA and temporal SPCA were significantly higher in glaucomatous eyes as compared to the contralateral normal eyes ($p<0.001$). In the OA the RIs were not significantly different, in the glaucomatous and in the paired normal eyes ($p<0.05$). At the time of color Doppler imaging examination the mean IOPs of both the glaucomatous and normal eyes were not significantly different ($p<0.05$).

Discussion

The results of this study clearly demonstrate that there are quantitative hemodynamic changes in the retrobulbar circulation associated with chronic glaucoma, specifically, the mean RI in both the CRA and temporal SPCA of the unilateral glaucomatous eyes was significantly greater than that of the paired normal eyes. Other studies have also shown quantitative retrobulbar hemody-

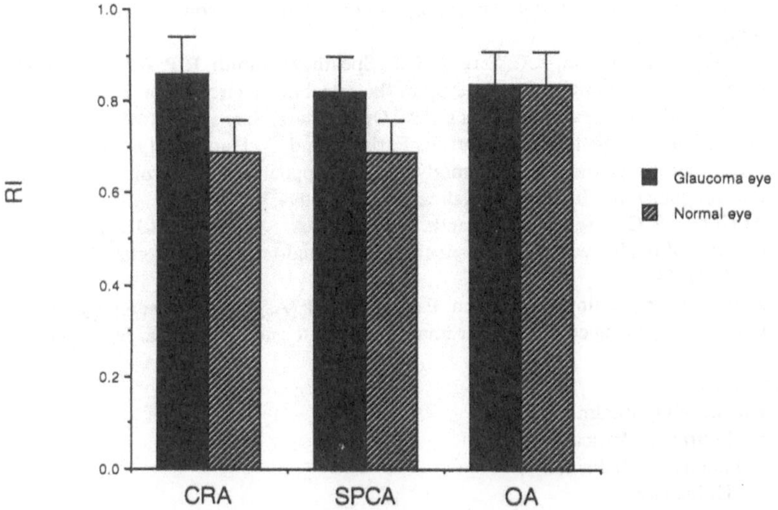

Fig. 1. The mean (SE) resistance index (RI) of the central retinal artery (CRA), short posterior ciliary artery (SPCA) and ophthalmic artery (OA) of the glaucomatous and paired normal eyes of 10 patients with unilateral pseudoexfoliation glaucoma. Note a significant change in the RI between the normal and glaucomatous eyes in the CRA and SPCA ($p<0.001$), but no difference in the OA ($p<0.05$).

namic changes in glaucomatous eyes [2–6]. Our study differs from earlier studies since it consists of patients with unilateral pseudoexfoliation glaucoma having a contralateral normal eye. We were thus able to eliminate the bias of systemic hemodynamic parameters, such as cardiac output, blood pressure and systemic disease, which inevitably can affect even the best matched controls.

Since the IOP of the glaucomatous eyes in our group was controlled and was not significantly different from that of the normal eyes, it is most unlikely that the retrobulbar hemodynamic changes in the glaucomatous eyes were pressure related.

Our data indicate that altered ocular circulation may have a role in the damage seen in pseudoexfoliation glaucoma. However, it is not yet known whether such injury is primary or secondary.

References

[1] S.S. Hayreh. Blood flow supply to the optic nerve head and its role in optic atrophy, glaucoma and edema of the optic disc. Br. J. Ophthalmol. 1969;53:721–6.

[2] F. Galassi, G. Nuzzacci, A. Sodi, P. Casi and A. Vielmo. Color Doppler imaging in evaluation of optic nerve blood supply in normal and glaucomatous subjects. Int. Ophthalmol. 1992;16:273.

[3] J.R. Trible, V.P. Costa, R.C. Sergott, G.L. Speath, M. Smith, R.P. Wilson et al. The influence of primary open angle glaucoma upon the retrobulbar circulation: baseline, postoperative, and reproducibility analysis. Trans. Am. Ophthalmol. Soc. 1993;91:245.

[4] W.E. Lieb, W. Gobel, R.C. Sergott, R. Farhoumand, A. Harris and F. Grehn. Color Doppler investigations of the orbital hemodynamics in patients with chronic open angle and low tension glaucoma. Invest. Ophthalmol. Vis. Sci. 1994;35:2712.

[5] A. Harris, R.C. Sergott, G.L. Spaeth. J.L. Katz, J.A. Shoemaker, B.J. Martin. Color Doppler analysis of ocular vessel blood velocities in normal-tension glaucoma. Am. J. Ophthalmol. 1994;118:642.

[6] Z. Butt, G. McKillop, C. O'Brien, P. Allan and P. Aspinall. Measurements of ocular blood flow velocity using color Doppler imaging in low tension glaucoma. Eye 1995;9:29.

M. Neudorfer
Department of Ophthalmology
Tel-Aviv Sourasky Medical Center
Sackler Faculty of Medicine
Tel-Aviv University
Tel-Aviv, Israel

[1]Department of Radiology
Tel-Aviv Sourasky Medical Center
Sackler Faculty of Medicine
Tel-Aviv University
Tel-Aviv, Israel

70. Color Doppler imaging in orbital and ocular tumors

J. NÉMETH,[1] K. SÉNYI,[1] B. TAPASZTÓ,[1] Z. HARKÁNYI,[2] R. KOVÁCS,[2]
Z. MORVAY[3] and E. NAGY[3]
([1,2]Budapest and [3]Szeged, Hungary)

Abstract

Forty-two patients with a suspected orbital and intraocular tumor were examined using color Doppler imaging (CDI) to evaluate the clinical impact of the method. The age of the patients varied from six months to 86 years. Patients were divided into two groups according to histopathological diagnosis (24 cases) or to the clinical course of the disease (18 cases). The tumor group consisted of patients with choroidal melanoma (n = 19), choroidal (n = 1) and orbital (n = 3) haemangioma, leiomyoma (n = 1), retinoblastoma (n = 1), carcinoma (n = 3), fibrous histiocytoma (n = 1) and 3 unverified tumors. The non-tumor group (n = 9) was comprised of patients with tumor-like lesions such as haematomas, inflammations, macular degeneration and mucocele. A- and B-scan ultrasound was performed with Ultrascan Digital B 2000 equipment. The Acuson 128 and Ultramark-9 HDI systems were used for CDI. Color velocity imaging (CVI) was performed with Philips P-700 system.

In most cases of choroidal melanomas, CDI recorded low resistance arterial signals inside the masses. In other types of intraocular and orbital tumors, CDI also revealed blood flow inside the masses. No Doppler signs (false negative result) were obtained in a case of choroidal melanoma and in one case of orbital cavernous haemangioma. There was a false positive CDI result in a patient with severe posterior scleritis mimicking choroidal melanoma and in another with a not recent choroidal haemorrhage and vitreoretinal proliferation. In all types of tumors, flow velocities were increased over normal values in the ophthalmic artery.

From this study it appears that CDI is helpful in the differential diagnosis in cases of intraocular tumors when the optical media are not clear, and in all cases of orbital tumors.

Key words: Color Doppler imaging, color velocity imaging, tumor diagnosis

G Cennamo and N. Rosa (eds.), Ultrasonography in Ophthalmology 15, pp. 549–555.

Introduction

In cases of suspected orbital or intraocular tumor, ophthalmic A- and B-scan ultrasound is the first imaging approach. Although ultrasound is a fast and cost-effective method for differential diagnosis, in certain cases additional radiological studies are needed. Since the introduction of color Doppler imaging (CDI) in ophthalmology [1], various publications have dealt with the use of the method in the diagnosis of ocular and orbital tumors [2–10] and in the follow-up of choroidal melanomas after irradiation [4,5,7].

We used CDI in addition to conventional B-scan ultrasound, to examine 42 cases of suspected orbital and intraocular tumor. The goal of our study was to determine the impact of CDI in differentiating cases of intraocular and orbital masses, and to analyze Doppler waveforms from the masses and intraorbital vessels.

Methods

A- and B-scan ultrasound was performed using Ultrascan Digital B equipment with a 10 MHz probe. Color Doppler imaging was performed with the Acuson 128 and ATL Ultramark-9, HDI systems with 5–10 MHz linear array and with 7 MHz phased array sector probes.

As a preliminary investigation, color velocity imaging (CVI) was performed in eight normal subjects and in five patients using Philips P-700 system equipped with a 5–10 MHz linear transducer. Color velocity imaging or the 'time domain correlation method' is based on a different principle than color Doppler [11–13].

We first localized the area of interest using the B-scan grey scale technique and then used CDI to find signs of circulation. We then measured blood flow velocities with the duplex technique after angle correction in the following vessels: ophthalmic artery, central retinal artery and vein, ciliary arteries, superior ophthalmic vein and tumor vessels.

Patients

Over the past 5 years, we examined 42 patients (17 male and 25 female) who had a diagnosis of known or suspected tumor of the eye or the orbit. The final diagnosis was confirmed by histology in 24 cases. In the other 18 cases, the diagnosis was supported by regular clinical observations and ultrasound follow-up. The age of the patients was between 6 months and 86 years (average: 51.5 22.9 years). Seventeen healthy volunteers (age from 12 to 81 years, average: 50.0 23.1 years) served as control group.

Results

Blood flow velocities in the ophthalmic artery were increased in both intraocular and orbital tumors with respect to the normal control values (Table 1); these differences were not significant, possibly because of the low number of patients.

Doppler signals were detected inside the tumor masses in 31 of the 33 tumor patients (Table 2, Figs. 1 and 2). A low resistance arterial Doppler signal was obtained in 27 cases of ocular tumors. However, we also detected a series of atypical waveforms. A high resistance arterial Doppler waveform was obtained in two melanoma cases. We detected high resistance arterial and venous flow signals in the leiomyoma of the ciliary body. Intraocular haemangiomas yielded

Table 1. Blood flow velocities in normal controls and in intraocular and orbital tumor patients (SP: systolic peak, ED: end-diastolic velocities in cm/sec.)

Groups (No. of patients)	Ophthalmic artery SP	Ophthalmic artery ED	Central retinal artery SP	Central retinal artery ED	Central retinal vein max.	Superior ophthalmic vein max.
Control (n = 17)	35.5	8.3	13.1	4.2	4.7	13.9
Intraocular tumor (n = 10)	44.3	15.0	13.0	4.5	5.8	13.6
Orbital tumor (n = 4)	44.7	11.3	15.7	4.7	6.2	11.5

Table 2. Detectable Doppler signals in tumor patients (n = 33)

Diagnosis	No Doppler signals No. of patients	Positive Doppler signal No. of patients
Malignant melanoma	1	18
Melanocytoma	0	1
Choroideal haemangioma	0	1
Retinoblastoma	0	1
Leiomyoma	0	1
Other ocular tumors	0	3
Orbital haemangioma	1	2
Carcinoma	0	3
Fibrous histiocytoma	0	1
Total	2	31

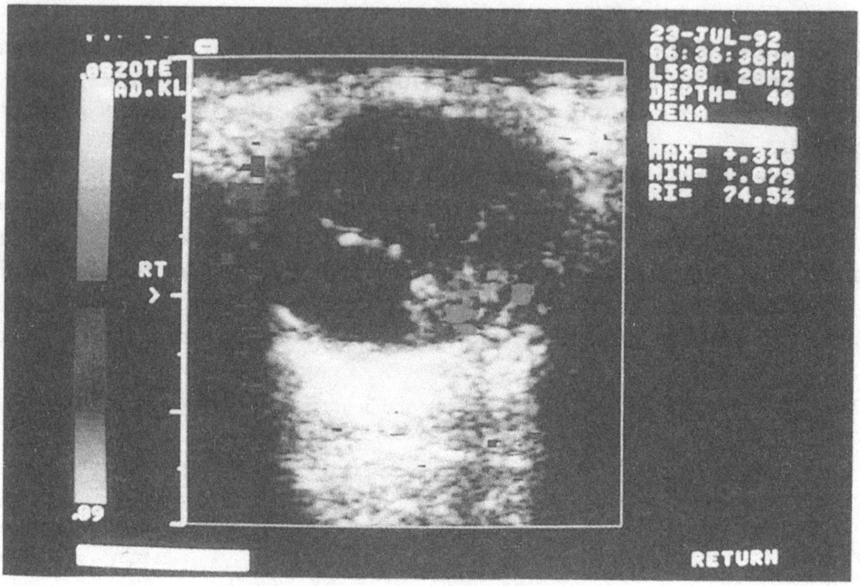

Fig. 1. Color Doppler imaging of an intraocular malignant melanoma

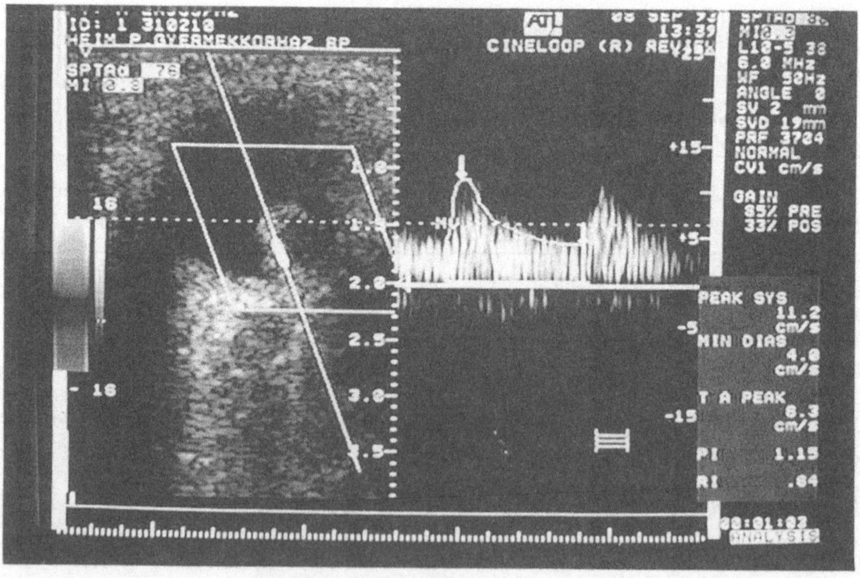

Fig. 2. Combined picture of color Doppler imaging and Doppler spectra of an intraocular choroidal malignant melanoma. Note the flow parameters at the lower right corner of the picture (peak systolic, end diastolic and time averaged mean velocities, pulsatility and resistivity indices)

Table 3. Detectable Doppler signals in non-tumor patients (n = 9)

Diagnosis	No Doppler signal No. of patients	Positive Doppler signal No. of patients
Haemorrhage (subchoroid., subret.)	4	0
Uveitis	1	1
Age-related macular degeneration	1	0
Posterior scleritis	0	1
Mucocele of frontal sinus	1	0
Total	7	2

low velocity flow and low resistance Doppler signals. In one case of cavernous haemangioma of the orbit, we did not detect any Doppler signal inside the mass. In a case of orbital carcinoma of the Meibomian gland, we found venous Doppler signals only inside the tumor. In a case of orbital fibrous histiocytoma, the mass was hypervascular as compared with the surrounding tissues and the waveform corresponded to low resistance arterial circulation.

In two of the cases of choroidal malignant melanoma of the posterior pole, we observed a direct connection between the tumor vessels and the posterior short ciliary artery. In a histologically not verified tumor localized above the optic disc, the central retinal artery and vein were seen to 'feed' the tumor tissue. In a case of extraocular extension of an intraocular malignant melanoma of the choroid, the CDI revealed flow signals not only in the intraocular but also in the orbital part of the tumor mass.

No Doppler signals were detected inside the mass in cases of choroidal or vitreous haemorrhages, uveitis, age-related macular degeneration and mucocele (Table 3).

A false-positive CDI result was obtained in a patient with severe posterior scleritis mimicking choroidal melanoma both on B-scan and clinically. In another patient with high intraocular pressure, clinical signs of intraocular inflammation and a B-scan echogram resembling intraocular tumor and haemorrhage, we detected venous flow signals inside the eye, in the suspected intraocular mass. Histopathology revealed an old subchoroidal haemorrhage and praeretinal and vitreous proliferative membranes.

Discussion

In 18 of the 19 choroidal melanoma cases, CDI revealed arterial Doppler signals inside the mass. The spectrum showed low resistance flow in 17 of the

19 cases. In other tumors (haemangioma, melanocytoma, retinoblastoma, leiomyoma, histiocytoma and carcinomas of the eye and the orbit), CDI also revealed blood flow inside the masses. In our cases, the presence of Doppler signals inside the suspected tumor mass was decisive for the diagnosis.

Using CDI and CVI, we were able to determine flow signals in small ocular and orbital masses (the smallest size was 1.9 mm). The detection of flow signals obtained with CVI, CDI or duplex, suggests the diagnosis of tumor (malignant or benign), even if this finding cannot be considered specific of tumors. Flow signals can also be detected in some benign processes. On the other hand, the absence of Doppler signals inside a mass does not exclude the possibility of a malignant tumor. As shown earlier [5,7,14], Doppler signals were not found in a low percentage (2–17%) of malignant melanoma and metastatic carcinoma cases.

The detection of flow signals is highly dependent on the technical performance of the study and the operator's skill. Several technical and biological factors determine the detectability of circulation in tissues. Such technical factors are spatial and temporal resolution, Doppler sensitivity, angle dependency, and spontaneous movements of the examiner. In case of small orbital vessels, low velocity range and low filter are the most appropriate settings. The biological factors are: the size of vessels, the direction of vessels, blood flow velocity, the eye movements of the patients, tissue movements synchronous with heart rate and breathing.

Because the color sign is usually larger than the actual size of the vessels, especially in the case of small vessels, color Doppler signs of superficial vessels (retinal-choroideal vessels or vessels of cyst walls) can cover the area of the whole suspected mass if the mass is very small. In that case it is impossible to differentiate between the superficial and the inside circulation of the mass.

The detection of low velocity flow and small volume flow is significantly enhanced by new ultrasound systems and software. The detection rate of flow can be further increased with the introduction of ultrasound contrast agents.

In conclusion, we found that CDI and CVI are helpful differential diagnostic methods in cases of intraocular tumors when the optical media are not clear, and in all cases of orbital tumors. The knowledge of tumor vasculature is also essential for therapy because the vasculature of tumors plays a role in the response to conservative treatment [5].

Acknowledgement

CVI and part of the CDI studies were performed in the Health Care Centre of Ferencváros, Budapest. The study was supported by the Hungarian Ministry of Health, ETT Project N. T-07 289/93.

References

[1] S.J. Erickson, L.E. Hendrix, B.M. Massaro, et al. Color Doppler flow imaging of the normal and abnormal orbit. Radiology 1989;173:511–516.

[2] R.W. Berger, R. Guthoff, K. Helmke and P. Winkler. Doppler ultrasonography in the follow-up of malignant melanoma of the choroid. In R. Sampaolesi (ed.), Ultrasonography in ophthalmology. Dordrecht: Kluwer Academic Publishers, 1990;327–331.

[3] L. Falco, S. Esente, S. Fanfani, N. Pasarelli and S. Utari. Our experience in the diagnosis of intraocular tumours by a B-scan computerized system and angiodynography (Doppler). Preliminary results. Acta Ophthalmol. 1992;70(204):76–80.

[4] R.F. Guthoff, R.W. Berger, K. Helmke and P. Winkler. Dopplersonographische Befunde bei intraocularen Tumoren. Fortschr. Ophthalmol. 1989;86:239–241.

[5] R.F. Guthoff, R.F. Berger, P. Winkler, K. Helmke and L.C. Chumbley. Doppler ultrasonography of malignant melanomas. Arch. Ophthalmol. 1991;109:537–541.

[6] R. Jain, S. Sawhney and M. Berry. Real-time sonography of orbital tumours, Colour Doppler characterization: Initial experience. Acta Ophthalmol. 1992;70(204):46–49.

[7] W.E. Lieb, J.A. Shields, S.M. Cohen, D.A. Merton, D.G. Mitchell, C.L. Shields, and B.B. Goldberg. Color Doppler imaging in the management of intraocular tumors. Ophthalmology 1990;97:1660–1664.

[8] W.E. Lieb, P.M. Flaharty, A. Ho and R.C. Sergott. Color Doppler imaging of the eye and orbit. A synopsis of a 400 case experience. Acta Ophthalmol. 1992;70(204):50–54.

[9] J. Németh, Z. Morvay, Z. Horóczi and E. Nagy. A színkódolt Doppler ultrahang vizsgálat szemészeti alkalmazása Szemészet 1992;129:43.

[10] P.G. Wolff-Korman, B.A. Kormann, G.C. Hasenfratz and F.A. Spengel. Duplex and color Doppler ultrasound in the differential diagnosis of choroidal tumors. Acta Ophthalmol. 1992;70(204):66–70.

[11] O. Bonnefous and P. Pesque. Time domain formulation of pulse Doppler ultrasound and blood velocity estimation by cross correlation. Ultrasonic Imaging 1996;8:73–85.

[12] Z. Harkányi, J.B. Liu, D. Merton and B.B. Goldberg. Color Velocity Imaging: új ultrahang módszer a vérkeringés vizsgálatában. Lege Artis Medicinae 1992;2:646–651.

[13] C.H. Tegeler, F.W. Kremkau and L.P. Hitchings. Color Velocity Imaging: introduction to a new ultrasound technology. J. Neuroimaging 1991;1:85–90.

[14] O. Berges and E. Nau. High resolution B mode echography and color Doppler (CDFI) of the macula. Acta Ophthalmol. 1992:70(204):74–75.

[1]Dr. J. Németh
Semmelweis Medical University
1st Department of Ophthalmology
Tömö u. 25-29
H-1083 Budapest, Hungary

[2]Pál Heim Children's,
Dept. of Radiology
Budapest, Hungary

[3]Albert Szent-Györgyi Medical University
Dept. of Radiology
Szeged, Hungary

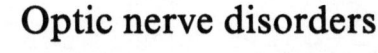

Optic nerve disorders

71. Optical pits and (other) acoustic fistulas. True B-scan findings or artifacts? An ultrasonic report on six patients

H.C. FLEDELIUS
(Hillerød, Denmark)

Abstract

We report the ultrasonically demonstrated 'fistulas' on B-scans obtained in six patients with various ophthalmic disorders. Four patients presented with minor structure changes, as verified ophthalmoscopically: three had optic pit, one had optic nervehead coloboma. In addition, we present ultrasound images from two patients where optical verification was not possible: one had a conjunctival cyst, later to be surgically removed; and one was evaluated immediately after birth, for small leukomatous eyes and the ultrasound diagnosis was microphthalmus with orbital cyst.

The patients were evaluated ultrasonically with standard equipment, NIDEK 2500 and 3000. It appears that axial and lateral resolution are important for imaging small anatomical structures. The reliability of the findings is discussed. Are we dealing with true imaging or with artifacts?

Key words: Optical pits, coloboma, B-scan echography, microphthalmus with orbital cyst

Introduction

Examining the eye and the orbit by ultrasound is a dynamic process. A large number of scans appear on the screen from various directions and must be interpreted by the examiner, who will provide the diagnosis for the referring colleague, often accompanied by selected frozen scans.

As part of the work-up, ultrasonic findings without obvious anatomical correlations are sometimes observed – and usually discarded on the spot as being irrelevant or artifacts. In this report six patients are discussed, all showing 'acoustic fistulas' on B-scans. Four were associated with optic disc lesions, one was a simple conjunctival cyst, and a blind newborn presented with microphthalmos with orbital cyst.

G Cennamo and N. Rosa (eds.), Ultrasonography in Ophthalmology 15, pp. 559–564.

Table 1. Ultrasound findings obtained in the six patients studied

Diagnosis	Sex, Age	Ultrasound findings
1. Optic pit	f, 39	Acoustic channel on disc (Fig. 1)
2. Optic pit	m, 73	Acoustic channel on disc
3. Optic pit	f, 58	Pit difficult to demonstrate
4. Optic nervehead coloboma	m, 50	A broader notch at the site of the disc
5. Conjunctival cyst	m, 23	A fistula between eye and cyst,artifact
6. Microphthalmus with orbital cyst	m, newborn	Diagnosed by A- & B-scan at age days. Channel between eye and cyst?

Case description and discussion

The ultrasound findings obtained in the six patients are reported in Table 1. In the first two patients the optic pits were occasional findings. The third referral was due to suspicion of glaucomatous disc change. Associated retinal changes were not detected in the three patients. All had normal corrected visual acuity.

Acoustically, a channel or a 'fistula' leading down into the optic nerve shadow was detected in two of the three patients affected by optic pit; it was less obvious in patient no. 3, although pit size appeared at least equal to those of cases no. 1 and 2.

The optimum resolution of the equipment indicated by the manufacturer is: 0.1 mm axially and 0.2 mm laterally. The optic nervehead diameter being about 1.5 mm; the above optic pits should thus have been (more) readily demonstrated. Likewise, using the optic nervehead as a routine reference point during B-scanning, large physiological cups and glaucomatous disc excavations should be (more) commonplace findings during routine examinations. From a practical point of view, the resolution of most commercially available ultrasound scanners thus appears poorer than for instance given by the above specifications.

Patient no. 4, a 50-year-old male, was seen only on the occasion of an examination of his daughter aged 12 who dramatically developed blindness. She suffered from Recklinghausen's disease, complicated by severe epilepsy, difficult to control. Normal computerized tomographic scans suggested that her blindness was cortical, a sequel to repeated prolonged epileptic episodes. The father noticed one blind eye himself, and neurofibromatosis was suspected, but ophthalmoscopy merely revealed a coloboma of the optic nerve head. B-scan demonstrated a notch in the posterior pole contour, leading down into the acoustic optic nerve shadow (Fig. 2).

Patient no. 5 came to have an epipulbar conjunctival cyst under the upper lid removed. The lesion was well demonstrated by ultrasound as solitary and well-defined. Acoustically, however, in a transbulbar projection there was an open

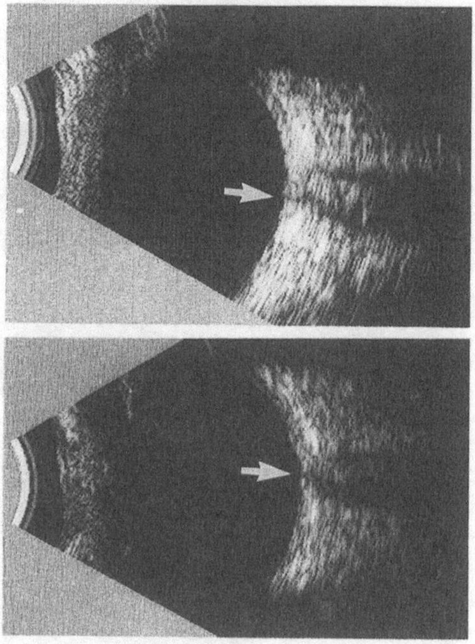

Fig. 1. Scans at tumour sensitivity setting, patient No. 1. White arrow indicates the tiny acoustic gap in the optic nervehead, cf. text

channel connecting the lumen of the eyeball proper with that of the conjunctival cyst (Fig. 3). Clearly this had no anatomical correlate, but the artifact cannot be easily explained.

Patient no. 6 was a newborn male, from a consanguineous marriage. He had deep-set leukomatous eyes. The initial A-scan gave the diagnosis of microphthalmos with orbital cyst, amply verified by the B-scan imaging (Fig. 4). A lumen was demonstrated behind the small eyeball, on the right side in particular. The appearance is similar to a case presented in Guthoff's textbook [1], except that a 'connecting channel' between the two lumina is suggested in the present case. The acoustic section being on mid-eye level, it is unlikely that this finding is due to an acoustical shadowing resulting from a non perpendicular approach at equatorial level. Anyhow, we need a histological examination of the orbital contents to evaluate the importance of the ultrasound imaging: true finding [2] or artifact?

I saw him again at the age of 18 months. He had severe mental retardation and was totally blind in both eyes. The eyes were a little smaller than at birth, and the cyst was smaller and more difficult to demonstrate. Involutive changes are thus suggested.

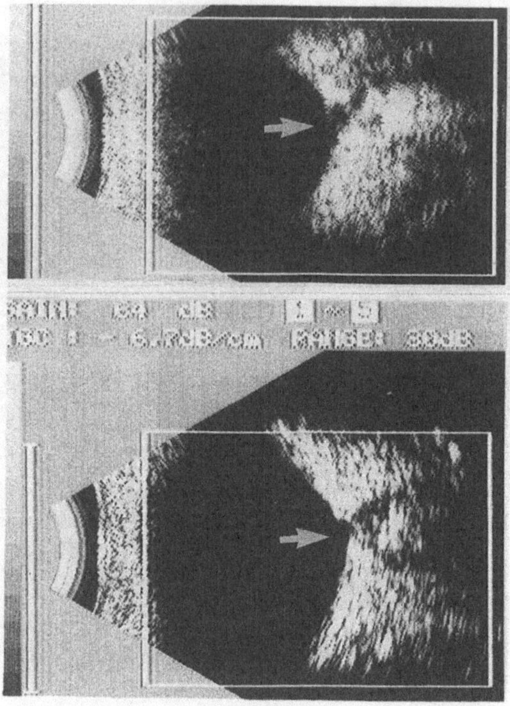

Fig. 2. **Optic nervehead coloboma, patient No. 4, depicted as an acoustical notch (white arrow). Tumour sensitivity (top), -10 db (at bottom)**

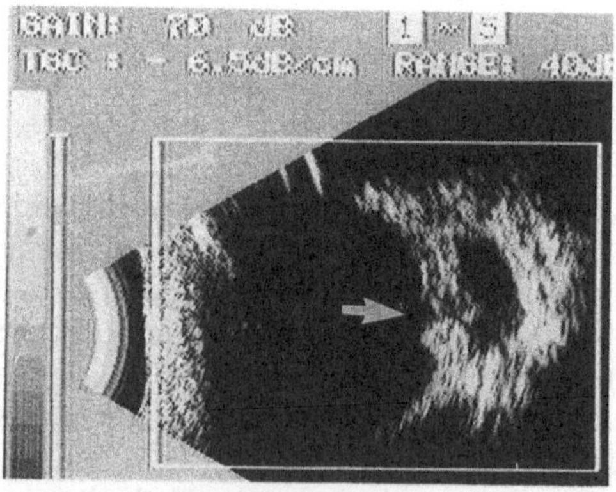

Fig. 3. **A transocular B-scan, from below and upwards-temporally, depicting the conjunctival cyst with the false acoustic fistula (arrow) to the eyebulb, cf. text**

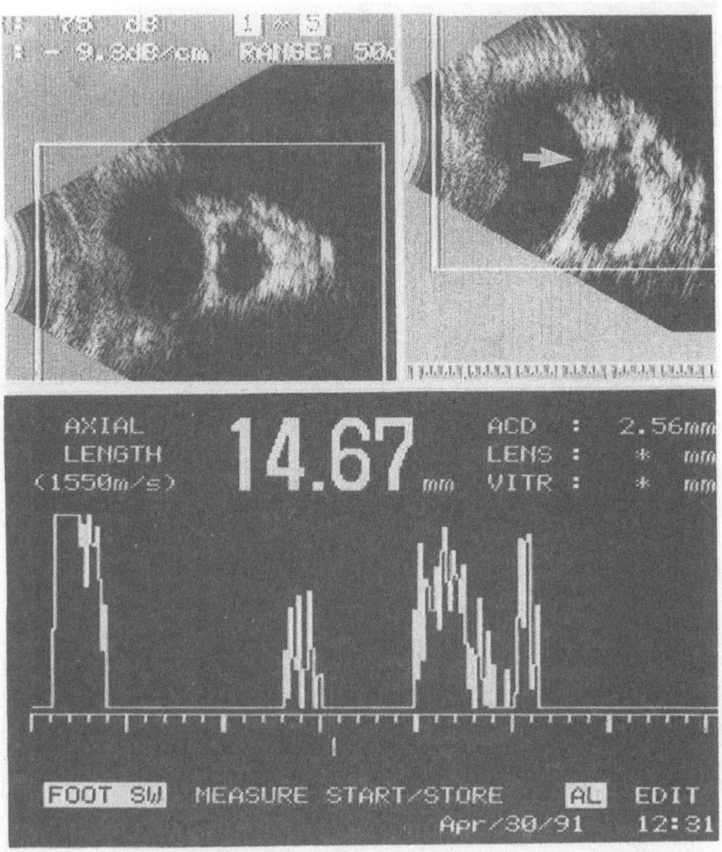

Fig. 4. Eye size 14.7 mm in a 2 days old boy with leukomatous cornea. Behind the microphthalmic eye a cyst-like structure is shown, on A- and B-scan. At top, right, a channel from eye to retrobulbar cyst (arrow) is strongly suggested

Conclusion

In our routine ultrasound examinations we sometimes encounter unexpected structures on the B-scan as positive or negative findings. Evaluating such cases, we usually omit or disregard these unexpected findings in the answer to the referring colleague. In the present article based on six patients, such small ultrasonic changes are discussed, with a view to: a) equipment resolution; and b) discriminating between true findings and acoustic artifacts.

References

[1] R. Guthoff. Ultraschall in der ophthalmologischen Diagnostik. Bücherei des Augenarztes. Vol. 116. Stuttgart: Enke, 1988;48.

[2] S. Duke Elder. Microphthamus with cyst. In System of Ophthalmology. Vol. 3 part 2. London: Kimpton, 1964;481.

Hans C. Fledelius
Eye Department
Hillerød Hospital
Hillerød, Denmark

72. Combination of increased intracranial pressure and optic nerve compression in a patient with multiple meningiomas detected with standardized echography

P. TILL and M. TILL[1]
(Vienna and [1]St. Pölten, Austria)

Abstract

We describe the case of a 54-year-old female with bilateral papilledema and vision field depression with unilateral exophthalmos. Standardized echography revealed bilateral optic nerve sheath distension by increased subarachnoidal fluid and differentiated increased intracranial pressure (caused by intracranial parietal dura-meningioma) combined with optic nerve compression caused by sphenoid wing meningioma. Standardized echography is a rapid and reliable test which enables us to differentiate papilledema caused by increased intracranial pressure from paplledema caused by compressive optic neuropathy.

Key words: Standardized echography, multiple meningiomas, compressive optic neuropathy

Case report

A 53-year-old female presented with a seven-year history of increasing exophthalmos of her left eye with bilateral visual impairment (Fig. 1). The neurosurgeon admitted the patient to our echographic department to clarify the bilateral vision field depression (Fig. 2) and the 5-mm exophthalmos. Computed tomographic findings suggested Paget syndrome was the cause for the protrusion and revealed an intracranial dural meningioma of the parietal region (Fig. 3). Ophthalmoscopy showed mild chronic bilateral papilledema.

Standardized echography of the left orbit differentiated a sphenoid wing meningioma with irregularly structured, high reflective tissue in the orbital apex and posterior orbital roof with pathological extraorbital echosignals (Fig. 4).

Standardized echography of the optic nerves in initial straight gaze demonstrated marked fluid sheath distension with a maximal arachnoidal diameter (normal values: 3.1–4.5 mm) of 6.29 mm of the right and 7.16 mm of the left optic nerve (Fig. 5 top echograms). With exercise and the 30 degree test the arachnoidal diameter of the right optic nerve decreased to 5.42 mm (Fig. 5 left

G Cennamo and N. Rosa (eds.), Ultrasonography in Ophthalmology 15, pp. 565–570.

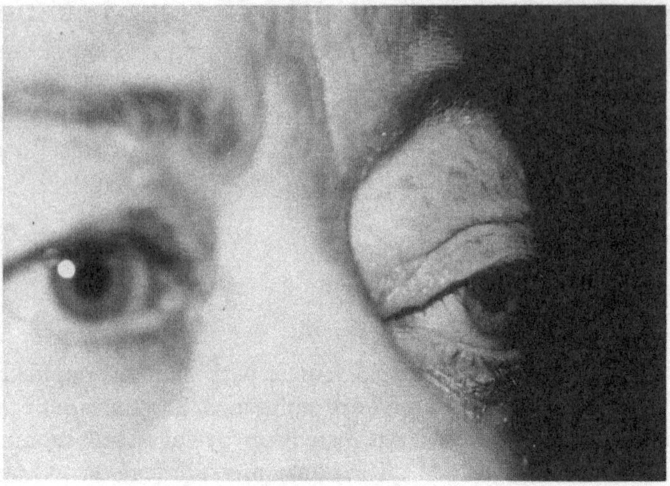

Fig. 1. 53-year-old female with a seven-year history of increasing exophthalmos of her left eye

(a) (b)

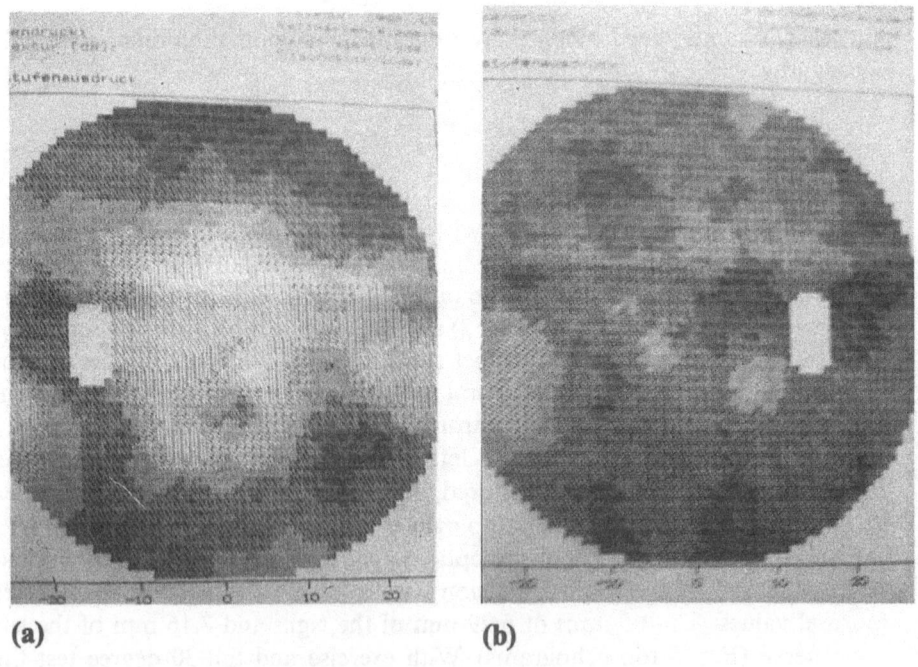

Fig. 2. Vision field depression of the right (a) and of the left eye (b)

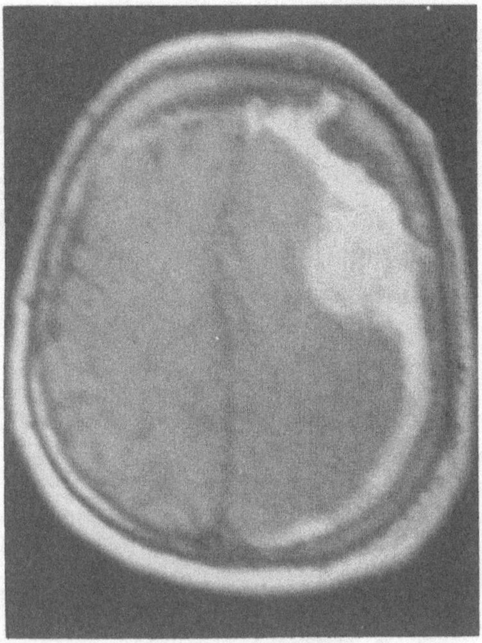

Fig. 3. Computed tomography demonstrates an intracranial dural meningioma of the pariental region

center echogram) and a few seconds after the rest, the diameter increased to 6.17 mm (Fig. 5 left bottom echogram): this immediate return of the subarachnoidal fluid is typical sign of IIP (caused by the intracranial meningioma).

With exercise and the 30 degree test the arachnoidal diameter of the left optic nerve decreased to 6.05 mm (Fig. 5 right center echogram), after two more exercises and 30 degree tests, it decreased to 5.36 mm; no more fluid was expelled. Also after rest the arachnoidal diameter remained at 5.36 mm (Fig. 5 right bottom echogram).

Compressive optic neuropathy (CON) is proven when orbital subarachnoidal fluid decreases during exercises and when the expelled fluid fails to fully return or to return at all during the resting period of at least 3 minutes, which follows the exercise. The failure of the displaced fluid to return spontaneously indicated that there is a lack of free communication between the intracranial and orbital subarachnoidal space, i.e., compression of the optic nerve because of the sphenoid wing meningioma.

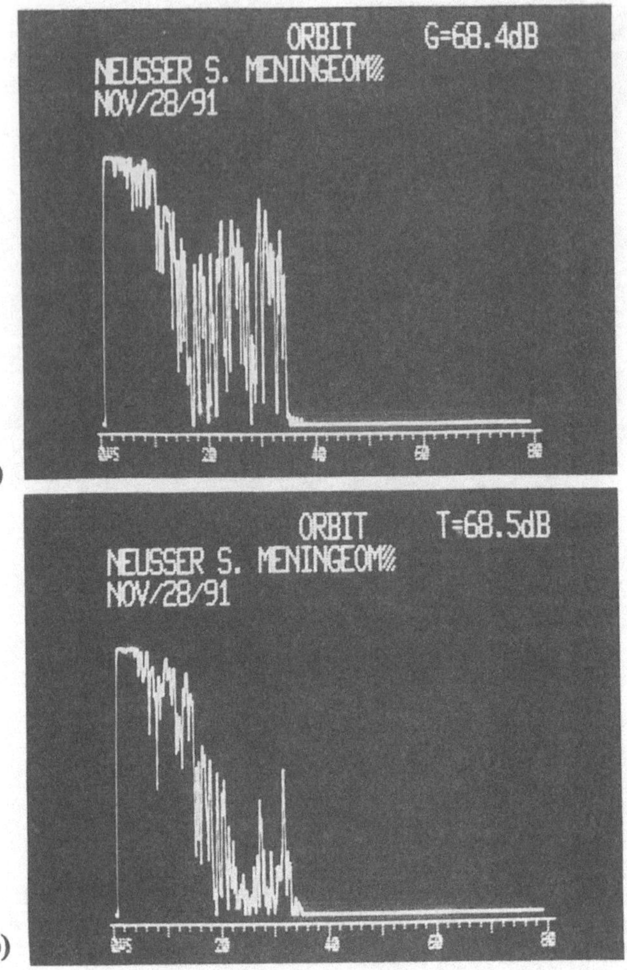

(a)

(b)

Fig. 4. Standardized A-scan echograms of the left orbit demonstrate a sphenoid wing meningioma with irregularly structured high reflective echospikes in the orbital apex and posterior orbital roof (a) with extraocular echosignals (b)

Fig. 5 (opposite page). Bilateral papilledema: A-scan measurements of maximal diameters of both optic nerves recorded in straight gaze before exercise: the right arachnoidal diameter measured 6.29 mm (top left echogram) and 7.16 mm in the left optic nerve (top right echogram). In 30 degree gaze after exercise right optic nerve decreased to 5.42 mm (left center echogram) and in straight gaze after exercise there was an increase of the maximal arachnoidal diameter to 6.17 mm (left bottom echogram). It is typical for IIC that the subarachnoidal fluid promptly returns into the orbit after exercise. The proof of CON in the left optic nerve (LON) required two courses of exercise after which the arachnoidal diameter was reduced to 6.05 mm (right center echogram) and only after a third course of exercise to the LON did the diameter decrease to 5.36 mm (right bottom echogram). The post exercise arachnoidal diameter was still 5.36 mm and no subarachnoidal fluid returned into the orbit: Typical sign for CON

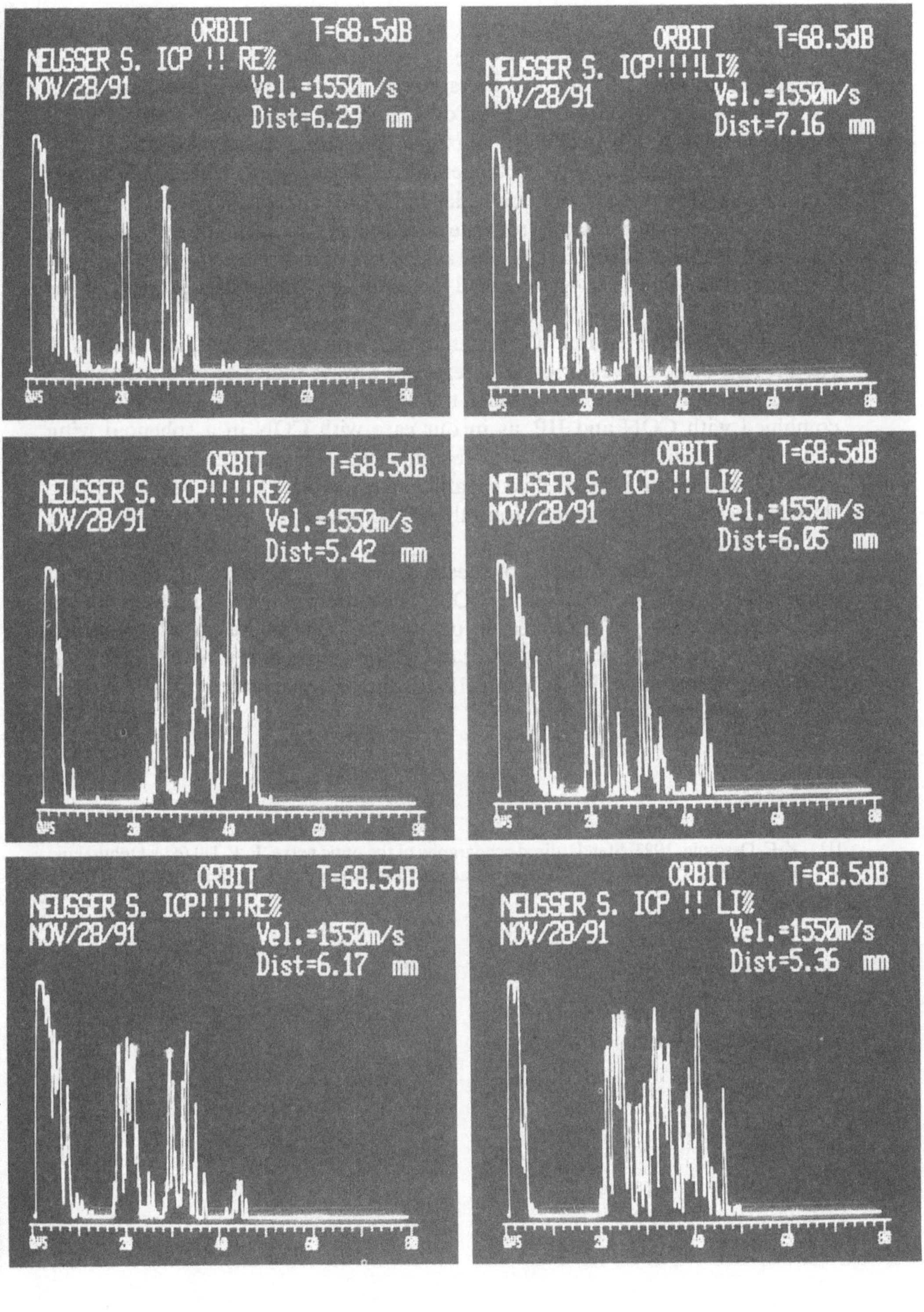
ORBIT T=68.5dB
NEUSSER S. ICP !! RE%
NOV/28/91
Vel.=1550m/s
Dist=6.29 mm
ORBIT T=68.5dB
NEUSSER S. ICP!!!!LI%
NOV/28/91
Vel.=1550m/s
Dist=7.16 mm
ORBIT T=68.5dB
NEUSSER S. ICP!!!!RE%
NOV/28/91
Vel.=1550m/s
Dist=5.42 mm
ORBIT T=68.5dB
NEUSSER S. ICP !! LI%
NOV/28/91
Vel.=1550m/s
Dist=6.05 mm
ORBIT T=68.5dB
NEUSSER S. ICP!!!!RE%
NOV/28/91
Vel.=1550m/s
Dist=6.17 mm
ORBIT T=68.5dB
NEUSSER S. ICP !! LI%
NOV/28/91
Vel.=1550m/s
Dist=5.36 mm

Discussion

In cases of increased intracranial pressure (IIP) not all the orbital subarachnoidal fluid may be displaced from the orbit into the intracranial region during exercise even through prolonged maximal abduction or any other mode of exercise. The stretching of the optic nerve and the pressure exerted by both the stretched and the contracted extraocular muscle are insufficient in such cases to overcome the counterpressure from the intracranial subarachnoidal fluid. In our case the reduction of the arachnoidal diameters during the 30 degree test was limited and the optic nerves remained wet even after prolonged exercise of the nerves.

Ossoinig [1] reported that a great amount of subarachnoidal fluid present in compressed optic nerves prior to an exercise always indicates severe compression. Ossoinig found an exception to this rule in a case of Graves orbitopathy combined with CON and IIP, as in our case with CON in a sphenoid wing meningioma and IIP because of intracranial parietal dura-meningioma. Both optic nerves showed marked fluid sheath distension prior to exercise. Following the exercise, the fluid returned promptly and completely in one nerve, whereas it did not return to the other.

In this case the large amount of sheath distension was caused by the IIP and did not necessarily indicate severe CON. The extremely slow fluid exchange in the compressed nerve (as proven, in our case, by the failure of fluid to return after exercise) may be a valid indicator of CON. In cases of severe IIP, no fluid at all will result from exercise. In plain IIP, the fluid always returns to the orbits in a matter of seconds.

Reference

[1] K.C. Ossoinig. 1993. Standardized echography of the optic nerve. In P. Till (ed.), Ophthalmic Echography 13. Dordrecht: Kluwer Academic Publishers. Doc. Ophthalmol. Proc. Series 1993;3–99.

Prof. Dr. P. Till
University Eye Clinic
Dept. A
Waehringer Guertel 18-20
A-1090 Vienna, Austria

73. Compressive optic neuropathy: echographic study in retrobulbar optic neuritis

N. ROSA and G. CENNAMO

(Naples, Italy)

Abstract

Optic neuritis can be a challenging diagnostic and therapeutic problem. Recovery can be obtained with steroid therapy, although a recurrence-free follow-up has been obtained without steroid therapy. This suggests that a mechanism other than simple inflammation is involved in this disease. We examined 60 patients who had a clinical diagnosis of retrobulbar optic neuritis with digitalized A-scan equipment in an attempt to clarify this other mechanism. Interestingly, among these patients we found seven cases of compressive optic neuropathy. Even though further studies are required to correlate this condition to the recovery of visual acuity, compressive optic neuropathy is an important negative prognostic factor. In addition, the finding of compressive optic neuropathy in patients affected by optic neuritis might have a bearing on why recovery or not of visual acuity in patients with optic neuritis occurs regardless of steroid therapy. Should this be the case, steroid therapy could be administered according the presence of this condition.

Key words: Standardized echography, optic nerve, optic neuritis, compressive optic neuropathy

Introduction

The pathogenesis of retrobulbar optic neuritis is varied: inflammation, vascular diseases, degenerations and some cases could be due to an external compression [1]. The histopathology of optic neuritis varies widely because the pathologic response depends on whether the cause is inflammatory (with predominant inflammatory cell infiltration), ischemic or degenerative [2]. Optic neuritis caused by inflammation is classified according to the topographic location: "perineuritis" if the leptomeninges around the nerve are involved, or "axial neuritis" if the central portion of the optic nerve is involved.

This inflammation will cause a swelling of the optic nerve and/or of its sheaths. Swelling in the mid-posterior orbit or in the optic canal could cause compression of the nerve and consequently an increased amount of the

G Cennamo and N. Rosa (eds.), Ultrasonography in Ophthalmology 15, pp. 571–573.

subarachnoidal fluid in the optic nerve sheaths in the retrobulbar area. In 1989 we started to study the optic nerves in patients with retrobulbar neuritis to look for compressive optic neuropathy [3].

Material and methods

Sixty patients with a clinical diagnosis of retrobulbar neuritis were studied to check the presence of compressive optic neuropathy. All patients first underwent a complete orbital examination to exclude external compression on the optic nerve, to detect compressive optic neuropathies and to measure the pial diameter in lateral gaze position. The optic nerve examination was performed in the primary gaze position, in extreme lateral gaze position and with the so-called "exercise" [4].

Results

We found no change in the overall optic nerve diameter in 37 patients. Of these patients, 30 presented an increased pial diameter at extreme lateral gaze position, and seven were normal. Twenty-three patients had an increased optic nerve diameter. Among these, 18 presented pial diameter thickening, and five sheath thickening. Among these 18 patients, we found seven patients with a compressive optic neuropathy.

Discussion

In the early 1970s Karl C. Ossoinig showed how to detect and to measure the optic nerve diameter in its intraorbital portion using standardized A-scan echography [5]. Later, a method was devised to distinguish solid optic nerve thickenings due to increased intracranial pressure [6], and Cennamo *et al.* demonstrated that the optic nerve diameter was correlated with intracranial pressure [7]. In 1987 Ossoinig studied the possibility of detecting compressive optic neuropathies using standardized A-scan. With new digitalized A-scan equipment [8] it is possible to distinguish the spikes coming from the pial, arachnoidal and dural surfaces and to measure them with an electronic accuracy of 0.03 mm [9]. Therefore, optic nerve diseases can be detected using standardized A-scan echography with a better resolution compared to computerized tomography and magnetic resonance imaging [10], and consequently this technique is the only imaging method with which to verify *in vivo* whether the inflammation is a perineuritis or an axial neuritis.

Thus the finding of increased arachnoidal or pial diameter could help to clarify the pathogenetic mechanism underlying optic neuritis. A case in point is the demyelinization process which involves the axial portion of the optic nerve. There are three successive histologic changes: demyelinization, microglial reaction and astrocytic proliferation. In the early stage, the degenerative changes are associated with vascular congestion, and a mild peripheral infiltrate of lymphocytes and plasma cells. The older lesions are characterized by a dense glial network, so that the age of the lesion can be determined by the presence or absence of inflammation and swelling, and the degree of gliosis.

Further studies are needed to evaluate if the different echographic patterns can be correlated to different steps of optic neuritis. For instance, an overall increase of the optic nerve could be due to an active phase of the disease, and a normal optic nerve diameter with an increased pial diameter and a normal-sized optic nerve could represent a successive phase.

Compressive optic neuropathy is a very important finding in patients affected by optic neuritis and may explain why recovery or not of visual acuity in patients with optic neuritis occurs regardless of steroid therapy [11]. Perhaps the response or non response to steroid treatment could be related to the presence or absence of associated compressive optic neuropathy. Should this be the case, steroid therapy could be administered according the presence of this condition.

References

[1] G. Cennamo, N. Rosa, S. Bianco and M.A. Breve. Studio ecografico della patologia infiammatoria del nervo ottico. Cl. Ocul. e Pat. Ocul. 1994;15:153–155.

[2] D.J. Apple and M.F. Rabb. Clinicopathologic correlation of ocular disease. II Ed. St. Louis: The C.V. Mosby Co., 1978.

[3] G. Cennamo, N. Rosa and A. La Rana. Biomicroscopia ad ultrasuoni del nervo ottico. Cl. Ocul. e Pat. Ocul. 1991;4:269–273.

[4] K.C. Ossoinig. Standardized echography of the optic nerve. In P. Till (ed.), Ophthalmic echography. Proc. 13th SIDUO Congress, Doc. Ophthalmol. Proc. Series 55. 1993;13:3–99.

[5] K.C. Ossoinig. Standardized echography: basic principles, clinical applications and results. Intern. Ophthalmol. Clin. 1979;19:4.

[6] K.C. Ossoinig, F.S. Byrne and G. Cennamo. Echographic differential diagnosis of optic nerve lesions. Doc. Ophthal. Proc. series, vol. 29. Ultrasonography in ophthalmology, Dr. W. Junk Publ., 1981.

[7] G. Cennamo, G. Gangemi and L. Stella. The correlation between endocranial pressure and optic nerve diameter: an ultrasonographic study. Proc. X SIDUO Congress. Doc. Ophthalmol. Proc. Series 48, 1987.

[8] G. Cennamo, N. Rosa, F. Tranfa and G. Bonavolontà. Ruolo dell'ecografia nella diagnostica della otticopatia compressiva. Proc. LXXIII SOI Congress, 1993.

[9] G. Cennamo, N. Rosa, A. La Rana and B. Pastena. Standardized A-scan echography and the normal optic nerve: experience with the new Mini A equipment. Acta Ophthalmol. 1992;204: 87–89.

[10] A. Camera, G. Piccirillo, G. Cennamo, F. Tranfa, N. Rosa, F. Frigeri, V. Martinelli and B. Rotoli. Optic nerve involvement in acute lymphoblastic leukemia. Leukemia and Lymphoma 1993;11:153–155.

[11] R.W. Beck and J.D. Trobe. What we learned from the optic neuritis treatment trial. Ophthalmology 1995;102:1504–1508.

Giovanni Cennamo
Istituto di Oftalmologia, Università di Napoli Federico II
Via S. Pansini 5, 80131 Naples, Italy

74. Standardised echography in optic neuritis

H.R. ATTA, R. BUIMER, A.D. DICK and C. DEES
(Aberdeen, Scotland, UK)

Abstract

A pilot echographic study was conducted to determine the incidence and severity of optic nerve swelling in acute 'idiopathic' optic neuritis and to examine cerebrospinal fluid dynamics in the subarachnoid space, employing the method of standardised echography and the '30 degree test'. An attempt was made to correlate the degree of nerve swelling with the initial visual loss and with the rate and extent of recovery of vision. The visual function and echographic features of the optic nerve in 27 patients with the diagnosis of acute idiopathic optic neuritis were assessed with standardised echography. A significant increase in nerve diameter was found in 74% of cases. Nerve swelling was associated with more severe initial visual loss and a higher incidence of slow or incomplete visual recovery. The authors conclude that standardised echography is a useful tool in the diagnosis of optic neuritis and may play a role in predicting the visual outcome and in selecting patients likely to benefit most from medical or surgical nerve decompression.

Key words: Standardised echography, optic neuritis, ultrasound

Introduction

Idiopathic optic neuritis is an acute demyelinating disease of the optic nerve which is clinically diagnosed [1–3] with a rapid onset of loss of both visual acuity and colour vision, retrobulbar pain worse on ocular movement, and a relative afferent pupillary defect. This is followed by spontaneous recovery over a few weeks or months, but many patients are left with some permanent impairment of visual acuity, colour vision or contrast sensitivity [4,5]. The Optic Neuritis Treatment Trial has shown that treatment with high dose intravenous corticosteroids speeds the recovery of visual function in some patients but does not improve the longterm visual outcome [6]. This study however did not employ an imaging modality to assess the degree of optic nerve swelling and was not designed to evaluate the effects of treatment in subgroups and therefore does not identify patients with optic neuritis who may derive longterm benefit from steroid treatment.

G Cennamo and N. Rosa (eds.), Ultrasonography in Ophthalmology 15, pp. 575–585.

Little is known aout the pathology of acute optic neuritis [7], partly because of the paucity of pathological specimen. Three factors have been put forward as an explanation for optic nerve swelling in acute optic neuritis: (a) oedema of the nerve proper similar to swelling of white matter in acute demyelination in the central nervous system [8]; (b) an increase in perineural subarachnoid fluid [9,10]; (c) reduction of axoplasmic flow by an acute demyelinating plaque in the optic canal [11].

Standardised echography is a non-invasive easily accessible imaging technique which aids the diagnosis of optic nerve lesions [12,13]. Echography enables accurate measurements of the optic nerve because of the nerve's low reflectivity, abutting the highly reflective perineural sheath and heterogeneous reflectivity of the orbital fat. If an increased optic nerve diameter is found, differentiation between fluid and solid lesions as a cause of the swelling can be achieved by repeating the measurement with the globe in 30 degrees of abduction. If increased subarachnoid fluid is present, stretching of the nerve sheath in abductions causes redistribution of fluid and net reduction of nerve diameter; this is termed a positive 30 degree test [14,15] and occurs for example in raised intracranial pressure [16].

Absence of a reduction in width (negative 30 degree test) indicates solid thickening of the nerve (e.g. glioma) or its sheath (e.g. meningioma) or, in optic neuritis, either oedema of the nerve proper or a blockage of redistribution of fluid from intracanalicular lesion [10]. Intracanalicular demyelinating plaques were associated with slower or poorer visual recovery in a series of patients examined with magnetic resonance imaging (MRI) [11].

We undertook a pilot study to image the optic nerve with standardised echography in acute idiopathic optic neuritis with the aim to (a) determine the incidence of increased nerve diameter, (b) perform the 30 degree test to assess cerebrospinal fluid dynamics in optic neuritis, and (c) correlate these echographic findings with (i) the severity of initial visual loss and (ii) the rate and extent of visual recovery.

Patients and methods

All patients who presented to the eye department of Aberdeen Royal Infirmary between May 1991 and August 1993 with the clinical diagnosis of optic neuritis as described in the introduction [1,2] were invited to enter the study. Inclusion and exclusion criteria are listed in Table 1. The history and clinical examination included Snellen visual acuity, colour vision score with Ishihara pseudoisochromatic plates, pupillary reaction and fundoscopy. Subsequent echography of the optic nerve and Dicon suprathreshold visual fields were performed. B-scan and standardised A-scan ultrasound assessment of the optic nerve was performed by a single observer (HRA) as described previously [13]. Both optic nerve diameters were assessed without knowledge of which eye was affected, followed by a 30 degree test on any nerve that was found to be swollen. Figure 1

Table 1

Inclusion criteria	Exclusion criteria
Typical clinical presentation of acute idiopathic optic neuritis	Age over 55 years Bilateral disease
Age below 55 years	Suspected ischemic optic neuropathy
Presentation less than 14 days following onset of visual loss	Recurrent optic neuritis
Willing to undergo echographic examination	

shows an example of B-scan and standardised A-scan display in a normal optic nerve versus optic neuritis. Nerve swelling was present if it measured at least 0.3 mm larger than the contralateral one [15]. The 30 degree test was taken to be positive if the swelling decreased by at least 10% on abduction [14,15]. Figure 2 shows an example of reduction in echographic nerve diameter on 30 degree testing. Patients were divided, according to the echographic findings, into three groups: Group I, those with normal optic nerve; Group II, those with swollen nerve and positive 30 degree test; and Group III, those with swollen nerve and negative 30 degree test. Patients were then followed up with repeat assessments of visual acuity, colour vision and fundoscopy until their condition resolved or stabilised.

Results

Clinical details

Thirty-one patients were initially referred for the study. Three did not fulfill diagnostic criteria of optic neuritis and one was excluded from analysis because of bilateral involvement. Twenty-seven were included in the initial clinical and echographic analysis, and 25 completed the study. Clinical features are summarised in Table 2. Female to male ratio was 2: 1 (18 females, 9 males). Mean age was 35 years, range 13 to 50. A relative afferent pupillary defect was present in all cases (100%), and reduced colour vision, defined as missing 2 or more out of 17 pseudo-isochromatic plates, was present in 22 of 27 cases (81%). Pain on ocular movements was present in 23 of 27 patients (85%).

Mean delay from onset of symptoms to performing ultrasound was 12 days. Fundoscopy revealed swelling of the optic disc in 10 of 27 cases (37%), normal disc in 15 (56%), and equivocal in 2 cases (7%).

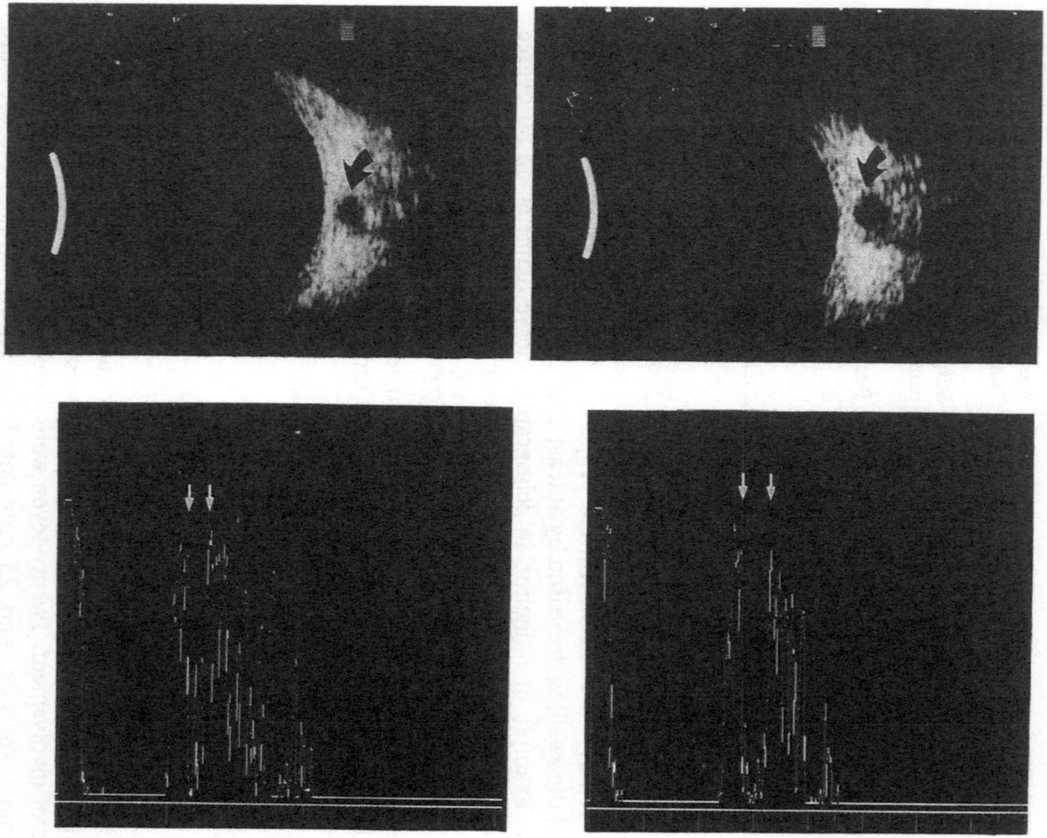

Fig. 1. Echographic display of normal optic nerve versus optic neuritis.
Top left: Transverse B-scan of normal optic nerve (black arrow). Top right: Transverse B-scan in optic neuritis. Note widening of the nerve void (black arrow). Bottom left: A-scan of normal optic nerve. Bottom right: A-scan in optic neuritis. White arrows indicate optic nerve (sheath) diameter. Note increased diameter in optic neuritis (3.91 mm versus 2.85 mm)

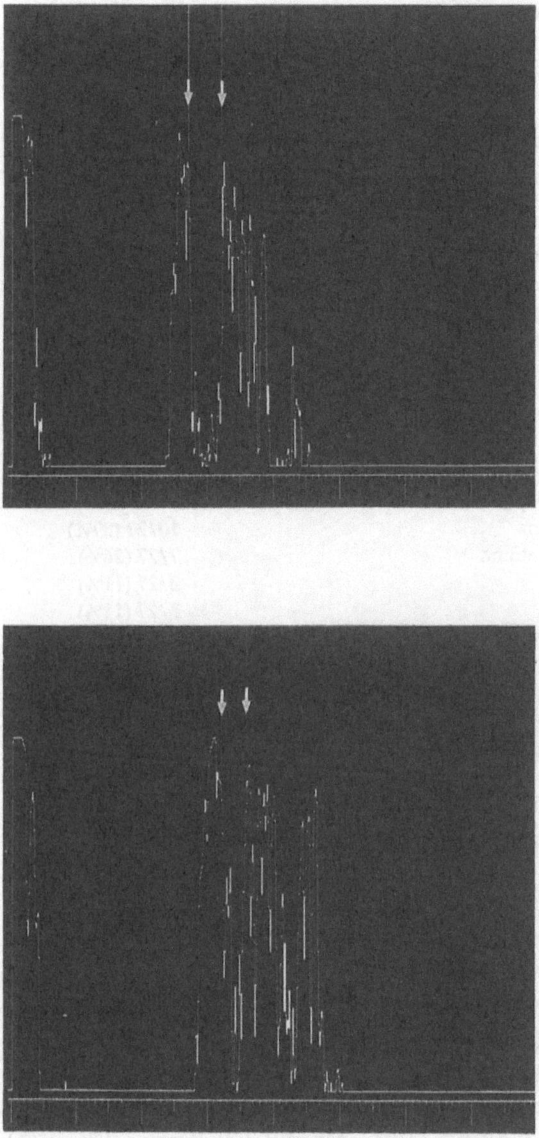

Fig. 2. **Example of swollen nerve and positive 30 degree test. Arrows indicate optic nerve sheaths Top: Measurement in primary position of gaze = 3.91 mm. Bottom: Measurement with globe in 30 degree of abduction; note reduction in optic nerve (sheath) diameter = 2.94 (a 25% reduction)**

Table 2. Optic neuritis: Clinical features in 27 cases

Female: male ratio	2: 1
Mean age	35 years (range 13–50)
Relative afferent Pupillary defect	27/27 (100%)
Orbital pain	23/27 (85%)
Initial visual acuity	
Hand Movements (HM)	5/27 (19%)
Counting Fingers (CF)	6/27 (22%)
6/18 – 6/60	9/27 (33%)
6/6 – 6/12	7/27 (26%)
Impaired colour vision (Ishihara)	22/27 (81%)
Visual field (Dicon)	
Central scotoma	10/27 (37%)
Paracentral scotoma	7/27 (26%)
Other	3/27 (11%)
Normal field	3/27 (11%)
No test performed	4/27 (15%)
Disc swelling	10/27 (37%)
Good recovery (VA 6/9)	24/27 (89%)

Echography (See Table 3)

Twenty of 27 cases (74%) had swelling of the affected optic nerve on standardised 'A-scan' ultrasound. In this group the average diameter of affected nerves was 3.63 mm (range 3.0–4.4), whereas the average diameter of contralateral unaffected nerves was 2.84 mm (range 2.5–3.1). The increase in diameter of the affected nerve compared to unaffected contralateral nerve was 0.8 mm (range 0.4–1.3). Of those cases with swollen nerves, 11 of 27 (41%) had a positive 30 degree test, where the average decrease in nerve diameter on abduction was 0.61 mm (17%), range 0.3–0. 9 mm (10%–25%). Nine of 27 cases (33%) had a swollen nerve with negative 30 degree test. Seven of 27 cases (26%) had no discernible swelling on echography, where the average affected nerve diameter was 2.93 mm (range 2.7–3.1), compared to a contralateral unaffected nerve diameter of 2.87 mm.

The average time interval between onset of symptoms of optic neuritis and performing echography in this group was similar (11 days) to the overall average (12 days).

Table 3. Average optic nerve diameter in acute optic neuritis (mm)

	Diameter of affected optic nerve	mm larger than contralateral	Percentage decrease on 30 degree test
Group I (n = 7)	2.93	0.04	0.3%
Group II (n = 11)	3.64	0.75	17%
Group III (n = 9)	3.63	0.86	4% *

Group I: nerve not swollen

Group II: Nerve swollen, positive 30 degree test

Group III: Nerve swollen, negative 30 degree test

* Denotes that the nerve diameter increases on 30 degree testing, an observation similarly noted before [10]

Visual acuities versus echography (See Table 4)

In the group of patients with echographically normal nerves (n = 7), 3 had VA 6/6 to 6/12 and 4 had VA 6/24 to 6/36 on presentation. In cases with echographically swollen nerve (n = 20), 4 had VA 6/6 to 6/12, 5 had VA 6/24 to 6/36, and 11 had a VA of count fingers or hand motion on presentation. This distribution was the same whether the 30 degree test was positive or negative. Of patients who completed the study (n = 25), 22 recovered 6/9 or better vision. The period of follow up varied from 6 weeks in patients who recovered quickly to 6 months in patients who recovered more slowly. Two recovered to no better than 6/12, and one recovered 6/18. All three with poorer visual outcome had had a swollen optic nerve on presentation. No patient with an echographically normal nerve had an initial VA of worse than 6/36 or a final VA of less than 6/9 (Figs. 3 and 4). Figure 5 correlates initial VA with the affected optic nerve diameter without reference to the contralateral nerve or the 30 degree test.

Table 4. Initial visually acuity in optic neuritis and echographic features of the optic nerve

	6/6–6/12	6/18–6/36	6/60 or worse
Normal nerve(n = 7)	3	4	0
Enlarged nerve, positive 30′ test	2	3	6
Enlarged nerve, negative 30′ test	2	2	5

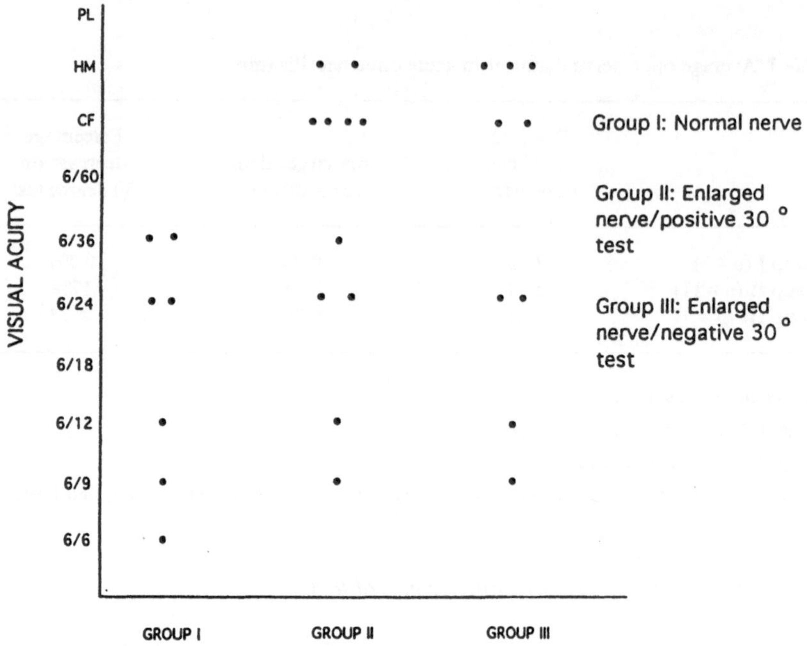

Fig. 3. Initial visual acuity and echographic features of optic nerve

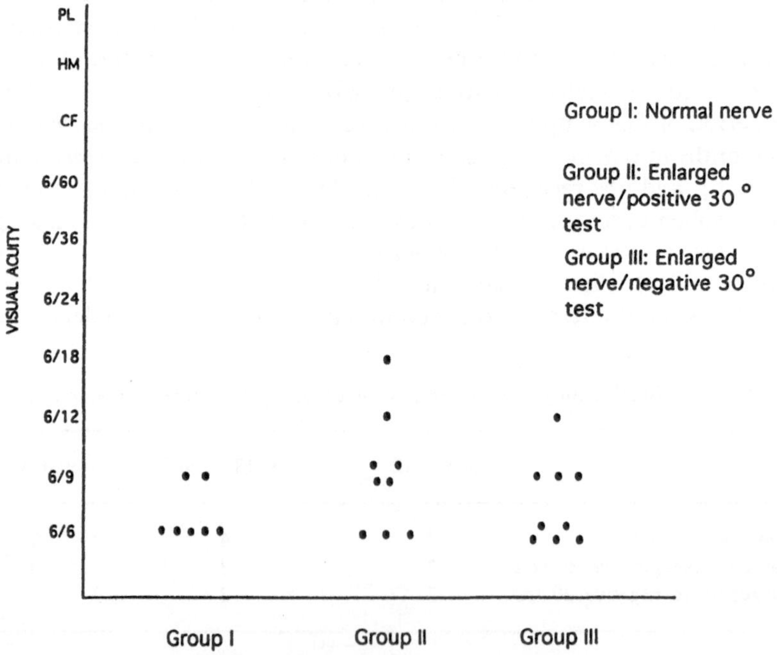

Fig. 4. Final visual acuity and initial echographic features of optic nerve

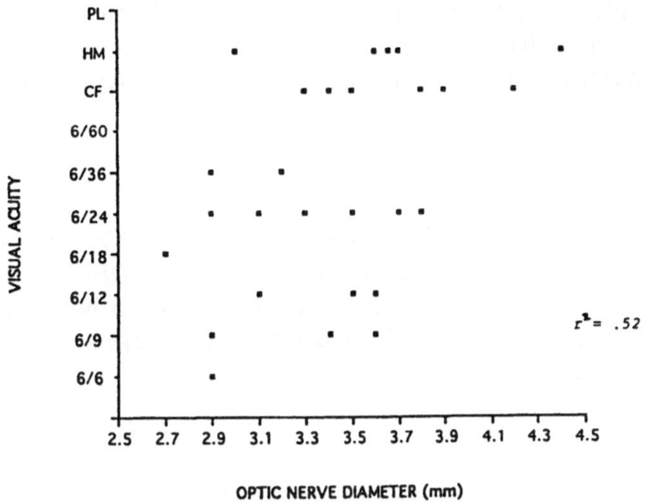

Fig. 5. Visual acuity and optic nerve diameter on initial presentation

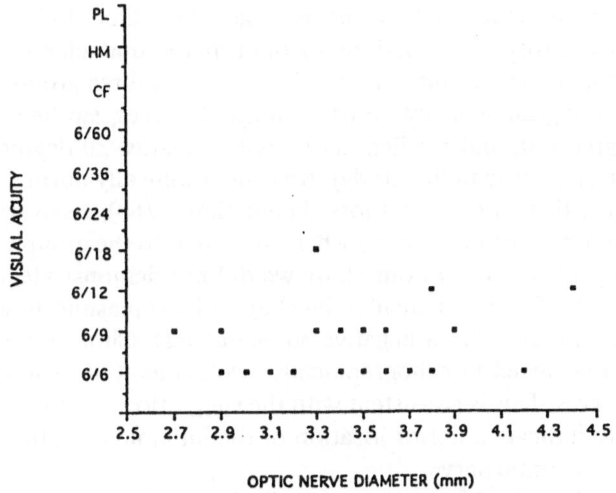

Fig. 6. Visual acuity after recovery and initial optic nerve diameter

The correlation is weak ($r^2 = 0.52$), but there is a tendency for more severely swollen nerves to be associated with more profound initial loss of vision. There is no correlation between initial nerve diameter and visual outcome except that final VA of less than 6/9 only occurred with an initial nerve diameter of more than 3.2 mm (Fig. 6). The rate of visual recovery, expressed as the average length of time required to recover a VA of 6/9 or better was 4 weeks in cases with echographically normal nerves (range 2–6); 4.7 weeks in cases with swollen nerves and positive 30 degree test (range 3–6) and 5 weeks in cases with swollen nerve and negative 30 degree test (range 1–13) (differences not statistically significant).

Disc oedema

Of cases with an echographically normal optic nerve (n = 7), 2 had clinical disc oedema. Moreover, of cases with an echographically swollen optic nerve, 8 had disc oedema. Although the range of initial VA was similar in patients with and without disc oedema (6/18 – HM and 6/9 – HA, respectively), the average initial VA did differ: 6/48 and 6/24, respectively.

Discussion

Standardised echography can provide valuable information in the diagnosis and management of acute idiopathic optic neuritis. Echographically detectable swelling of the optic nerve in optic neuritis has been described before [9,10,17,18] with variable results of the 30 degree test. Our study provides the first quantitative, prospective analysis of optic nerve diameter in acute idiopathic optic neuritis. The results suggest that there are three groups of patients with different echographic characteristics: normal nerves, swollen nerves with positive 30 degree test, and swollen nerves with negative 30 degree test (26%, 41% and 33% respectively in this study). An echographically normal optic nerve was associated with limited visual loss (better than 6/60), recovery to 6/9 or better and a higher speed of recovery when compared to the group with swollen optic nerve on presentation. In our study we did not demonstrate, as one may postulate because of intracanalicular blockage of axoplasmic flow, a poorer visual outcome in cases with a negative 30 degree test. Clinical swelling of the optic disc head occurred in echographically swollen as well as in echographically normal nerves. This is consistent with the suggestion [11] that disc oedema is more likely to indicate anterior location of the inflammation than a generalised swelling of the optic nerve.

Although numbers in this study are small, the results showed a correlation between the clinical course and the echographic appearance of the optic nerve. Further investigations are required, both to confirm our findings and to determine if there is any prognostic indication from the echographic appearance of the optic nerve.

Future echographic investigations in acute optic neuritis need to take into account any temporal changes in echographic appearance of the optic nerve that may occur during the course of the disease and the effect the location of the acute demyelinating plaque within the optic nerve has on the echographic appearance.

Our study demonstrated a role for echography in the diagnosis and management of optic neuritis. Echography will help confirm the diagnosis, exclude other (compressive) lesions as a cause of optic nerve dysfunction, and may provide a prognostic indication of visual recovery and help select subgroups of patients who may benefit most from intensive steroid therapy or surgical nerve sheath decompression.

References

[1] N.R. Miller (ed.). Walsh & Hoyt's Clinical Neurophthalmology, 4th ed. Baltimore: Williams and Wilkins, 1982:227.
[2] Optic Neuritis Study Group. The clinical profile of optic neuritis. Arch. Ophthalmol. 1991; 109:1673–1678.
[3] G.D. Perkin and F.C. Rose. Optic neuritis and its differential diagnosis. Oxford Medical Publications, 1979:91–101.
[4] W.G. Bradley and C.M.W. Whitty. Acute optic neuritis: its clinical features and their relation to prognosis for recovery of vision. J. Neurol. Neurosurg. Psychiat. 1967;30:531.
[5] T.L. Slamovits et al. Visual recovery in patients with optic neuritis and visual loss to no light perception. Am. J. Ophthalmol. 1991;111:209–214.
[6] R.W. Beck et al. A randomised, controlled trial of corticosteroids in the treatment of acute optic neuritis. N. Eng. J. Med. 1992;326:581–588.
[7] D. Toussaint et al. Clinicopathological study of the visual pathways eyes and cerebral hemispheres in 32 cases of disseminated sclerosis. J. Clin. Neuro-Ophthalmol. 1983;3:211.
[8] C.W.M. Adams et al. Inflammatory vasculitis in multiple sclerosis. J. Neuorol. Sci. 1985;69:269–283.
[9] S.F. Byrne and R.L. Green. Ultrasound of the eye and orbit. St. Louis: Mosby-Year Book. 1992:405–409.
[10] K.C. Ossoinig. Standardised echography of the optic nerve. In P. Till (ed.), Doc. Ophthalmol. Proc. Ser. 55. Dordrecht: Kluwer Academic Publishers. 1990:75–77.
[11] D.H. Miller *et al.* Magnetic resonance imaging of the optic nerve in optic neuritis. Neurology 1988;38:175–179.
[12] K.C. Ossoinig. Standardised echography: basic principals, clinical applications and results. Int. Ophthalmol. Clin. 1979;19:127–210.
[13] H.R. Atta. Imaging of the optic nerve with standardised echography. Eye 1988;2:358–366.
[14] S.F. Byrne. Evaluation of the optic nerve with standardised echography. In J.L. Smith (ed.), Neuro-Ophthalmology Now. 1986:45-66.
[15] K.C. Ossoinig, G. Cennamo and S.F. Byrne. Echographic differential diagnosis of optic nerve lesions. Doc. Ophthalmol. Proc. Ser. 1981;29:327–331.
[16] S.L. Hupp, J.S. Glaser and S.F. Byrne. Optic nerve sheath decompression. Arch. Ophthalmol. 1987;105:386–389.
[17] S.F. Byrne and R.L. Green. Orbital Echography. In W. Tasman and E.A. Jaeger (eds), Duane's Clinical Ophthalmology. Lippincott Company, Revised Ed.. 1991;1:Chap. 26.
[18] M.S. Gans, S.F. Byrne and J.S. Glaser. Standardised A-scan echography in optic nerve disease. Arch. Ophthalmol. 1987;105:1232–1236.

H.R. Atta
Eye Department
Aberdeen Royal Infirmary
Aberdeen, Scotland, UK

75. New results about the echographic examination of the optic nerve. Experimental and clinical investigations.

G. HASENFRATZ, M.D.J. DE LA TORRE and W. HAIGIS

(Würzburg, Germany)

Abstract

The optic nerve can be displayed *in vivo* by A- and B-scan techniques. To correlate the anatomical structures of the optic nerve with the echograms, and to determine whether the diameter of the nerve can be measured by routine examination techniques, we conducted experimental studies on bovine optic nerve *in vitro* with the A-scan technique, and measured the sound velocity in bovine optic nerves. We also compared the two A-scan techniques most frequently used to display the optic nerve *in vivo* in 47 normal persons and in 35 patients with changes of the optic nerve. The experimental studies showed that the orbital fat and the outer sheaths of the optic nerve cause refraction of the soundbeam. The sound velocity of ultrasound in bovine optic nerves was 1567 ± 25 m/s. The two most widely used *in vivo* examination techniques showed no differences in healthy subjects, but significant differences in patients with increased subarachnoidal fluid.

Key words: Standardized echography, optic nerve

Introduction

A- and B-scan can be used for echographic examination of the optic nerve. With both examination techniques two questions arise: which morphologic structures of the optic nerve are represented by the echogram (mainly by A-scan); and: is it possible to measure the real thickness of the optic nerve? This is a long-debated topic and different groups have reached different conclusions.

Also under discussion is how to examine the optic nerve. Schröder and Guthoff [1,2] suggested it be examined by placing the sound probe on the temporal conjunctiva while the globe is in maximal abduction, because this technique will most likely result in a perpendicular approach of the sound beam towards the optic nerve. In A-scans, in their opinion, the inner surface of the dura and the surface of the fasciculus opticus are represented by two echosignals.

G Cennamo and N. Rosa (eds.), Ultrasonography in Ophthalmology 15, pp. 587–596.

Ossoinig *et al.* and Byrne *et al.*, as well as own studies [3,4,6,7] recommended the optic nerve be examined with standardized echography with the globe in primary position and with the probe placed on the temporal conjunctiva. Experimental studies on bovine optic nerves have supported the clinical experiences that the optic nerve can be displayed and examined very well by this technique [6]. When the standardized A-scans, in cases in which the display of the optic nerve is optimal *in vivo* and *in vitro*, are analyzed, three echosignals on both sides of the optic nerve can be distinguished. These signals have been correlated to the interface between the dura and the surrounding fat tissue, to interface between the arachnoidea and the subarachnoidal fluid (liquor cerebrospinalis) and the surface of the fasciculus.

The basic problem still remained with both these examination techniques how can the surface(s) of the optic nerve be displayed and recognized with the A-scan even though the sound beam hits the optic nerve at an oblique angle.

Method

We have conducted further *in vitro* examinations of the bovine optic nerve under improved conditions with respect to our earlier studies. Moreover, the sound velocity of ultrasound in the bovine optic nerve has been determined [5] and we studied the two main examination techniques (see above) *in vivo* in normal subjects and in patients with changes of the optic nerve.

Measurement of the sound velocity in the bovine optic nerve

The distance between the tip of an A-scan sound probe and the bottom of a water bath was measured (distilled water 21°C). A part of a bovine optic nerve without surrounding fat tissue was placed between the sound probe and the bottom, and the distance between the probe and the upper surface of the optic nerve was measured. Using the sound velocity of ultrasound (8 MHz) in water (1,492 m/s) the calculation was performed using the formula shown in Fig. 1.

Examination of the bovine optic nerve in vitro

The globes of slaughtered cows together with a large part of the optic nerve and the orbital fat were exenterated. The material was examined on the day of exenteration. We prepared the material in three different ways:

A: Sutures (Vicryl 6–0) were attached to the exenterated material at the muscle insertions and at the distal end of the optic nerve. The entire preparation was fixed, with the sutures, to a plastic frame, and examined in a water bath (20°C). By attaching the sound probe to a device, it was possible to immerse the instrument into the water and to control the angle between the direction of the probe and the specimen towards the approximate direction of the optic nerve within the fat tissue.

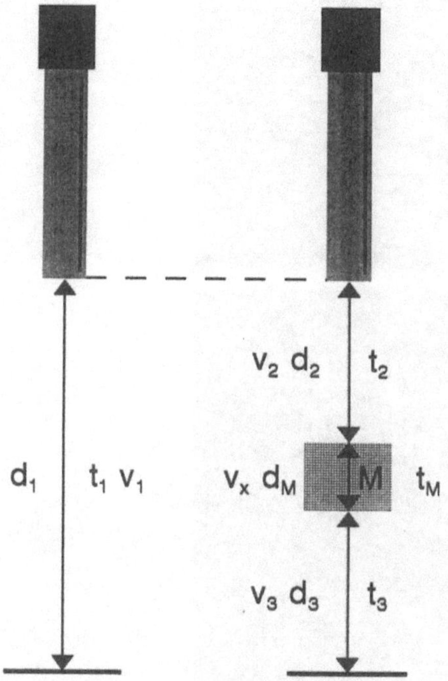

$$d_1 = d_2 + d_M + d_3$$

$$d = t\,v$$

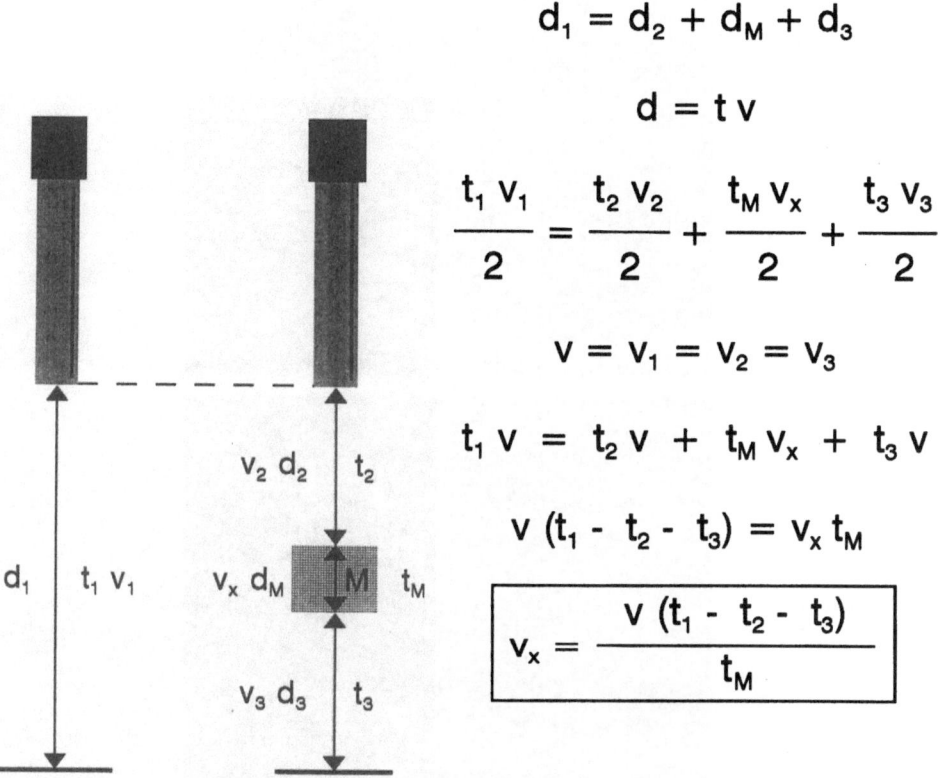

$$\frac{t_1 v_1}{2} = \frac{t_2 v_2}{2} + \frac{t_M v_x}{2} + \frac{t_3 v_3}{2}$$

$$v = v_1 = v_2 = v_3$$

$$t_1 v = t_2 v + t_M v_x + t_3 v$$

$$v\,(t_1 - t_2 - t_3) = v_x\, t_M$$

$$\boxed{v_x = \frac{v\,(t_1 - t_2 - t_3)}{t_M}}$$

Fig. 1. **Measurement of the sound-velocity: d_1/t_1 = distance/sound-travelling-time between the sound probe and the bottom of the water-bath, d_2/t_2 = distance/sound-travelling-time between the sound probe and the specimen (M), d_3/t_3 = distance/sound-travelling-time between the specimen and the bottom of the water-bath, d_M/t_M = thickness/sound-travelling-time of the specimen, V_1, V_2, V_3 = known sound-velocities (water), V_x = sound-velocity to determine**

B: After removing the fat tissue completely, the specimen (globe and optic nerve) was placed in the water bath within the plastic frame and the examination was performed according to A.

C: After removing the dura mater and the arachnoidea, the specimen (the optic nerve with the surrounding pia mater) was placed in the water bath and examined as indicated in A.

The B and C specimens were then checked by histopathological examinations.

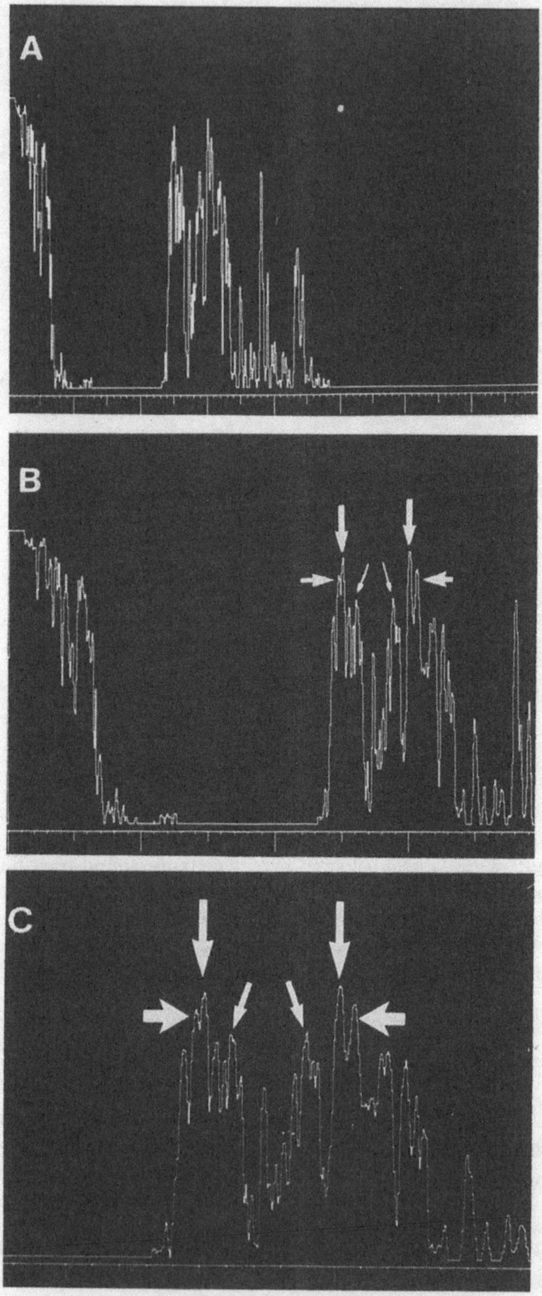

Fig. 2. A–C: Display of the optic nerve with standardized A-scan (perpendicular sound-beam, procedure A 1): A normal display with horizontal-extension for, 'orbit', B zoom 2: 1 (normal display with horizontal-extension for 'globe'), C zoom 4: 1. Large arrows = interface between arachnoid/subarachnoidal space (points of measurement), little arrows = interface between orbital fat tissue/dura mater, thin arrows = interface between subarachnoidal space/pia mater

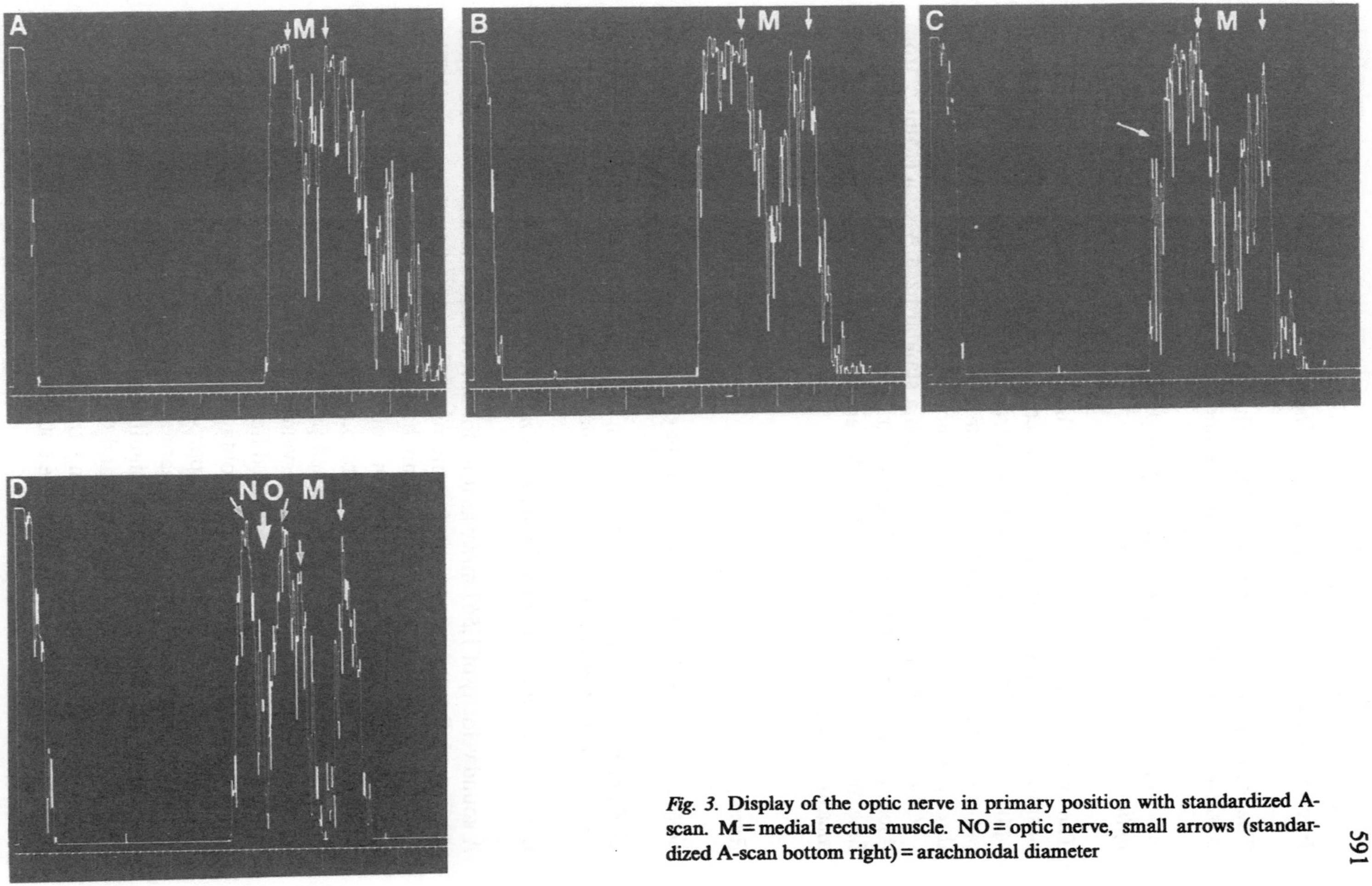

Fig. 3. Display of the optic nerve in primary position with standardized A-scan. M = medial rectus muscle. NO = optic nerve, small arrows (standardized A-scan bottom right) = arachnoidal diameter

In vivo *examination of the optic nerve of healthy persons with two techniques*

The examinations were performed with the eye in the primary and in abductive position; 47 normal subjects were examined.

In vivo *examination of the optic nerve in patients with different diseases of the optic nerve*

The examinations were performed with the eye in the primary and in abductive position; we examined 16 patients affected by Graves' disease with compressive optic neuropathy, six patients with intracranial hypertension, six glaucoma patients with excavation of the disc, four patients with optic nerve glioma and three patients with optic nerve meningioma.

All examinations were performed with a standardized A-scan (Mini-A from Alcol Biophysics®; 8 MHz). The highest reflective echosignals from the interface between the arachnoid and the subarachnoidal space were used for measurements.

Results

Determination of the sound velocity in bovine optic nerves

To determine the velocity of ultrasound in bovine optic nerves, four sequences of measurements were made. The mean sound velocity was 1567 (25) m/s.

In vitro *examinations of the bovine optic nerve*

A sound velocity of 1,567 m/s was used for *in vitro* examinations of bovine optic nerve and the measurements in microsec were transferred into mm. The measurements with an oblique sound beam were compared with theoretical values calculated using the rules for sound beam deflection and the known values for the sound velocity of ultrasound in water and in the bovine optic nerve, when the optic nerve is reached perpendicularly. The theoretical values were subtracted from the measured values, and the means and the standard deviations were determined from the differences (Tables 1–3).

A comparison of the mean values obtained with the three different specimens and with each type of sound beam approach (Student's t test: $p<0.01$) showed that the measurements at a sound beam angle of 15° and 30° between A and B were not significantly different. A significant difference, however, was found between A and C with respect to B and C. This means that after removing the orbital fat tissue and after removing the dura mater and the arachnoid, a significantly higher mean value of the optic nerve diameter was measured.

Table 1. Measurement of the bovine optic nerve with surrounding fat tissue

Sound beam incidence	90°	75°	60°
Mean value (mm) (n = 20)	4.52	4.58	4.65
Theoretical value (mm)		4.69	5.30
Difference		0.13 (0.02)	0.66 (0.02)

Table 2. Measurement of the bovine optic nerve without surrounding fat tissue and with complete optic nerve

Sound beam incidence	90°	75°	60°
Mean value (mm) (n = 20)	4.49	4.60	4.75
Theoretical value (mm)		4.66	5.27
Difference		0.07 (0.01)	0.51 (0.02)

Table 3. Measurement of the bovine optic nerve without surrounding fat tissue and without dura mater and arachnoidea (fasciculus opticus with pia mater)

Sound beam incidence	90°	75°	60°
Mean value (mm) (n = 20)	4.52	4.58	4.65
Theoretical value (mm)		4.69	5.30
Difference		0.13 (0.02)	0.66 (0.02)

Measurement of the diameter of the optic nerve in normal subjects

Two methods were used to measure the optic nerve diameter in normal individuals: with the globe in primary position (technique A) and with globe abduction (technique B). The sound probe was placed on the temporal conjunctiva in both techniques, 47 normal persons were examined, and the results are shown below:

Right eye: (mean value/mm)	technique A:	3.6
	technique B:	3.6
Left eye: (mean value/mm)	technique A:	3.7
	technique B:	3.6

The values were not significantly different.

Measurement of the diameter of the optic nerve in patients

Techniques A and B were used to measure the diameter of the optic nerve in the patients, and the results were the following:

- Compressive neuropathy of the optic nerve in patients with Grave's disease (n = 16):
  mean value/mm — technique A: 6.3; technique B: 5.8

  The values were significantly different.

- Thickened optic nerve in patients with cranial hypertension (n = 6):
  mean value/mm — technique A: 5.6; technique B: 5.0

  The values were significantly different.

- Excavation of the disc in patients with glaucoma (n = 6)
  mean value/mm — technique A:3.8; technique B: 3.7

  The values were not significantly different.

- Optic nerve glióma (n = 4):
  mean value/mm — technique A: 6.2; echnique B: 6.2

  The values were not significantly different.

- Optic nerve meningioma (n = 3):
  mean value/mm — technique A: 6.4; technique B: 6.3

  The values were not significantly different.

Discussion

The basis of this study of the optic nerve by A-scan was the consideration that when examining the optic nerve clinically, it is not possible to direct a perpendicular sound beam towards the optic nerve. In general, a perpendicular sound beam approach is required to obtain optimal echosignals from a surface with respect to the interface between two media, and this is not possible or at least very difficult when it comes to the display of the optic nerve *in vivo*. Nevertheless, with A-scan clear surface echosignals can be obtained from both sides of the optic nerve and thus the nerve can be easily differentiated from the surrounding orbital fat tissues.

In this study we obtained clear echosignals from the surface of the optic nerve. This was true for the controlled examination of the optic nerve under perpendicular sound beam direction and when the sound probe was tilted to a sound beam angle of 15° and 30°.

The results obtained with a perpendicular and with a tilted sound beam approach were not significantly different in preparations in which the fat-tissue still surrounded the optic nerve and in those with the fat-tissue removed. Only when we also removed the dura mater and the arachnoid (procedure C), i.e., when the optic nerve with surrounding pia mater was examined, did we find significantly larger diameters when examining the specimen with an oblique angle. To confirm this difference, we compared these measurements with the theoretical values calculated with the rules for reflection and refraction of the sound beam, taking into account the known sound velocity in both media (water and optic nerve) without any other additional refraction. A comparison of these two values indicates that there is additional refraction of the sound beam caused by the fat tissue and/or by the layers of the dura mater/arachnoid. This hypothesis is supported by the measurements of the diameter of the optic nerve with pia mater which were almost exactly identical to the theoretical values. The slightly smaller value obtained when tilting the sound probe to 30° (see Results) could be due to another refraction at the surface of the pia mater/optic nerve; however, we were unable to verify this in our study.

The measurements of the optic nerve *in vivo* with respect to the measurements of the thickness of the optic nerve in normal subjects and in patients with various diseases of the optic nerve showed that, to demonstrate optic nerve dilatation due to increased subarachnoidal fluid, the examination of the optic nerve should be performed with the globe in the primary position. In cases of Graves' disease and of intracranial hypertension, which are associated with increased subarachnoidal fluid, there were significantly different values with the two examination techniques described. On the contrary, no significant differences were found between the two techniques in normal optic nerves and in optic nerve tumors.

In summary, our experimental and clinical examinations showed that correct measurements of the diameter of the optic nerve can be made even with the sound beam in an oblique direction which is the situation encountered during clinical evaluation of the optic nerve with standardized A-scan. Our results support the recommendation that the optic nerve be examined with the eye in primary position in cases of suspected subarachnoidal fluid increase and where echography is used to detect or rule out this change.

References

[1] W. Schröder and R. Guthoff. Modellversuche zur Messung des Sehnerven. In H. Gernet (Hrsg.), Diagnostica Ultrasonica in Ophthalmologia, SIDUO VII, Münster 1978. Münster: Remy Verlag, 1979;3–4.

[2] W. Schröder and R. Guthoff. Ultrasonography of the optic nerve. In J.M. Thijssen and A.M. Verbeek (eds.), Ultrasonography in Ophthalmology. Doc. Ophthalmol. Proc. Ser. 29. The Hague: Dr. W. Junk, Publ., 1981;359–362.

[3] S.F. Byrne. The echographic measurement and differential diagnosis of optic nerve lesions. In K.C. Ossoinig (ed.), Ophthalmic echography. SIDUO X, St. Petersburg, USA. Doc. Ophthalmol. Proc. Ser., 48. Dordrecht: Dr. W. Junk Publ., 1987;571–585.

[4] S.F. Byrne and R. Green. Ultrasound of the eye and the orbit. St. Louis: The C.V. Mosby Co., 1992.

[5] W. Haigis. Akustische Daten der Gewebe und Flüssigkeiten des menschlichen Körpers (insbesondere von Auge und Orbita). In W. Buschmann and H.G. Trier (Hrsg.). Berlin: Springer, 1989; Kap. 8.10.

[6] G. Hasenfratz. Experimental studies on the display of the optic nerve. In K.C. Ossoinig (ed.), Ophthalmic echography. SIDUO X, St. Petersburg, USA. Doc. Ophthalmol. Proc. Ser. 48. Dordrecht: Dr. W. Junk Publ., 1987;587–602.

[7] K.C. Ossoinig, G. Cennamo and S.F. Byrne. Echographic differential diagnosis of optic nerve lesions. Doc. Ophthalmol. Proc. Ser. 29, 1981; 327–332.

Prof. Dr. G. Hasenfratz
Universitäts-Augenklinik Würzburg
Josef-Schneider-Str., 11
97080 Würzburg
Germany

Index

G Cennamo and N. Rosa (eds.), Ultrasonography in Ophthalmology 15, pp. 597–599.

Documenta Ophthalmologica Proceedings Series

21. J. François, E. Maumenee & I. Esente (eds.): *First International Congress on Cataract Surgery* (Florence, Italy, 1978). 1979 ISBN 90-6193-162-2
22. E.L. Greve (ed.): *Glaucoma Symposium.* Diagnosis and Therapy (Amsterdam, The Netherlands, 1979). 1980 ISBN 90-6193-164-9
23. E. Schmöger & J.H. Kelsey (eds.): *Visual Electrodiagnosis in Systemic Diseases.* Proceedings of the 17th ISCEV Symposium (Erfurt, GDR, 1979) 1980 ISBN 90-6193-163-0
24. A. Hamburg (ed.): *Symposium on Uveal Melanomas.* On the Occasion of the Snellen Medal Presentation to Dr W.A. Manschot (Utrecht, The Netherlands, 1979). 1980 ISBN 90-6193-722-1
25. H. Zauberman (ed.): *Proceedings of the Conference on Subretinal Space* (Jerusalem, Israel, 1979). 1981 ISBN 90-6193-721-3
26. E.L. Greve & G. Verriest (eds.): *4th International Visual Field Symposium* (Bristol, UK, 1980). 1981 ISBN 90-6193-165-7
27. H. Spekreijse & P.A. Apkarian: *Visual Pathways: Electrophysiology and Pathology.* 18th ISCEV Symposium (Amsterdam, The Netherlands, 1980). 1981 ISBN 90-6193-723-X
28. H.C. Fledelius, P.H. Alsbirk & E. Goldschmidt (eds.): *3rd International Conference on Myopia* (Copenhagen, Denmark, 1980). 1981 ISBN 90-6193-725-6
29. J.M. Thijssen & A.M. Verbeek (eds.): *Ultrasonography in Ophthalmology.* Proceedings of the 8th SIDUO Congress (Nijmegen, The Netherlands). 1981 ISBN 90-6193-724-8
30. L. Maffei (ed.): *Pathophysiology of the Visual System.* Proceedings of a Workshop (Pisa, Italy 1980). 1981 ISBN 90-6193-726-4
31. G. Niemeyer & Ch. Huber (eds.): *Techniques in Clinical Electrophysiology of Vision.* 19th ISCEV Symposium (Horgen-Zürich, Switzerland, 1981). 1982 ISBN 90-6193-727-7
32. A.Th.M. van Balen & W.A. Houtman (eds.): *Strabismus Symposium* (Amsterdam, The Netherlands, 1981). 1982 ISBN 90-6193-728-0
33. G. Verriest (ed.): *Colour Vision Deficiencies VI.* Proceedings of the 6th Symposium of the International Research Group on Colour Vision Deficiencies (Berlin- Steglitz, Germany, 1981). 1982 ISBN 90-6193-729-9
34. A. Roucoux & M. Crommelinck (eds.): *Physiological and Pathological Aspects of Eye Movements.* Proceedings of a Workshop (Pont d'Oye Castle, Habay-la-Neuve, Belgium, 1982). 1982 ISBN 90-6193-730-2
35. E.L. Greve & A. Heijl (eds.): *5th International Visual Field Symposium* (Sacramento, Calif., USA, 1982). 1983 ISBN 90-6193-731-0
36. R. Birngruber & V.-P. Gabel (eds.): *Laser Treatment and Photocoagulation of the Eye.* Proceedings of an International Symposium (Munich, Germany, 1982). 1984 ISBN 90-6193-732-9
37. H.E.J.W. Kolder (ed.): *Slow Potentials and Microprocessor Applications.* 20th ISCEV Symposium (Iowa City, USA, 1982). 1983 ISBN 90-6193-733-7

Documenta Ophthalmologica Proceedings Series

38. J.S. Hillman & M.M. Le May (eds.): *Ophthalmic Ultrasonography.* Proceedings of the 9th SIDUO Congress (Leeds, UK, 1982). 1984 ISBN 90-6193-734-5
39. G. Verriest (ed.): *Colour Vision Deficiencies VII.* Proceedings of the 7th Symposium of the International Research Group on Colour Vision Deficiencies (Geneva, Switzerland, 1983). 1984 ISBN 90-6193-735-3
40. J.R. Heckenlively (ed.), G.H.M. van Lith & T.Lawwill (ass. eds): *Pattern Electroretinogram, Circulatory Disturbances of the Visual System and Pattern-Evoked Responses.* 21st ISCEV Symposium (Budapest, Hungary, 1983). 1984 ISBN 90-6193-503-2
41. E.C. Campos (ed.): *Sensory Evaluation of Strabismus and Amblyopia in a Natural Environment.* In Honour of Prof. Bruno Bagolini. 1984 ISBN 90-6193-508-3
42. A. Heijl & E.L. Greve (eds.): *6th International Visual Field Symposium* (Santa Margherita Ligure, Italy, 1984). 1985 ISBN 90-6193-524-5
43. E.L. Greve, W. Leydhecker & C. Raitta (eds.): *2nd European Glaucoma Symposium* (Hyvinkää, Finland, 1984). 1985 ISBN 90-6193-526-1
44. P.C. Maudgal & L. Missotten (eds.): *Herpetic Eye Diseases.* Proceedings of an International Symposium (Leuven, Belgium, 1984). 1985 ISBN 90-6193-527-X
45. B. Jay (ed.): *Detection and Measurement of Visual Impairment in Pre-Verbal Children.* Proceedings of a Workshop (London, UK, 1985). 1986 ISBN 0-89838-789-2
46. G. Verriest (ed.): *Colour Vision Deficiencies VIII.* Proceedings of the 8th Symposium of the International Research Group on Colour Vision Deficiencies (Avignon, France, 1985). 1987 ISBN 0-89838-801-5
47. P.L. Emiliani (ed.): *Development of Electronic Aids for the Visually Impaired.* Proceedings of a Workshop on the Rehabilitation of the Visually Impaired (Florence, Italy, 1984). 1986 ISBN 0-89838-805-8
48. K.C. Ossoinig (ed.): *Ophthalmic Echography.* Proceedings of the 10th SIDUO Congress (St. Petersburg Beach, Florida, USA, 1984). 1987 ISBN 0-89838-873-2
49. E.L. Greve & A. Heijl (eds.): *7th International Visual Field Symposium* (Amsterdam, The Netherlands, 1986). 1987 ISBN 0-89838-882-1
50. D. BenEzra, S.J. Ryan, B.M. Glaser & R.P. Murphy (eds.): *Ocular Circulation and Neovascularization.* Proceedings of the First International Symposium (Jeruzalem, Israel, 1986). 1987 ISBN 0-89838-892-9
51. J.M. Thijssen, J.S. Hillman, P.E. Gallenga & G. Cennamo (eds.): *Ultrasonography in Ophthalmology 11.* Proceedings of the 11th SIDUO Congress (Capri, Italy, 1986). 1988 ISBN 0-89838-378-1
52. B. Drum & G. Verriest (eds.): *Colour Vision Deficiencies IX.* Proceedings of the 9th Symposium of the International Research Group on Colour Vision Deficiencies (Annapolis, Md., USA, 1987). 1989 ISBN 0-89838-403-6

Documenta Ophthalmologica Proceedings Series

53. R. Sampaolesi (ed.): *Ultrasonography in Ophthalmology 12.* Proceedings of the 12th SIDUO Congress (Iguazú Falls, Argentina, 1988). 1990 ISBN 0-7923-0765-8
54. B. Drum, J.D. Moreland & A. Serra (eds.): *Colour Vision Deficiencies X.* Proceedings of the 10th Symposium of the International Research Group on Colour Vision Deficiencies (Cagliari, Italy, 1989). 1991 ISBN 0-7923-0948-0
55. P. Till (ed.): *Ophthalmic Echography 13.* Proceedings of the 13th SIDUO Congress (Vienna, Austria, 1990). 1993 ISBN 0-7923-1808-0
56. B. Drum (ed.): *Colour Vision Deficiencies XI.* Proceedings of the 11th Symposium of the International Research Group on Colour Vision Deficiencies (Sydney, Australia, 1991). 1993 ISBN 0-7923-1864-1
57. B. Drum (ed.): *Colour Vision Deficiencies XII.* Proceedings of the 12th Symposium of the International Research Group on Colour Vision Deficiencies (Tübingen, Germany, 1993). 1995 ISBN 0-7923-2889-2
58. J.M. Thijssen, H.C. Fledelius & S. Tane (eds.): *Ultrasonography in Ophthalmology 14.* Proceedings of the 14th SIDUO Congress (Tokyo, Japan, 1992). 1995 ISBN 0-7923-3475-2
59. C.R. Cavonius (ed.): *Colour Vision Deficiencies XIII.* Proceedings of the International Symposium (Pau, 1995). 1997 ISBN 0-7923-4224-0
60. V. Lakshminarayanan (ed.): *Basic and Clinical Applications of Vision Science.* The Professor Jay M. Enoch Festschrift Volume. 1997 ISBN 0-7923-4348-4
61. G. Cennamo (ed.): *Ultrasonography in Ophthalmology 15.* Proceedings of the 15th SIDUO Congress (Cortina, Italy, 1994). 1997 ISBN 0-7923-4464-2

KLUWER ACADEMIC PUBLISHERS – DORDRECHT / BOSTON / LONDON